NEW DIRECTIONS IN VESTIBULAR RESEARCH

W9-CHC-256

ANNALS OF THE NEW YORK ACADEMY OF SCIENCES
Volume 781

NEW DIRECTIONS IN VESTIBULAR RESEARCH

*Edited by Stephen M. Highstein, Bernard Cohen,
and Jean A. Büttner-Ennever*

The New York Academy of Sciences
New York, New York
1996

Cover art: A single cochlear hair cell isolated from the turtle basilar papilla that has been incubated with the cell-permeant indicator fluo-3 AM. Photo courtesy of Miriam Goodman and Jonathan Art, Committee on Neurobiology, University of Chicago, Illinois.

Library of Congress Cataloging-in-Publication Data

New directions in vestibular research / edited by Stephen M. Highstein, Bernard Cohen, and Jean A. Büttner-Ennever.
    p. cm. — (Annals of the New York Academy of Sciences ; v. 781)
    Includes bibliographical references and index.
    ISBN 1-57331-006-9 (cloth : alk. paper). — ISBN 1-57331-007-7 (paper : alk. paper)
    1. Vestibular apparatus—Congresses. I. Highstein, Stephen M. II. Cohen, Bernard, 1929– . III. Büttner-Ennever, Jean A. IV. Series.
Q11.N5 vol. 781
[QP471]
500 s—dc20
[596'.01825]
                                96-15560
                                CIP

SP
Printed in the United States of America
ISBN 1-57331-006-9 (cloth)
ISBN 1-57331-007-7 (paper)
ISSN 0077-8923

ANNALS OF THE NEW YORK ACADEMY OF SCIENCES

Volume 781
June 19, 1996

NEW DIRECTIONS IN VESTIBULAR RESEARCH[a]

Editors and Conference Organizers
STEPHEN M. HIGHSTEIN, BERNARD COHEN, AND JEAN A. BÜTTNER-ENNEVER

CONTENTS

[a]This volume contains papers presented at a conference entitled New Directions in Vestibular Research, which was sponsored by the New York Academy of Sciences and held on June 25–27, 1995 in New York City.

Part VII. Spatial Orientation

Part VIII. Mechanism of Vestibular Action

Part IX. Motor Learning and the Vestibulo-Ocular Reflex

Part X. Vestibular and Cerebellar Interactions

Poster Papers

Financial assistance was received from:

Major Funder
- NATIONAL INSTITUTE ON DEAFNESS AND COMMUNICATION DISORDERS, NATIONAL INSTITUTES OF HEALTH

Supporters
- NATIONAL AERONAUTICS AND SPACE ADMINISTRATION
- NATIONAL INSTITUTE OF NEUROLOGICAL DISORDERS AND STROKE, NATIONAL INSTITUTES OF HEALTH
- NATIONAL SCIENCE FOUNDATION
- OFFICE OF NAVAL RESEARCH

Introduction

STEPHEN M. HIGHSTEIN,[a] BERNARD COHEN,[b]
AND JEAN A. BÜTTNER-ENNEVER[c]

[a]Department of Otolaryngology
Washington University School of Medicine
4566 Scott Avenue
St. Louis, Missouri 63110

[b]Department of Neurology
Mount Sinai School of Medicine
One Gustave Levy Place
New York, New York 10029

[c]Institute of Neuropathology
University of Munich
Pettenkoferstrasse 12
80336 Munich, Germany

Although the vestibular system was the last of the sensory systems to be discovered, it was one of the earliest sensory systems to have evolved, and it continues to be a focus of active research. During the four years that have elapsed since the meeting Sensing and Controlling Motion[a] was held in Palo Alto, California, major advances have been made in the application of the basic sciences to vestibular research. Cellular and molecular techniques have been utilized in the study of the peripheral and central vestibular systems; advances have been made in understanding the function of the peripheral labyrinth and its hair cells; mathematical models of vestibular function have been refined; and new data is available on learning and memory in the vestibulo-ocular reflex.

Thus, it seemed timely to provide an update in several focused areas where there had been significant advances and to explore newly developing areas. This was the first goal of the meeting on New Directions in Vestibular Research, held at the Rockefeller University in New York City from June 25–27, 1995 and sponsored by the New York Academy of Sciences. The organizers also wanted to offer young scientists an opportunity to present their results and to give them a chance to interact with more established workers in the field. This was accomplished by having them chair sessions and speak both from the platform and at poster sessions. Significant support came from the National Institute on Deafness and Other Communication Disorders and the National Science Foundation, which provided a large number of fellowships for graduate students and postdoctoral fellows to attend the meeting. We also hoped that new information that was emerging quickly in various subdisciplines could be made available in a timely fashion so that it might influence ongoing research and foster new lines of work. The New York Academy of Sciences has promoted this effort by the prompt publication and wide dissemination of the results of the conference.

"New Directions" includes studies of central and peripheral development, hair cell regeneration, and molecular and cellular mechanisms utilized in transduction. A

---

[a]Proceedings published as volume 656 of the *Annals* of the New York Academy of Sciences.

developing area that is explored is how composite otolith and canal inputs are sensed in the central nervous system, leading to a greater appreciation of the contribution of the otoliths and linear acceleration to spatial orientation. Considerable new information on the coding of vestibular adaptive mechanisms in the flocculus and paraflocculus is presented, as well as new data on the interaction between the vestibular nuclei and the nodulus and the uvula of the vestibulocerebellum. An exciting new area with far-reaching results is the introduction of single-cell recording in head-free animals. Three groups have reported that brain stem neurons, monosynaptically innervated by the VIIIth nerve, modify their signal content related to head movement depending upon the animal's behavioral state or intent. For example, vestibular nucleus neurons that encode head velocity during passive gaze shifts, including enforced head rotation, decrease or cancel the signal related to head velocity during gaze shifts involving active head movement. Since the vestibular system functions to sense and control movement in the active state, the import of these studies is that the function of the system will only be fully understood if it is examined in that state.

We would like to acknowledge the generous support of the National Institute on Deafness and Other Communication Disorders, the National Institute of Neurological Disorders and Stroke, the National Aeronautics and Space Administration, the National Science Foundation, and the Office of Naval Research. We thank our advisory committee, which included Victor Wilson, John I. Simpson, Daniel Sklare, Frank Sulzman, Joel Davis, Chris Platt, Jay M. Goldberg, and Theodore Raphan, for their wise advice. We are particularly grateful to New York Academy of Sciences for sponsoring the conference, and give special thanks to Renée Wilkerson and her staff for efficiently organizing and running the meeting, and to Marion Garry and Bill Boland for their fine editorial work, without which this volume could not have been published.

Afferent Calyces and Type I Hair Cells during Development

A New Morphofunctional Hypothesis[a]

ALAIN SANS[b] AND ERIC SCARFONE

Neurobiologie et Développement du Système Vestibulaire
Inserm U432–Université Montpellier II
34095 Montpellier Cedex 5, France

Higher vertebrates have vestibular sensory cells (type I) that have the particularity of being totally surrounded by a nerve calyx. This anatomic disposition poses a conceptual problem because it is difficult to understand why afferent terminals that contact type I hair cells do not limit themselves to effecting synaptic contact at the base of the cell. Instead, they totally surround these cells up to their apical part despite the fact that no synaptic bodies can be found at this location.

An ontogenetic approach can be used to good effect in this situation to examine the remodeling process and interrelations that temporally and spatially affect nerve fibers and their targets before they obtain their adult structure. We have, therefore, spent the last few years studying the development in the human fetus of nerve endings, synaptogenesis, the development of surface receptors, and the onset of different calcium-binding proteins.[1-4] Furthermore, we have studied the appearance and the migration of proteins linked to synaptic microvesicles during their development in the mouse.[5]

In this study we focus on the development and vesicular content of nerve fibers invading the vestibular epithelium, with a large part of our study devoted to the human fetus. It is important that the critical periods of sensory receptor development in man be understood. That ontogenetic processes in humans are very slow compared to those of small mammals enables the relation between morphological differentiation of sensory cells and nerve fibers to be more clearly identified. Inner ear tissues were obtained from fetuses after legal abortions, in accordance with current regulations of the French National Ethics Committee.

By studying the differentiation and maturation of vestibular sensory cells and their afferents, we show the probable influence of a nerve calyx feedback loop on the type I cell—interactions which could regulate both physiological and metabolic mechanisms.

[a]This work was supported in part by the CNES (Grant No. 95.0271).
[b]E-mail: Neuros@crit.univ-montp2.fr

1

GROWTH OF NERVE FIBER INTO THE VESTIBULAR EPITHELIUM

In the human embryo fibers start to penetrate the epithelium during week 7 of gestation. At this stage the great majority of cells are not differentiated; their nuclei are distributed on several layers. However, nascent hair bundles can be seen in the central zone of cristae and macula indicating that a few sensory cells began their differentiation. In the same central zone, rare nerve fibers penetrate the epithelium up to its juxta-luminal part. During weeks 8–9 nerve fibers massively invade the epithelium, thus establishing a dense horizontal network (FIG. 1A) at the base of the most externally situated cell layer. These cells will develop into sensory cells. Nerve fibers then project between these cells towards the luminal surface, emitting digitations with varicosities (FIG. 1B and C). This process of nerve fibers growing along vertical and horizontal axes can be clearly seen by confocal microscopy, using immunocytochemical labeling of thick sections (50 μm) by an antibody directed against synaptophysin (FIG. 1).

The freeze-fracture study of a vestibular epithelium taken from a 9-week-old fetus ampullaris cristae confirms this transversal growth of fibers towards the luminal surface, and also shows the establishment of passing contact with differentiating sensory cells (FIG. 2). It should be emphasized that in the initial stages the first fibers to arrive at the epithelium make contact with the cells situated at the central part of the cristae ampullaris (FIG. 1), or the maculae striola. In later stages the newly arrived fibers reach the base of the cristae and the macula periphery.

During ontogenesis, the colonization process of vestibular epithelia by nerve fibers is thus effected in two ways: transversal growth of fibers towards the luminal surface after establishing a horizontal network underneath the sensory cells, and lateral growth following an apex-base gradient for the cristae, and a striola-peripheral gradient for macula.

ESTABLISHMENT OF FIRST SYNAPTIC CONTACTS

The contact between nerve fibers and sensory cells is characterized by the appearance of multiple synaptic bodies in sensory cells and by an increase in membrane density, especially that of the nerve fiber. Numerous floating synaptic bodies can also be seen in the sensory cell, attaching themselves to cell membranes at the point where nerve fibers make contact with the cell (FIG. 3A–C). Coated vesicle (FIG. 3A–C) and microtubules (FIG. 3D) can be distinguished in the vicinity of synaptic bodies. This overexpression of synaptic bodies in the presynaptic element corresponds to intense vesicular traffic on the postsynaptic side. Vestibular fibers mostly contain dense cored vesicles (FIG. 4), co-located with small clear vesicles (FIG. 5). These vesicles could be the equivalent of synaptic vesicles, since we have demonstrated the presence of synaptophysin (FIG. 1), a constituent protein of synaptic microvesicle membranes. This result prompts one to pose the questions: Are the fibers afferent or efferent? If they are afferent, then why do they contain synaptic microvesicles? If they are efferent, then why do they face synaptic bodies? (FIG. 5).

The analysis of nerve calyx growth shows that in reality these small clear vesicles are principally found in the terminal parts of afferent nerve fibers during growth

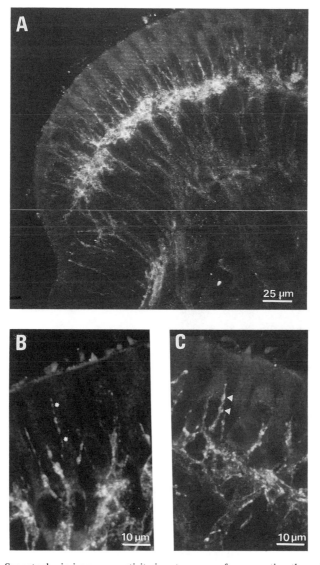

FIGURE 1. Synaptophysin immunoreactivity in a transverse frozen section through a cristae ampullaris. (**A**) Synaptophysin is present in nerve fibers, forming a dense plexus underlining the base of sensory cells. Individual afferent fibers emerge from this layer and penetrate into the upper part of the sensory epithelia. Note the small number of fibers. (**B** and **C**) High magnification of the sensory cell area. In **B**, a slender vertical immunoreactive neurite is indicated by *white asterisks*. In **C**, varicosities along a neurite are indicated by *white triangles* (see also FIG. 2).

NOTE: This illustration and those that follow are of vestibular epithelia from 9-week-old human fetuses.

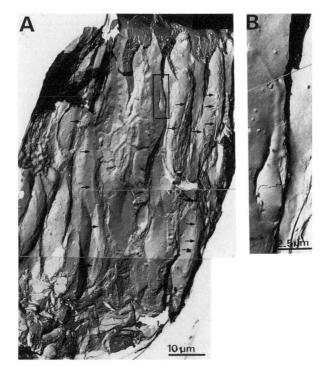

FIGURE 2. Freeze fracture of a crista ampullaris. **(A)** The lower part of the picture shows a transverse fracture of nerve fibers. The vestibular epithelium has several layers of cells. Hair bundles can be clearly seen at the upper part of the sensory cells. Numerous nerve fibers can be detected (*arrows*) running from the base to the apex of the epithelium. **(B)** High magnification of a nerve fiber shown in **A,** establishing a bouton *en passant* that could correspond to the varicosities in FIGURE 1C. Note the thin terminal digitation.

(FIG. 6A), and are limited in mature calyces to the area surrounding the apical part of cells (FIG. 6B). Other nerve endings have very few dense cored vesicles and contain a dense and homogenous population of clear microvesicles; these nerve endings are efferent (FIG. 7).

NERVE FIBERS AND MICROVESICLES DURING ONTOGENESIS OF THE MOUSE VESTIBULE

The slow development in humans enables a high level of spatiotemporal accuracy to be achieved when analyzing the first stages of maturation. We also conducted a similar analysis[5] in the mouse, from day 14 of gestation up to postnatal day 12. The period encompasses total development of the peripheral labyrinth in this small mammal. Synapsin I and synaptophysin are two proteins associated with the membrane of the synaptic vesicles in axonal endings. In the peripheral vestibular system, we localized these proteins in ganglion neurons and their peripheral extensions at a

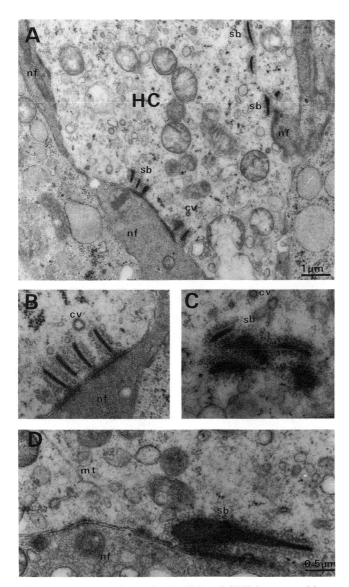

FIGURE 3. First stages of synaptogenesis. **(A)** Hair cell (HC) is contacted by several nerve fibers (nf). Multisynaptic bodies are facing the nerve terminal; free-floating synaptic bodies (sb) can also be seen (right side). Multisynaptic bodies **(B)** and free-floating synaptic bodies (sb) **(C)** coexist with coated vesicles (cv) and microtubules (mt) **(D).**

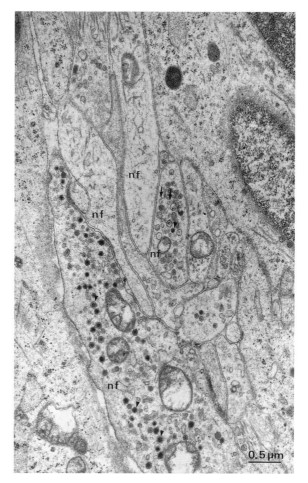

FIGURE 4. Growing vestibular nerve fibers and microvesicles. Some nerve fibers (nf) contain numerous dense core microvesicles (*arrowheads*) and clear microvesicles (*arrows*).

very early stage, during ontogenesis (GD14). At this time neurites have not yet massively invaded the epithelium. This localization persists during later stages of embryogenesis and during the perinatal period. The development processes studied in the human fetus between weeks 9 and 11 are very similar to those studied in the mouse between GD14 and birth. After birth the two vesicle proteins were subject to relocation. During postnatal maturation, synapsin I and synaptophysin disappeared from the fibers, and were only detected by immunocytochemistry in the vestibular ganglion neurons and the terminal parts of afferent and efferent endings. In adults, synapsin I and synaptophysin labeling coexist in the terminal parts of afferent fibers (FIG. 8) where clear microvesicles can be observed by electronic microscopy.

DISCUSSION

Critical stages of nerve fiber synaptogenesis are similar in the human species and in other mammals. The slower development in humans as compared to other mammals made it possible to ascertain that nerve fibers invading the epithelium first establish a network underneath the layer of future sensory cells, then penetrate toward the juxta-luminal surface while establishing *en passant* contacts with the cells. The main result contributed by these ontogenetic studies concerns the massive

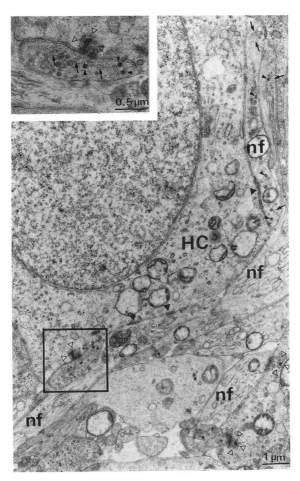

FIGURE 5. Afferent or efferent nerve fibers? Hair cells (HC) are contacted by several nerve fibers (nf) which have in their terminal parts mostly numerous clear (*arrows*) or dense core (*arrowheads*) microvesicles. Some of them make contact opposite synaptic bodies (indicated by three *open triangles*) or membrane densification (*filled triangle*). **Inset:** Detail of a synaptic body facing a vesiculated terminal.

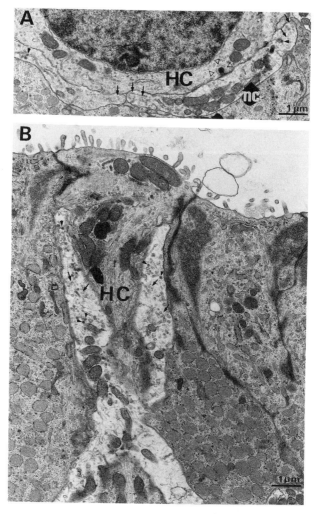

FIGURE 6. Afferent nerve calyces and synaptic microvesicles. (**A**) Transverse section of growing nerve calyces (nc) surrounding a type I sensory hair cell (HC). Numerous clear microvesicles (*arrows*) in the terminal part of the calyx are colocalized with dense core vesicles (*arrowhead*). Note the synaptic body (indicated by triangles). (**B**) Longitudinal section of a vesicle-containing nerve calyx surrounding the apical part of an immature hair cell (HC).

presence of vesicles in afferent fibers. Part of the vesicles has characteristics resembling synaptic vesicles of axonal endings: they are clear, small in size (40 to 50 nm), and coexist in afferent fibers with proteins specifically associated with the membrane of synaptic vesicles.[5] These observations suggest that the afferent endings that do receive sensory information have, in addition, the capability to release neurotransmitters, in the same way as do axonal endings. This poses two questions:

(1) Are microvesicles prone to exocytosis during development and (2) what is their physiological role in the adult?

During development the growing axons are capable of neurotransmitter release. Xie and Poo[6] demonstrated, using muscle membrane patches attached to a recording pipette, acetylcholine release by embryonic motoneurons. This release is vesicular, as demonstrated by Matteoli *et al.* [7] in cultured hippocampal neurons. Synaptic vesicles have been shown to have a very high turnover, with multiple exoendocytic cycles all along the neurite membranes developing independently of all synaptic contact. The view of these authors is that release of neurotransmitters during neuronal development could play an important role in establishing neuronal networks and in the interactions between axons and innervated non-neuronal tissues.

During the differentiation of vestibular sensory cells, it seems that a correlation existed between the timing of nerve fibers invading into the epithelium and the acquisition of morphological characteristics specific to cells. This cell differentiation could be influenced by the release by afferent fibers of a neurotransmitter playing a

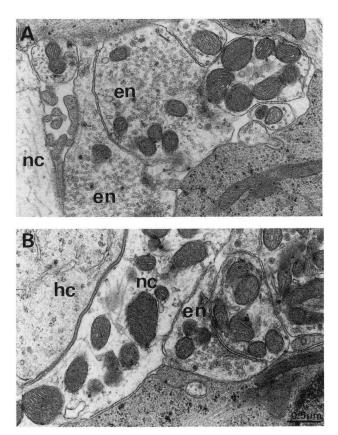

FIGURE 7. Efferent nerves and synaptic microvesicles. (**A** and **B**) Efferent nerves (en) are densely filled with small clear microvesicles. nc, nerve calyx; hc, hair cell.

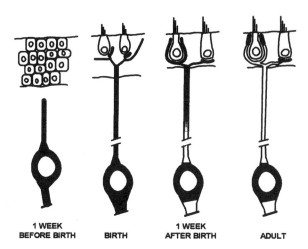

FIGURE 8. Schematic diagram of the segregation of synaptic vesicle-specific proteins in the afferent fibers during development in the mouse. Distribution of the proteins is indicated by a dark filling.

trophic role. The multiplication of synaptic bodies at this time in the hair cell suggests an increased release of the neurotransmitter, which could in turn influence the growth and the direction taken by axons. At the mature stage the interrelation between vestibular nerve fibers and sensory cells is essential for the maintenance of hair cell phenotype, inasmuch as an experimental denervation of receptors provoked a dedifferentiation of sensory cells.[8] In the adult, microvesicles are concentrated in afferent bouton endings contacting type II cells, as well as in the terminal part of calyces surrounding the apex of type I cells.

Even though we have not proved that synaptic microvesicles are indeed secretory, it is tempting to propose[9] a new hypothesis concerning the functioning of vestibular receptors. Hair cells are strongly polarized from a morphofunctional point of view: the apical pole is devoted to the mechanoelectrical transduction of the sensory signal, whereas the basal pole contains formations specialized in synaptic transmission. Furthermore, the appearance in the higher vertebrates of type I cells surrounded by a nerve calyx could signify a phylogenetic gain as compared to animal species that only have type II cells. In addition, type I hair cells present motor properties[10] that suggest adaptation capacities.

With regard to type II cells, the release of the neurotransmitter by afferent boutons can only affect the basal pole of the cell because of their position. From a functional point of view, afferent feedback-control is thus exercised on the synaptic transmission of the sensory signals.

Concerning type I cells, the presence of the nerve calyx enables feedback-control to be transported to the apical pole of the cell. This retrocontrol can therefore be exercised directly at the input end of the cell (FIG. 9), and the neurotransmitter released by the calyx can participate in the regulation of adaptive processes that affect mechanical transduction. This makes it possible to realize a rapid and subtle adjustment of cellular sensitivity at the very point where the sensory message originates.

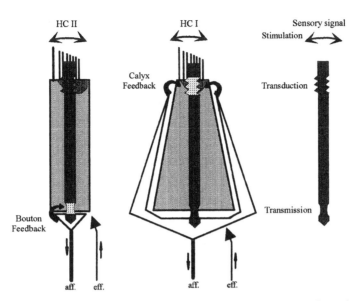

FIGURE 9. Reciprocal interactions between nerve fibers and sensory cells: a functional hypothesis. All hair cells (HC) have a highly polarized organization. Mechanoelectrical transduction of sensory stimuli occurs at the apical pole (hair bundle/cuticular plate), and synaptic transmission of the resulting sensory signal occurs at the basal pole (synaptic bodies/afferent endings). If, as we postulate, reciprocal interactions occur between hair cells and afferent endings, the feedback action of bouton endings at the output end of type II hair cells can only affect the last stage of sensory signal processing: synaptic transmission. In the case of type I hair cells, however, the existence of the nerve calyx makes it possible to bring this feedback action to the input end of the cell, where the first stages of sensory signal processing occur: mechanoelectrical transduction. This would result in a far more efficient method for controlling hair cell function, by modulating active processes that occur during transduction (see text).

ACKNOWLEDGMENTS

Antibodies directed against synaptophysin have been kindly donated by R. Jahn (Howard Hughes Medical Institute, BCMM, New Haven, CT). The authors thank B. Arnaud for photographic work, and J. Boyer, M. Renaudin, and Denis Orcel for editorial work.

REFERENCES

1. SANS, A. & C. J. DECHESNE. 1987. Afferent nerve ending development and synaptogenesis in the vestibular epithelium of human fetuses. Hear. Res. **28:** 65–72.
2. DECHESNE, C. J., P. ESCUDERO, N. LAMANDE, M. THOMASSET & A. SANS. 1987. Immuno-histochemical identification of neuron-specific enolase and calbindin in the vestibular receptors of human fetuses. Acta Otolaryngol. (Stockh.) **436(Suppl.):** 69–75.
3. DECHESNE, C. J. & A. SANS. 1985. Development of vestibular receptor surfaces in human fetuses. Am. J. Otolaryngol. **6:** 378–387.

4. DECHESNE, C. J. 1992. Development of vestibular organs in the human. *In* Development of Auditory and Vestibular Systems 2. Romand, Ed.: 419–447. Elsevier Science Publishers. New York.

5. SCARFONE, E., D. DEMEMES & A. SANS. 1991. Synapsin I and synaptophysin expression during ontogenesis of the mouse peripheral vestibular system. J. Neurosci. **11:** 1173–1181.

6. XIE, Z. P. & M. M. POO. 1986. Initial events in the formation of neuromuscular synapse: Rapid induction of acetylcholine release from embryonic neuron. Proc. Natl. Acad. Sci. USA **83:** 7069–7073.

7. MATTEOLI, M., K. TAKEI, M. PERIN, T. SUDHOF & P. DE CAMILLI. 1992. Exo-endocytotic recycling of synaptic vesicles in developing processes of cultured hippocampal neurons. J. Cell Biol. **117:** 849–861.

8. FAVRE, D. & A. SANS. 1991. Dedifferentiation phenomenons after denervation of mammalian adult vestibular receptors. Neuroreport **2:** 501–504.

9. SCARFONE, E., D. DEMEMES, R. JAHN, P. DE CAMILLI & A. SANS. 1988. Secretory function of the vestibular nerve calyx suggested by presence of vesicles, synapsin I and synaptophysin. J. Neurosci. **8:** 4640–4645.

10. GRIGUER, C., J. LEHOUELLEUR, J. VALAT, A. SAHUQUET & A. SANS. 1993. Voltage dependent reversible movements of the apex in isolated guinea pig vestibular hair cells. Hear. Res. **67:** 110–116.

Development of Second-Order Vestibular Projections in the Chicken Embryo[a]

JOEL C. GLOVER[b]

Department of Anatomy
Institute of Basic Medical Sciences
University of Oslo
P.B. 1105–Blindern
0317 Oslo, Norway

INTRODUCTION

The vestibulospinal and vestibulo-ocular reflexes incorporate the dependable stereotypy of a hard-wired system and the adaptive plasticity of a malleable system. On the one hand, the speed, accuracy, and robust phylogenetic maintenance of the reflexes imply developmental mechanisms that ensure precise synaptic recognition. On the other hand, the existence of adaptive gain modulation and metamorphic transformations demand a substantial capacity for synaptic plasticity and reorganization. How these attributes are combined during the development of the brain presents an intriguing challenge to the neuroembryologist. Here I review recent studies my colleagues and I have made on the development of vestibulospinal and vestibulo-ocular projections in the chicken embryo. These studies focus on the way vestibular interneurons are selectively coupled to their appropriate synaptic targets.

FUNCTIONAL NEUROANATOMY OF THE VESTIBULAR PROJECTIONS

When we began our investigations, the functional anatomy of avian vestibular projections was not described well enough to provide a sufficient basis for developmental studies. Our first task therefore was to map the location of vestibulospinal and vestibulo-ocular neurons and to determine their functional relationships in the chicken embryo at 11 days of embryonic development, at which stage many projection systems in the hindbrain and spinal cord are fairly mature. Although this task is still not finished, we have obtained enough information to show that the vestibulospinal and vestibulo-ocular axonal projections and the pattern of connections from vestibulo-ocular neurons to oculomotor and trochlear motoneurons are organized along the general vertebrate plan. (Vestibulo-ocular projections to the abducens nucleus have not yet been included in our studies). A finding of particular significance from a developmental perspective is a feature of vestibular organization that appears not to have been elucidated fully in other species: namely, that vestibular interneurons are compartmentalized into a hodological mosaic in much the same way as are their motoneuron targets in the spinal cord and mesencephalon.

To obtain our description of these projections in the 11-day embryo, we used four main techniques: (1) retrograde axonal tracing to determine the location of vestibu-

[a]This work was supported by grants from the Norwegian Medical Research Council, the Nansen Fund, and the Jahre Fund.
[b]E-mail: joel@pons.uio.no

13

lar interneurons that project to particular targets; (2) anterograde axonal tracing to determine the patterns of synaptic termination exhibited by defined groups of vestibular interneurons; (3) neurotransmitter immunohistochemistry; and (4) retrograde transport of radiolabeled neurotransmitters or neurotransmitter analogues to determine the potential neurotransmitter phenotypes of the vestibular interneurons. Since some of these studies have been reviewed recently,[1] I present here only an overview of the main features. These are illustrated schematically in FIGURE 1.

Retrograde axonal tracing using differentiable tracers has shown that vestibulo-spinal and vestibulo-ocular neurons are organized into coherent, segregated clusters, each of which has a characteristic spatial domain and axonal projection pathway.[2,3] There are three vestibulospinal clusters, all located at about the level of the VIIIth cranial nerve root. These give rise to the lateral and medial vestibulospinal tracts

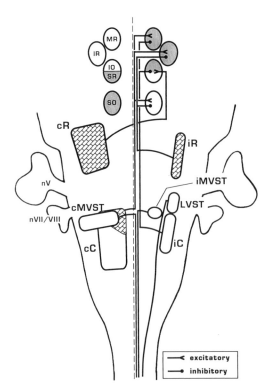

FIGURE 1. The organization of vestibulospinal and vestibulo-ocular neurons and their projections in the 11-day-old embryo. Hatching represents neuron groups for which direct evidence of potential neurotransmitter phenotype has been obtained. See text for definitions of abbreviations.

(LVST and MVST), the former being exclusively ipsilateral whereas the latter has distinct ipsilateral and contralateral components. Because these three groups of vestibular interneurons are the separate origins of the three distinct vestibulospinal projections, they have been named the LVST, the ipsilateral MVST (iMVST), and the contralateral MVST (cMVST) groups, respectively. None of these vestibulospinal groups has yet been studied with anterograde axonal tracing or with methods that reveal potential neurotransmitter phenotype. Thus we cannot make any statements yet about their functional relationships in the chicken.

The vestibulo-ocular projections have a more complex origin. Here there are four major clusters of interneurons, two of which lie rostral to and two of which lie generally caudal to the vestibulospinal groups.[1,2] For each of the rostral and caudal pairs of clusters, one cluster projects ipsilaterally and one projects contralaterally. We refer to these clusters as the ipsilateral and contralateral rostral (iR and cR) vestibulo-ocular groups, and the ipsilateral and contralateral caudal (iC and cC) vestibulo-ocular groups (FIG. 1). The iR and cR groups appear to be relatively homogeneous in terms of their functional connections (see below), whereas the iC and cC groups may consist of two or more functional subgroups. For example, the cC group includes the interneurons of the abducens nucleus as well as a larger subpopulation of neurons that is partially segregated into dorsal and ventral components (cf. ref. 3).

It is important to realize that these groups of vestibular interneurons do not correspond directly to any of the classically defined vestibular nuclei. They are defined exclusively on the basis of location and axonal trajectory, making each of them topographically unique within the system of second-order vestibular projections. They represent a separate level of organization that is not related to cytoarchitectonics but that is probably more closely tied to functional relationships.

The termination patterns of the major vestibulo-ocular groups have been examined with anterograde axonal tracing. The picture is fairly straightforward. The iR group terminates predominantly in the ipsilateral superior oblique and inferior rectus motoneuron pools, whereas the cR group terminates predominantly in the contralateral inferior oblique and superior rectus pools[4] (FIG. 1). The rostral portion of the cC group terminates predominantly in the contralateral superior oblique and inferior rectus pools, that is, in register with the termination from the iR group on the opposite side.

The projections from the cC and iC groups, when traced in combination, terminate in all five oculomotor and trochlear motoneuron pools.[5] Subtracting the termination pattern of the rostral part of the cC group described above suggests that the iC group and the remainder of the cC group in combination terminate, ipsilaterally and contralaterally, respectively, in the inferior oblique, superior rectus, and medial rectus pools (FIG. 1).

In general, the ipsilateral and contralateral vestibulo-ocular projections in mammals are, respectively, inhibitory and excitatory, although there are some exceptions.[6] This would suggest that in the chicken the iR and iC groups are inhibitory and the cR and cC groups are excitatory. Indeed, our neurotransmitter studies have provided evidence that the iR group is GABAergic, whereas the cR group and at least the abducens interneurons and rostral portion of the cC group are glutamatergic.[1,7] If we assume this relationship to hold for the iC group and the remainder of the cC group, and combine this with the anterograde tracing results, we can propose the simple connectivity scheme shown in FIGURE 1. In this scheme, at least some of the hodologically defined vestibulo-ocular groups have termination patterns consistent with a potentially specific function. For example, the cR group excites the inferior oblique and superior rectus motoneurons innervating their respective muscles in opposite eyes, whereas the iR group inhibits the superior oblique and inferior rectus motoneurons innervating their respective muscles in opposite eyes. Likewise, the rostral portion of the cC group excites the superior oblique and inferior rectus motoneurons innervating their respective muscles in opposite eyes, an action opposing that of the iR group. Each of these actions can be considered partially synergistic for animals with laterally positioned eyes.

The remaining projections shown in FIGURE 1 are more difficult to classify functionally, both because the termination patterns of the iC group and the remainder of the cC group have not been labeled separately, and because they may each represent the aggregate termination from different subgroups. For example, the cC group as a whole excites the contralateral superior oblique, inferior rectus, and medial rectus motoneurons. The simultaneous excitation of superior oblique and inferior rectus is a potentially synergistic action in vertical or rotatory eye movements. The excitation of the medial rectus motoneurons, on the other hand, must be a component of horizontal eye movements, and is likely to derive from the abducens interneurons. Likewise, the iC group inhibits the inferior oblique, superior rectus, and medial rectus motoneurons. The inhibition of the inferior oblique and superior rectus motoneurons specifically opposes the excitation of the same motoneurons by the cR group, both of which actions must be involved in vertical or rotatory eye movements. The inhibition of the medial rectus motoneurons, on the other hand, must be a component of horizontal eye movements and specifically opposes the presumed action of the abducens interneurons. Thus, the iC and cC groups are each likely to consist of subgroups of neurons with different functions. The extent to which these subgroups are spatially segregated remains to be determined.

As indicated in FIGURE 1, the vestibular interneurons are clustered into spatially segregated groups, each of which has a specific axonal trajectory and a specific termination pattern. Moreover, if we allow the dualism of contralateral and ipsilateral projections being equivalent, respectively, to excitatory and inhibitory actions to hold, then all motoneuron pools receive both an excitatory and an inhibitory input, and at least some of the vestibulo-ocular groups acquire potentially specific functions. The picture is more complex, however. Only the most predominant termination patterns are indicated. In many cases a minority of terminal branches extend beyond the confines of the principal motoneuron pool target; whether these innervate motoneurons in other pools or dendrites of the principal target motoneurons is not known. Moreover, we have observed some commissural collateral branches at the level of the oculomotor complex whose targets remain to be determined. These are not indicated. It is unclear to what extent individual neurons in each group provide concerted or separate innervation to the motoneuron pools innervated by the group. Also unclear is the pattern by which the neurons in each group are recruited by the different vestibular end organs. Until these issues are resolved, the functional specificity of each group cannot be defined unambiguously.

DEVELOPMENT OF THE VESTIBULAR PROJECTIONS

We are studying the development of the vestibulospinal and vestibulo-ocular projections from two different angles. First, we are trying to correlate the emerging spatial domains of the hodologically defined vestibular groups with patterns of gene expression and other mechanisms contributing to pattern formation in the hindbrain neural tube. The aim here is to discover the mechanisms that determine axon pathway choice. Second, we are trying to follow the patterns of synaptic termination made by the vestibular axons as they grow into target areas. The aim here is to find out whether each group terminates selectively within the available target neuron populations from the outset.

Retrograde tracing studies at earlier embryonic stages is facilitated by two features of the hindbrain neural tube. First, longitudinal axons are organized into two distinct bilaterally symmetrical bundles with stereotyped locations: the medial longitudinal fascicle (MLF), coursing along either side of the midline floor plate, and the lateral longitudinal fascicle (LLF), coursing along the ventrolateral margin of the alar plate on each side.[8] Second, the hindbrain neural tube is partitioned into transient but morphologically overt neuromeres, termed rhombomeres.[9] The boundaries between rhombomeres provide landmarks by which axonal tracers can be targeted precisely to one or the other longitudinal axon bundles at specific axial levels. Thus it is possible to label vestibular interneurons as their axons are growing towards their targets. Such labeling has shown that by 4 to 5 days of development, certain of the vestibulospinal and vestibulo-ocular interneuron groups described above are present as distinct, segregated clusters that are delimited by rhombomere boundaries.[8,10,11] For example, the LVST vestibulospinal group is located in a lateral domain lying within rhombomere 4, whereas the iC vestibulo-ocular group lies in the same lateral domain in rhombomeres 5 and 6. Immediately medial to the iC group lies the cC group, also neatly confined longitudinally within the domain of rhombomeres 5 and 6.

That these groups can be identified by retrograde labeling at such early stages of axon outgrowth demonstrates the selective nature of that outgrowth: the axons from a given group do not extend into inappropriate pathways, a behavior that would necessitate a later phase of retraction to establish the ultimate pattern of projections. For example, the iC vestibulo-ocular axons destined to project ipsilaterally in the MLF do so from the outset, and the cC axons destined to project contralaterally in the MLF also do so from the outset, apparently ignoring the ipsilateral MLF. The selective anterograde labeling required to assay axon behavior as the axons initially contact the available pathways is technically difficult at these early stages. Although we cannot rule out a certain degree of trial and error at first contact, any indecisiveness on the part of the axons must be resolved well before they have projected any distance longitudinally.

The rhombomeres have been shown to be developmental pseudocompartments whose boundaries restrict the movement of cells within the plane of the neural tube and whose domains are characterized by unique patterns of regulatory gene expression, which, moreover, exhibit dynamic changes along the mediolateral axis (reviewed in ref. 12). Thus, neurons lying within different rhombomeres and at different mediolateral positions within a given rhombomere must experience stereotypically different patterns of gene expression at some stage of their genesis and differentiation. This suggests that the spatiotemporal disposition of vestibular interneurons regulates their differentiation, potentially specifying such properties as axon pathway choice, termination pattern, and neurotransmitter phenotype.

Curiously, some of the vestibular interneuron groups appear to differentiate much later than the others. Although the LVST group and the various vestibulo-ocular groups can be identified by retrograde labeling by 4 to 5 days of development, the two vestibulospinal groups comprising the MVST cannot be identified until several days later.[11] Thus it is not yet possible to place their genesis and differentiation within the context of the rhombomeric organization of the hindbrain.

To determine whether the vestibulo-ocular groups establish specific termination patterns as selectively as they do their axon trajectories, we performed anterograde labeling at early stages, prior to and during the innervation of the extraocular motoneuron targets. Anterograde labeling of the iR and cR groups has demonstrated a selective innervation of the appropriate motoneuron pools at least as early as day 9, shortly after the axons reach the target area.[4] The process has been followed more closely for the iC and cC groups.[5] In this study, the oculomotor nerve was retrogradely labeled, and the vestibulo-ocular projection anterogradely labeled, differentially, with fluorescent tracers. This allows the simultaneous visualization of the axon terminal collaterals and their potential motoneuron targets. The iC and cC axons reach the level of the oculomotor complex by about day 5, at which time a substantial number of immature motoneurons can be labeled retrogradely from the oculomotor nerve. The ensuing process of innervation is highly dynamic, owing to several dramatic changes in the motoneurons. These are initially organized in a single cluster ipsilateral to the labeled nerve, and have not yet differentiated dendrites. Over the next several days, this single cluster gradually resolves into subgroups corresponding to the separate oculomotoneuron pools; some of the motoneurons migrate across the midline to establish the contralaterally projecting superior rectus pool; and all of the motoneurons begin to elaborate dendrites that extend beyond the confines of the pools of origin. On this dynamic backdrop, the vestibulo-ocular axons make their entrance by the extension of collateral branches. The temporal sequence is illustrated schematically in FIGURE 2. Terminal collaterals

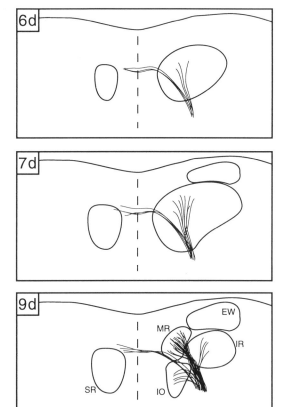

FIGURE 2. The sequence of events during the development of the termination pattern of iC and cC vestibulo-ocular axons in the oculomotor complex. Abbreviations are defined in the text.

first appear late on day 6, at which time they extend obliquely toward the dorsomedial pole of the still coherent motoneuron cluster, with some veering across the midline in the vicinity of the migrating superior rectus motoneurons. By the next day, the ipsilateral collateral projection is strengthened, and the motoneurons are beginning to separate into pools. By day 9 the region to which the collaterals first extended resolves into the medial rectus pool. This pool is now heavily invested with terminal collaterals, and additional collaterals extend into the inferior rectus and the overlapping inferior oblique and superior rectus pools. This establishes the predominant features of the mature pattern of termination for the combined iC and cC axons (FIG. 1).

The early extension of these terminal collaterals is clearly selective. They aim initially for a specific region of the developing motoneuron cluster, focusing on that region even as later collaterals to neighboring regions arise. The region corresponding to the Edinger-Westphal nucleus is essentially ignored at all stages. A reasonable interpretation of the sequence of events is that iC and cC axons predetermined to innervate medial rectus motoneurons establish the first collaterals, which are either selectively attracted by or selectively recognize the differentiating medial rectus motoneurons. Somewhat later, iC and cC axons predetermined to innervate the other motoneuron pools extend collaterals into these.

Although by appearances the initially selective innervation pattern exhibited by these axons suggests a process of selective attraction or recognition, it is important to realize that alternative nonselective mechanisms may exist. For example, if the extension of any collateral is contingent on the release of a general chemoattractant common to all motoneurons, then a careful timing of the onset of the ability of different motoneurons to release the attractant, the arrival of different vestibulo-ocular axons at the target area, and the onset and termination of their capacity to respond to the attractant could produce the observed behavior. Experimental manipulations are required to resolve this issue.

CONCLUSIONS

The results reviewed here demonstrate that vestibulospinal and vestibulo-ocular interneurons in the chicken embryo are organized into coherent clusters, each of which occupies a unique spatial domain and has a characteristic axon trajectory. Moreover, the vestibulo-ocular clusters have specific termination patterns in the extraocular motoneuron pools and may to some extent have specific functions. The axon trajectories and termination patterns are established accurately during early development. This suggests the presence of selective mechanisms that ensure the generation of an appropriately specific connectivity pattern. The correlation of cluster domains with unique fields of regulatory gene expression at early stages suggests a mechanistic link between the position of a vestibular interneuron and the differentiation of its axon trajectory, termination pattern, and neurotransmitter phenotype.

ACKNOWLEDGMENTS

I thank my co-workers Gudrun Petursdottir, Jan Jansen, Jon Storm-Mathisen, and Asborg Rinde for collaboration and for sharing unpublished results.

REFERENCES

1. GLOVER, J. G. 1994. The organization of vestibulo-ocular and vestibulospinal projections in the chicken embryo. Eur. J. Morphol. **32:** 193–200.
2. GLOVER, J. C. & G. PETURSDOTTIR. 1988. Pathway specificity of reticulospinal and vestibulospinal projections in the 11-day chicken embryo. J. Comp. Neurol. **270:** 25–38.

3. PETURSDOTTIR, G. 1990. Vestibulo-ocular projections in the 11-day chicken embryo: Pathway specificity. J. Comp. Neurol. **297:** 283–297.
4. JANSEN, J. K. S. 1991. A note on the development of the vestibulo-ocular pathway in the chicken. Anat. Embryol. **184:** 305–311.
5. GLOVER, J. G. & A. RINDE. 1995. Initially selective termination patterns exhibited by vestibulo-ocular projections in the chicken embryo. Soc. Neurosci. Abstr. **21:** 803.
6. PRECHT, W. 1979. Vestibular mechanisms. Annu. Rev. Neurosci. **2:** 265–289.
7. STORM-MATHISEN, J., J. K. S. JANSEN, J. C. GLOVER & B. O. FISCHER. 1990. The vestibulo-ocular (V-O) pathway in the chick embryo. Soc. Neurosci. Abstr. **16:** 903.
8. GLOVER, J. C. 1993. The development of brain stem projections to the spinal cord in the chicken embryo. Brain Res. Bull. **30:** 265–271.
9. LUMSDEN, A. & R. KEYNES. 1989. Segmental patterns of neuronal development in the chick hindbrain. Nature **337:** 424–428.
10. GLOVER, J. C. 1989. Rhombomeres and longitudinal boundaries in the chicken embryo brainstem subdivide vestibular neurons according to axonal pathway. Soc. Neurosci. Abstr. **15:** 959.
11. GLOVER, J. C. & G. PETURSDOTTIR. 1991. Regional specificity of developing reticulospinal, vestibulospinal, and vestibulo-ocular projections in the chicken embryo. J. Neurobiol. **22:** 353–376.
12. KEYNES, R. & R. KRUMLAUF. 1994. Hox genes and regionalization of the nervous system. Annu. Rev. Neurosci. **17:** 109–132.

Development of the Labyrinthine Efferent System[a]

BERND FRITZSCH[b]

Department of Biomedical Sciences
Creighton University
Omaha, Nebraska 68178

INTRODUCTION

The existence of efferents to the vertebrate ear has been an enigmatic and controversial issue for many years.[1] Earlier studies relied on the problematic ultrastructural identification (which may have confused efferents with reciprocal synapses known to exist in the ear of many vertebrates, particularly during development),[2,3] degeneration techniques (which resulted in the false identification of cerebellar Purkinje cells as being efferent to the frog ear)[4] or histochemical reactions (which relies on the false assumption of histochemical uniformity of these cells). Modern tracing techniques have clarified most of these controversies, and there is undeniable evidence for the existence of an efferent system to the ear of vertebrates.[5,6] These tracers have also clarified the distribution of efferents to the vestibular sense organs and auditory receptors in most vertebrate classes. The data show that labyrinthine efferent cells are predominantly found in a single nucleus that is associated with the facial motoneurons (FIG. 1), in particular, the branchiomotor component, which is found in the brain stem of vertebrates.[1,7]

Modern tract tracing data may have settled the question of the existence and distribution of labyrinthine efferents in adult vertebrates, but unsettled disputes over the development of efferents remain. For example, until six years ago efferents to the mammalian ear were presumed to arrive later than afferents.[8] This suggestion was based on electron microscopic data that described only afferent terminals in the vestibular[9] and cochlear epithelia.[8] This assumed late arrival of efferents to the mouse inner ear was thus based predominantly on a lack of criteria to identify these fibers by electron microscopic techniques at early stages; the data from more recent immunocytochemical studies have been interpreted only in this context[10] without even discussing the possibility that efferent fibers may be present and labeled by antibodies otherwise specific for axons.

In contrast to this suggested neonatal arrival of efferents at the labyrinthine periphery, data exist on the final mitosis of presumed cochlear efferent cells in the trapezoid nucleus of the rat.[11] These data suggest that some cochlear efferent cells become postmitotic about the same time as facial branchiomotor motoneurons[11] and may be among the first neurons to become postmitotic within the brain stem. Given the known trophic dependence of all these efferent neurons on their periphery, one may ask how these cells are trophically supported from embryonic days 9 to 11, when they become postmitotic in the mouse until postnatal day 2 or more when they start to form synapses.[3]

[a] This work was supported in part by National Institutes of Health Grant No. P50 DC 00215.
[b] E-mail: Fritzsch@creighton.edu

These conflicting data and the open questions arising from them prompted us to reinvestigate the time of arrival of labyrinthine efferent fibers in the developing ear, as well as the distribution of labyrinthine efferent perikarya over time in the developing mouse and chicken. To accomplish these goals we used two recent techniques, the diffusion of the lipophylic dye, DiI, in fixed tissue[12] and the rapid diffusion of low molecular tracers in *in vitro* brain-stem preparations.[13] In addition, we used a combination of detailed analysis of transgenic mice and correlated studies of *in situ* gene expression in conjunction with fluorescent tracers[14,15] to test alternate hypotheses about the molecular governance of fiber outgrowth.

METHODS

Staged chicken and mouse embryos were obtained as previously described.[16,17] Briefly, the application of dyes was done at identical sites, but animals were either (1) fixed in 4% paraformaldehyde in 0.1 M phosphate buffer (for DiI) or (2) brain-stem preparations were made for the *in vitro* application of fast diffusing dyes. The

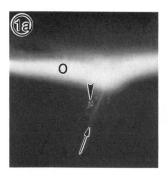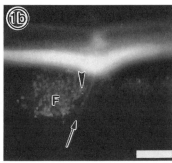

FIGURE 1. Labyrinthine efferents in juvenile lamprey, *Ichthyomyzon unicuspis.* Afferent (O) and efferent neurons (*arrowhead*) of the inner ear (**a**) and the facial nerve (**b**) are filled through application of Texas Red dextran amine to the octaval branches inside the otic capsule (**a**) and of fluoresceine dextran amine to the facial nerve (**b**). Flat-mounted whole brain, anterior is to the right, medial is down. The Mauthner cell (*arrow*) is weakly stained by some transcellular transfer of dye and serves as a landmark in both micrographs. Note the large population of facial motoneurons (F; **b**) of which the labyrinthine efferent cells (*arrowhead* in **a** and **b**) appear to be only a small fraction. Labyrinthine efferent cells were not double labeled but appear so because of incomplete filter segregation. Bar indicates 100 μm.

applications were aimed either peripherally or centrally to target selectively efferent cells or axons alone, or in combination with facial motoneurons and axons. After appropriate diffusion times, the animals were prepared and viewed either as whole mounts or sectioned and viewed with an epifluorescent microscope and a conventional light microscope.

SEGREGATION OF VESTIBULAR AND COCHLEAR EFFERENT CELLS FROM FACIAL BRANCHIOMOTOR MOTONEURONS

Mouse

Application of either dye to the VII/VIIIth nerve complex in 10.5-day-postcoitus (dpc)-old mice results in anterograde labeling of afferents and a few retrogradely labeled cells within rhombomere 4. Similar applications in 11-dpc mice reveal two distinct populations of cells within rhombomeres 4 and 5, adjacent to the floor plate. Most of the cells in rhombomere 4 extend secondary processes parallel to the floor plate, and a few cells apparently translocate caudally within this secondary process to rhombomere 6 by 11–11.5 dpc (FIG. 2a and b). Here these caudally translocating cells change direction and migrate ventrolaterally to form the branchiomotor nucleus of the facial nerve at about 12.5 dpc, while their trailing axons become the internal genu of the facial branchiomotor nerve.

Other cells in rhombomere 4 show axonal branches that enter and traverse the floor plate at 11.5 dpc and yet another group of cells that extends secondary processes laterally within rhombomere 4 or caudolaterally into rhombomere 5. At first (11.5 dpc) some, and subsequently (12 dpc; FIG. 2c) many, cells appear rather suddenly on the contralateral side. Selective labeling of the VIIIth cranial nerve around 12.5–13 dpc reveals two more-or-less segregated ipsilateral and contralateral populations of inner ear efferent cells (FIG. 2c). Thus, on both sides of the hindbrain there are populations of labyrinthine efferent cells that are bilateral along the floor plate, with a number of cells dispersing more laterally (FIG. 2c and d). However, on the ipsilateral side a much larger population of efferent cells is found which forms an elongated column extending through rhombomeres 4 and 5 (FIG. 2d). Even later (14 dpc; FIG. 2e and f) individual cells can be distinguished near the ventricle and next to the efferent fiber tracts in addition to the more meningeally displaced cells.

Comparison with the known adult distribution of ipsilateral efferents in rodents suggests that the large, ipsilateral ventrolateral population represents the predominantly ipsilateral population of cochlear efferents in the lateral superior olive (LSO)[18,19] and the smaller population of ipsilateral cochlear efferents located in the ventral nucleus of the trapezoid body (VNTB).[18] The smaller, contralateral population in a similar position should represent the contralateral component of VNTB olivocochlear efferent cells.[18] The bilateral population near the floor plate and the bilateral cells more lateral and closer to the ventricle (FIG. 2e and f) may represent the bilaterally distributed vestibular efferents.[20] These cells closely resemble the distribution of vestibular efferents around the internal facial genu and the more ventral vestibular population in the caudal pontine reticular formation.[20] In contrast to this dynamic segregation of efferent neurons differentiating within rhombomere 4, the population of efferent neurons in rhombomere 5 does not show any caudal translocation, but does translocate laterally within the primary process.

Chicken

In chicken, the first cells in the hindbrain can be filled through application to the VII/VIIIth nerve complex as early as 2.5 days of incubation (E2.5). All retrogradely labeled efferent cells are unilaterally distributed, predominantly in rhombomere 4, but also in rhombomere 5 (FIG. 3a and b). Only one-half a day later many more cells are labeled in both rhombomeres and some additional cells appear in rhombomere 3. At E3 many cells in both rhombomeres undergo a lateral translocation within the primary process (FIG. 3c and d). There is no caudal extension parallel to the floor plate. However, a large number of cells in rhombomere 4 and a few cells in rhombomere 5 extend a secondary process into the floor plate.[17,21,22] The latter cells apparently translocate within this process first closer to the floor plate and eventually appear inside the floor plate at about 3–3.5 days (FIG. 3d and e) and a few hours later on the contralateral side (FIG. 3f). An *in vitro* analysis showed that cells do migrate through the floor plate within about 24 hours,[23] apparently by translocating their perikarya through the leading processes as suggested for other efferent neurons of

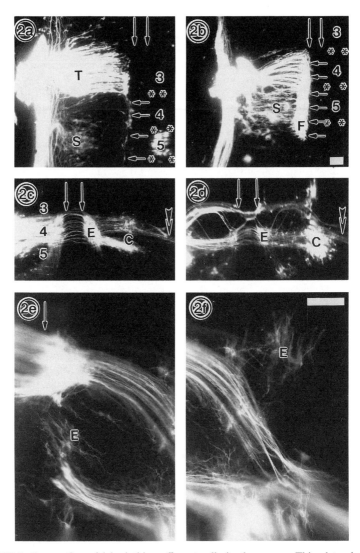

FIGURE 2. Segregation of labyrinthine efferent cells in the mouse. This plate shows the organization of facial motoneurons and labyrinthine efferents in 10.5 dpc (**a**), 11 dpc (**b**), 12 dpc (**c**), 13 dpc (**d**), and 14 dpc (**e** and **f**) old mice. Flat-mounted brains, anterior is top. Rhombomeres are indicated by numbers, boundaries by asterisk. In early stages DiI application to the trigeminal/greater petrosal (T; **a**) and facial/octaval nerve (**b**) labels the afferent projections along the alar plate and also the efferent cells near the floor plate (*large arrow*). Trigeminal motoneurons (T; **a**) and visceromotor motoneurons of the superior salvatory nucleus (S; **a** and **b**) translocate laterally within the primary process. Facial branchiomotor motoneurons (F; **b**) translocate within a secondary process parallel to the floor plate from rhombomere 4 into rhombomere 6 (*small arrows;* **a** and **b**) bypassing the abducent motoneurons in rhombomere 5 (5; **a**). Labyrinthine efferents disperse from rhombomere 4 into rhombomere 5 and eventually segregate into vestibular efferent (E; **c–f**) and cochlear (C; **c** and **d**) populations. Note that efferent axons cross the floor plate only in rhombomere 4 (**c** and **d**) and extend bilaterally to the contralateral ear (double arrowhead; **c** and **d**). Bar in **b** indicates 100 μm for **a–d**; bar in **f** indicates 100 μm for **e** and **f**.

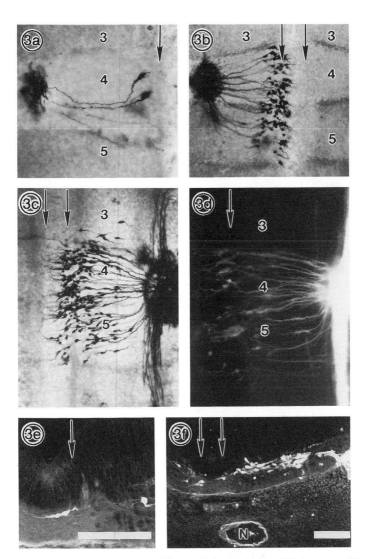

FIGURE 3. Segregation of labyrinthine efferent cells in the chicken. Whole-mounted (anterior is up, **a–d**) and sectioned (**e** and **f**) chicken brains in which the facial and labyrinthine efferents and afferents were filled with biotinylated (**a–c**) or Texas Red conjugated (**e** and **f**) dextran amines, or with DiI (**d**). Applications were to the facial/octaval nerve proximal to the ganglion on the right (**c–f**) or the left side (**a** and **b**). The earliest efferent cells are to be found in rhombomere 4 (E2.5; **a**), but are soon joined by cells in rhombomere 5 (E2.5; **b**). Some of these cells extend a secondary process into the floor plate (*large arrows;* **b–d**) and will eventually translocate the perikaryon first into the floor plate (E3; **c** and **e**) and then to the contralateral side (E3.5; **d** and **f**). Note that most cells translocate through rhombomere 4 but a substantial fraction does this in rhombomere 5. N, notochord. Bar in **f** indicates 100 μm for **b, c, d,** and **f**; bar in **e** indicates 100 μm for **a** and **e**.

the brain stem.[24,25] Further segregation leads to the well-described distribution of efferents in a column extending from the floor of the IVth ventricle to the meninges medial of the facial motor nucleus.[26,27]

In summary, chicken and mice both have facial motoneurons and labyrinthine efferent cells that become postmitotic around the same developmental time and overlap initially within the brain stem. Although chickens do have the equivalent of the superior salivatory nucleus of mammals, it is unclear whether these cells become postmitotic exclusively in rhombomere 5, as in the mouse. Thus, branchiomotor and visceromotor motoneurons derive from two distinct rhombomeres in the mouse, but may actually overlap in both rhombomeres in birds. Clearly, labyrinthine efferents form in both rhombomere 4 and the anterior portion of rhombomere 5 in the chicken, but only in rhombomere 4 in the mouse and overlappingly with the branchiomotor motoneurons.

Subsequently, labyrinthine efferents and facial branchiomotor motoneurons segregate through differential migration within primary or secondary processes. The pathways taken are, however, very different. The facial branchiomotor motoneurons of the mouse migrate caudally along the floor plate, trailing their axons to form the facial genu as previously suggested.[11,28] By contrast, visceral motoneurons of rhombomere 5 and labyrinthine efferents of rhombomere 4 migrate predominantly laterally away from the floor plate, but in either secondary processes (labyrinthine efferents) or in their axons (visceral motoneurons). In the chicken, all motoneurons follow the same pattern of lateral migration within primary processes, except for the contralaterally migrating labyrinthine efferents that translocate across the floor plate through secondary processes. Thus, substantial differences exist in the mode of dispersal of motoneurons generated in rhombomeres 4 and 5 both within a species and between species. It is only recently that some of the putative mechanisms that may guide these behaviors have become apparent.

POSSIBLE MOLECULAR BASIS FOR DIFFERENTIAL CELLULAR MIGRATION IN HINDBRAIN MOTONEURONS

It is possible that the floor plate releases substances that mediate the (1) lateral migration of motoneurons in chicken and mice, (2) medial migration of labyrinthine efferents in chicken, and (3) longitudinal migration of facial branchiomotor motoneurons in mice. Netrin 1 is one possible candidate that mediates this; it is expressed in the floor plate and has a bivalent action: it repels some axons while attracting others.[29] Thus, different neurons can react in a different manner to the same signal, and it is conceivable that a given neuron may change its behavior toward the same signal during development. Given that neuronal migration is nothing more than translocation within a leading axonal process, it can be assumed that the guiding principles for neuronal migration and axonal steering are, in principle, comparable. Changing the trajectories of migration in a given population could thus involve a simple switch in gene activation. Instead of receptors that use a given molecule for a repulsing action, another kind of receptor is expressed that uses the same signal for attracting actions of the migrating cell. In the mouse, it is possible that the migration of facial branchiomotor motoneurons along the floor plate is mediated by a balance between attraction and repulsion generated by two different kinds of substances such as the semaphorins and the netrins.[30]

PATHWAYS OF EFFERENT FIBERS ARE DIFFERENT
IN THE CHICKEN AND MOUSE

Dil or dextran application to rhombomeres 4 and 5 in the chicken and mouse reveals that the first fibers exit the brain stem by E2.5 and 10 dpc, respectively. At this early stage a distinction does not yet exist between the branchiomotor and labyrinthine efferent projection. This could be due to the lack of available criteria that can distinguish the two sets of fibers.

Mouse

In the mouse, fibers emanating from neurons within rhombomere 4 segregate within the brain stem into two fascicles by 11 dpc (FIG. 4a). One fascicle extends in the same plane from the cells of origin near the floor plate to the vestibular root, the labyrinthine efferents. The second, much larger bundle is fan shaped and converges on a point halfway between the perikarya and the vestibular root. Here the fibers change direction and run toward the facial branchiomotor root. Thus, a segregation of branchiomotor fibers and labyrinthine efferent fibers already is present in the brain stem of mouse embryos as is also found in the adult system.[19,28] In addition, a third fascicle emanates from the visceromotor motoneurons in rhombomere 5 and forms the intermediate nerve which exits between the labyrinthine efferent and the branchiomotor motoneuron axons (FIG. 4a).

Fibers crossing the floor plate are found to emanate from cells exclusively within rhombomere 4 (FIG. 3b and c). Many of these fibers appear to be collaterals that can be traced to the contralateral VIIIth nerve root as early as 12 dpc (FIG. 2c and d). This bilateral distribution of fibers agrees with the known bilateral projection of the vestibular efferents and the cochlear efferents in the VNTB.[20] Peripherally, these fibers can be traced toward the various differentiating sensory epithelia where they end in growth cones by 13 dpc (FIG. 4b). Only a rare filopodium from these growth cones appears to reach into the sensory epithelia by this stage. However, by 14 dpc, many fibers have extended filopodia and growth cones into the sensory epithelia (FIG. 4c), and by 14.5 dpc individual efferent fibers branch underneath the hair cells to form processes around several hair cells (FIG. 4d). Verification of the early stages of synapse formation requires electron microscopic analysis.

Chicken

In embryonic chicken, no distinction exists among the pathways taken by branchiomotor, visceromotor or labyrinthine efferent fibers in rhombomeres 4 and 5. All fibers converge in a more-or-less pronounced arc toward the facial root. Although efferent fibers extend only 100 μm into the VII/VIIIth complex by E2.5, they extend about 200–300 μm by E3. It is around E3.5 that the labyrinthine efferent fibers can be identified: they leave the brain along with facial efferent fibers, but reorganize and diverge as two discrete fascicles to enter the dorsal and ventral subdivision of the VIIIth nerve, respectively (FIG. 5d). The fact that only efferent fibers behave in this manner has been proven by applying fast-diffusing dextrans to the cut midline of E3.5 chicken embryos.[17] These applications revealed only fibers rerouting from the facial root into the VIIIth nerve, which is consistent with the interpretation that all crossing cells are in fact efferent to the ear (FIG. 5a and c). Anterograde filling of efferent

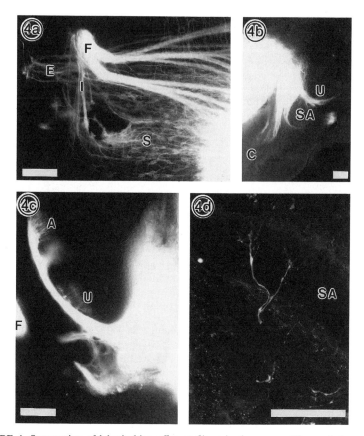

FIGURE 4. Segregation of labyrinthine efferent fibers in the mouse. These whole-mounted brain (**a**) and sections (**b–d**) show the segregation of facial branchiomotor (F; **a**) and labyrinthine efferent fibers (E) lateral to the facial root (F) as revealed by application of DiI (**a–c**) or Texas Red dextran amine (**d**) to the basal plate of the brain stem. Note the labeling of superior salvatory neurons (S) which project through the intermediate nerve (I) by 11 dpc (**a**). By 13 dpc all sensory epithelia of the ear have efferent fibers adjacent to them (**b**). By 14 dpc these fibers invade the sensory epithelia (**c**), and by 14.5 dpc growth cones branch underneath the future hair cells and filopodia extend between them (**d**). A, anterior vertical canal; C, cochlea; F, facial nerve or root; SA, saccule; U, utricle. Bar indicates 100 μm.

fibers from the brain stem shows them to be underneath the respective sensory epithelium by E4.5. At E6, the fibers extend into the sensory epithelia and branch profusely (FIG. 5d).

The differences in behavior of efferent fibers between the mouse and the chicken could be best explained by assuming (1) either a diffusible factor released from the otocyst that attracts the efferents much as it has been suggested for afferents[31] or (2) through a specific interaction with cells and/or matrix at decision points that make efferent fibers radically change their course and stir away from facial branchiomotor fibers. Given that the pathway selection in the developing mouse and chicken efferents, with respect to the point where they deviate from facial motoneurons, is different (inside the brain in the mouse and in the VII nerve root in the chicken), it appears reasonable to assume that a diffusible substance is the more likely candidate for mediating efferent axonal behavior.

POSSIBLE MOLECULAR BASIS FOR DIFFERENTIAL AXONAL PROJECTIONS OF FACIAL MOTONEURONS AND LABYRINTHINE EFFERENTS

In order to test for possible diffusible substances released from the developing ear, we checked whether efferent fibers arrive at areas of neurotrophin expression at

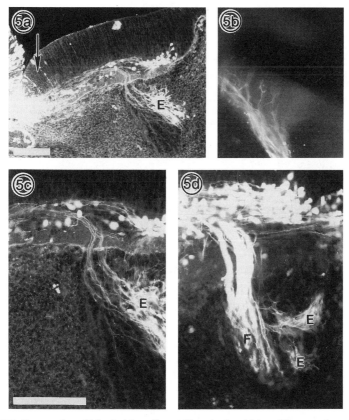

FIGURE 5. Segregation of labyrinthine efferent fibers in the chicken. These sections show the segregation of facial branchiomotor (F; **d**) and labyrinthine efferent fibers (E; **a, c,** and **d**) outside the brain as revealed by application of Texas Red dextran amine (**a, c,** and **d**) or DiI (**b**) to the basal plate (**d** and **d**) or the floor plate (**a** and **c**) of the brain stem. By E3.5 labyrinthine efferents form two fascicles within the anterior and posterior subdivision of the octaval nerve (**d**). Evidence that at least all cells that translocate across the floor plate project to the ear is obtained after dye application to longitudinally cut in the floor plate (*large arrow;* **a**). By six days the efferent fibers have started to ramify within the sensory epithelia of the horizontal canal (**b**). Bar in **c** indicates 100 μm for **b–d;** bar in **a** indicates 100 μm for **a**.

the otocyst and whether they express the appropriate receptor. The first likely candidate we investigated was brain-derived neurotrophic factor (BDNF) and its receptor tyrosine kinase B (trkB). The reason for choosing this neurotrophin from several possible candidates was based on the suggestions that BDNF may be the neurotrophin that supports facial motoneurons[32] and that a mutant lacking a functional trkB allele loses a substantial number of facial branchiomotor motoneurons,[33] a claim that has recently been refuted (Silos-Santiago, in preparation).

For the study of efferent arrival areas, we examined the distribution of efferent fibers at the developing chicken ear at E4.5, employing the anterograde transport of fast-diffusing fluorescent dextran amines in combination with in situ hybridization for BDNF and trkB.[15] In agreement with previous data on rodents,[34] these data showed areas of high BDNF expression in the otocyst of the chicken and that efferents first reach the otocyst at these areas. Unfortunately, we could not detect appreciable concentrations of trkB mRNA in the labyrinthine efferent or facial motoneuron perikarya. By contrast, afferent fibers are typically not as close to the sensory epithelia as efferents, but express a strong trkB signal, again in agreement with data on rodents.[35] Important for our further analysis was the finding that efferent axons are always next to differentiated afferent dendrites when we labeled both fiber types simultaneously with neuronal tracers. These data were more consistent with the idea that labyrinthine efferents use differentiated labyrinthine afferents to home toward sensory epithelia. However, it appears likely that a signal other than BDNF may play a further role in navigation near the sensory epithelia.

We next examined the role played by BDNF and trkB in transgenic mice, through a targeted disruption of the BDNF receptor gene, trkB.[33] Our data showed a remarkable loss of afferent innervation to the semicircular canals between 12.5 dpc and 13.5 dpc and a reduction of the afferent innervation to the saccule and the utricle,[14] in general agreement with an earlier report of extensive loss of vestibular ganglion cells in BDNF knockout mutants.[36] Even more striking were the effects on the vestibular efferents. The fibers reached the utricle with about a one-day delay and very sparingly compared to normal litter mates. By contrast, neither cochlear afferents nor efferents were apparently affected by this gene disruption, at least until P0.

Although a direct action of the trkB receptor cannot be ruled out, the two sets of data combined tend to agree more with a scenario where only viable afferents can guide efferents to sensory epithelia. It is reasonable to assume that the first afferents growing out to sensory epithelia at 12.5 dpc are the first to depend on the neurotrophins sequestered from the target and their neurotrophin receptors. These afferent vestibular ganglion cells should consequently be the first cells to degenerate. Apparently the other signals released from the ear, which guide afferents to sensory epithelia,[31] are either shut down very early or else do not diffuse far enough to guide afferents in older stages of development. As a consequence, there is no further fiber extension toward the sensory epithelia despite the fact that new ganglion cells do become postmitotic until 14 dpc.[37] A detailed comparison of afferent and efferent innervation in sensory epithelia, with a reduced innervation in these mutants, showed in fact a detailed match in distribution in support of the above-outlined scenario.[14]

Examination of a second receptor (trkC) of a neurotrophin known to play a role in spiral ganglion survival[38] showed no appreciable effect on the vestibular system.[14] However, a double mutant lacking both trkB and trkC had no innervation at all to the ear, which nevertheless developed normally until birth.[14] It appears that neither afferents nor efferents are necessary for ear development and a certain degree of hair cell maturation. However, it needs to be shown in these double mutants whether labyrinthine efferent fibers, as well as afferents, extend to the ear at all earlier in development. If the above-outlined interpretation is correct, one would not expect any efferent extension toward the sensory epithelia at any time in these double mutants.

SUMMARY

The data presented here show that labyrinthine and facial branchiomotor efferent cells in the chicken and the mouse become postmitotic overlappingly, both spatially and temporally. Differential migration of labyrinthine efferents and facial motoneurons leads to the already described distinct distribution of labyrinthine efferents and facial motoneurons in adult brains. Differences exist between the chicken and the mouse with respect to the origin of labyrinthine efferents (rhombomere 4 and 5 for the chicken; rhombomere 4 alone for the mouse) and the way contralateral labyrinthine efferents form (migration across the floor plate in the chicken; extension of an axon across the floor plate in the mouse). The different routes taken by migrating motoneurons may all be mediated by substances released from the floor plate, some of which were recently characterized.

Labyrinthine efferent axons and facial motoneuron axons segregate at distinctly different areas in the chicken and mouse: outside the brain in the former and inside the brain in the latter. Examination of the possible basis for pathway selection tends to support the idea that efferents use intact afferent fibers as highways for their navigation to distinct sensory epithelia.

ACKNOWLEDGMENTS

I wish to thank J. D. Kingsley for streamlining my English and Maria Christensen for technical assistance. I also wish to acknowledge the delightful collaboration with Drs. I. Silos-Santiago, A. Fagan, R. Smeyne, M. Barbacid, and F. Hallböök on knockout mice and in situ hybridization in the chicken.

REFERENCES

1. ROBERTS, B. L. & G. E. MEREDITH. 1992. The efferent innervation of the ear: Variations on an enigma. In The Evolutionary Biology of Hearing. D. B. Webster, A. N. Popper & R. R. Fay, Eds.: 182–210. Springer. New York.
2. FRITZSCH, B., H. H. ZAKON & D. Y. SANCHEZ. 1990. The time course of structural changes in regenerating electroreceptors of a weakly electric fish. J. Comp. Neurol. 300: 386–404.
3. SOBKOWICZ, H. M. 1992. The development of innervation in the organ of Corti. In Development of Auditory and Vestibular Systems 2. R. Romand, Ed.: 59–100. Elsevier. Amsterdam.
4. PRECHT, W. 1976. Physiology of the peripheral and central vestibular system. In Frog Neurobiology. R. Llinas & W. Precht, Eds.: 452–480. Springer. New York.
5. FRITZSCH, B. & U. WAHNSCHAFFE. 1987. Electron microscopical evidence for common inner ear and lateral-line efferents in urodeles. Neurosci. Lett. 81: 48–52.
6. HIGHSTEIN, S. M. 1992. The efferent control of the organs of balance and equilibrium in the toadfish, Opsanus tau. Ann. N.Y. Acad. Sci. 656: 108–123.
7. PERACHIO, A. A. & G. A. KEVETTER. 1989. Identification of vestibular efferent neurons in the gerbil: Histochemical and retrograde labelling. Exp. Brain Res. 78: 315–326.

8. PUJOL, R. 1986. Synaptic plasticity in the developing cochlea. *In* The Biology of Change in Otolaryngology. R. W. Ruben, T. R. Van de Water & E. W Rubel, Eds.: 47–54. Elsevier. Amsterdam.

9. FAVRE, D. & A. SANS. 1978. The development of vestibular efferent nerve endings during cat maturation: Ultrastructural study. Brain Res. **142**: 333–337.

10. SCARFONE, E., D. DEMEMES & A. SANS. 1991. Synapsin I and synaptophysin expression during ontogenesis of the mouse peripheral vestibular system. J. Neurosci. **11**: 1173–1181.

11. ALTMAN, J. & S. A. BAYER. 1980. Development of the brainstem in the rat. III. Thymidine-radiographic study of the time of origin of neurons of the vestibular and auditory nuclei of the upper medulla. J. Comp. Neurol. **194**: 877–904.

12. GODEMENT, P., J. VANSELOV, S. THANOS & F. BONHOEFFER. 1987. A study in developing visual systems with a new method of staining neurones and their processes in fixed tissue. Development **101**: 687–713.

13. FRITZSCH, B. 1993. Fast diffusion of 3000 molecular weight dextran amines. J. Neurosci. Methods **50**: 95–103.

14. FRITZSCH, B., I. SILOS-SANTIAGO, D. SMEYNE, A. FAGAN & R. BARBACID. 1995. Reduction and loss of inner ear innervation in *trk*B and *trk*C receptor knockout mice: A whole mount DiI and SEM analysis. Auditory Neurosci. **1**: 401–417.

15. HALLBÖÖK, F. & B. FRITZSCH. 1995. The distribution of BDNF and *trk*B mRNA in the otic region of 4.5 day chicken as revealed with a combination of *in situ* hybridization and tract tracing. Hear. Res. Submitted.

16. FRITZSCH, B. & D. H. NICHOLS. 1993. DiI reveals a prenatal arrival of efferents at developing ears of mice. Hear. Res. **65**: 51–60.

17. FRITZSCH, B., M. A. CHRISTENSEN & D. H. NICHOLS. 1993. Fiber pathways and positional changes in efferent perikarya of 2.5 to 7 day chick embryos as revealed with DiI and dextran amines. J. Neurobiol. **24**: 1481–1499.

18. CAMPBELL, J. P. & M. M. HENSON. 1988. Olivocochlear neurons in the brainstem of the mouse. Hear. Res. **35**: 271–274.

19. BROWN, M. C. 1993. Fiber pathways and branching patterns of biocytin-labeled olivocochlear neurons in the mouse brainstem. J. Comp. Neurol. **337**: 600–613.

20. ASCHOFF, A. & J. OSTWALD. 1988. Distribution of cochlear efferents and olivocollicular neurons in the brainstem of rat and guinea pig. Exp. Brain Res. **71**: 241–251.

21. MARSH, E., K. UCHINO & R. BAKER. 1992. Cranial efferent neurons extend processes through the floor plate in the developing hind brain. Biol. Bull. **183**: 354–356.

22. GILLAND, E. & R. BAKER. 1992. Longitudinal and tangential migration of cranial nerve efferent neurons in the developing hind brain of *Squalus acanthias*. Biol. Bull. **183**: 356–358.

23. SIMON, H. & A. LUMSDEN. 1993. Rhombomere-specific origin of the contralateral vestibuloacoustic efferent neurons and their migration across the embryonic midline. Neuron **11**: 209–220.

24. FRITZSCH, B. & R. G. NORTHCUTT. 1993. Origin and migration of trochlear, oculomotor and abducent motoneurons in *Petromyzon marinus* L. Dev. Brain Res. **74**: 122–126.

25. GILLAND, E. & R. BAKER. 1993. Conservation of neuroepithelial and mesodermal segments in the embryonic vertebrate head. Acta Anat. **148**: 110–123.

26. WHITEHEAD, M. C. & D. K. MOREST. 1981. Dual populations of efferent and afferent cochlear axons in the chicken. Neuroscience **6**: 2351–2365.

27. CODE, R. A. & C. A. CARR. 1994. Choline acetyltransferase-immunoreactive cochlear efferent neurons in the chick auditory brainstem. J. Comp. Neurol. **340**: 161–173.

28. GUINAN, J. J., M. P. JOSEPH & B. E. NORRIS. 1989. Brainstem facial-motor pathways from two distinct groups of stapedius motoneurons in the cat. J. Comp. Neurol. **287**: 134–144.

29. COLAMARINO, S. A. & M. TESSIER-LAVIGNE. 1995. The axonal chemoattractant Netrin-1 is also a chemorepellent for trochlear motor axons. Cell **81**: 621–631.

30. DODD, J. & A. SCHUCHARDT. 1995. Axon guidance: A compelling case for repelling growth cones. Cell **81**: 471–475.

31. BIANCHI, L. M. & C. S. COHAN. 1993. Effects of the neurotrophins and CNTF on developing statoacoustic neurons: Comparison with an otocyst-derived factor. Dev. Biol. **159**: 353–365.
32. OPPENHEIM, R. W., Y. QIN-WEI, D. PREVETTE & Q. YAN. 1992. Brain-derived neurotrophic factor rescues developing avian motoneurons from cell death. Nature **360**: 755–757.
33. KLEIN, R., R. J. SMEYNE, W. WURST, L. K. LONG, B. A. AUERBACH, A. L. JOYNER & M. BARBACID. 1993. Targeted disruption of the *trk*B neurotrophin receptor gene results in nervous system lesions and neonatal death. Cell **75**: 113–122.
34. PIRVOLA, U., J. YLIKOSKI, J. PALGI, E. LEHTONEN, U. ARUMAE & M. SAARMA. 1992. Brain-derived neurotrophic factor and neurotrophin 3 mRNAs in the peripheral target fields of developing inner ear ganglia. Proc. Natl. Acad. Sci. USA **89**: 9915–9919.
35. PIRVOLA, U., U. ARUMAE, M. MOSHNYAKOV, J. PALGI, M. SAARMA & J. YLIKOSKI. 1994. Coordinated expression and function of neurotrophins and their receptors in the rat inner ear during target innervation. Hear. Res. **75**: 131–144.
36. ERNFORS, P., K. F. LEE & R. JAENISCH. 1994. Mice lacking brain-derived neurotrophic factor develop with sensory deficits. Nature **368**: 147–150.
37. RUBEN, R. J. 1967. Development of the inner ear of the mouse: A radioautographic study of terminal mitosis. Acta Oto-Laryngol. **220**: 1–44.
38. FARINAS, I., K. R. JONES, C. BACKUS, X.-Y. WANG & L. F. REICHARDT. 1994. Severe sensory and sympathetic deficits in mice lacking neurotrophin-3. Nature **369**: 658–661.

Hair Cell Generation in Vestibular Sensory Receptor Epithelia

ELIZABETH C. OESTERLE[a] AND EDWIN W RUBEL

*Virginia Merrill Bloedel Hearing Research Center and
Department of Otolaryngology-HNS
University of Washington
Seattle, Washington*

INTRODUCTION

The functions of the ear depend largely on sensory hair cells, which transduce mechanical stimuli into electrical signals that can be conducted to the brain. Vestibular hair cells, the primary receptors of the vestibular end organs, are neuroepithelial cells characterized by apical hair bundles composed of a single kinocilium and a large number of actin-filled stereocilia. In the otolith end organs, the kinocilium is coupled to the otolithic membrane, transmitting movement of this membrane to the displacement-sensitive stereocilia. Vestibular hair cells are typically classified into two types based upon cell body and synapse morphology. Type I hair cells are flask-shaped and innervated by specialized calyceal endings (FIG. 1). Type II hair cells are cylindrical and receive multiple bouton-type endings. Type II hair cells are found in all vertebrates, whereas type I cells are usually considered to be unique to higher vertebrates. A type I-like hair cell has been detected in fish.[1,2] The vestibular sensory receptor epithelium is composed of the vestibular hair cells, glia-like supporting cells, and the terminals of afferent and efferent neurons.

WHEN DO VESTIBULAR HAIR CELLS ORIGINATE?

Vestibular hair cells are produced during embryogenesis and, in many animals, postnatally. Postembryonic production of hair cells occurs throughout life in cold-blooded vertebrates including elasmobranchs,[3–5] bony fishes,[6–8] and amphibians.[9–10] In contrast, hair cell production in warm-blooded vertebrates (e.g., birds and mammals) was thought to be limited to the period of embryogenesis,[11] and any postnatal hair cell loss was considered to be irreversible and associated with a permanent functional deficit. This thinking was challenged in 1988 when Jørgensen and Mathiesen[12] discovered the ongoing production of new vestibular hair cells in the normal adult budgerigar, a warm-blooded vertebrate. Using tritiated-thymidine autoradiography, they demonstrated the mitotic production of new vestibular hair cells in adult avian vestibular sensory epithelia. The findings of Jørgensen and Mathiesen were later replicated by Roberson *et al.*[13] who demonstrated the postnatal production of vestibular hair cells in normal chicks. Both type I and type II hair cells are produced on an ongoing basis in the mature avian inner ear,[14] and they are

[a] Address correspondence to Elizabeth C. Oesterle, Ph.D., Virginia Merrill Bloedel Hearing Research Center, University of Washington, Box 356515, Seattle, Washington 98195. E-mail: Oesterle@otomail.u.washington.edu

thought to arise from mitotic divisions of supporting cells within the sensory epithelium.[13–16]

The reasons for the continued postnatal production of vestibular hair cells are not fully understood. In several species the new hair cells are primarily added to the outer edges of the receptor epithelium,[3,17–20] whereas in some fish and in the avian inner ear the new cells are added throughout the receptor epithelium.[8,12–13] Continued postembryonic hair cell production in lower vertebrates (e.g., lampreys, sharks, skates, bony fish) results in ever-increasing numbers of hair cells as the body size of the animal increases.[3,4,7,10] In avian vestibular end organs, hair cell numbers do not appear to increase markedly as the bird ages, and the production may be related to a continual hair cell turnover.[12,14,21] Cell proliferation in the normal avian vestibular epithelium most likely replaces elements that are lost due to "normal turnover" and as a result of aging, trauma, or disease.

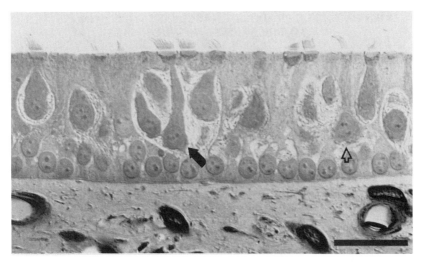

FIGURE 1. Photomicrograph of the vestibular sensory epithelium of a 10-day-old chicken. Hair cell nuclei are located in the lumenal portion of the sensory epithelium. Several rows of supporting cell nuclei lie next to the basal lamina. The structural organization of the avian vestibular sensory epithelium is almost identical to that of mammals. *Solid arrow:* Type I hair cell; these cells are flask-shaped and enclosed in the nerve ending. *Open arrow:* Type II hair cell. Calibration bar = 20 μm.

The story regarding the mammalian inner ear is unclear. In an autoradiographic investigation of the developing inner ear of the mouse, Ruben[11] did not find mitoses in the vestibular sensory epithelia after a few days postpartum. However, several recent studies indicate that the long-held assumption that hair cell production in the mammalian inner ear occurs only during embryogenesis needs to be reevaluated. Forge et al.[22] and Rubel et al.[23] examined the vestibular sensory epithelium of the normal mature guinea-pig ear with scanning electron microscopy and detected a few hair cells with immature stereociliary bundles. The bundles displayed the same morphological characteristics as those seen in embryonic chickens—short stereocilia, uniformly sized, and clumped around a single, centrally located kinocilium. Moreover, the apical surfaces of the cells were smaller than those of normal, mature hair cells. These findings raise the possibility that there may be a limited postnatal production of new hair cells in the mature mammalian vestibular sensory epithelium. Alternatively, some hair cells may get injured, lose their stereocilia bundle, and then repair that structure by the growth of a new sensory surface.[24] Recent studies, where a cell proliferation marker was continuously infused into the normal rodent ear for periods ranging from 4 days up to 6 weeks,[23,25] suggest that cells with immature stereociliary bundles do not arise via a proliferative mechanism. Proliferating sensory epithelial cells were not detected in the normal, undamaged vestibular sensory epithelium in these studies. Rubel et al.[23] suggest that hair cells with immature bundles may have been derived from a process of cellular transformation wherein another cell type in the sensory epithelium was converted to a hair cell without going through mitosis. Alternatively, immature hair cell bundles may be the result of hair cells repairing their stereociliary bundles.

DOES HAIR CELL PRODUCTION INCREASE FOLLOWING INSULT TO THE SENSORY EPITHELIUM?

A correlation frequently exists between continued or recent neurogenesis and regeneration (reviewed in ref. 26). Tissues or organs that show constant turnover or ongoing production of sensory elements also possess the capacity to rapidly increase the production of sensory elements in response to insult. For example, the gustatory and olfactory systems of all vertebrate classes show an ongoing production of sensory elements and possess the capacity to proliferate rapidly in response to lesions.[27-28] Inner ear vestibular sensory epithelia also appear to follow this trend. In birds, fish and amphibians, where there is a continual postnatal production of new vestibular hair cells, mitotic activity and hair cell production are rapidly up-regulated after ototoxic antibiotic treatment[14,29,30] (FIG. 2). The new hair cells are at first recognizably immature. Later, they differentiate to become indistinguishable from mature hair cells. Both type I and type II hair cells are regenerated such that virtually all the damaged and lost hair cells are replaced.[14] The new hair cells have been shown to be functional and contribute to the recovery of vestibular function[31,32] (see Carey et al.[33]). Supporting cells that lie within the vestibular sensory receptor epithelium are thought to serve as progenitor cells for the regenerated hair cells.[15,16,34,35]

With regard to the mammalian inner ear, as previously discussed, it is uncertain as to whether any ongoing hair cell proliferation occurs in the normal undamaged vestibular sensory epithelium. Recent studies in rodents and humans have shown a limited increase in DNA synthesis after aminoglycoside-induced hair cell loss.[23,35,36] Although investigators agree that a small number of new supporting cells are produced after ototoxic insult, it is still unresolved as to whether any new hair cells can arise via a proliferative regenerative mechanism in the mature mammalian vestibular sensory epithelium. Using scanning electron microscopy, Forge et al.[22] report increased numbers of cells with immature stereociliary bundles following ototoxin-induced hair cell death. These findings were confirmed by Rubel et al.[23] Given the absence of new hair cells arising via a proliferative route,[23] it is reasonable to speculate that the immature hair cell bundles seen by Forge and collaborators may arise via nonproliferative mechanisms. These nonmitotic mechanisms might include hair cell migration from undamaged macular regions, hair bundle repair in partially damaged hair cells, or cellular transformation of undamaged supporting cells into hair cells. Some support for the existence of nonmitotic mechanisms of hair cell regeneration comes from several recent reports. As discussed in detail in an accompanying paper,[37] hair cell recovery (after drug-induced insult) in bullfrog

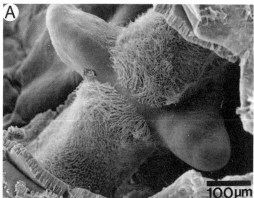
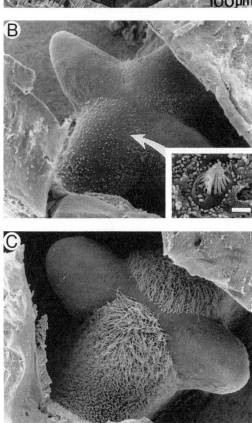

FIGURE 2. Scanning electron micrograph of superior ampullae. (**A**) Crista ampullaris from a 10-day-old normal chicken. (**B**) Crista ampullaris from a chicken injected daily with 600 mg/kg streptomycin (i.m.) for 7 days. The animal was killed immediately after the completion of the injection series. Note the almost complete absence of stereocilia. (**C**) Crista ampullaris of a chicken allowed to survive 60 days after the completion of the streptomycin injections. The sensory epithelium has recovered most of its normal appearance. (From Weisleder and Rubel.[14] Reproduced, with permission, from the *Journal of Comparative Neurology*.)

vestibular otolith organs appears to occur largely by the direct transformation of supporting cells into hair cells without any mitotic divisions.[38] Direct transformation of supporting cells into hair cells is also thought to play a role in the regeneration of avian auditory hair cells after ototoxin-induced hair cell death.[39,40]

HOW DO HAIR CELLS ORIGINATE?

What controls the production of new hair cells? For a mitotic regenerative repair mechanism: What initiates precursor cell proliferation, and what stimulates hair cell differentiation? For a nonmitotic mechanism such as direct transformation: What stimulates supporting cell transformation? Studies of the cultured inner ear suggest that the molecules or factors that trigger hair cell production and differentiation are endemic to the end organ. Warchol and Corwin[41] and Oesterle et al.[42] noted the production of new supporting cells and hair cells in explants of mature vestibular sensory epithelium taken from normal chickens that were cultured in serum-free medium. Abdouh et al.[43] report an overproduction of hair cells in developing rat cochlea that were cultured in serum-free medium. Tsue and colleagues[44] demonstrated that utricles taken from the mature avian inner ear and grown in culture release a substance into their environment that alters levels of cell proliferation in co-cultured normal vestibular sensory epithelium. These studies all suggest that the molecules or factors that trigger hair cell production are produced within the end organ itself. We do not yet know what the signals are. The cellular events that result in all forms of postembryonic addition of hair cells are likely to depend on the binding of specific growth factors to receptors expressed on surfaces of progenitors that either divide to give rise to hair cells or convert directly into hair cells.

Growth Factors Stimulating Progenitor Cell Proliferation

The specific factors that regulate the proliferation of cells in the sensory epithelia of the inner ear have not been conclusively identified. Several growth factors are known to be mitogenic for the developing otocyst as a whole, but little is known regarding factors mitogenic for hair-cell progenitors specifically, in either developing, renewing, or regenerating inner ears. Epidermal growth factor (EGF), platelet-derived growth factor (PDGF), and bombesin are mitogenic for the whole chicken embryo otocyst. Several of these factors are potentiated by insulin.[45] Basic fibroblast growth factor (bFGF) has a mitogenic effect and role in inducing the invagination of the chick otic vesicle *in vitro,*[46] and antisense oligonucleotides and antibodies targeted against *int*-2, a FGF-related proto-oncogene, inhibit proliferation and formation of the otic vesicle.[46] In a controversial study, Lefebvre et al.[47] suggest that retinoic acid may act synergistically with serum to stimulate proliferation in the developing auditory sensory epithelium (the organ of Corti) of drug-damaged neonatal rats. Chardin and Romand,[48] in contrast, were unable to find any stimulation of hair-cell progenitor proliferation by retinoic acid.

In the mature inner ear, insulin-like growth factor-I (IGF-I) stimulates the proliferation of precursor cells in the mature avian vestibular sensory epithelium (FIG. 3) in a dose-dependent manner.[49] Utricles from normal postnatal chickens were isolated and grown in culture. Tritiated [³H]thymidine, a cell proliferation marker, was added to the cultures at the start of the culture period. IGF-I was added to the experimental cultures only. After two days of *in vitro* growth, the explants were fixed, and the numbers of [³H]thymidine-labeled cells were assessed. A dose-dependent increase in proliferation occurs in response to IGF-I. A threefold increase in sensory epithelial cell proliferation is produced by the addition of 100 ng/mL of IGF-I.

The hormone insulin also stimulates cell proliferation in cultured vestibular sensory epithelium taken from the normal postnatal chicken[49] (FIG. 4). Insulin concentrations equal to or greater than 100 ng/mL are effective in stimulating mitosis in the mature avian vestibular epithelium. A twofold increase in proliferation is produced by the addition of 100 ng/mL insulin.

IGF-I, insulin, and insulin-like growth factor-II (IGF-II) are members of the insulin-like growth factor family of peptides that regulate metabolic pathways, mitogenesis, and cell differentiation. IGF-I shares about 50% sequence identity with proinsulin.[50] IGF-I is synthesized by a number of tissues in the body, including the central nervous system and muscle, but the majority of circulating IGF-I is secreted

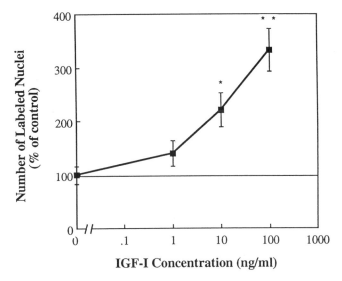

IGF-I Concentration (ng/ml)

FIGURE 3. The effects of IGF-I on [³H]thymidine incorporation in cultured avian vestibular sensory epithelium. Normal utricles were taken from postnatal chickens and grown in culture for 2 days. IGF-I was added to experimental cultures, but not to control cultures, at the start of the culture period. [³H]thymidine was present during the entire incubation period. [³H]thymidine is taken up by the DNA of dividing cells during the S phase of the cell cycle, allowing the identification of proliferating cells. IGF-I up-regulates cell proliferation in the normal vestibular sensory epithelium in a dose-dependent manner. Each data value represents the mean value (±SEM) of at least 16 specimens. The mean number of [³H]thymidine-labeled cells in the sensory epithelium of the IGF-I supplemented cultures was expressed as a percentage of the control cultures. The control mean is indicated in the figure by the solid line. Single asterisks indicate a significant difference at the .05 level. A double asterisk indicates that the growth factor mean is significantly different from the control mean at the .01 level. (From Oesterle et al.[49])

from the liver.[51,52] Cell types known to express IGF-I include hepatocytes, neurons, astrocytes, renal tubular cells, fibroblasts, vascular smooth and skeletal muscle satellite cells,Schwann cells, macrophages, and neutrophils (reviewed in ref. 53). Although circulating IGF-I proteins can act in an endocrine mode, most tissues synthesize IGF proteins, which then can act locally in an autocrine/paracrine manner.[53] Proliferation of a variety of cell types, at least in culture, requires the presence of IGF-I. These include many human tumor cell lines, fibroblasts, neuroblasts, myoblasts, keratinocytes, smooth muscle cells, osteoblasts, chondrocytes,

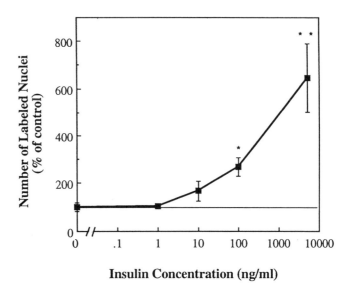

Insulin Concentration (ng/ml)

FIGURE 4. The effects of insulin on [³H]thymidine incorporation in cultured avian vestibular sensory epithelium. Normal utricles were taken from postnatal chickens and grown in culture for 2 days. [³H]thymidine was present during the entire incubation period. Insulin increases cell proliferation in a dose-dependent manner. Each data value represents the mean value (±SEM) of at least 11 specimens. The solid line represents the control mean. Single asterisks indicate a significant difference at the .05 level. A double asterisk indicates that the growth factor mean is significantly different from the control mean at the .01 level. (From Oesterle et al.[49])

hemopoietic cells, astroglia, satellite cells, fetal brown adipocytes, granulosa cells, neuronal cells, and retinal pigment epithelial cells (see refs. 54–56 for reviews).

Actions of IGF-I are mediated by the IGF-I receptor (type I IGF receptor), which is a membrane-bound tyrosine kinase receptor, homologous to the insulin receptor.[57] IGF-I receptors bind IGF-I, IGF-II, and insulin (at supraphysiological concentrations) (reviewed in refs. 58 and 59). In the inner ear, IGF-I first reliably stimulates mitosis in the mature vestibular sensory epithelium at a concentration of 10 ng/mL, whereas 100 ng/mL of insulin—10 times more—is required to significantly stimulate mitosis in the cultured vestibular sensory epithelium. Given that the IGF-I receptor binds IGF-I and insulin with different affinities, the higher required concentration of insulin suggests that insulin is probably exerting its mitogenic effects in the mature avian vestibular sensory epithelium by binding to the IGF-I receptors.[49]

Several lines of evidence suggest an involvement of EGF and transforming growth factor α (TGF-α) in regulating cell proliferation in the mammalian inner ear. TGF-α and EGF are members of the EGF family of growth factors. They are known to affect epithelial and mesenchymal cell proliferation, migration, and differentiation (reviewed in ref. 60), and to regulate epithelial cell proliferation during wound healing.[61] They are mitogens for developing retinal neuronal progenitor cells[62,63] and stimulate proliferation of multipotent cells isolated from the adult mouse brain.[64] All known actions of EGF and TGF-α appear to be mediated by the EGF receptor (EGF-R), and no evidence exists for a distinct receptor (reviewed in ref. 65). TGF-α mRNA has been shown to be present at high levels in the otic vesicle of the mouse fetus,[66] and EGF receptors have been detected on supporting cells of the organ of Corti in the neonatal rat[67] and mature rodent.[68] EGF receptors have also been localized to vestibular hair cells and supporting cells in the mature rat (Oesterle and Debel, unpublished). Proteins with TGF-α-like and EGF-like immunoreactivity are expressed in the mature avian cochlea.[69,70] Regarding the possible actions of EGF and TGF-α in the ear, EGF has been shown to stimulate proliferation in the growth-arrested chick otocyst, and insulin can potentiate this effect.[45] TGF-α stimulates a low level of proliferation in normal[71,72] and drug-damaged[36] murine vestibular sensory epithelium grown in culture. As shown in FIGURE 5, the mitogenic effect of TGF-α is potentiated by insulin.[72] EGF, when supplemented with insulin, also stimulates a low level of proliferation *in vitro* in the normal mature murine vestibular sensory epithelium.[72] TGF-α is more potent in increasing proliferation of hair-cell progenitors than EGF. Both act synergistically with insulin. The enhanced potency of TGF-α in the inner ear may be the result of higher receptor affinity and perhaps differential trafficking of internalized TGF-α/EGF-R versus EGF/EGF-R complexes.[73] Recent work of Kuntz and Oesterle[25] demonstrates that TGF-α plus insulin significantly stimulates a low level of proliferation *in situ* in the normal rat vestibular sensory epithelium.

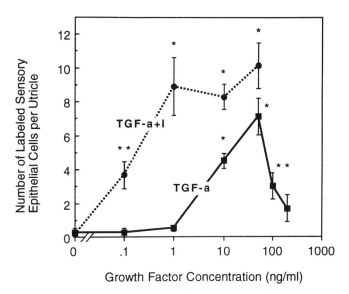

FIGURE 5. The effect of TGF-α on DNA synthesis in mouse vestibular sensory epithelium. Utricles of normal adolescent mice were isolated and grown in culture for 3 days. [^{3}H]thymidine was present during the entire incubation period. TGF-α or TGF-α plus insulin was added at the start of the culture period. Concentrations of TGF-α varied from 0.1 to 200 ng/mL, whereas the concentration of insulin was held constant at 5 μg/mL. TGF-α or TGF-α plus insulin up-regulate cell proliferation in the normal vestibular sensory epithelium in a dose-dependent manner. Results are expressed as the mean number of [^{3}H]thymidine-labeled cells in the sensory epithelium per organ $\pm$ SEM. *$p \leq .01$ vs. control, **$p \leq .05$ vs. control. The TGF-α alone function was significantly different ($p \leq .01$) from the TGF-α plus insulin function. (From Yamashita & Oesterle.[72] Reproduced, with permission, from the *Proceedings of the National Academy of Sciences USA*.)

Differences between Mammalian and Avian Vestibular Sensory Epithelia

As discussed previously, TGF-α stimulates cell proliferation in normal murine vestibular sensory epithelium, but not in normal avian vestibular sensory epithelium. IGF-I stimulates proliferation in normal avian vestibular sensory epithelium, but not in murine vestibular sensory epithelium.[49,72] The origin of these differences is unknown at present. Substantial differences in sensory epithelial cell proliferation do exist between avian and mammalian inner ears. Hundreds of new cells are produced daily in the vestibular sensory epithelium of the normal, undamaged avian inner ear.[12-14,74] In contrast, proliferation is a very rare event, at best, in the normal mammalian vestibular sensory epithelium.[23,25,35,72] Given the substantial ongoing proliferation in the avian vestibular sensory epithelium, it is conceivable that TGF-α is present *in situ* at levels high enough to mask any mitogenic effects produced by an exogenous addition of TGF-α. Alternatively, the overall growth factor milieu or expression of growth factor receptors may differ between mammals and birds.

Factors Affecting Hair Cell Differentiation

The specific factors that regulate the differentiation of hair cells in the sensory epithelium of the inner ear have not been identified. To understand what makes a cell become a hair cell, much of the research to date has been directed at the expression and function of transcription factors in the inner ear. Receptors for retinoic acid and thyroid hormone have received most of the attention because they are well understood and because alterations in retinoic acid or thyroid hormone during development are known to cause inner ear defects (reviewed in ref. 75). Both are members of the steroid/hormone receptor superfamily. Several lines of evidence have implicated the intracellular receptors for retinoic acid and thyroid hormone in controlling critical steps of cochlear differentiation. The addition of retinoic acid, a derivative of vitamin A, to cultured otic vesicles results in the precocious differentiation of the sensory receptor epithelium and the secretory and supporting epithelium.[76] Addition of retinoic acid to explants of developing cochlea from embryonic day 13–16 (E13–E16) mice results in the development of extra hair cells.[77] By also adding [³H]thymidine, Kelly and co-workers showed that most of the extra hair cells were born before E14, suggesting that retinoic acid increases hair cell number by altering the fate of the existing cells, rather than by stimulating proliferation of the precursor cells. *In situ* hybridization analysis of mRNAs encoding proteins involved in mediating the retinoic acid response reveals that some types of retinoic acid receptors (retinoic acid receptor-β) are strongly expressed in the sensory epithelium of the developing ear.[78] Cytoplasmic retinoic acid binding protein II (CRABP II), a ligand-binding protein that is thought to control intracellular levels of free retinoic acid, is expressed in the cochlear epithelium during development.[79] By culturing cochlear explants from developing or adult mice on the F9 reporter cell line, which responds to retinoic acid by expressing β-galactosidase, Kelley et al.[77] showed that developing mouse cochleas, but not adult cochleas, contain retinoic acid. Similar experiments with adult murine vestibular organs, adult avian sacculus, and adult avian basilar papillas suggest that they too contain retinoic acid. These findings led Kelley et al.[77] to speculate that high levels of retinoic acid in adult inner ear epithelia may be related to tissues that are capable of producing new hair cells throughout the life of the organism.

Another critical transcriptional regulator for the inner ear appears to be the receptor for thyroid hormone. As reviewed in Corey and Breakefield,[75] hearing loss is often associated with hypothyroidism or syndromes that disrupt signaling by thyroid hormone. Bradley and co-workers[80] have used *in situ* hybridization to locate thyroid hormone receptors in the developing ear. Both β-forms of the thyroid hormone receptors are expressed in the cochlear portion of the developing cochlea, whereas the α-form appears in both cochlear and vestibular regions of the developing rat inner ear. The localization of thyroid hormone receptor mRNA to specific regions of the cochlea is intriguing.

Further work needs to be done to elucidate the role thyroid hormone and retinoic acid play in the developing ear and possibly in hair cell differentiation. The homeobox genes, members of the Pax family, and the role of growth factors in hair cell differentiation also remain to be examined. This provides an enormous and exciting challenge for the future. Identification of the molecular factors involved in promoting hair cell genesis and differentiation should assist in the eventual development of therapies to treat sensorineural hearing and balance disorders.

REFERENCES

1. CHANG, J. S. Y., A. N. POPPER & W. M. SAIDEL. 1992. Heterogeneity of sensory hair cells in a fish ear. J. Comp. Neurol. **324:** 621–640.
2. POPPER, A. N., W. M. SAIDEL & J. S. Y. CHANG. 1993. Two types of sensory hair cell in the saccule of a teleost fish. Hear. Res. **64:** 211–216.
3. CORWIN, J. T. 1981. Postembryonic production and aging of inner ear hair cells in sharks. J. Comp. Neurol. **201:** 541–553.
4. CORWIN, J. T. 1983. Postembryonic growth of the macula neglecta auditory detector in the ray, *Raja clavata*: Continual increases in hair cell number, neural convergence, and physiological sensitivity. J. Comp. Neurol. **217:** 345–356.
5. CORWIN, J. T. 1985. Auditory neurons expand their terminal arbors throughout life and orient toward the site of postembryonic hair cell production in the macula neglecta in elasmobranchs. J. Comp. Neurol. **239:** 445–452.
6. PLATT, C. 1977. Hair cell distribution and orientation in goldfish otolith organs. J. Comp. Neurol. **172:** 283–297.
7. POPPER, A. N. & B. HOXTER. 1984. Growth of a fish ear. I. Quantitative analysis of sensory hair cell and ganglion cell proliferation. Hear. Res. **15:** 133–142.
8. POPPER, A. N. & B. HOXTER. 1990. Growth of a fish ear. II. Locations of newly proliferated sensory hair cells in the saccular epithelium of *Astronotus ocellatus.* Hear. Res. **45:** 33–40.
9. LI, C. W. & E. R. LEWIS. 1979. Structure and development of vestibular hair cells in the larval bullfrog. Ann. Otol. Rhinol. & Laryngol. **88:** 427–437.
10. CORWIN, J. T. 1985. Perpetual production of hair cells and maturational changes in hair cell ultrastructure accompany postembryonic growth in an amphibian ear. Proc. Natl. Acad. Sci. USA **82:** 3911–3915.
11. RUBEN, R. J. 1967. Development of the inner ear of the mouse: A radioautographic study of terminal mitoses. Acta Otolaryngol. Suppl. **220:** 1–44.
12. JØRGENSEN, J. M. & C. MATHIESEN. 1988. The avian inner ear: Continuous production of hair cells in vestibular sensory organs, but not in the auditory papilla. Naturwissenschaften **75:** 319–320.
13. ROBERSON, D. W., P. WEISLEDER, P. S. BOHRER & E. W. RUBEL. 1992. Ongoing production of sensory cells in the vestibular epithelium of the chick. Hear. Res. **57:** 166–174.
14. WEISLEDER, P. & E. W RUBEL. 1993. Hair cell regeneration after streptomycin toxicity in the avian vestibular epithelium. J. Comp. Neurol. **331:** 97–110.
15. TSUE, T. T., D. L. WATLING, M. D. COLTRERA & E. W RUBEL. 1994. Identification of hair cell progenitors and intermitotic migration of their nuclei in the normal and regenerating avian inner ear. J. Neurosci. **14:** 140–152.

16. WEISLEDER, P. W., T. T. TSUE & E. W. RUBEL. 1995. Hair cell replacement in avian vestibular epithelium: Supporting cell to Type I hair cell. Hear. Res. **82:** 125–133.
17. GEISLER, C. D., W. A. VAN BERGEIJK & L. S. FRISHKOPF. 1964. The inner ear of the bullfrog. J. Morphol. **114:** 43–58.
18. LI, C. W. & E. R. LEWIS. 1974. Morphogenesis of auditory receptor epithelia in the bullfrog. In Scanning Electron Microscopy III.: 791–798. ITT Research Institute. Chicago, IL.
19. LEWIS, E. R. & C. LI. 1973. Evidence concerning the morphogenesis of saccular receptors in the bullfrog (*Rana catesbeiana*). J. Morphol. **139:** 351–362.
20. LEWIS, E. R. & C. LI. 1975. Hair cell types and distribution in the otolithic and auditory organs of the bullfrog. Brain Res. **83:** 35–50.
21. JØRGENSEN, J. M. 1981. On a possible hair cell turn-over in the inner ear of the Caecilian *Ichthyophis glutinosus* (Amphibia: Gymnophiona). Acta Zool. **62**(3): 171–186.
22. FORGE, A., L. LI, J. T. CORWIN & G. NEVILL. 1993. Ultrastructural evidence for hair cell regeneration in the mammalian inner ear. Science **259:** 1616–1622.
23. RUBEL, E. W., L. A. DEW & D. W. ROBERSON. 1995. Mammalian vestibular hair cell regeneration. Science **267:** 701–703.
24. SOBKOWICZ, H. M., B. K. AUGUST & S. M. SLAPNICK. 1992. Epithelial repair following mechanical injury in the developing organ of Corti in culture: An electron microscopic and autoradiographic study. Exp. Neurol. **115:** 44.
25. KUNTZ, A. L. & E. C. OESTERLE. 1996. TGFα induces hair cell production in mature mammalian sensory epithelia in vivo. Assoc. Res. Otolaryngol. Abstr. 19.
26. HOLDER, N. & J. D. W. CLARKE. 1988. Is there a correlation between continuous neurogenesis and directed axon regeneration in the vertebrate nervous system? Trends Neurosci. **11:** 94–99.
27. ZALEWSKY, A. A. 1969. Regeneration of taste buds after reinnervation by peripheral or central sensory fibers of vagal ganglia. Exp. Neurol. **25:** 429–437.
28. GRAZIADEI, P. P. C. 1973. Cell dynamics in the olfactory mucosa. Tissue & Cell **5:** 113–131.
29. LOMBARTE, A., H. Y. YAN, A. N. POPPER, J. S. CHANG & C. PLATT. 1993. Damage and regeneration of hair cell ciliary bundles in a fish ear following treatment with gentamicin. Hear. Res. **64:** 166–174.
30. BAIRD, R. A., M. A. TORRES & N. A. SCHUFF. 1993. Hair cell regeneration in the bullfrog vestibular otolith organs following aminoglycoside ototoxicity. Hear. Res. **65:** 164–174.
31. JONES, T. A. & R. C. NELSON. 1992. Recovery of vestibular function following hair cell destruction by streptomycin. Hear. Res. **62:** 181–186.
32. CAREY, J. P., E. W RUBEL & A. F. FUCHS. 1994. Recovery of the VOR parallels hair cell regeneration in the aminoglycoside-damaged chicken vestibular system. Assoc. Res. Otolaryngol. **17:** 132.
33. CAREY, J. P., A. F. FUCHS & E. W RUBEL. 1996. Hair cell regeneration and recovery of the vestibulo-ocular reflex in the avian vestibular system. J. Neurophysiol. Submitted.
34. WEISLEDER, P. & E. W RUBEL. 1992. Hair cell regeneration in the avian vestibular epithelium. Exp. Neurol. **115:** 2–6.
35. WARCHOL, M. E., P. R. LAMBERT, B. J. GOLDSTEIN, A. FORGE & J. T. CORWIN. 1993. Regenerative proliferation in inner ear sensory epithelia from adult guinea pigs and humans. Science **259:** 1619–1622.
36. LAMBERT, P. R. 1994. Inner ear hair cell regeneration in a mammal: Identification of a triggering factor. Laryngoscope **104:** 701–718.
37. BAIRD, R. A., P. S. STEYGER & N. R. SCHUFF. 1995. Mitotic and non-mitotic hair cell regeneration in the bullfrog vestibular otolith organs. Ann. N.Y. Acad. Sci. This volume.
38. BAIRD, R. A., S. BALES, C. FIORILLO & N. R. SCHUFF. 1995. In vivo and in vitro evidence for non-mitotic hair cell regeneration in the bullfrog vestibular otolith organs. Assoc. Res. Otolaryngol Abstr. **18:** 45.
39. ROBERSON, D. W., S. KREIG & E. W RUBEL. 1996. Light microscopic evidence that direct transdifferentiation gives rise to new hair cells in regenerating avian auditory epithelium. Aud. Neurosci. In press.

40. ALDER, H. J. & Y. RAPHAEL. 1995. New hair cells in the acoustically damaged chick inner ear following cytosine arabinoside application. Assoc. Res. Otolaryngol Abstr. **18:** 45.
41. WARCHOL, M. E. & J. T. CORWIN. 1993. Supporting cells in avian vestibular organs proliferate in serum-free culture. Hear. Res. **71:** 28–36.
42. OESTERLE, E. C., T. T. TSUE, T. A. REH & E. W RUBEL. 1993. Hair-cell regeneration in explant cultures of the postnatal chick inner ear. Hear. Res. **70:** 85–108.
43. ABDOUH, A., G. DESPRES & R. ROMAND. 1993. Hair cell overproduction in the developing mammalian cochlea in culture. Neuroreport **5(1):** 33–36.
44. TSUE, T. T., E. C. OESTERLE & E. W RUBEL. 1993. Diffusible factors regulate hair cell regeneration in the avian inner ear. Proc. Natl. Acad. Sci. USA **91:** 1584–1588.
45. REPRESA, J. J., C. MINER, E. BARBOSA & F. GIRALDEZ. 1988. Bombesin and other growth factors activate cell proliferation in chick embryo otic vesicles in culture. Development **102:** 87–96.
46. REPRESA, J., Y. LEON, C. MINER & F. GIRALDEZ. 1991. The *int*-2 proto-oncogene is responsible for induction of the inner ear. Nature **353:** 561–563.
47. LEFEBVRE, P. P. *et al.* 1993. Retinoic acid stimulates regeneration of mammalian auditory hair cells. Science **260:** 692–695.
48. CHARDIN, S. & R. ROMAND. 1995. Regeneration and mammalian auditory hair cells. Science **267:** 707–709.
49. OESTERLE, E. C., T. T. TSUE & E. W RUBEL. 1995. Induction of cell proliferation in avian inner ear sensory epithelia by insulin-like growth factor-I and insulin. J. Comp. Neurol. Submitted.
50. ROTWEIN, P. 1991. Structure, evolution, expression and regulation of insulin-like growth factors I and II. Growth Factors **5:** 3.
51. DAUGHADAY, W. H. & P. ROTWEIN. 1989. Insulin-like growth factors I and II: Peptide, messenger ribonucleic acid and gene structures, serum, and tissue concentrations. Endocrinol. Rev. **10:** 68–91.
52. RECHLER, M. M. & S. P. NISSLEY. 1990. The nature and regulation of the receptors for insulin-like growth factors. Annu. Rev. Physiol. **47:** 425–442.
53. LEWIS, M. E., N. T. NEFF, P. C. CONTRERAS, D. B. STONG, R. W. OPPENHEIM, P. E. GREBOW & J. L. VAUGHT. 1993. Insulin-like growth factor-I: Potential for treatment of motor neuronal disorders. Exp. Neurol. **124:** 73–88.
54. BASERGA, R. & R. RUBEN. 1993. Cell cycle and growth control. Crit. Rev. Eukaryotic Gene Exp. **3:** 47–61.
55. GOLDRING, M. B. & S. R. GOLDRING. 1991. Cytokines and cell growth control. Crit. Rev. Eukaryotic Gene Exp. **1:** 301–326.
56. MACAULAY, V. M. 1992. Insulin-like growth factors and cancer. Br. J. Cancer **65:** 311–320.
57. CZECH, M. P. 1989. Signal transduction by the insulin-like growth factors. Cell **59:** 235–238.
58. WERNER, H., C. T. ROBERTS, JR., M. K. RAIZADA, C. A. BONDY, M. ADAMO & D. LEROITH. 1992. *In* Receptors in the Developing Nervous System. I. S. Zagon & P. J. McLaughlin, Eds.: 109–127. Chapman and Hall Ltd., London.
59. LOWE, W. L. 1991. *In* Insulin-like Growth Factors: Molecular and Cellular Aspects. D. LeRoith, Ed.: 49. CRC Press Inc. Boca Raton, FL.
60. CARPENTER, G. & M. I. WAHL. 1990. *In* Peptide Growth Factors and Their Receptors. M. B. Sporn & A. B. Roberts, Eds.: 69–171. Springer-Verlag. Berlin.
61. SCHULTZ, G. S., M. WHITE, R. MITCHELL, G. BROWN, J. LYNCH, D. R. TWARDZIK & G. J. TODARO. 1987. Epithelial wound healing enhanced by transforming growth factor-alpha and vaccinia growth factor. Science **235:** 350–352.
62. ANCHAN, R. M., T. A. REH, J. ANGELLO, A. BALLIET & M. WALKER. 1991. EGF and TGF-alpha stimulate retinal neuroepithelial cell proliferation in vitro. Neuron **6:** 923–936.
63. LILLIEN, L. & C. CEPKO. 1992. Control of proliferation in the retina: Temporal changes in responsiveness to FGF and TGF alpha. Development **115:** 253–266.
64. REYNOLDS, B. A. & S. WEISS. 1992. Generation of neurons and astrocytes from isolated cells of the adult mammalian central nervous system. Science **255:** 1707–1710.

65. MASSAGUÉ, J. 1990. Transforming growth factor-alpha. A model for membrane-anchored growth factors. J. Biol. Chem. **265:** 21393–21396.
66. WILCOX, J. H. & R. DERYNCK. 1988. Developmental expression of transforming growth factors alpha and beta in mouse fetus. Mol. Cell. Biol. **8:** 3415–3422.
67. LEFEBVRE, P. P., H. STAECKER, B. MALGRANGE, G. MOONEN & T. R. VAN DE WATER. 1994. Transforming growth factor alpha acts with retinoic acid to stimulate the regeneration of mammalian auditory hair cells. Assoc. Res. Otolaryngol. Abstr. **17:** 115.
68. WRIGHT, C. G., K. S. ROBINSON & S. A. COMERFORD. 1995. Transforming growth factor alpha in the adult mammalian inner ear. Assoc. Res. Otolaryngol. Abstr. **18:** 109.
69. XU, X. M. & J. T. CORWIN. 1992. Soc. Neurosci. Abstr. **18:** 1401.
70. XU, X. M. & J. T. CORWIN. 1993. Soc. Neurosci. Abstr. **19:** 1401.
71. YAMASHITA, H. & E. C. OESTERLE. 1994. Mitogenic effects of EGF and TGF-alpha on cultured vestibular sensory epithelium from the mammalian inner ear. Assoc. Res. Otolaryngol. Abstr. **17:** 131.
72. YAMASHITA, H. & E. C. OESTERLE. 1995. Induction of cell proliferation in mammalian inner-ear sensory epithelial by transforming growth factor α and epidermal growth factor. Proc. Natl. Acad. Sci. USA **92:** 3152–3155.
73. EBNER, R. & R. DERYNCK. 1991. Epidermal growth factor and transforming growth factor-alpha: Differential intracellular routing and processing of ligand-receptor complexes. Cell Regul. **2:** 599–612.
74. KIL, J., M. E. WARCHOL & J. T. CORWIN. 1995. On-going and aminoglycoside-induced apoptotic cell death in the vestibular epithelia of chicks. Assoc. Res. Otolaryngol. Abstr. **18:** 82.
75. COREY, D. P. & X. O. BREAKEFIELD. 1994. Transcription factors in inner ear development. Proc. Natl. Acad. Sci. USA **91:** 433–436.
76. REPRESA, J., A. SANCHEZ, C. MINER, J. LEWIS & F. GIRALDEZ. 1990. Retinoic acid modulation of the early development of the inner ear is associated with the control of c-fos expression. Development **110:** 1081–1090.
77. KELLY, M. W., X.-M. XU, M. A. WAGNER, M. E. WARCHOL & J. T. CORWIN. 1994. The developing organ of Corti contains retinoic acid and forms supernumerary hair cells in response to exogenous retinoic acid in culture. Development **119:** 1041–1055.
78. DOLLE, P., E. RUBERTE, P. LEROY, G. MORRISS-KAY & P. CHAMBON. 1990. Retinoic acid receptors and cellular retinoid binding proteins. I. A systematic study of their differential pattern of transcription during mouse organogenesis. Development **110:** 1133–1151.
79. RUBERTE, E., V. FRIEDERICH, G. MORRISS-KAY & P. CHAMBON. 1992. Differential distribution patterns of CRABP I and CRABP II transcripts during mouse embryogenesis. Development **115:** 973–987.
80. BRADLEY, D. J., H. C. TOWLE & W. S. YOUNG III. 1994. α and β thyroid hormone receptor (TR) gene expression during auditory neurogenesis: Evidence for TR isoform-specific transcriptional regulation *in vivo.* Proc. Natl. Acad. Sci. USA **91:** 439–443.

Hair Cell Regeneration and Vestibulo-Ocular Reflex Recovery[a]

JOHN P. CAREY,[b,c] ALBERT F. FUCHS,[b,d–f]
AND EDWIN W RUBEL[b,c,e]

[b]Virginia Merrill Bloedel Hearing Research Center
[c]Department of Otolaryngology/Head and Neck Surgery
[d]Regional Primate Research Center, and
[e]Department of Physiology and Biophysics
University of Washington
Seattle, Washington 98195

INTRODUCTION

Hair cells in the avian ear can regenerate after noise damage[1–3] or ototoxic aminoglycoside damage.[4–6] Moreover, afferent connections are reestablished on regenerated hair cells in both the auditory[7–9] and vestibular[6] epithelia. Numerous studies have documented recovery of avian auditory function after hair cell regeneration,[10–17] but to our knowledge only one study has documented the recovery of avian vestibular function. Jones and Nelson reported that compound action potentials from the vestibular nerve of chickens treated with streptomycin exhibited an immediate sixfold decrease in sensitivity to linear horizontal accelerations.[18] The thresholds of compound action potentials returned to normal within two weeks, but the amplitudes and latencies of the responses required eight weeks to normalize. Jones and Nelson did not correlate the electrophysiological measurements of the vestibular recovery with hair cell regeneration. Furthermore, the existence of compound action potentials in the vestibular nerve is no guarantee that behaviorally useful information is communicated to the brain stem.

To determine whether a direct relationship exists between hair cell regeneration and vestibular reflex recovery, we tested the horizontal vestibulo-ocular reflex (VOR) in chickens during the course of hair cell regeneration induced by treatment with streptomycin. The VOR produces eye movements that compensate for head movements to prevent the visual scene from slipping across the retina. The efficacy of the vestibular hair cells is reflected by the size of the compensatory eye movement velocity ($\dot{E}$) in response to head movement velocity ($\dot{H}$), that is, the VOR gain ($\dot{E}/\dot{H}$). By inducing a profound loss of hair cells in the semicircular canal cristae and then testing the horizontal VOR throughout the course of hair cell regeneration, we were able to determine that the loss and recovery of vestibular hair cells is associated with changes in the gain of the VOR.

[a]This study was supported by NIH grants EY00745 and RR00166, NIDCD training grant DC00018, NIDCD 00395, funds from NOHR, and the Virginia Merrill Bloedel Hearing Research Center.

[f]Address correspondence to Albert F. Fuchs, Ph.D., Regional Primate Research Center, Box 357330, University of Washington, Seattle, WA 98195-7330. E-mail: fuchs@u.washington.edu

METHODS

Experimental Subjects

White Leghorn chicks (*Gallus domesticus*) were administered streptomycin sulfate (Sigma) in normal saline, 1200 mg/kg/day intramuscularly, for 5 days beginning 4–8 days posthatching. Injected chicks were allowed to recover for 1–4 days ($n = 8$), 1 week ($n = 6$), 2 weeks ($n = 8$), 3 weeks ($n = 10$), or 8–9 weeks ($n = 4$) before they were tested with rotational stimuli. We refer to experimental groups and their age-matched controls by their recovery periods, not chronologic ages; for example, "1–4-day chicks," "1-week controls," and so on.

Surgical Preparation

Eye movements were measured by the magnetic search coil technique.[19] A post was affixed to the surgically exposed superior pole of the globe in a manner similar to that described by Wallman *et al.*[20] A prefabricated search coil (9 mm diameter, 3 turns of Teflon-coated AWG 38 wire with 15 strands per turn) was fastened to the other end of the post. A second post was attached to the skull with dental cement so that the head could be coupled to the turntable. Surgery was performed under ketamine anesthesia. Chicks then were allowed to recover until they could walk without difficulty, generally 2–4 h later.

Rotational Stimulation

The alert chick was put in a restraining cylinder, placed on a turntable, and subjected to passive whole-body horizontal (yaw) rotation. Bars fixed to the turntable held the beak and the head post, thereby ensuring that the rotational stimuli were delivered directly to the head. The head was positioned at the center of rotation with the beak pitched slightly down to minimize vertical eye movements during horizontal rotation.

All chicks were rotated sinusoidally in the dark at frequencies of 0.1, 0.3, 0.5, 0.8, 1.0, and 1.4 Hz presented in a random order. The amplitude of the table excursion was ± 10°. Alertness was maintained with occasional auditory stimuli, flashes of light between periods of rotation, and unexpected bursts of high-frequency rotation. Rotational testing generally required 15–60 min. All procedures were approved by the Animal Care and Use Committee at the University of Washington and conformed to the National Institutes of Health's Guide for the Care and Use of Laboratory Animals.

Eye Movement Measurement

An alternating magnetic field centered at the animal's head was generated by orthogonal pairs of 14-inch-diameter coils built into the rotary table. Horizontal and vertical eye position signals were extracted from the eye coil by phase-sensitive detectors, amplified, and filtered at 500 Hz. Turntable position was simultaneously measured by a potentiometer. The signals were digitized at a sampling rate of 1 kHz.

At each session the eye coil was calibrated to ± 10° pitch and yaw displacements. Measurements of angular displacement were accurate to within ± 0.5° over a range of $\pm$ 30°. The entire system was also checked at each session by simulating a perfect VOR with the coil fixed in space at the center of rotation. Under these conditions the analysis program yielded a VOR gain and phase relative to head velocity of 1.00 $\pm$ 0.02 and 180.0° $\pm$ 0.5°.

VOR Data Analysis

An interactive analysis program for Macintosh computers displayed single cycles of sinusoidal head position and the associated horizontal eye movement. Saccades were deleted manually. The program produced digital derivatives of the desaccaded eye position and head position and fit each with a least-squares sine wave. The gain of the VOR for each cycle was calculated as the ratio of the amplitude of the fitted horizontal eye velocity (E) to the amplitude of the head velocity (H). The phase shift of the VOR was calculated as the difference in the phases of horizontal eye and head velocities. A phase between 0 and 180° indicates that the eye leads head movement; a phase between 180 and 360°, that it lags. Average gains and phases were calculated from 10 or more cycles in which $\geq$ 60% of the data points remained after desaccading. We considered 0.1 the lowest measurable gain. In cycles with higher gains, $\geq$ 60% of the eye velocity variance could be attributed to sinusoidal behavior (i.e., r^2 for the least-squares sine wave was $\geq$ 0.6). In cycles with lower gains, only ~ 20% of the variance was sinusoidal. The efficacy of the VOR for different ages and treatments is presented as Bode plots, i.e., average gains and phase shifts $\pm$ their standard deviations as a function of stimulus frequency.[21]

Histologic Preparation and Analysis

Within 24 h of rotational testing, chicks were sacrificed with pentobarbital intraperitoneally. The labyrinthine tissues were fixed by transcardiac and otic perfusion of 2% paraformaldehyde, 2.5% glutaraldehyde, 0.1 M sucrose, and 0.1 M phosphate buffer, pH 7.4. Cristae were dissected, osmicated, and dehydrated in ethanol. To prepare specimens for scanning electron microscopy (SEM), we removed the ampulla and cupula before critical-point drying and gold-palladium coating. The specimens were viewed with a JEOL 63005 electron microscope at 15 kV accelerating voltage. Specimens for light microscopy were embedded in Spurr's resin and sectioned transversely at 2 μm. Elements were counted as hair cells only if they contained a nucleus (with a visible nucleolus) situated above the row of supporting cell nuclei at the basement membrane, had a cell body that extended to the luminal surface of the sensory epithelium, and contacted underlying neural elements. A cell was typed on the basis of the morphology of its afferent ending.[22] An afferent with a complete calyx was considered to innervate a type I hair cell. An afferent ending that did not completely surround the hair cell was considered a bouton afferent, and the hair cell it innervated was identified as a type II hair cell. The length of the basement membrane underlying the sensory epithelium was measured in sections imaged on a Macintosh IIfx computer by means of the National Institutes of Health Image morphometric program, version 1.57.[23] Hair cell "density" was defined as the number of hair cells per 100-μm length of basement membrane.[6] Densities of type I, type II, and total hair cells were averaged from six to eight sections spaced regularly along the length of each crista.

RESULTS

Functional Damage and Recovery

VOR Gains

Streptomycin eliminated any measurable VOR gain for up to one week after treatment (FIG. 1, solid lines). In contrast, age-matched control birds all had measurable VOR gains (FIG. 1, dashed lines). Gains were quite variable in these young control birds, but exceeded 0.1 at all but the lowest frequency tested.

VOR recovery was first measurable two weeks after streptomycin treatment (FIG. 2, top panels). Two of eight treated chicks had VOR gains in the control range (shaded areas), suggesting complete recovery. Six had gains below the average control values (dashed line), and three of these had gains of < 0.1 (indistinguishable from 0) across the entire frequency range. Recovery was more apparent three weeks after treatment, when all 10 tested birds showed some recovery; five had VOR gains in the control range at three or more frequencies. Two of four 8–9-week treated chicks showed normal VOR gains, and two even showed greater than normal gains.

VOR Phase Shifts

For treated and control birds, eye velocity generally led perfect compensation, that is, 180° (FIG. 2, lower panels). The mean phase lead of the VOR in control birds (dashed lines) was relatively constant (13° ± 3° SD) over the frequency range 0.3–1.4 Hz. At 0.1 Hz, control birds showed a larger mean phase lead (43° ± 7° SD) for all ages.

Treated chicks at 2 and 3 weeks after injection had greater mean VOR phase leads than those of control birds at all frequencies, although the phase leads of some individuals fell within the control range (shaded areas). Like the control chicks,

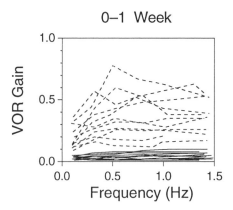

FIGURE 1. Vestibulo-ocular reflex (VOR) gain as a function of the frequency of horizontal sinusoidal rotation during the first week after treatment with streptomycin. Data are from five control and eight treated birds tested 1–4 days after treatment (*solid lines*) and from six control and six treated birds tested 6–8 days after treatment (*dashed lines*).

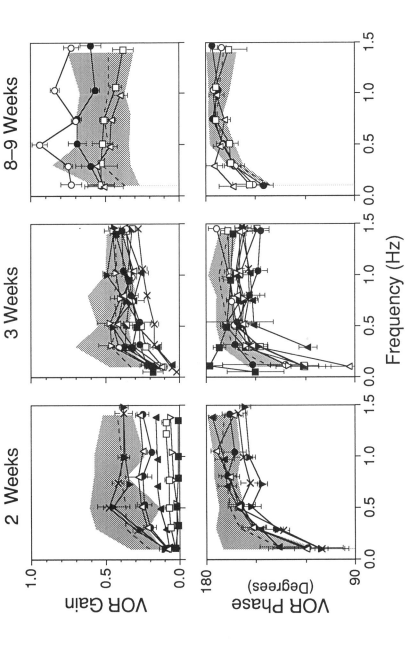

FIGURE 2. Vestibulo-ocular reflex (VOR) gain and phase as a function of the frequency of horizontal sinusoidal rotation at 2, 3, and 8–9 weeks after treatment with streptomycin. Each symbol represents the mean response of the same streptomycin-treated individual in both gain and phase plots. Error bars are standard deviations. Means from control birds are represented by dashed lines, and the range of control values is shaded. Phase data are shown only for cycles where VOR gain ≥ 0.1. Like symbols in different recovery periods do *not* represent the same individual; each bird was tested at only one time point.

treated chicks had greater phase leads at lower frequencies. As VOR gains increased during the 2–9 weeks after treatment with streptomycin, both VOR phase leads and their variability decreased and returned to control values by 8–9 weeks post-treatment.

Anatomic Recovery

The scanning electron micrograph shown in FIGURE 3B demonstrates the destruction typically seen after treatment with streptomycin. In contrast to the dense mat of stereocilia covering the normal crista (FIG. 3A), only a small band of residual stereocilia is found at the edges of the epithelium (FIG. 3B). SEMs from cristae recovered 6–8 days after intoxication showed loss of even this band as new stereocilia appeared (FIG. 3C). Finally, SEMs from cristae taken 8–9 weeks following treatment with streptomycin were indistinguishable from those of the normal crista (FIG. 3A).

Hair cell densities in the horizontal cristae were evaluated by light microscopy for each recovery period; the results are summarized in FIGURE 4. The density of total hair cells in cristae examined in the first week after streptomycin treatment (top panel, bars) was about 40% of control values (triangles and dashed lines). There was no difference in the density of hair cells at 1–4 days and at 6–8 days after treatment. We made no attempt to determine whether these hair cells were new or residual cells not eradicated by the streptomycin treatment. The average density of total hair cells increased between the first and third weeks after the injection; the largest part of this increase was attributable to type II cells. The average density of type II hair cells (middle panel) was 52% of the average control density in the first week of recovery and increased to normal by 3 weeks post-treatment. In contrast, the density of type I hair cells (bottom panel) in the first week post-treatment was essentially zero and did not recover significantly until after 8–9 weeks, at which time type I hair cells were still less numerous than normal (64% of control value). Only a modest recovery of type I cells was seen in 2- and 3-week subjects (10% and 12% of control values, respectively).

DISCUSSION

The major finding of this study is that the regenerated avian vestibular epithelium is functional. The VOR, a reflex whose input arises from hair cells on the crista ampullaris of the semicircular canals, had normal characteristics after the streptomycin-damaged hair cells had recovered or been replaced. Our conclusion that VOR integrity depends on hair cell recovery is supported by two major correlations. First, a streptomycin-induced reduction of 60% in the total number of hair cells in the crista ampullaris of the horizontal semicircular canal was associated with virtual abolition of the horizontal VOR. Second, as hair cell density increased in this vestibular epithelium, there was a parallel return of the VOR to its normal gain and phase.

One might predict that hair cell density would determine the gain of the VOR. Indeed, following the first week after treatment with streptomycin, a monotonic rise in VOR gain is found at both high and low frequencies as well as a monotonic rise in average total hair cell density (FIG. 5). However, correlations between VOR gain and total hair cell density were rather poor (FIG. 6, upper). The lack of correlation between the density of total hair cells and VOR gain is especially obvious in the first week after treatment (FIG. 5), when the VOR consistently was abolished even though ~ 40% of the normal hair cell density was present. The absence of the VOR

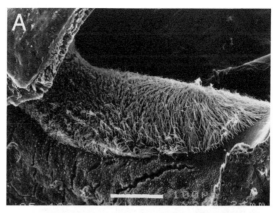

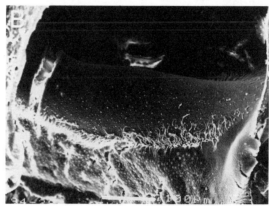

FIGURE 3. Scanning electron micrographs (SEMs) of cristae from horizontal semicircular canals. (**A**) Control bird. (**B**) Treated bird one day after streptomycin. (**C**) Treated bird one week after streptomycin. Bars = 100 μm.

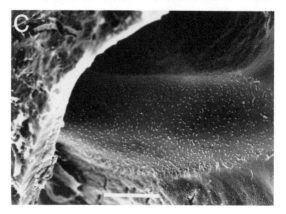

in the presence of so many hair cells suggests that the surviving hair cells were not functional. Perhaps they remained intoxicated for a time after streptomycin treatment. Or they may have temporarily lost their stereocilia, leaving them uncoupled from the dynamics of the endolymph and cupula. Alternatively, they may have been

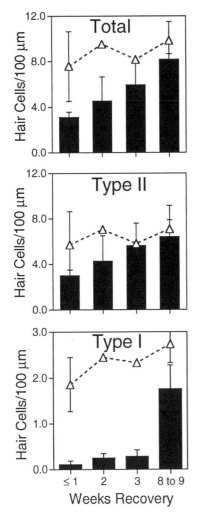

FIGURE 4. Hair cell density from light microscopy of horizontal cristae in treated (*bars*) and age-matched control (*triangles*) chickens at several recovery times after aminoglycoside intoxication. Different panels indicate relations for total hair cells and types I and II separately.

new hair cells that were not yet capable of signal transduction. Light microscopic data do not allow us to decide whether any or all these possibilities apply here.

VOR gain was best correlated with the percentage of type I cells. For example, at 1.0 Hz VOR gain was linearly correlated with type I hair cell density with $r^2 = 0.70$ (FIG. 6, lower). Correlations for the other frequencies tested were similarly good ($r^2 = 0.58$–0.82). In contrast, attempts to linearly correlate VOR gain at 1.0 Hz with type II hair cell density yielded $r^2 = 0.27$ (FIG. 6, middle). Correlation at other frequencies was also poor ($r^2 = 0.25$–0.32). FIGURE 5 demonstrates the relationship between type I hair cell density and VOR gain. Type I hair cell density was low 7 days after treatment and remained low 21 days after treatment, when the VOR had not yet fully recovered. However, the density of type I hair cells was only slightly less than normal after 8–9 weeks, when the VOR was completely normal.

The correlation of VOR recovery with the presence of type I hair cells was unexpected. In mammals, a variety of evidence converges on the suggestion that regularly discharging vestibular afferents and their prominent inputs from type II hair cells are largely responsible for the VOR.[24,25] Therefore, recovery of type II hair cells should underlie the recovery of VOR gain. We did not find this to be the case in our chicks. However, in contrast to the situation in mammals, Yamashita and Ohmori found that type I hair cells in the isolated crista of the chicken had greater input to afferents with regular response dynamics.[26] Therefore, perhaps in birds type I hair cells preferentially contribute to the VOR.

It also is possible that VOR recovery has a large central component. In this scenario, the input signal from regenerated, repaired, or even remaining hair cells would be adequate to drive the VOR if their signals were amplified by compensation in central pathways. VOR gain could increase if afferent signals from a constant number of hair cells were made more effective by a gradual increase in efficacy of central synapses. If 40% of the initial complement of hair cells did survive the streptomycin treatment, they might provide sufficient input for the VOR after central amplification. However, FIGURE 3B and C suggests that many of the hair cells seen in light microscopy sections may not have intact stereocilia at the surface. Therefore, immediately after treatment there may be little, if any, peripheral signal for central processes to amplify.

In conclusion, VOR recovery probably involves a number of events, including replacement of hair cells by regeneration, the attendant growth of stereocilia on new and surviving cells, the establishment of new afferent contacts, and compensation by brain-stem circuits for changes in afferent signals. Although we cannot sort out the

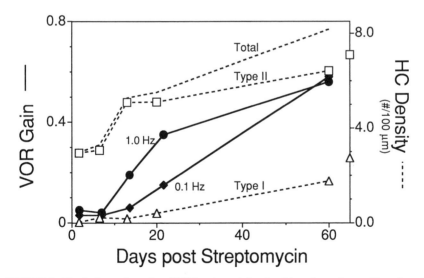

FIGURE 5. Vestibulo-ocular reflex (VOR) gain and the densities of type I, type II, and total hair cells as a function of the recovery time after treatment with streptomycin. Solid lines show VOR gains at 0.1 Hz (*filled diamonds*) and 1.0 Hz (*filled circles*). Dashed lines show densities of type I (*triangles*), type II (*squares*), and total (no symbols) hair cells. Symbols on right ordinate are mean control densities of type I (*triangle*) and type II (*square*) hair cells from the oldest controls.

relative contributions of each of these events, they clearly are very effective because they restore an initially absent VOR to its normal characteristics within 8–9 weeks. Our data suggest that repair or regeneration of hair cells plays the pivotal role in VOR recovery.

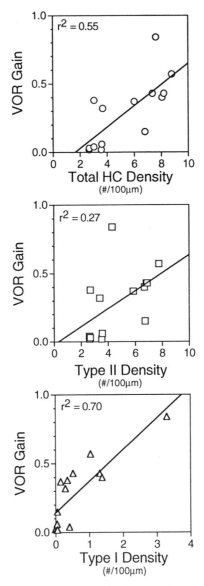

FIGURE 6. Scatter plots of vestibulo-ocular reflex (VOR) gain at 1.0 Hz versus total, type II, and type I hair cell densities. Data are from streptomycin-treated birds at all recovery periods. Least-squares linear fits with their squared correlation coefficients (r^2) are shown for the data in each panel.

ACKNOWLEDGMENTS

We gratefully acknowledge Ed Grossman and Robert Cent for writing the analysis program, Robert Schor for programming assistance, and Shawn Kreig and Dale Cunningham for histology.

REFERENCES

1. COTANCHE, D. A. 1987. Regeneration of hair cell stereociliary bundles in the chick cochlea following severe acoustic trauma. Hear. Res. **30:** 181–195.
2. CORWIN, J. T. & D. A. COTANCHE. 1988. Regeneration of sensory hair cells after acoustic trauma. Science **240:** 1772–1774.
3. RYALS, B. M. & E. W RUBEL. 1988. Hair cell regeneration after acoustic trauma in adult Coturnix quail. Science **240:** 1774–1776.
4. CRUZ, R. M., P. R. LAMBERT & E. W RUBEL. 1987. Light microscopic evidence of hair cell regeneration after gentamycin toxicity in chick cochlea. Arch. Otolaryngol. Head Neck Surg. **113:** 1058–1062.
5. LIPPE, W. R., E. W. WESTBROOK & B. M. RYALS. 1991. Hair cell regeneration in the chicken cochlea following aminoglycoside toxicity. Hear. Res. **56:** 203–210.
6. WEISLEDER, P. & E. W RUBEL. 1993. Hair cell regeneration after streptomycin toxicity in the avian vestibular epithelium. J. Comp. Neurol. **331:** 97–110.
7. DUCKERT, L. G. & E. W RUBEL. 1993. Morphological correlates of functional recovery in the chicken inner ear after gentamycin treatment. J. Comp. Neurol. **331:** 75–96.
8. RYALS, B. M. & E. W. WESTBROOK. 1994. TEM analysis of neural terminals on autoradiographically identified regenerated hair cells. Hear. Res. **72:** 81–88.
9. RYALS, B. M., E. W. WESTBROOK, S. STOOTS & R. F. SPENCER. 1992. Changes in the acoustic nerve after hair cell regeneration. Exp. Neurol. **115:** 18–22.
10. NORTON, S. J. & E. W RUBEL. 1990. Active and passive ADP components in mammalian and avian ears. *In* The Mechanics and Biophysics of Hearing. P. J. Dallos, C. D. Geisler, J. W. Matthews, M. A. Ruggero & C. R. Steele, Eds.: 219–226. Springer-Verlag. New York.
11. SALVI, R. J., S. S. SAUNDERS, E. HASHINO & L. CHEN. 1994. Discharge patterns of chicken cochlear ganglion neurons following kanamycin-induced hair cell loss and regeneration. J. Comp. Physiol. **174:** 351–369.
12. MCFADDEN, E. A. & J. C. SAUNDERS. 1989. Recovery of auditory function following intense sound exposure in the neonatal chick. Hear. Res. **41:** 205–215.
13. TUCCI, D. L. & E. W RUBEL. 1990. Physiologic status of regenerated hair cells in the avian inner ear following aminoglycoside ototoxicity. Otolaryngol. Head Neck Surg. **103:** 443–450.
14. GIROD, D. A., D. L. TUCCI & E. W RUBEL. 1991. Anatomical correlates of functional recovery in the avian inner ear following aminoglycoside ototoxicity. Laryngoscope **101:** 1139–1149.
15. HASHINO, E. & M. SOKABE. 1989. Kanamycin induced low-frequency hearing loss in the budgerigar (*Melopsittacus undulatus*). J. Acoust. Soc. Am. **85:** 289–294.
16. MAREAN, G. C., J. M. BURT, M. D. BEECHER & E. W RUBEL. 1993. Hair cell regeneration in the European starling (*Sturnus vulgaris*): Recovery of pure-tone detection thresholds. Hear. Res. **71:** 126–136.
17. NIEMIEC, A. J., Y. RAPHAEL & D. B. MOODY. 1994. Return of auditory function following structural regeneration after acoustic trauma: Behavioral measures from quail. Hear. Res. **75:** 209–224.
18. JONES, T. A. & R. C. NELSON. 1992. Recovery of vestibular function following hair cell destruction by streptomycin. Hear. Res. **62:** 181–186.
19. ROBINSON, D. A. 1963. A method of measuring eye movements using a scleral search coil in a magnetic field. IEEE Trans. Biomed. Eng. **10:** 137–145.
20. WALLMAN, J., J. VELEZ, B. WEINSTEIN & A. E. GREEN. 1982. Avian vestibuloocular reflex: Adaptive plasticity and developmental changes. J. Neurophysiol. **48:** 952–967.

21. MELVILL JONES, G. & J. H. MILSUM. 1965. Spatial and dynamic aspects of visual fixation. IEEE Trans. Biomed. Eng. **12:** 54–62.
22. WERSÄLL, J. 1956. Studies on the structure and innervation of the sensory epithelium of the cristae ampullaris in the guinea pig. A light and electron microscopic investigation. Acta Oto-Laryngol. Suppl. **126:** 1–85.
23. NATIONAL INSTITUTES OF HEALTH IMAGE PROGRAM. Developed at the NIH and available from the Internet by anonymous FTP from zippy.nimh.nih.gov or on floppy disk from the National Technical Information Service. Part No. PB95-500195GEI. Springfield, VA.
24. HIGHSTEIN, S. M., J. M. GOLDBERG, A. K. MOSCHOVAKIS & C. FERNANDEZ. 1987. Inputs from regularly and irregularly discharging vestibular nerve afferents to secondary neurons in the vestibular nuclei of the squirrel monkey. II. Correlation with output pathways of secondary neurons. J. Neurophysiol. **58:** 719–738.
25. MINOR, L. B. & J. M. GOLDBERG. 1991. Vestibular-nerve inputs to the vestibulo-ocular reflex: A functional-ablation study in the squirrel monkey. J. Neurosci. **11:** 1636–1648.
26. YAMASHITA, M. & H. OHMORI. 1990. Synaptic responses to mechanical stimulation in calyceal and bouton type vestibular afferents studied in an isolated preparation of semicircular canal ampullae of chicken. Exp. Brain Res. **80:** 475–488.

Mitotic and Nonmitotic Hair Cell Regeneration in the Bullfrog Vestibular Otolith Organs[a]

R. A. BAIRD,[b] P. S. STEYGER, AND N. R. SCHUFF

R. S. Dow Neurological Sciences Institute
Legacy Good Samaritan Hospital
Portland, Oregon 97209

INTRODUCTION

Hair cells, the primary receptors of the auditory and vestibular organs, are neuroepithelial cells characterized by apical hair bundles composed of a single true cilium—the kinocilium—and a large number of actin-filled stereocilia.[1,2] These specialized cells are highly susceptible to damage by noise, infections, and ototoxic drugs.[3–5] Until recently, it was generally accepted that hair cells in mammals could only be produced during embryonic development and that, once lost in mature animals, were gone forever (but see refs. 6–8). Many studies have shown, however, that the vestibular organs of amphibians, fish, and birds continue to produce new hair cells at a low level throughout adult life.[9–12] Moreover, the amphibian vestibular organs, like those in birds[13–17] and fish,[18] retain the capacity to rapidly regenerate new hair cells following the elimination of existing hair cells by gentamicin ototoxicity.[19]

Using complementary *in vivo* and *in vitro* approaches, we have recently shown that new hair cells in the bullfrog vestibular otolith organs are created by a combination of mitotic and nonmitotic mechanisms.[20–22] As in the lateral line organs,[23] some regenerated hair cells appear to arise from the progeny of proliferating supporting cells.[11,24–27] Progenitor cells, originally located near the basement membrane, migrate apically, and undergo mitotic division at the lumenal surface.[28–32] It is not yet clear whether these progenitor cells are uncommitted stem cells[33] or result from the dedifferentiation of mature supporting cells.[34] Marginal cells outside the sensory macula may also contribute to hair cell regeneration.[35] Our own results strongly suggest that supporting cells can also convert, or transdifferentiate, into hair cells without an intervening cell division.[20–22] This important new finding sheds new light on the process of hair cell regeneration in lower vertebrates and may ultimately provide the means by which deafness and peripheral vestibular disorders in higher vertebrates can be alleviated through the replacement of lost hair cells.

METHODS

For *in vivo* experiments, bullfrogs received twice-daily intraperitoneal injections of 5-bromo-2'-deoxyuridine (BrdU) (10 mg BrdU/kg body weight), a thymidine

[a] This work was supported by NIDCD grant 02040, NASA grant NCC 2-651, and the Oregon Lions Sight and Hearing Foundation.
[b] Address correspondence to Richard A. Baird, Ph.D., R. S. Dow Neurological Sciences Institute, Legacy Good Samaritan Hospital, 1120 NW 20th Avenue, Portland, Oregon 97209. E-mail: bairdr@ohsu.edu

analogue taken up by the DNA of mitotic cells,[36] for periods ranging from 2 to 9 days.[21-22] Two days after beginning systemic BrdU injections, experimental animals were anesthetized by immersion in 0.2% MS-222, and their right ears were intraotically injected with 200 μM gentamicin sulfate and allowed to survive for 1–7 days. Bullfrogs were then re-anesthetized with 0.2% MS-222, and their saccular and utricular maculae were removed from the membranous labyrinth.

For *in vitro* experiments,[20] excised maculae from normal animals were incubated in 200–500 μL of modified amphibian culture medium (GIBCO) supplemented with 1 μM BrdU and 100 μg/mL ciprofloxacin, a non-ototoxic antibiotic.[37] Gentamicin-treated cultures were preincubated for 6–18 h in culture medium supplemented with 200–250 μM gentamicin sulfate and subsequently incubated in normal culture medium. To block cell proliferation, control and gentamicin-treated cultures were incubated in culture medium supplemented with 25 μM aphidicolin, a blocker of mitotic division in eukaryotic cells.[38] Cultures were maintained at room temperature (25 °C) in a 5% CO_2 environment for 7–9 days, replacing half the appropriate culture medium with fresh medium every two days.

Saccular and utricular maculae from *in vivo* and *in vitro* experiments were fixed in 4% paraformaldehyde, rinsed in phosphate buffer, and labeled with Texas Red-conjugated phalloidin to study the process of scar formation and repair in normal and gentamicin-treated end organs.[20,22] Phalloidin-labeled maculae were then processed for BrdU immunocytochemistry to study the relationship between cell proliferation and hair cell regeneration.[22-22] In gentamicin-treated animals, morphological changes in hair cells and supporting cells were examined at varying times following gentamicin treatment. We also measured hair cell and supporting cell density in wholemount and sectioned end organs to determine whether (1) hair bundle density accurately reflected cellular damage to hair cells, (2) hair cells migrated from undamaged into damaged macular regions, and (3) supporting cell density was maintained in gentamicin-treated animals.

RESULTS

In normal phalloidin-labeled organs, saccular hair cells were uniformly distributed within a kidney-shaped macula (FIG. 1A). Intraotic gentamicin injections resulted in the uniform destruction of the hair bundles (FIG. 1B) and, at later times, the cell bodies of saccular hair cells. In the utriculus, hair cells in the striola, a narrow zone with specialized morphology,[18,19] were selectively damaged while hair cells outside of this zone were relatively unaffected.[19-22] Regenerating hair cells, identified by their short, well-formed hair bundles, were seen in both maculae as early as 1–2 days after gentamicin treatment. Extensive restoration of hair bundle density was seen in both the sacculus (FIG. 1C) and the utricular striola (data not shown) by 7–9 days after gentamicin treatment.

Mitotic Hair Cell Regeneration

In vivo *Studies*

The *in vivo* appearance of small cells with mitotic figures in preliminary studies[19] suggested that hair cell regeneration in amphibians might involve, as in other species,[11,24-27] the mitotic division of a progenitor cell population. Cell proliferation, measured with BrdU immunocytochemistry, was seen in both normal and gentamicin-treated material and increased at later survival times.[21] In gentamicin-treated animals, cell proliferation was suppressed at early survival times and did not attain the levels seen in normal animals. Cell proliferation was greater in the saccular than the utricular macula in both normal and gentamicin-treated animals.

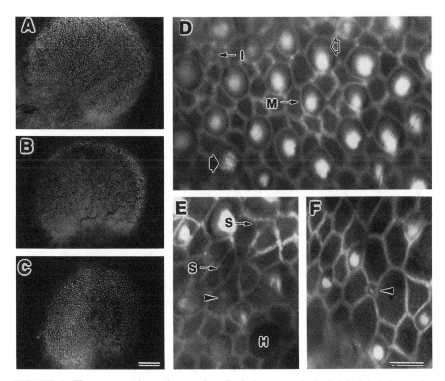

FIGURE 1. Fluorescent photomicrographs of whole-mounted phalloidin-labeled saccular maculae in a normal animal (**A**) and in animals sacrificed 1 day (**B**) and 7 days (**C**) after receiving a 200 μM gentamicin sulfate injection. Note the extensive loss of hair bundles and the presence of large epithelial holes immediately after gentamicin treatment (**B**) and the reappearance of hair bundles at later survival times (**C** and **D**). (**D–F**) Computer-assisted fluorescent images of wholemount phalloidin-labeled saccular maculae in a normal animal (**D**) and in animals sacrificed 5 days after receiving a 200 μM gentamicin sulfate injection (**E** and **F**). In normal animals (**D**), phalloidin-labeled cuticular plates (*open arrow*) and hair bundles (*solid arrow*) are seen. Mature (**M**) and immature (**I**) hair cells with round lumenal surfaces are surrounded by supporting cells with smaller polygonal lumenal surfaces. In gentamicin-treated animals, round epithelial holes (**H**) left by extruded hair cells are filled by the expanding processes of surrounding supporting cells to form scar formations (**S**). During scar repair, a single supporting cell participating in scar formation develops a cuticular plate (*arrowhead,* **E**), migrates towards the center of the scar, and develops an immature hair bundle (*arrowhead,* **F**). Bars, 100 μm (**A–C**); 10 μm (**D–F**).

BrdU-labeled cells had either a *condensed* (FIG. 2A–C) or *diffuse* (FIG. 2D–F) appearance. At early survival times, condensed BrdU-labeled cells were seen in both the peripheral macular margins and, within the maculae, immediately adjacent to the basement membrane (FIG. 2A). These cells had round cell bodies and, unlike mature

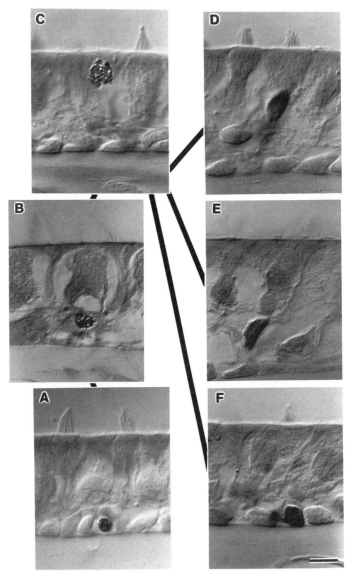

FIGURE 2. Condensed BrdU-labeled cells (**A–C**) and diffuse BrdU-labeled hair cell (**D**), supporting cell (**E**), and basal cell (**F**) in normal and gentamicin-treated saccular maculae at early and late survival times. Bars, 10 μm (**A–F**).

hair cells or supporting cells, did not contact the lumenal surface. At later survival times, cells with similar cellular morphology were seen at more apical positions (FIG. 2C and D). These cells often displayed mitotic figures, suggesting that proliferating cells migrated vertically from basal levels, with mitotic division occurring at the lumenal surface (FIG. 2C). Diffuse BrdU-labeled cells were seen only at late survival times, did not exhibit mitotic figures, and were typically clustered in cell pairs, indicating that they had left the cell cycle as the progeny of dividing cells. In normal animals, diffusely labeled cell pairs typically had similar cellular morphology and were most often supporting cells. Diffusely labeled cells were seldom seen in gentamicin-treated animals, even at late survival times.

Ongoing proliferation in both the sacculus and utriculus was seen in all macular regions. Gentamicin-induced proliferation, by contrast, was clustered about the reversal of hair cell polarization, a central region in the sacculus or utricular striola that typically sustained the highest levels of cellular damage. Surprisingly, cell proliferation within 7 days of gentamicin treatment was too low to account for the amount of hair cell recovery seen in gentamicin-treated animals.[21,22] Moreover, hair cells with immature hair bundles were seldom BrdU-labeled, suggesting that hair cell recovery following gentamicin ototoxicity might be due to nonmitotic mechanisms.

In vitro *Studies*

We considered the possibility that BrdU, because it was not continuously administered, was not equally available to all proliferating cells. To rule out this possibility, we repeated our *in vivo* experiments in organ cultures of the vestibular otolith organs.[20] Saccular and utricular maculae incubated in amphibian culture medium had normal cellular morphology, and cell proliferation in both normal and gentamicin-treated cultures was similar to their *in vivo* counterparts (FIG. 3A). Gentamicin-treated cultures incubated in normal culture medium produced hair cells with immature hair bundles, demonstrating that hair cell regeneration was also supported by our culture conditions (FIG. 3B). Hair cells with immature hair bundles were seldom BrdU-labeled, and cell proliferation, as in *in vivo*, was too low within 7 days of gentamicin treatment to account for the amount of hair cell recovery seen in gentamicin-treated cultures. Gentamicin-treated cultures incubated in aphidicolin, a blocker of nuclear DNA replication,[38] displayed normal levels of hair cell regeneration with near-zero levels of cell proliferation, demonstrating that mitotic division was not required for hair cell regeneration (FIG. 3C).

Nonmitotic Hair Cell Regeneration

To further explore the contribution of nonmitotic mechanisms to hair cell regeneration, we used Texas Red-conjugated phalloidin to label filamentous actin in immature hair bundles and to study the process of scar formation and repair in gentamicin-treated animals.[22] We also measured hair cell and supporting cell density and examined morphological changes in hair cells and supporting cells at varying times following gentamicin treatment.

In normal animals, the apical surfaces of hair cells and supporting cells in the saccular (FIG. 1D) and utricular (data not shown) maculae formed a complex mosaic, with hair cells seldom in contact with other hair cells. The apical surfaces of hair cells were circular whereas those of supporting cells were polygonal in shape, ranging from four to six sides. Hair cells in the central sacculus, although all of the same phenotype, differed markedly in the size of their hair bundles. Most ($\sim 90\%$) saccular hair cells had uniformly large hair bundles; a small minority ($\sim 10\%$) had significantly smaller hair bundles that were assumed to be less mature than those of larger hair cells.

Immediately after gentamicin treatment, small epithelial holes, presumably left by individual extruded hair cells, were observed throughout the saccular macula

BRDU-LABELED   **SACCULAR CULTURES**   HAIR BUNDLE
CELLS   DENSITY

990   0.013

949   0.009

                                                 0.008

15 —

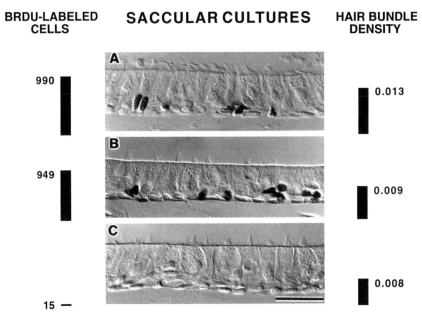

FIGURE 3. Cross-sectioned control (**A**) and gentamicin-treated (**B** and **C**) saccular culture incubated for 7 days in normal (**A** and **B**) and aphidicolin-supplemented (**C**) culture medium. Number of diffuse BrdU-labeled cells and hair bundle density are shown to the left and right, respectively. Note the presence of diffuse BrdU-labeled cells in normal medium (**A** and **B**) and the loss of these cells in aphidicolin-supplemented medium (**C**). In gentamicin-treated cultures (**B** and **C**), note the presence of immature hair bundles and the partial restoration of cellular organization. Note the abundance of basal nuclei in normal medium (**B**) and the relative paucity of such nuclei in aphidicolin-supplemented medium (**C**). Bars, 100 μm (**A–C**).

(FIG. 1E). Epithelial holes were rapidly filled in by the expanding apical processes of neighboring supporting cells to form wedge-shaped scar formations (FIG. 1E). Scar formations in the bullfrog vestibular otolith organs, unlike those in the organ of Corti[39,40] and mammalian vestibular organs[41] (but see also refs. 6–8), were not permanent fixtures but were rapidly replaced by immature hair cells. The first step in this process appeared to be the development of a cuticular plate in one of the supporting cells participating in a scar formation (arrow, FIG. 1E). Small cells with cuticular plates were also observed in or near the center of scar formations and were often associated with immature hair bundles (arrow, FIG. 1F), suggesting that single supporting cells migrated inward and converted into hair cells.

Consistent with the above scenario, hair cells with immature hair bundles in normal and gentamicin-treated animals were, on average, surrounded by fewer supporting cells than more mature hair cells.[22] Mature hair cells, for example, typically had five neighboring supporting cells, although they could be surrounded by from four to seven supporting cells. Immature hair cells, by contrast, were typically surrounded by only four supporting cells, indicating that a single supporting cell in each scar formation underwent conversion into a hair cell.

Gentamicin treatment, although it did not damage supporting cells, did result in rapid changes to supporting cell morphology in regions of hair cell loss (FIG. 4A and B). These changes included the rapid expansion of the apical processes of supporting cells (arrowheads, FIG. 4A) and, at later times, the development of hair cell-like characteristics in supporting cells (arrows, FIG. 4A and B). These developments included the appearance of cuticular plates and immature hair bundles in supporting cells and the apical migration of supporting cell nuclei in damaged macular regions. Early morphological changes in supporting cells presumably reflect the process of scar formation whereby supporting cells expand to fill the epithelial holes left by extruded hair cells and help to maintain the integrity of the lumenal surface. Later morphological changes, on the other hand, suggest a process of direct phenotypic conversion, or transdifferentiation, in supporting cells (see DISCUSSION).

We measured hair bundle and nuclear density at varying times subsequent to gentamicin treatment to determine whether supporting cell density was maintained in gentamicin-treated animals.[22] The density of mature hair cells in gentamicin-treated animals was markedly decreased immediately after gentamicin treatment but

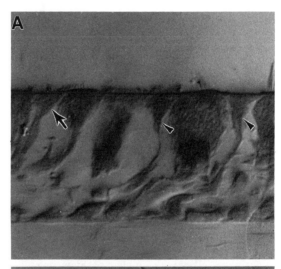

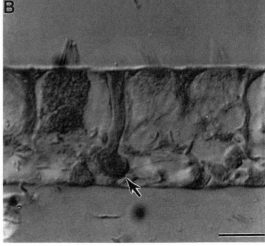

FIGURE 4. Cross-sectioned saccular maculae in animals sacrificed 2 days (**A**) and 3 days (**B**) after receiving a 200 μM gentamicin sulfate injection. In **A,** arrow and pointers indicate, respectively, supporting cells with and without immature hair bundles in regions of local hair cell loss. In **B,** arrow indicates converting cell with basal cell nucleus and immature hair bundle. Bars, 10 μm (**A** and **B**).

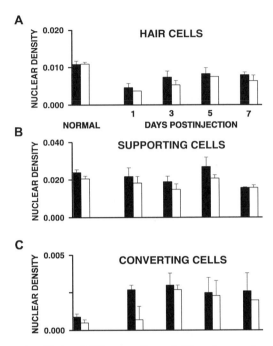

FIGURE 5. Bar graphs of hair cell (**A**), supporting cell (**B**), and converting cell (**C**) density in the neural (*solid bars*) and abneural (*open bars*) saccular macula plotted against postinjection time for eight animals receiving a 200 μM gentamicin injection. Values for four normal animals are plotted to the left. Values, means ± SDs.

steadily *increased* at later survival times (FIG. 5A). Supporting cell density, on the other hand, steadily *decreased* with survival time except for a transient increase 5 days after gentamicin treatment (FIG. 5B). These data suggest that the number of new hair cells was linked to the number of supporting cells. The density of *converting* cells, that is, supporting cells with hair cell-like characteristics (see above), is plotted in FIGURE 5C. Converting cell density, low in normal animals, rapidly increased after gentamicin treatment to the level predicted by our earlier phalloidin-labeling experiments. The number of converting cells at any survival time was also consistent with the suggestion that supporting cells underwent a phenotypic conversion, or transdifferentiation, to hair cells, with converting cells representing a necessary morphological intermediate between the supporting cell and hair cell phenotypes (see DISCUSSION).

DISCUSSION

The results of our studies indicate that both mitotic and nonmitotic processes contribute to hair cell recovery in the bullfrog vestibular otolith organs. There are at least two possible origins of new hair cells in the inner ear involving mitotic division: (1) proliferation and differentiation of stem cells[33] and (2) proliferation and *indirect transdifferentiation* of supporting cells.[21,28–32] In the first process (FIG. 6A), uncommitted stem cells are induced to undergo mitotic division by trauma, with the progeny of these cells becoming committed precursor cells that terminally differentiate as hair cells and supporting cells. *Indirect* transdifferentiation, by contrast, implies that a differentiated cell reverts to a less differentiated state and proliferates to give rise to cells of a new phenotype (FIG. 6B). Indirect transdifferentiation has been demonstrated in several cell types. In amphibian and chick retina, cells in the retinal pigment epithelium, when stimulated by basic fibroblast growth factor, have been shown to proliferate and ultimately transdifferentiate into either lens epithelium or neural progenitors.[42,43] In teleost fish, rod precursor cells, after retinal destruction, are able to reenter the cell cycle and differentiate into a variety of retinal cell types not normally associated with rod precursors during embryonic development.[42] Thus, rod precursors normally committed to the rod phenotype become pluripotent after cellular or mechanical damage. Indirect transdifferentiation has also been shown to occur in rat pancreatic cells[44] and in mammalian mammary cells.[45]

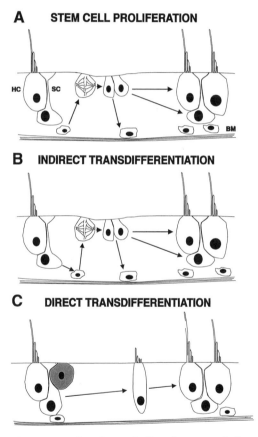

FIGURE 6. Schematic representation of two mitotic and one nonmitotic mechanisms by which new hair cells might be produced in the vestibular otolith organs. (**A**) Pre-existing stem cells migrate from the basement membrane, divide at the lumenal surface, and differentiate into new basal cells, supporting cells, and hair cells. (**B**) Mature supporting cells de-differentiate and re-enter the mitotic cycle, with their progeny transdifferentiating into mature hair cells. (**C**) Mature supporting cells directly transdifferentiate into mature hair cells without an intervening cell division. BM, basement membrane; LS, lumenal surface; HC, hair cell; SC, supporting cell.

Mature hair cells in the vestibular otolith organs did not undergo mitotic division. Rather, mitotic progenitors had distinctive cell morphology and, as in other inner ear organs,[24–27] were located immediately adjacent to the basement membrane. These progenitors, as in previous studies,[28–32] underwent interkinetic migration, moving from basal levels to more apical positions, with mitotic division and differentiation occurring at the lumenal surface. It is not clear whether progenitor cells in the vestibular organs are true stem cells[33] or supporting cells that have dedifferentiated and subsequently reentered the cell cycle.[34] It is also possible that only a subset of supporting cells is able to undergo mitosis or that supporting cells may alternate between mitotic and nonmitotic states.[33] These possibilities not only increase the difficulty of distinguishing between these two cell populations, but also blur the distinction between stem cell proliferation and indirect transdifferentiation.

The results of our *in vitro* aphidicolin studies demonstrate that hair cell regeneration does not require cell proliferation.[20,21] We considered three possible nonmitotic mechanisms for hair cell regeneration, including hair bundle replacement in damaged hair cells, hair cell migration from undamaged macular regions, and phenotypic conversion (or *direct transdifferentiation*) of supporting cell into hair cells without an intervening cell division (FIG. 6C). In the sacculus, gentamicin treatment produced large numbers of epithelial holes in the sensory epithelium (FIG. 1B and E). Moreover, hair bundle and apical nuclear density were well correlated at all times,[22] indicating that damaged hair cells were rapidly extruded after gentamicin treatment and that hair bundle replacement did not occur in damaged hair cells. Hair cell migration from undamaged macular regions was unlikely to be responsible for hair cell recovery in the sacculus, where gentamicin treatment produced a near-complete destruction of saccular hair cells. In the utriculus, no changes in hair cell density were seen in extrastriolar regions after gentamicin treatment, indicating that migration of hair cells from undamaged macular regions was also not responsible for hair cell recovery in this organ.

Our phalloidin-labeling experiments suggest that at least some supporting cells were able to undergo direct transdifferentiation into hair cells without an intervening cell division.[22] The number of supporting cells surrounding immature hair cells was less than that surrounding mature hair cells, suggesting that some supporting cells involved in scar formation were able to convert directly into hair cells. Consistent with this suggestion, supporting cells with hair cell-like characteristics, including cuticular plates and immature hair bundles, were commonly observed in regions of hair cell loss. Moreover, coordinated shifts in the numbers of hair cell and supporting cell nuclei were observed following gentamicin treatment, indicating that the number of new hair cells was inversely correlated with the number of supporting cells. This correlation would be expected of direct, but not indirect, transdifferentiation.

Direct transdifferentiation without concomitant cell division has recently been recognized as a possible pathway to cell differentiation. This process, although rare in vertebrates, is known to occur in glial cells, sympathetic neurons, and both smooth and skeletal muscle (44). We can only speculate what advantages direct transdifferentiation may have for hair cell recovery in the inner ear. Our studies do demonstrate that direct transdifferentiation can more rapidly create new hair cells than cell proliferation. Moreover, direct transdifferentiation can produce new hair cells without the metabolic cost of maintaining a quiescent stem cell population or the cellular disruption associated with mitotic division. The primary function of this nonmitotic process thus appears to be the restoration of lost hair cells, whereas that of slower mitotic process(es) is the replacement of supporting cells. The presence of both mitotic and nonmitotic mechanisms for hair cell regeneration may permit inner ear organs a high degree of flexibility, allowing them to maintain normal function in the face of small and large degrees of cellular and mechanical damage. In summary, our studies demonstrate that nonmitotic, as well as mitotic, mechanisms can be used to produce new hair cells. This exciting finding increases the likelihood that peripheral deafness and vestibular disorders can ultimately be alleviated in higher vertebrates through the replacement of lost hair cells.

REFERENCES

1. CORWIN, J. T. & M. E. WARCHOL. 1991. Auditory hair cells: Structure, function, development, and regeneration. Annu. Rev. Neurosci. **14:** 301–333.
2. CORWIN, J. T., M. E. WARCHOL & M. T. KELLEY. 1993. Hair cell development. Curr. Opin. Neurobiol. **3:** 32–37.
3. COTANCHE, D. A., K. H. LEE, J. S. STONE & D. A. PICARD. 1994. Hair cell regeneration in the bird cochlea following noise damage or ototoxic drug damage. Anat. Embryol. **189:** 1–18.
4. COTANCHE, D. A. & K. H. LEE. 1994. Regeneration of hair cells in the vestibulocochlear system of birds and mammals. Curr. Biol. **4:** 509–513.
5. TSUE, T. T., E. L. OESTERLE & E. W. RUBEL. 1994. Hair cell regeneration in the inner ear. Otolaryngol. Head Neck Surg. **111:** 281–301.
6. FORGE, A., L. LI, J. T. CORWIN & G. NEVILL. 1994. Ultrastructural evidence for hair cell regeneration in the mammalian inner ear. Science **259:** 1616–1619.
7. WARCHOL, M. E., P. R. LAMBERT, B. J. GOLDSTEIN, A. FORGE & J. T. CORWIN. 1994. Regenerative proliferation in inner ear sensory epithelia from adult guinea pigs and humans. Science **259:** 1619–1622.
8. RUBEL, E. W., L. A. DEW & D. W. ROBERSON. 1995. Mammalian vestibular hair cell regeneration. Science **267:** 701–703.
9. LEWIS, E. R. & C. W. LI. 1973. Evidence concerning the morphogenesis of saccular receptors in the bullfrog (*Rana catesbeiana*). J. Morphol. **139:** 351–362.
10. CORWIN, J. T. 1985. Perpetual production of hair cells and maturational changes in hair cell ultrastructure accompany postembryonic growth in an amphibian ear. Proc. Natl. Acad. Sci. USA **82:** 3911–3915.
11. POPPER, A. N. & B. H. HOXTER. 1990. Growth of a fish ear. II. Locations of newly proliferated hair cells in the saccular epithelium of *Astronotus ocellatus*. Hear. Res. **45:** 33–40.
12. JORGENSEN, J. M. & C. MATHIESEN. 1988. The avian inner ear: Continuous production of hair cells in vestibular sensory organs, but not in the auditory papilla. Naturwissenschaften **75:** 319–320.
13. CRUZ, R. M., P. R. LAMBERT & E. W. RUBEL. 1987. Light microscopic evidence of hair cell regeneration after gentamicin toxicity in chick cochlea. Arch. Otolaryngol. Head Neck Surg. **113:** 1058–1062.
14. GIROD, D. A., D. L. TUCCI & E. W. RUBEL. 1991. Anatomical correlates of functional recovery in the avian inner ear following aminoglycoside ototoxicity. Laryngoscope **101:** 1139–1149.
15. HASHINO, E., Y. TANAKA & M. SOKABE. 1991. Hair cell damage and recovery following chronic application of kanamycin in the chick cochlea. Hear. Res. **52:** 356–368.
16. LIPPE, W. R., E. W. WESTBROOK & B. M. RYALS. 1991. Hair cell regeneration in the chicken cochlea following aminoglycoside toxicity. Hear. Res. **56:** 203–210.
17. WEISLEDER, P. & E. W. RUBEL. 1993. Hair cell regeneration after streptomycin toxicity in the avian vestibular epithelium. J. Comp. Neurol. **331:** 97–110.
18. YAN, H. Y., W. M. SAIDEL, J. S. CHANG, J. C. PRESSON & A. N. POPPER. 1991. Sensory hair cells of a fish ear: Evidence of multiple types based on ototoxicity sensitivity. Proc. R. Soc. Lond. B **245:** 133–138.
19. BAIRD, R. A., M. A. TORRES & N. R. SCHUFF. 1993. Hair cell regeneration in the bullfrog vestibular otolith organs following aminoglycoside ototoxicity. Hear. Res. **65:** 164–174.
20. BAIRD, R. A., S. BALE, C. FIORILLO & N. R. SCHUFF. 1995. Hair cell regeneration does not require mitotic proliferation. Science. Submitted.
21. BAIRD, R. A., M. A. TORRES & N. R. SCHUFF. 1995. Ongoing and gentamicin-induced proliferation in the bullfrog vestibular otolith organs. I. Relationship to cellular proliferation. J. Comp. Neurol. Submitted.

22. BAIRD, R. A., M. A. TORRES & N. R. SCHUFF. 1995. Ongoing and gentamicin-induced proliferation in the bullfrog vestibular otolith organs. II. Contribution of non-mitotic mechanisms. J. Comp. Neurol. Submitted.
23. BALAK, K. J., J. T. CORWIN & J. E. JONES. 1990. Regenerated hair cells can originate from supporting cell progeny: Evidence from phototoxicity and laser ablation experiments in the lateral line system. J. Neurosci. **10:** 2502–2512.
24. KATAYAMA, A. & J. T. CORWIN. 1989. Cell production in the chicken cochlea. J. Comp. Neurol. **281:** 129–135.
25. RAPHAEL, Y. 1992. Evidence for supporting cell mitosis in response to acoustic trauma in the avian inner ear. J. Neurocytol. **21:** 663–671.
26. ROBERSON, D., P. WEISLEDER, P. BOHRER & E. W. RUBEL. 1992. Ongoing production of sensory cells in the vestibular epithelium of the chick. Hear. Res. **57:** 166–174.
27. OESTERLE, E. C. & E. W. RUBEL. 1993. Postnatal production of supporting cells in the chick cochlea. Hear. Res. **66:** 213–224.
28. KATAYAMA, A. & J. T. CORWIN. 1993. Cochlear cytogenesis visualized through pulse labeling of chick embryos in culture. J. Comp. Neurol. **281:** 129–135.
29. STONE, J. S. & D. A. COTANCHE. 1993. Identification of the timing of S phase and the patterns of cell proliferation during hair cell regeneration in the chick cochlea. J. Comp. Neurol. **341:** 50–67.
30. RAPHAEL, Y., H. J. ADLER, Y. WANG & P. A. FINGER. 1994. Cell cycle of transdifferentiating supporting cells in the basilar papilla. Hear. Res. **80:** 53–63.
31. TSUE, T. T., D. L. WATLING, P. WEISLEDER, M. D. COLTRERA & E. W. RUBEL. 1994. Identification of hair cell progenitors and intermitotic migration of their nuclei in the normal and regenerating avian inner ear. J. Neurosci. **14:** 140–152.
32. WEISLEDER, P., T. T. TSUE & E. W. RUBEL. 1995. Hair cell replacement in avian vestibular epithelium: Supporting cells to type I hair cells. Hear. Res. **82:** 125–133.
33. PRESSON, J. C. & A. N. POPPER. 1990. Possible precursors to new hair cells, supporting cells, and Schwann cells in the ear of a postembryonic fish. Hear. Res. **46:** 9–22.
34. CORWIN, J. T., J. E. JONES, A. KATAYAMA, M. W. KELLEY & M. E. WARCHOL. 1991. Hair cell regeneration: The identities of progenitor cells, potential triggers, and instructive cues. *In* Regeneration of Vertebrate Sensory Receptor Cells. G. R. Bock & J. Whelan, Eds. CIBA Found. Symp. **160:** 103–120. Wiley. New York.
35. GIROD, D. A., L. G. DUCKERT & E. W. RUBEL. 1989. Possible precursors of regenerated hair cells in the avian cochlea following acoustic trauma. Hear. Res. **42:** 175–194.
36. BAGGER-SJOBACK, D., L. LUNDMAN & I. NILSSON-EHLE. 1992. Ciprofloxacin and the inner ear—A morphological and round window membrane permeability study. ORL Otorhinolaryngol. **54:** 5–9.
37. SUGIHARA, M., T. HATTORI & M. FUKUDA. 1986. Immunohistochemical detection of BrdU in formalin tissues. Histochemistry **85:** 193–195.
38. HARRIS, W. A. & V. HARTENSTEIN. 1991. Neuronal determination without cell division in Xenopus embryos. Neuron **6:** 499–515.
39. RAPHAEL, Y. & R. A. ALTSCHULER. 1991. Reorganization of cytoskeletal and junctional proteins during cochlear hair cell degeneration. Cell Motil. Cytoskeleton **18:** 215–227.
40. RAPHAEL, Y. & R. A. ALTSCHULER. 1991. Scar formation after drug-induced cochlear insult. Hear. Res. **51:** 173–184.
41. MEITELES, L. Z. & Y. RAPHAEL. 1994. Scar formation in the vestibular sensory epithelium after aminoglycoside toxicity. Hear. Res. **79:** 26–38.
42. HITCHCOCK, P. F. & P. A. RAYMOND. 1992. Retinal regeneration. Trends Neurosci. **15:** 103–108.
43. RAO, M. S., D. G. SCARPELLI & J. K. REDDY. 1986. Transdifferentiated hepatocytes in rat pancreas. *In* Current Topics in Developmental Biology: Commitment and Instability in Cell Differentiation. T. S. Okada & H. Kondoh, Eds. Vol. **20:** 63–78. Academic Press. Orlando, FL.
44. BERESFORD, W. A. 1990. Direct transdifferentiation: Can cells change their phenotype without dividing? Cell Differ. Dev. **29:** 81–93.
45. EGUCHI, G. & R. KODAMA. 1993. Transdifferentiation. Curr. Opin. Cell Biol. **5:** 1023–1028.

Voltage Responses of Mouse Utricular Hair Cells to Injected Currents[a]

ALFONS RÜSCH AND RUTH ANNE EATOCK[b]

Department of Otorhinolaryngology and Communicative Sciences
Baylor College of Medicine
Houston, Texas 77030

INTRODUCTION

The vestibular organs of mammals, birds, and reptiles have two distinct hair cell types: type I and type II. Type II hair cells are evolutionarily older, as they are found in all hair cell organs. They are contacted by the bouton terminals of primary afferent neurons and efferent neurons. Type I cells occur only in the vestibular organs of amniotes and are enveloped by a single large afferent terminal called a calyx ending. Efferent nerve fibers form bouton terminals on the outer faces of the calyx endings. Although the presence of the calyx ending has been the defining characteristic of type I hair cells,[1] morphological features that distinguish the hair cells themselves have also been noted. Type I cells have an amphora shape, with a constricted neck between the nuclear region and cuticular plate, whereas type II cells tend to be more cylindrical.[1,2] Type I cells also tend to have larger hair bundles and larger subcuticular mitochondria than do adjacent type II cells.[3–5]

Recently, it has become clear that type I and II cells also differ electrophysiologically. Type I cells, but not type II cells, possess a large potassium (K^+) conductance that is activated at unusually negative voltages. We refer to this conductance as $g_{K,L}$, for low-voltage-activating K^+ conductance. This distinction holds in mammals and birds and in semicircular canal organs and utricles.[6–8] $g_{K,L}$ has predictable, marked effects on the voltage responses of type I hair cells to injected current, as we illustrate here using hair cells of the mouse utricle.

A fast, K^+-selective inwardly rectifying conductance, g_{K1}, appears to be expressed by hair cells from many preparations, including the mouse utricle.[9] Recently, an additional inwardly rectifying conductance, g_h, was described in leopard frog saccular cells.[10] g_h is readily distinguished from g_{K1} by its slow, sigmoidal kinetics and its permeance to both K^+ and Na^+. In the mouse utricle, we find that almost all mature type II cells and about one-third of type I cells express g_h. Therefore g_h may be, like g_{K1}, a common feature of vertebrate vestibular hair cells. Here we show that despite its small size, g_h may substantially modulate the receptor potentials of mouse utricular hair cells.

The effects of basolateral conductances on the receptor potential are tested by using the whole-cell patch-clamp technique to record the voltage responses of single cells to injected current steps. Bypassing the mechanoelectrical transduction process in this way has the advantage that the voltage response of the hair cell to currents is not convolved with the current response of the cell to mechanical deflections. Nevertheless, it is important to demonstrate that the injected currents are in the

[a] This research was supported by NIDCD grant R01 DC02290.
[b] Corresponding author. E-mail: eatock@bcm.tmc.edu

71

physiological range. We begin, therefore, by showing transducer currents, which have not previously been reported in mammalian vestibular hair cells.

METHODS

Tissue Preparation

Utricles were obtained from albino mice (ICR outbred strain, Harlan Sprague Dawley, Inc., Indianapolis, IN). Some utricles were explanted on collagen-coated coverslips on postnatal day (PD) 1 and grown in organotypic cultures at 37 °C until they were studied between PD 4 and PD 8. At the time of explantation, the utricular nerve was cut distal to Scarpa's ganglion, so that the nerve fibers degenerated. Most nerve calyces *in vivo* form during the first postnatal week, and therefore never formed in the cultures. Other utricles were excised from 1- to 17-day-old mice and studied immediately. Culturing and recording techniques were based on those used for the mouse cochlea.[11]

Cell Identification

Mature vestibular hair cells can be identified morphologically in the light microscope as type I or type II by the presence or absence of a constricted neck. Evidence from various sources[6-8] shows that $g_{K,L}$ is a distinctive property of mature type I hair cells. In a subset of 17 mouse utricular hair cells studied after the first postnatal week, we found that all 12 cells with constricted necks expressed $g_{K,L}$. The remaining five cells did not have necks and did not express $g_{K,L}$. This confirms for the mouse utricle that cells with $g_{K,L}$ are type I hair cells.

In recordings made during the first postnatal week, however, hair cell identification by either light microscopy or electrophysiology was not always possible because of the immature state of the epithelium. In the mouse utricle, type I cells acquire both their amphora shape and $g_{K,L}$ during the first week (ref. 12 and Lysakowski, Rüsch and Eatock, unpublished observations). Because a cylindrical hair cell with no $g_{K,L}$ may be either a type II cell or an immature type I cell, we avoid the type I and II nomenclature and refer instead to "cells with $g_{K,L}$" and "cells without $g_{K,L}$."

Solutions

The sensory epithelium was superfused at a rate of ~10 ml h^{-1} with an extracellular solution that contained (mM): 144 NaCl, 0.7 NaH$_2$PO$_4$, 5.8 KCl, 1.3 CaCl$_2$, 0.9 MgCl$_2$, 5.6 D-glucose, 10 Hepes-NaOH, vitamins and amino acids as in Eagle's MEM, pH 7.4, ~320 mmol kg^{-1}. The standard pipette (internal) solution comprised (mM): 140 KCl, 0.1 CaCl$_2$, 5 EGTA-KOH, 3.5 MgCl$_2$, 2.5 Na$_2$ATP, 5 Hepes, pH 7.4, ~290 mmol kg^{-1}.

Recording

Recordings were done in the whole-cell voltage- or current-clamp mode of the patch-clamp technique and, in most experiments, with the Axopatch 200A amplifier

(Axon Instruments, Foster City, CA). The remaining experiments were done with the List EPC-7 amplifier (Adams and List Associates, Darmstadt, Germany), which provides a better current clamp.

Depending on whether the goal was to study the mechanoelectrical transduction or voltage-gated conductances, the utricles were prepared in two different ways.

1. For transduction experiments, the otolithic membrane was removed after bathing the cut-open utricle in 100 μg/ml of Protease XXVII (Sigma, St. Louis, MO) for 30 min at room temperature. This enzyme treatment is likely to have disabled a fraction of the transducer conductance, but the removal of the otolithic membrane by purely mechanical means left all hair bundles dysfunctional. A patch pipette was pushed into the sensory epithelium ~ 10–30 μm from the recording site at a low angle. A strong efflux of fluid from the pipette kept the tip clean while simultaneously expanding the intercellular spaces between the hair cells. The pipette was then guided through the intercellular spaces onto the basal part of the target cell body. In this way, damage to the hair bundles at the recording site was avoided. The efflux of high-K^+ solution from the patch pipette transiently depolarized hair cells close to the recording site, but the resting membrane potential of the target cell had usually recovered by the time the whole-cell recording configuration was established.

2. For voltage- and current-clamp recordings of the basolateral conductances, enzymes were avoided and the otolithic membrane was removed mechanically, causing damage to the hair bundles but sparing the basolateral membranes from enzymatic digestion. A tear was made in the sensory epithelium to expose the basolateral surfaces of the hair cells. The cell bodies were cleaned with a stream of extracellular solution, and then patch pipettes were sealed onto the membrane in the region of the nucleus.

Series resistances were between 2.5 and 11 MΩ, 40–90% of which was electronically compensated. Voltages have been corrected for uncompensated series resistances and liquid junction potentials (-4 mV). Data were filtered by 8-pole Bessel filters (Frequency Devices, Haverhill, MA) at 1–20 kHz and digitized at twice the corresponding frequency. The temperature was between 23 and 25 °C. Values are expressed as means ± standard deviations.

RESULTS

To investigate how receptor potentials differ between hair cells with different voltage-gated conductances, we bypassed the mechanoelectrical transduction process and recorded voltage changes in response to current injection. To demonstrate that the injected currents are in the physiological range, we begin by showing mechanoelectrical transduction currents recorded from mouse utricular hair cells.

Transduction Currents

Force stimuli from a fluid jet evoked robust transduction currents in utricular hair cells, as illustrated for two hair cells in FIGURE 1. The stimulus traces in FIGURE 1A and the stimulus axis in FIGURE 1B show the voltage applied to the piezoelectric disc of the stimulator. We assume that the deflecting force applied to the hair bundles is a linear function of the driving voltage (see ref. 11). Cells were held at -84

mV, where most conductances are deactivated. As described later, the inward rectifier, g_h, would be partly activated at this voltage, but g_h was not expressed in the cells of FIGURE 1. In FIGURE 1A, saturating deflections of the hair bundle away from

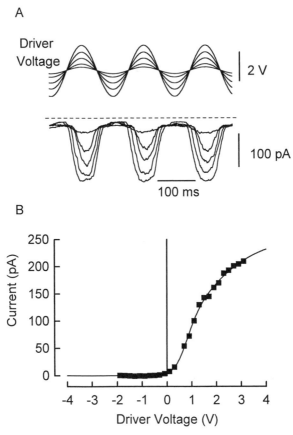

FIGURE 1. Mechanoelectrical transduction in hair cells in mouse utricles. The stimulus was a fluid jet delivered by a pipette with a tip diameter of ~ 20 μm, positioned 10–30 μm from the hair bundle. External (bath) fluid was driven in and out of the pipette by the voltage-controlled motion of a piezoelectric disc mounted at the back of the pipette. (**A**) Superimposed transducer currents (*lower traces*) evoked by an amplitude series of sinusoidal fluid-jet stimuli at 6 Hz (*upper traces*). The dashed line shows 0 pA. Hair cell in an acutely studied utricle, PD 1. As was the case for all mouse utricular hair cells on PD 1, the cell did not express $g_{K,L}$. The stimulus traces show the driving voltage to the piezoelectric disc. (**B**) Mechanoelectrical transfer function for a hair cell with no $g_{K,L}$ from an acutely studied utricle on PD 4. The cell was stimulated with 100-ms force steps and the transduction currents were measured 80 ms after the step onset. The data (■) are well fitted by a second-order Boltzmann function (curve) (see text, equation 1). I_{max}: 253 pA; k_1: 0.82 V^{-1}; k_2: 3.41 V^{-1}; DV_1: 1.13 V; DV_2: 0.86 V.

the kinocilium (negative deflections) reduced the inward holding current from ~ -20 pA to ~ -10 pA. Positive deflections induced inward currents of up to -150 pA.

In FIGURE 1B the peak currents evoked by step stimuli in a different cell are plotted as a function of the driving voltage. This transfer function had a saturating, nonlinear form that was well fitted by a second-order Boltzmann equation (equation 1).

$$I(DV) = \frac{I_{max}}{1 + e^{k_1(DV_1 - DV)}(1 + e^{k_2[DV_2 - DV]})} \tag{1}$$

$I(DV)$ is the transduction current, DV is the driving voltage to the piezoelectric disc, and k_1, k_2, DV_1 and DV_2 are constants. In this cell, about 4% of the maximally available conductance was activated at rest and the maximal inward current was ~ -250 pA.

In the current-clamp experiments that follow, we injected currents between -600 and $+600$ pA in order to bracket the range of recorded transducer currents.

A Low-Voltage Activating Delayed Rectifier Conductance, $g_{K,L}$

$g_{K,L}$ shares many properties with delayed rectifier conductances,[7,13] but has an unusually negative voltage range of activation, activating positive to -100 mV in some cells. As a result, at a holding potential of -64 mV, $g_{K,L}$ was substantially activated, producing a standing outward current (FIG. 2A). Moreover, voltage steps away from -64 mV evoked large instantaneous current jumps as the driving force for current flow through the open $g_{K,L}$ channels changed. Strongly hyperpolarizing steps deactivated $g_{K,L}$, causing the instantaneous current to decay. Depolarizing steps positive to -50 mV evoked delayed activation of a second conductance similar to the delayed rectifier conductance in cells with no $g_{K,L}$, as described next.

By contrast, cells with no $g_{K,L}$ had little standing current at -64 mV and little current at the onset of voltage steps (FIG. 2B). Steps positive to -50 mV activated, with a sigmoidal delay, a delayed rectifier K$^+$ conductance with sigmoidal kinetics, which we will call g_{DR}. The activation range of g_{DR} is typical of outwardly rectifying K$^+$ conductances in hair cells. FIGURE 2C compares the activation curves of $g_{K,L}$ and g_{DR}. Both were fitted with first-order Boltzmann functions (equation 2).

$$I(V) = \frac{I_{max} - I_{min}}{1 + e^{(V - V_{1/2})/s}} + I_{min} \tag{2}$$

$I(V)$ is membrane current, V is membrane voltage, I_{max} and I_{min} are the maximum and minimum current levels, $V_{1/2}$ is the voltage corresponding to half-maximal activation and s is the voltage step that evokes an e-fold change in current. $V_{1/2}$ values for $g_{K,L}$ ranged from ~ -90 to -60 mV in 57 cells. Such variability is unusual among delayed rectifier conductances, and may indicate that the voltage dependence of $g_{K,L}$ is under second-messenger control.[14] $V_{1/2}$ values for g_{DR}, in contrast, were both more positive and more tightly clustered, ranging from -25 to -36 mV for 35 cells. Arrows in FIGURE 2C point to the mean resting potentials of the two hair cell types in the mouse utricle: -77 ± 3.1 mV for 62 cells with $g_{K,L}$ and -65 ± 5.2 mV for 98 cells without $g_{K,L}$. This illustrates that $g_{K,L}$ is appreciably activated at the cells' resting potentials, whereas g_{DR} is not. For example, in the cells of FIGURE 2C, -77 mV corresponds to $\sim 30\%$ activation of $g_{K,L}$, whereas g_{DR} is $<0.5\%$ activated at -65 mV.

The voltage responses of hair cells with and without $g_{K,L}$ were strikingly different, as illustrated by the examples in FIGURE 3. Typically, cells with $g_{K,L}$ had small responses that faithfully reproduced the waveform of the injected current (FIG. 3A). These properties are expected given the appreciable activation of $g_{K,L}$ at the cells'

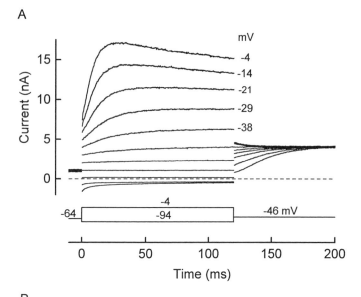

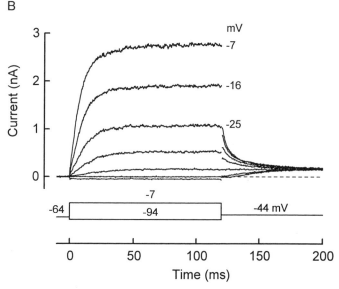

FIGURE 2. Voltage-gated currents in hair cells of the mouse utricle reveal two distinct potassium conductances, $g_{K,L}$ and g_{DR}. The holding potential (V_H) was -64 mV. (**A**) Hair cell with $g_{K,L}$, from a cultured utricle, PD 6. $g_{K,L}$ was substantially activated at V_H, producing the standing outward current at V_H and the large instantaneous jumps in current at the onset of the voltage steps. Resting potential (V_r): -80 mV; input resistance (R_{in}) at -64 mV: 11 MΩ; series resistance after electronic compensation (R_s): 0.7 MΩ; cell capacitance (C_m): 5.4 pF. (**B**) Hair cell with no $g_{K,L}$ from a cultured utricle, PD 3. g_{DR} was not activated at V_H, but activated with a delay during depolarizing voltage steps. V_r: -73 mV; R_{in} at -64 mV: 384 MΩ; R_s: 1.2 MΩ; C_m: 4.1 pF. (**C**) Activation curves for $g_{K,L}$ (●) and g_{DR} (■), from two other cells. Arrows point to the activation curve values at the mean resting potentials of cells with $g_{K,L}$ (-77 mV) and cells without $g_{K,L}$ (-65 mV). The curves were generated by stepping the membrane potential for 800 ms to various values, then stepping to -54 mV ($g_{K,L}$) or -44 mV (g_{DR}) to elicit tail currents. At -44 mV a larger driving force is provided, but -54 mV was chosen for the cell with $g_{K,L}$ to avoid activating the second delayed rectifier conductance. The tail currents at -54 mV or -44 mV were fitted, and the fits were extrapolated to their values at the instant of the step change in voltage. These values were divided by the maximum current and plotted as a function of prepulse potential. The smooth curves are fits of equation 2. $g_{K,L}$ curve, I_{max}: 3.99 nA; $V_{1/2}$: -73 mV; s: 5.1 mV. g_{DR} curve, I_{max}: 728 pA; $V_{1/2}$: -27 mV; s: 7.3 mV. $g_{K,L}$ data are from a cell in an acutely studied utricle, PD 9. g_{DR} data are from a cell in an acutely studied utricle, PD 4.

C

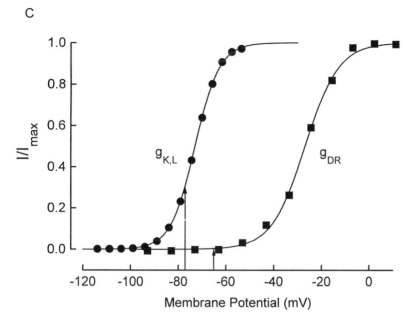

FIGURE 2 (*continued*).

resting potentials. The resulting low input resistance (R_{in}) means that input currents produce small voltage changes and that the cell has a short membrane time constant. For the cell of FIGURE 3A and C, in which R_{in} was 14 MΩ, a 100-pA step changed the membrane potential by only 1.4 mV. Such small changes did not significantly alter the activation level of voltage-gated conductances. As a consequence, the input resistance and the membrane voltage remained approximately constant after the onset of the current step. The speed of the voltage response to the onset of the current step is determined by the membrane time constant. For the cell of FIGURE 3A, C_m was 4.7 pF (mean C_m for cells with $g_{K,L}$: 3.5 ± 0.7 pF, $n = 82$), giving a time constant of only 66 μs.

Cells without $g_{K,L}$, by contrast, had relatively high input resistances because their resting potentials were negative to the activation range of the major conductance (g_{DR}). For example, for the cell in FIGURE 3B and C, R_{in} was 1.44 GΩ for current injections of ± 25 pA. Thus, current steps evoked much larger voltage changes with slower rise times (FIG. 3B). Current steps that depolarized the cell positive to −50 mV activated g_{DR}, causing partial repolarization and a reduction in the slope resistance from 169 to 51 MΩ (FIG. 3C).

An Inwardly Rectifying Conductance, g_h

Many hair cells have a small, fast, inwardly rectifying K$^+$ conductance (g_{KI}) that has been intensively studied in other tissues. It is expected to contribute to the resting conductance and resting potential.[10] In many cells of the mouse utricle, a slow, inwardly rectifying conductance, g_h, was also observed. g_h was found in about

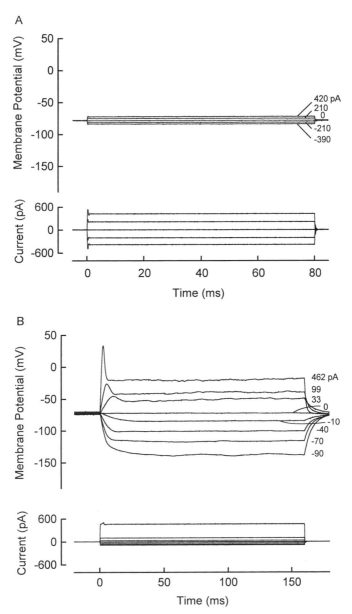

FIGURE 3. Voltage responses of a cell with $g_{K,L}$ (**A**) and a cell without $g_{K,L}$ (**B**) to injected currents (*bottom panels*; the sizes of the corresponding current steps are shown to the right of the voltage traces). (**A**) Hair cell from an acutely studied utricle, PD 9. V_r: −78 mV. (**B**) Hair cell from an acutely studied utricle, PD 1. V_r: −72 mV. (**C**) Voltage-current (V-I) relations for the cells shown in **A** and **B**, from families of voltage responses that include the data shown in **A** and **B**. For the cell with no $g_{K,L}$, peak (○) and steady-state (□) voltages are plotted separately. For the cell with $g_{K,L}$, peak and steady-state voltages are identical (■). For the cell with $g_{K,L}$, the slope of the linear regression fit (*solid line*) was 14 MΩ. For the cell without $g_{K,L}$, R_{in} was calculated to be 1.44 GΩ from the slope of the linear regression fit (not shown) through the three points centered on the zero-current value. The slope resistances for the peak and steady-state voltages evoked by positive currents > 100 pA were 169 and 51 MΩ, respectively.

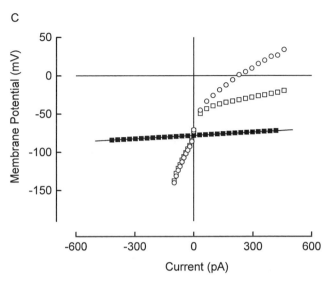

FIGURE 3 (*continued*).

30% of cells with $g_{K,L}$ and in all cells without $g_{K,L}$ after the first postnatal week. By this time, cells without $g_{K,L}$ are clearly type II hair cells rather than immature type I hair cells.[12]

g_h was originally described in photoreceptors[15] and heart cells[16] and has recently been characterized in frog saccular hair cells.[10] It is a mixed K^+/Na^+ conductance with a reversal potential in the solutions used here of -43.5 ± 1.8 mV ($n = 5$). It has slow sigmoidal activation and deactivation kinetics (FIG. 4A and ref. 10). g_h activated with increasing hyperpolarization negative to the mean resting potential of cells without $g_{K,L}$ (-65 mV; arrow in FIG. 4B). g_h activation curves were fitted with a Boltzmann function (equation 2), giving mean $V_{1/2}$ and s values of -101 ± 5 mV and 7.8 ± 1.2 mV ($n = 8$).

The effect of g_h on the voltage responses of hair cells to injected currents was readily apparent (FIG. 5). Strongly negative current steps evoked large hyperpolarizations with a pronounced transient component. The repolarization following the peak hyperpolarization had kinetics and voltage dependence consistent with activation of g_h.

DISCUSSION

Transducer Currents

Preliminary records of transducer currents from mouse utricular hair cells show that, as in other hair cells, the mechanoelectrical transfer function is saturating, nonlinear, and strongly asymmetric. Although the saturating current amplitudes were similar to or greater than those recorded from hair cells in most other preparations, they were just one-third to one-half the values obtained from cultured mouse cochlear hair cells.[11] This discrepancy may result primarily from a technical

A

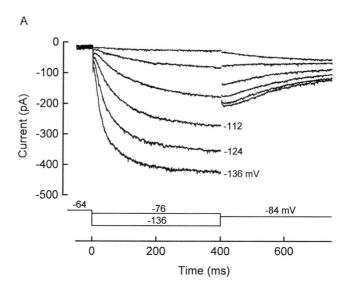

B

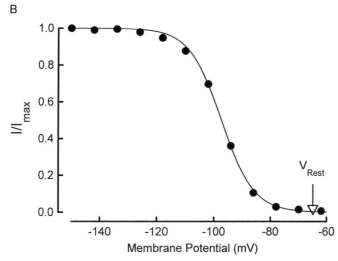

FIGURE 4. Properties of g_h, a slow, inwardly rectifying conductance in mouse utricular hair cells. (**A**) Currents evoked by a series of steps to voltages between -76 mV and -136 mV, in 12-mV steps. The presence of substantial tail currents at -84 mV, the equilibrium potential for K^+, illustrates that g_h is not exclusively K^+-selective. V_H: -64 mV. Ba^{2+} (1 mM) was added to the external medium to block the fast, inwardly rectifying potassium conductance, g_{K1}, that is also present in most mouse utricular hair cells. Cell without $g_{K,L}$, from a cultured utricle, PD 9. V_r (in standard solutions): -61 mV, R_s: 1.3 MΩ. (**B**) Activation curve of g_h of another cell. Tail currents at -84 mV, elicited by the protocol shown in **A**, were fitted and extrapolated to the onset of the step to -84 mV, normalized by the maximum current, and plotted as a function of the iterated voltage. The solid line shows the fit to the data of a Boltzmann function (equation 2). I_{max}: -102.8 pA; $V_{1/2}$: -97.3 mV; s: 5.7 mV. ^VRest (*arrow*): mean resting potential of cells without $g_{K,L}$.

difference between the utricular and cochlear preparations. In the cochlear cultures, no tectorial membrane ever formed, whereas in both cultured and acutely studied utricles, enzyme treatment was necessary to ease removal of the otolithic membrane in order to expose the hair bundles. The enzyme treatment is likely to have damaged the transduction apparatus. Therefore, to ensure coverage of the physiological range of transducer currents, we injected currents over a larger range ($\pm$ 600 pA) than we had recorded.

Effects of $g_{K,L}$ on Receptor Potential

$g_{K,L}$ has a profound impact on the voltage responses to injected currents within the physiological range. Its large size (average maximum value in mouse utricular hair cells: 75 nS at -54 mV, unpublished observations) essentially clamps the type I membrane near the equilibrium potential for E_K, preventing large voltage changes. As a corollary, the activation state of the cell's voltage-gated conductances, including $g_{K,L}$, cannot change substantially during the voltage response, leading to the very linear responses shown in FIGURE 3A. Only large negative current injections (exceeding 400 pA in FIGURE 5A) sufficed to deactivate $g_{K,L}$, thereby permitting large voltage excursions. It is difficult to imagine how input currents could drive the cell potential negative to E_K in vivo. Negative hair bundle deflections from rest turn off a rather small inward current, which would move the potential closer to E_K, but not negative to it. Thus, $g_{K,L}$ seems to restrict the type I cell to a small and linear receptor potential that does not deviate more than ~ 10 mV from E_K.

The small voltage responses and relatively negative resting membrane potential present a conundrum for conventional synaptic transmission from the type I hair cell to the calyx ending. Suppose that, as is presumed in other hair cells, transmitter release is mediated by calcium entry[17] through voltage-gated channels that activate positive to -60 mV.[18] $g_{K,L}$ would appear to prevent sufficient depolarization of the hair cell to allow significant transmitter release. We are forced to consider whether this puzzle is an artifact of the conditions common to experiments on voltage-gated currents in type I hair cells. In order to gain access to the cell membrane to form the whole-cell configuration, the cells have in all cases been isolated from their natural environment, either by enzymatic dissociation or by, in our experiments, widening the extracellular spaces by blowing the pipette solution onto the cells. In particular, the ability to enter the whole-cell configuration implies that the calyx membrane is either disturbed or, as in the cultured utricles and immature epithelia, not present. In an intact, mature system, $g_{K,L}$ might behave differently. The activation range of $g_{K,L}$ may be under second messenger control, and so could be quite different in vivo.[14] Additionally, the narrow synaptic cleft between the type I hair cell and the calyx ending may accumulate K^+, leading to substantial depolarization of the hair cell membrane (J. M. Goldberg, this volume).

If we neglect the problem of synaptic transmission, the current-clamp records from cells with and without $g_{K,L}$ argue that calyx afferents, which innervate type I hair cells, will have relatively low response gains to vestibular stimulation. In vivo recordings from nerve fibers innervating chinchilla semicircular canal organs provide some evidence for this.[19]

Effects of g_h on Receptor Potential

g_h has long been known to have a pronounced effect on the shape of the hyperpolarizing receptor potential of rods,[20] introducing a transient "nose" similar

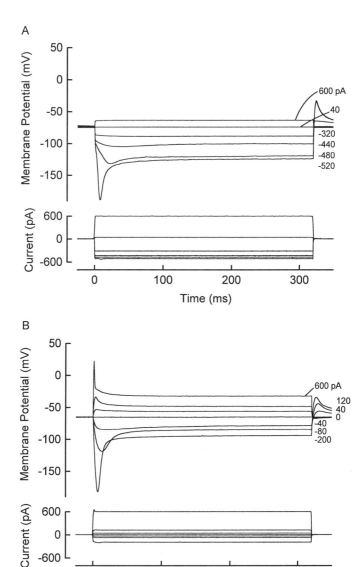

FIGURE 5. g_h introduces an initial transient component in the responses of cells with or without $g_{K,L}$ to injected negative currents. (**A**) Cell with $g_{K,L}$ and g_h, from a cultured utricle on PD 9. A transient component is evident in the most hyperpolarized responses (negative to -100 mV). The repolarization following the peak hyperpolarization is attributable to activation of g_h. V_r: -75 mV; R_{in}: 11 MΩ. (**B**) Cell with g_h and g_{DR}, but no $g_{K,L}$. Same cell as in FIGURE 4A; cultured utricle, PD 9. This cell shows transient components in both depolarizing and hyperpolarizing responses, reflecting activation of g_{DR} and g_h, respectively. R_{in}: 350 MΩ. (**C**) V-I relations for the cell in **A** (●, ■) and **B** (○, □). Peak (●, ○) and steady-state (■, □) voltages are plotted separately. The peak and steady-state relations diverge for small current injections of either polarity for the cell with no $g_{K,L}$, but diverge only for very large negative currents for the cell with $g_{K,L}$. The steady-state relations of the two cells converge at the very negative potentials at which $g_{K,L}$ is deactivated (negative to -100 mV).

C

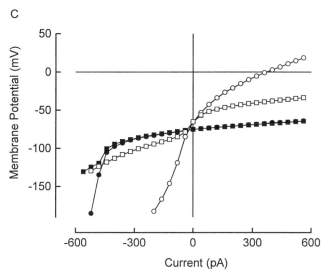

FIGURE 5 (*continued*).

to the waveforms in FIGURES 5A and 5B. g_h, and a similar effect of g_h in current clamp have recently been described in frog saccular hair cells.[10] The properties of g_h in mouse utricular hair cells agree closely with those of g_h in frog saccular hair cells. In both cases, g_h is a relatively small conductance with slow sigmoidal activation and deactivation kinetics. Its high incidence in these two rather different organs raises the possibility that g_h is relatively common in vestibular hair cells. g_h is much slower to activate than g_{Kl} and may, as a consequence, have escaped detection in some studies in which relatively short-duration voltage steps were used.

Despite its small size and slow kinetics, g_h may have sizable effects on the resting potential[10] and receptor potential (FIG. 5), depending on what other conductances are present. g_h activated just negative to the mean resting potential of mouse utricular cells without $g_{K,L}$. Because of the relatively high input resistances of these cells, fairly small, negative currents (50 pA or more for the cell of FIG. 5B and C) will induce large hyperpolarizations that will activate g_h and repolarize the cell. Such hyperpolarizations might occur *in vivo,* either mediated by efferent transmitters (which act directly on type II hair cells) or as a consequence of turning off a robust standing transducer current. Although preliminary results from the mouse utricular hair cells showed little transducer current at the resting bundle position, values in excess of 50 pA have been reported.[21] The physiological relevance of g_h in cells with $g_{K,L}$ (i.e., type I cells), however, is not evident in our data. Negative currents greater than 200 pA, which seem unrealistically large, were necessary to hyperpolarize the cell enough to deactivate $g_{K,L}$ and activate g_h (FIG. 5A and C). Smaller negative currents may suffice *in vivo* if $g_{K,L}$ has a more positive activation range, as suggested above.

In summary, current-clamp data suggest that the voltage-gated conductances, $g_{K,L}$ and g_h, are likely to contribute to differential processing of vestibular stimuli within the utricular macula. There is no doubt that such processing occurs because mammalian utricular afferents have diverse response patterns and types of spontaneous discharge (reviewed in ref. 22). The remaining challenge is to link specific voltage-gated conductances in the hair cell to specific patterns of afferent response.

REFERENCES

1. WERSÄLL, J. 1956. Studies on the structure and innervation of the sensory epithelium of the crista ampullares in the guinea pig. Acta Otolaryngol. **126(Suppl.):** 1–85.
2. WERSÄLL, J. & D. BAGGER-SJÖBÄCK. 1974. Morphology of the vestibular sense organ. *In* Handbook of Sensory Physiology. Vestibular System: Basic Mechanisms. H. H. Kornhuber, Ed.: 123–170. Springer-Verlag. New York.
3. LYSAKOWSKI, A. 1992. Possible morphological features to distinguish calyx vs. dimorphic type I vestibular hair cells in the chinchilla cristae. Soc. Neurosci. Abstr. **18:** 1400.
4. DiCAPRIO, L. L. & E. H. PETERSON. 1992. Differences in ciliary bundle morphology of type I and type II vestibular hair cells. Soc. Neurosci. Abstr. **18:** 509.
5. LIM, D. J. 1976. Morphological and physiological correlates in cochlear and vestibular sensory epithelia. Scanning Electron Microsc. **5:** 269–366.
6. CORREIA, M. J. & D. G. LANG. 1990. An electrophysiological comparison of solitary type I and type II vestibular hair cells. Neurosci. Lett. **116:** 106–111.
7. RENNIE, K. J. & M. J. CORREIA. 1994. Potassium currents in mammalian and avian isolated type I semicircular canal hair cells. J. Neurophysiol. **71:** 1–13.
8. EATOCK, R. A., W. Y. CHEN & M. SAEKI. 1994. Potassium currents in mammalian vestibular hair cells. Sens. Syst. **8:** 21–28.
9. RÜSCH, A. & R. A. EATOCK. 1994. Two types of inward rectifiers in hair cells of the mouse utricle. Soc. Neurosci. Abstr. **20:** 967.
10. HOLT, J. R. & R. A. EATOCK. 1995. The inwardly rectifying currents of saccular hair cells from the leopard frog. J. Neurophysiol. **73:** 1484–1502.
11. KROS, C. J., A. RÜSCH & G. P. RICHARDSON. 1992. Mechano-electrical transducer currents in hair cells of the cultured neonatal mouse cochlea. Proc. R. Soc. Lond. B **249:** 185–193.
12. RÜSCH, A. & R. A. EATOCK. 1994. Postnatal acquisition of a potassium conductance in hair cells of cultured mouse utricles. Assoc. Res. Otolaryngol. Abstr. **17:** 108.
13. RÜSCH, A. & R. A. EATOCK. 1995. A low-voltage-activating delayed rectifier in mammalian type I hair cells at different temperatures. Biophys. J. **68:** A392.
14. CHEN, W. Y. & R. A. EATOCK. 1994. Nitric oxide inhibits a low-voltage-activated potassium conductance in mammalian type I hair cells. Biophys. J. **66:** A430.
15. BADER, C. R., D. BERTRAND & E. A. SCHWARTZ. 1982. Voltage-activated and calcium-activated currents studied in solitary rod inner segments from the salamander. J. Physiol. **331:** 253–284.
16. DiFRANCESCO, D., A. FERRONI, M. MAZZANTI & C. TROMBA. 1986. Properties of the hyperpolarizing-activated current (I-f) in cells isolated from the rabbit sino-strial node. J. Physiol. **377:** 61–88.
17. KATAOKA, Y. & H. OHMORI. 1994. Activation of glutamate receptors in response to membrane depolarization of hair cells isolated from chick cochlea. J. Physiol. **477:** 403–414.
18. HUDSPETH, A. J. & R. S. LEWIS. 1988. Kinetic analysis of voltage- and ion-dependent conductances in saccular hair cells of the bull-frog, *Rana catesbeiana.* J. Physiol. **400:** 237–274.
19. BAIRD, R. A., G. DESMADRYL, C. FERNANDEZ & J. M. GOLDBERG. 1988. The vestibular nerve of the chinchilla. II. Relation between afferent response properties and peripheral innervation patterns in the semicircular canals. J. Neurophysiol. **60:** 182–203.
20. FAIN, G. L. & J. E. LISMAN. 1981. Membrane conductances of photoreceptors. Prog. Biophys. Mol. Biol. **37:** 91–147.
21. SHEPHERD, G. M. & D. P. COREY. 1994. The extent of adaptation in bullfrog saccular hair cells. J. Neurosci. **14:** 6217–6229.
22. GOLDBERG, J. M. 1991. The vestibular end organs: Morphological and physiological diversity of afferents. Curr. Opin. Neurobiol. **1:** 229–235.

Structural Variation in Ciliary Bundles of the Posterior Semicircular Canal

Quantitative Anatomy and Computational Analysis[a]

E. H. PETERSON,[b,c] J. R. COTTON,[d] AND J. W. GRANT[d]

[b]Department of Biological Sciences and Neurobiology Program
College of Arts and Sciences, College of Osteopathic Medicine
Ohio University
Athens, Ohio 45701-2979

[d]Department of Engineering Science and Mechanics
Virginia Polytechnic Institute
Blacksburg, Virginia 24061-0219

INTRODUCTION

Hair cells are mechanoreceptors; their function is to transduce mechanical stimuli into electrical signals that can be decoded by neurons. The mechanoreceptive organelle of the hair cell is its ciliary bundle, a cluster of modified microvilli (stereocilia; stereovilli[1]) that extend from the hair cell's apical surface into the cavity of the labyrinth. Graded deflection of the ciliary bundle (by otolithic membranes, cupula, or endolymph) modulates the receptor potential of the hair cell and the discharge of vestibular afferents (FIG. 1). Thus, understanding the mechanical factors governing this graded deflection is central to the understanding of peripheral vestibular signaling.

There are theoretical and empirical reasons for supposing that the magnitude of bundle deflection in response to an imposed force is strongly dependent on bundle structure (FIG. 1, shaded areas).[1–4] Thus, it is surprising that the relation between bundle structure and mechanics in vestibular hair cells has received so little rigorous attention. We address this issue here. Our goals in this report are (1) to begin a quantitative description of vestibular ciliary bundle structure in an amniote (note A), emphasizing possible differences between type I and type II receptors, and (2) to introduce a computational method for exploring the role that structure plays in ciliary bundle mechanics.

Our experimental preparation is a turtle, *Trachemys (Pseudemys) scripta;* considerable information is already available about the peripheral vestibular system in this species.[10–15] In this report we focus on hair cells from the posterior semicircular canal. Some of the present results have appeared previously in abstract form.[16–18]

[a]This work was supported by NIH NIDCD 00618, NSF IBN-9319630, and by the College of Osteopathic Medicine.

[c]Address correspondence to Ellengene H. Peterson, Department of Biological Sciences, Irvine Hall, Ohio University, Athens, OH 45701. E-mail: peterson@ouvaxa.cats.ohiou.edu

METHODS

Morphological Analysis

Scanning Electron Microscopy

We perfused deeply anesthetized (Nembutal™, 2 mL/kg) animals with oxygenated turtle Ringer's solution at 4 °C (pH 7.4),[19] 0.5 L of fixative (2% glutaraldehyde, 4% paraformaldehyde and 2 mM $MgCl_2$ in 0.1 M sodium phosphate buffer), postfixed the ampullae in fresh fixative (1 h) followed by 2% buffered osmium tetroxide (OsO_4; in 0.1 M sodium phosphate buffer; 1 h), saturated thiocarbohydrazide (10 min), and OsO_4 (1 h).[20] We dehydrated the ampullae in ethanol followed by

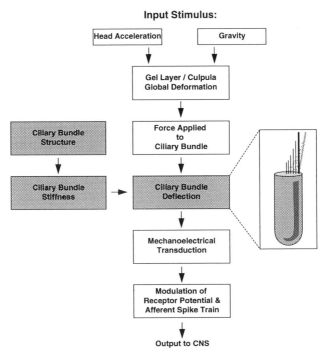

FIGURE 1. Steps by which hair cells transduce mechanical stimuli into neural signals. Shading indicates the focus of this report: how a ciliary bundle's structure shapes its stiffness and thus its deflection when forced.

critical point drying and gold-palladium sputter coating, and we inspected them under a JEOL JSM-840 scanning electron microscope. In some cases, we removed stereociliary bundles from the surface of the neuroepithelium by ultrasonication (15–30 s). We photographed the neuroepithelium at 2500× magnification and constructed complete montages of the sensory surface of four animals. For quantitative analysis of ciliary bundles we photographed the epithelium at 5000× and measured apical surface features and stereociliary numbers from the prints (10,000×

final magnification). We sampled the entire epithelium: the peripheral zone, which contains only type II hair cells, and the central zone, which contains both hair cell types. We report quantitative data from a single animal, which we confirmed by qualitative examination of the remaining three cases.

Differential Interference Contrast Microscopy

We visualized the ciliary bundles of identified type I and type II hair cells in cristae that had been fixed (4% glutaraldehyde), embedded in Epon, and sectioned transversely (at 30–40 μm) so that hair cells could be viewed normal to their long axis. We viewed the sections using a Zeiss Axioplan microscope equipped with a camera lucida attachment, drew each section at a final magnification of approximately 1,600×, and identified type I and type II hair cells by their shape and the presence or absence of a calyx. We measured the thickness of all complete bundles from the drawings (i.e., distance along the apical surface from the kinocilium to the shortest stereocilium). We analyzed all transverse sections through the central zone of three animals.

Finite Element Analysis

Finite element analysis (FEA) is a numerical method that uses information about the geometry and material properties of a mechanical system to solve a given boundary value problem. We are using this technique to approximate the mechanical response of forced ciliary bundles. Stereocilia were modeled using shear deformable (Timeshenko) beam theory. This is necessary because stereocilia exhibit large deformations due to shear[21] (see DISCUSSION), which classical (Euler-Bernoulli) beam theory does not accurately model. By modeling this radial anisotropy, we obtain biologically more accurate results than our previous work, which assumed the stereocilia to be isotropic.[22,23] Ciliary interconnections were modeled as uniaxial bars.

The linear finite element equations[24] were coded into a computer program that allows the user to define the structure and material properties of bundle elements (cilia and their interconnections) and then test the structure's deflection due to forces. The program was verified by comparing its results with those from analytical solutions of single stereocilia[23] and results from Algor, a commercially available finite element package. Element size was reduced until the solutions converged. In all our tests, force was applied to the top of the tallest stereocilium, parallel to the excitatory axis. Stiffness was defined as magnitude of applied force divided by magnitude of deflection of the tallest stereocilium.

Physical Assumptions

Stereocilia had shaft diameters of 0.20 μm, base diameters of 0.12 μm, taper heights of 1.0 μm, and center-to-center spacing of 0.24 μm.[25,26] Young's modulus was 3×10^9 N/m^2 (tensile modulus for actin). The shear modulus was 1×10^6 N/m^2 (see DISCUSSION).

Two kinds of links interconnected the cilia. Tip links connected cilia in each column. They were modeled as arising at a 45° angle from the radial edge of the top of one cilium and inserting into the radial edge of the next tallest cilium in the column. Shaft links connected each cilium to (1) adjacent cilia in the same column and (2) up to six lateral cilia (for full bundle simulations). They occurred every 0.25 μm over the top 2 μm of each cilium; earlier simulations suggested that lower lateral links will have minimal influence on bundle stiffness.[23] Stiffnesses of tip links and shaft links were 0.001499 N/m and 0.006361 N/m, respectively. These values are based on published dimensions of the links and the modulus for elastin; they are similar to values suggested for frog saccular hair cells.[4]

RESULTS

The neuroepithelium of the posterior canal comprises two triangular patches (hemicristae; FIG. 2).[12] Within each hemicrista there are two zones: an elliptical

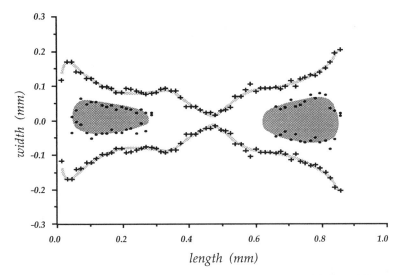

FIGURE 2. Schematic reconstruction of the posterior canal neuroepithelium. This sensory surface comprises two triangular hemicristae; their bases abut the canal walls (planum), and their apices are apposed at the canal center (torus). Each hemicrista has a central zone (*shaded*), which bears type I and type II hair cells, and a peripheral zone, which bears type II hair cells only. We measured the extent of the neuroepithelium (*crosses*) and the central zone (*dots;* defined by the presence of type I hair cells) from serial transverse sections through the posterior crista and combined them to produce this surface reconstruction.

central zone (shaded) and, surrounding it, a peripheral zone. The central zone bears type I and type II hair cells as well as bouton and calyx-bearing (calyceal and dimorphic) afferents; the peripheral zone bears only type II hair cells and bouton afferents.[12,15] Thus, *Trachemys* is unusual among amniotes in having a portion of the canal neuroepithelium devoted exclusively to one hair cell and one afferent type.

Scanning Electron Microscopy

In sonicated epithelia, the apical surfaces of hair cells are readily identifiable as elliptical profiles that bear a characteristic array of "stumps," that is, the remnants of kinocilia, stereocilia, and microvilli (FIG. 3). Ciliary remnants can usually be distin-

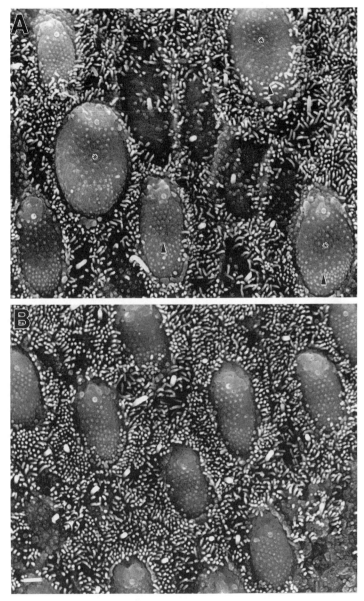

FIGURE 3. Scanning electron micrograph of the posterior crista; the tissue has been sonicated to reveal the apical surfaces of hair cells. Scale: 1 μm. (**A**) Central zone, which contains type I and type II hair cells. Profiles are either (1) large, with many stereocilia covering most of the surface (*asterisks*) or (2) smaller, with fewer stereocilia and narrower bundles (measured from kinocilium to row of shortest cilia; *arrowheads*). (**B**) Peripheral zone, which contains only type II hair cells. These apical surfaces resemble smaller profiles in the central zone.

guished from microvilli by their wider and more regular (approximately hexagonal) spacing; often they bear a central "pit." Such sonicated material can provide more accurate estimates of bundle dimensions (excluding heights) and geometry than is possible with intact epithelia.

Profiles in the central zone are markedly heterogeneous (FIG. 3A). They differ in the size and shape of apical surfaces, and in the number, dimensions, and spacing of their ciliary arrays. These structural features covary in orderly ways. On large, rounded profiles the ciliary bundle tends to cover much of the apical surface; it is *thick* (measured from the kinocilium to the shortest row of cilia, parallel to the excitatory/inhibitory (E/I) axis of the hair cell), relatively *wide* (measured perpendicular to the E/I axis), and bears a large number of stereocilia. In contrast, bundles on more elliptical profiles are smaller; they bear fewer stereocilia, which are sequestered toward the kinocilial end of the apical surface. Because the central zone contains both type I and type II hair cells, one hypothesis is that the different bundle morphologies belong to different hair cell types.

We can test this hypothesis by examining profiles in the peripheral zone, which contains only type II hair cells (FIG. 3B). In the periphery, profiles are homogeneous. Apical surfaces are narrow ellipses. Bundles are small and concentrated toward the kinocilium, with relatively few stereocilia. These profiles resemble the small profiles in the central zone (FIG. 3A).

FIGURE 4 compares ciliary number and bundle thickness for profiles in the central and peripheral zones. The scatterplot illustrates three points.

1. Peripheral profiles (diamonds) form a circumscribed cluster with relatively narrow ciliary bundles (thickness usually ≤ 2 μm) and 15–35 stereocilia. We know that these belong to type II hair cells.
2. Central profiles (squares) appear to fall into two clusters. One cluster has narrow bundles (thickness usually ≤ 3 μm) and less than 55–60 stereocilia; its distribution overlaps that of peripheral type II hair cells. The second cluster has thick ciliary bundles and 60 or more stereocilia. It also exhibits greater spread in ciliary number for a given bundle thickness, apparently because the number of ciliary columns in thick bundles can vary considerably (FIG. 3A; FIG. 7, compare cells b, c, and d).
3. A strong relation exists between bundle thickness and ciliary number ($r^2 = 0.79$; number of cilia = $-15.12 + 25.03 \times$ bundle thickness). Thus, if we know the thickness of a ciliary bundle, we can predict its complement of stereocilia with reasonable confidence.

Differential Interference Contrast Microscopy

Our scanning electron microscopy (SEM) material suggests that thick bundles in the central zone may belong to type I hair cells and narrower bundles to type II hair cells. We can test this idea in a second way by looking at transversely sectioned material in which the calyces that define type I hair cells are visible. In such material, we can characterize bundle thickness in identified type I hair cells and in type II hair cells from central and peripheral zones.

Differential interference contrast (DIC) micrographs of peripheral and central ciliary bundles are shown in FIGURE 5. In the peripheral zone (FIG. 5A), the type II ciliary bundle is very narrow when measured from the kinocilium to the shortest row of cilia (arrowheads). This is consistent with the appearance of these bundles in SEM material (FIG. 3B). In the central zone (FIG. 5B), type I and type II bundles differ in structure. Stereocilia on type I hair cells have larger diameters, and their height falloff is more gradual than that of type II hair cells. The type I bundle is also thick; it covers much of the apical surface of the hair cell, whereas the type II bundle is noticeably narrower.

Bundle thickness is shown quantitatively in FIGURE 6 for 444 hair cells from one animal. Two kinds of structural variation are evident. First, there is variation within a single hair cell type as a function of spatial position: peripheral type II hair cells have narrower bundles than those in the central zone. Second, there is variation between hair cell types: type I hair cells have thicker ciliary bundles than type II hair cells at the same location on the epithelium (for both comparisons, Mann-Whitney U test, $p < .001$). We observed comparable differences between bundle locations and types in two additional animals.

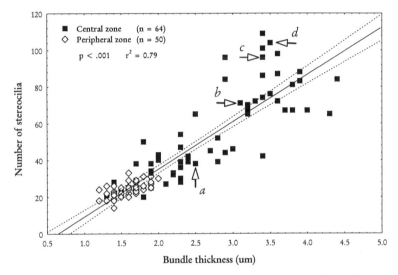

FIGURE 4. Ciliary number vs. bundle thickness for central and peripheral hair cells as seen in scanning electron micrographs. Profiles in the central zone (*squares*) appear to fall into two groups: one with thick bundles and > 60 stereocilia and one with narrow bundles and fewer stereocilia. The latter group overlaps the distribution of known type II hair cells in the periphery (*diamonds*). Arrows indicate the four bundles shown in FIGURE 7 (cells a, b, c, and d). We modeled cells a, b, and c in our finite element analysis (FIGS. 8–10).

Using the regression equation derived from our SEM material, we can estimate the number of stereocilia on type I, central type II, and peripheral type II hair cells. All but one of the 148 type I hair cells have estimated cilia counts greater than 50 (bundle thickness ≥ 2.6 μm), which corresponds reasonably well to the break between clusters seen in SEM samples from the central zone (FIG. 4). Thus, central profiles with 50 or fewer stereocilia are probably type II hair cells.

Finite Element Analysis

Our structural data indicate that posterior canal hair cells differ markedly in bundle thickness and width. To explore the mechanical sequelae of these structural

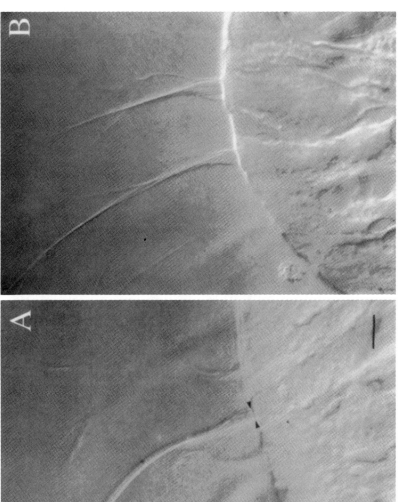

FIGURE 5. Differential interference contrast micrographs of transverse sections through the posterior crista. Scale: 5 μm. (**A**) Peripheral zone. The type II hair cell has a narrow ciliary bundle when measured from the kinocilium to the shortest cilium (*arrowheads*). This is consistent with the appearance of type II apical profiles in SEM material (FIG. 3B). (**B**) Central zone. Type I (*right*) and type II (*left*) hair cells can be distinguished by their characteristic cell body shapes. The type I hair cell has a thicker bundle, larger diameter stereocilia, and a more gradual falloff of ciliary heights than the adjacent type II.

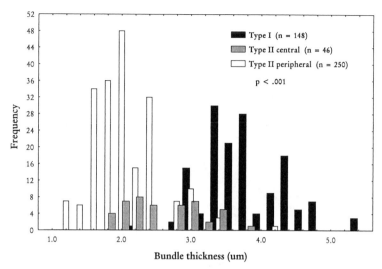

FIGURE 6. Bundle thickness measured in differential interference contrast material where type I hair cells can be identified by soma shape and the presence of a calyx (FIG. 5B). Central type II hair cells have significantly thicker bundles than peripheral type II hair cells and significantly narrower bundles than type I hair cells.

differences we modeled three arrays from the central zone (FIG. 7, cells a, b, c; FIG. 4, arrows; TABLE 1). Cell a falls within the cluster of profiles having few cilia and short columns (low thickness values); it is a putative type II receptor. Cells b and c fall at the border and in the center, respectively, of the cluster having many cilia and thick bundles (FIG. 7; FIG. 4, arrows); they are putative type I hair cells.

For the models we simplified the three arrays as follows.

1. If necessary, we made the arrays symmetrical with a single central column flanked on each side by 3, 4, or 5 lateral columns (TABLE 1). We forced the tallest cilium in the central column.
2. We assumed perfectly hexagonal arrays of cilia.
3. We assumed a "loose" packing configuration in which tip links are oriented parallel to the long axis of the apical surface.[27] This is so for cells a and b, and nearly so for c.
4. We set maximum ciliary height at 30 μm for all three arrays. This is a reasonable approximation of maximum height for central hair cells.[26]

Single Column Analysis

We modeled the central column in cells a and c to examine the effect of adding stereocilia at the short end of the column (up to a maximum of 7 and 11 cilia, respectively; TABLE 1). We did not model cell b because its central column is the same as that of cell a except for the absence of the eleventh (shortest) cilium; the effect of this last cilium is less than 0.05% (FIG. 8). Heights for stereocilia in each column (TABLE 2) are based on preliminary observations that maximum heights for bundles in this region are approximately 30 μm, minimum heights are 1–2 μm, and

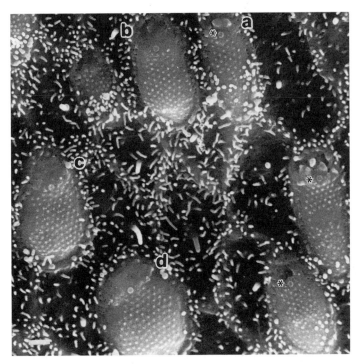

FIGURE 7. Scanning electron micrograph of sonicated hair cells from the central zone. On the right, asterisks mark three profiles with narrow bundles (putative type II hair cells). On the left, three profiles have thicker bundles (more stereocilia per column; cells b, c, and d, putative type I hair cells). The number of columns increases in the order b < c < d. Our modeled arrays are based on hair cells a, b, and c (FIGS. 8–10). Scale: 1 μm.

thick bundles have a more gradual height falloff than narrower bundles (cf. FIG. 5B). Cilia in each column were interconnected by shaft and tip links.

Modeled stiffness values for the two columns are shown in FIGURE 8, which illustrates the effect of adding successively shorter stereocilia to each column. With the assigned heights and only 7 cilia, column c had a stiffness of 0.4677×10^{-4} N/m. Sequential addition of cilia 8, 9, 10, and 11 yielded column stiffness values of 0.4699, 0.4714, 0.4720, 0.4722 $\times 10^{-4}$ N/m. Thus, the height difference alone increased column c stiffness over column a by 26.6% (0.3693 versus 0.4677×10^{-4} N/m, the

TABLE 1. Number of Stereocilia for Three Bundle Geometries

Array	Columns (n)	Column[a]										
		−5	−4	−3	−2	−1	0	1	2	3	4	5
a	7			5	5	6	7	6	5	5		
b	9		2	5	9	10	10	10	9	5	2	
c	11	3	5	8	9	10	11	10	9	8	5	3

[a]Column 0 = center column; ±1, ±2, etc. are lateral pairs.

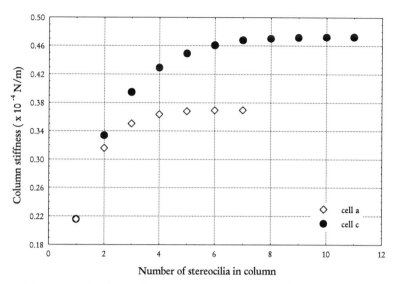

FIGURE 8. Calculated column stiffness depends on the number of stereocilia in the column. The number of stereocilia per column was set to resemble the central column of a narrow (putative type II) and a thick (putative type I) bundle (FIG. 7, cells a and c, respectively). Assigned heights of stereocilia are shown in TABLE 2. The effect of adding successively shorter stereocilia to the column diminishes rapidly when these stereocilia are less than 4–5 μm high (cilia 4ff and 7ff, in cells a and c, respectively).

7-cilia values for a and c, respectively). Adding the four shortest cilia contributed only 1.3% of the 27.9% difference in total stiffness between columns a and c.

The percent contribution of the last four cilia may depend on the rate of height falloff. To examine this, we assigned heights by the equation

$$h = a \cdot n^m + b$$

where h is stereocilia height, n is the order (row) of the stereocilium, a and b are constants determined by the height of the tallest and shortest stereocilia in the bundle, and m describes the height falloff. This equation was chosen over an exponential distribution because it allows the tallest and shortest cilia to remain constant while the falloff rate is manipulated by a single parameter, m. With m = 1, falloff is linear. With negative values of m, heights fall off more rapidly as m decreases (from −0.5 to −1.5; FIG. 9A). The tallest cilium was set at 30 μm and the shortest at 1.5 μm. With a linear height gradation column stiffness increases more

TABLE 2. Assigned Heights for Stereocilia in Central Columns[a]

Array	Row										
	1	2	3	4	5	6	7	8	9	10	11
a	30	10.5	5.75	4	2.75	2	1.5				
c	30	12.25	9.5	7.75	6.25	5.25	4.25	3.5	3.0	2.5	2.0

[a]Heights expressed in μm.

than 200% when column length increases from 4 to 12 stereocilia (TABLE 3). As m becomes increasingly negative, the effect of adding cilia diminishes rapidly (FIG. 9B; TABLE 3). Thus, the significance of bundle thickness (number of stereocilia per column) depends critically on ciliary height gradations within the column.

Array Analysis

We modeled partial or full arrays to examine the effects of adding lateral columns. The models were based on cells a, b, and c (FIG. 7); they had 7, 9, and 11 columns, respectively. Lateral columns have fewer cilia than the central column (TABLE 1); they were positioned to mimic the triangular configurations in FIGURE 7 (especially cells b and c; that is, short cilia rows wider than long cilia rows). Heights for lateral columns were matched to the central column (TABLE 2) so that they produced a biologically realistic bundle. Cilia in each column were interconnected by shaft and tip links; cilia in adjacent columns were interconnected by shaft links only.

We first modeled arrays by performing a single FEA on the whole configuration, starting with the central column and successively adding lateral column pairs. We refer to this as the "unit bundle method." Stiffness rises sharply with the addition of the first pair of lateral columns, but increasingly less with additional pairs (FIG. 10A). With the unit bundle approach, modeled stiffness values for arrays underestimate the contribution of lateral columns to total stiffness because of nonlinear deflections when the bundle is subjected to the 200 pN force (note B).

We also estimated the stiffness of arrays by modeling each lateral column individually to determine its stiffness, calculating the force required to deflect it parallel to the central column, summing these forces, and dividing by the deflection. We refer to this as the "per column method." Such simulations exhibit much greater increases in bundle stiffness with the addition of each lateral column pair (compared with the unit bundle method; FIG. 10B). This method overestimates both absolute bundle stiffness and the relative contribution of lateral columns because it assumes that shaft links are infinitely stiff.

DISCUSSION

We have used light and scanning electron microscopy to begin a quantitative description of ciliary bundles from the posterior semicircular canal. These data were incorporated into a finite element model that allowed us to examine the effect of bundle structure on the bundle's steady-state stiffness.

Morphological Analysis

Our anatomical studies to date have focused on the number and distribution of stereocilia on posterior canal hair cells. They reveal two distinct sources of variation in ciliary bundle structure: location-specific and type-specific.

1. Ciliary bundles vary with spatial position on the neuroepithelium. At the same longitudinal position along the crista (note C), peripheral type II hair cells have significantly narrower bundles than central type II hair cells (DIC material, FIG. 6). In sonicated SEM material, peripheral profiles (known type II) have significantly narrower bundles and fewer stereocilia than central

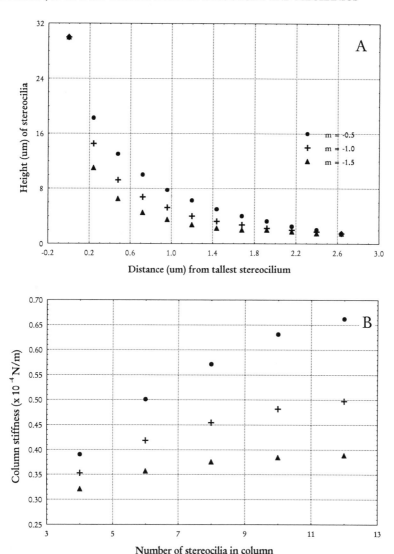

FIGURE 9. Calculated column stiffness depends on the rate at which stereocilia heights decrease. (**A**) Heights of stereocilia for the 12-column case. The number of stereocilia (12) and the heights of the tallest (30 μm) and shortest (1.5 μm) stereocilia are the same. The rate of height falloff (m) is varied. Heights fall off most steeply with the most negative values of m (*triangles*). (**B**) Calculated stiffness of the three columns. For these simulations, heights of the tallest and shortest stereocilia are the same as in **A**. The number of stereocilia in the column and the rate of height falloff (m) are varied. Data points at far right (number of stereocilia = 12) show column stiffness with a ciliary height distribution as shown in **A**. Stiffness increases with the addition of successively shorter stereocilia, but the magnitude of the increase depends strongly on the rate of height falloff within the column. With a steep height falloff (m = −1.5, *triangles*) column stiffness increases 21.2% with the addition of cilia 5–12. With the most gradual height falloff (m = −0.5, *circles*) column stiffness increases 69.6%. Symbols are the same as in **A**.

profiles; this is true whether the comparison is with all central profiles or the cluster of central profiles with relatively narrow bundles and few stereocilia (putative central type II hair cells; FIG. 4).

2. Ciliary bundles also vary with hair cell type. DIC material demonstrates that central type II hair cells have significantly narrower bundles than those of type I (FIGS. 5 and 6). Given the strong correlation between bundle thickness and ciliary number ($r^2 = 0.79$, FIG. 4), we conclude that type I bundles probably bear significantly more stereocilia than central type II hair cells.

SEM evidence for type-specific variation is indirect because we cannot visualize the calyces that define type I hair cells in such material, but two lines of evidence suggest that central profiles with narrow bundles and less than 50–60 stereocilia are type II hair cells. First, they strongly resemble peripheral profiles, which are known to belong to type II hair cells (FIGS. 3 and 4). Second, the different bundle thicknesses seen in central SEM samples (FIG. 4) parallel differences between identified type I and central type II hair cells in DIC material (FIG. 6). Nevertheless, more direct evidence is required before different arrays can be assigned to different hair cell types with complete confidence.

TABLE 3. Column Stiffness: Dependence on Ciliary Number and Height Falloff[a]

Stereocilia	Height Falloff			
(n)	m = 1	m = -0.5	m = -1.0	m = -1.5
4	0.5144	0.3903	0.3526	0.3208
6	0.7902	0.5008	0.4185	0.3568
8	1.058	0.5713	0.4545	0.3754
10	1.317	0.6311	0.4816	0.3843
12	1.572	0.6618	0.4972	0.3889

[a]Column stiffness expressed as $\times 10^{-4}$ N/m.

Finite Element Analysis

Our computational models predict the stiffness of different ciliary arrays. The absolute stiffness values are uncertain, because several physical parameter values are currently unknown. We rely on three sources for these values (in order of priority): our data from turtle hair cells; published data on bundle structure and material properties; and reasonable estimates, which are evaluated by comparisons with known values of similar materials and their apparent ability to produce biologically realistic model results. As our data base on turtle hair cells increases, we take fewer values from the other two sources. Where possible we report results of parametric analyses that explore the effects of these unknown values on bundle stiffness (FIGS. 8–10). Ultimately our model predictions must be tested experimentally.

Our current models incorporate two improvements over previous efforts.[22,23]

1. We model the stereocilia as radially anisotropic instead of isotropic. This is suggested by the core structure of stereocilia, which are bundles of parallel, cross-linked actin filaments, and experimental data suggesting that cilia undergo significant shear deformation during bending as the actin filaments slide relative to each other.[21] By using Timeshenko beam theory we can incorporate such shear deformable structures in our model. This approach requires us to specify a shear modulus for stereocilia that is independent of

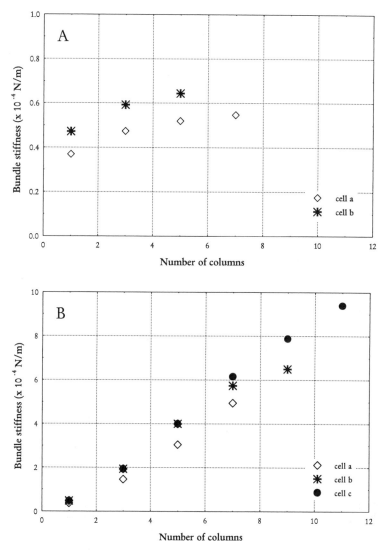

FIGURE 10. Calculated bundle stiffness increases with the addition of lateral columns. We built full or partial "bundles" by starting with the central column (number of columns = 1) and successively adding lateral pairs to produce 3-column, 5-column, etc., arrays. The simulated bundles (TABLE 1) are based on cells a, b, and c in FIGURE 7. (**A**) Unit bundle method. Bundle stiffness increases with the addition of lateral columns, but the successive increments diminish rapidly. This approach underestimates the effects of adding lateral columns. It is computationally intensive, which precluded us from modeling the full bundle on cell b. (**B**) Per column method. Bundle stiffness increases rapidly with the addition of successive lateral columns. This approach overestimates the effect of adding lateral columns, but it predicts the same pattern of stiffness change as seen in **A**: Adding lateral columns increases bundle stiffness, and the increase is greater when the additional columns are long (cells b and c).

Young's modulus. This has not been measured experimentally. We chose a shear modulus of 1×10^6 N/m because simulations suggest that increases beyond this value have little effect on stereociliary stiffness; decreasing the shear modulus below this value decreases stereociliary stiffness. The value we used appears to produce biologically realistic bundle deformations, but it needs to be refined.

2. We write our own code rather than relying on commercially available finite element packages. This greatly simplifies the task of incorporating anisotropic material properties into the model and changing parameter values in order to examine the effects of different structural variations.

Our simulations indicate that increasing the number of stereocilia in a column increases column stiffness, but the magnitude of this effect depends significantly on the rate at which ciliary heights decrease from the tallest to the shortest cilium (FIGS. 8 and 9). Adding successively shorter cilia increases column stiffness most dramatically when heights fall off linearly (TABLE 3); adding the same number of cilia has minimal effect when heights decrease very rapidly (FIG. 9, triangles). Thus, we need accurate measurements of ciliary heights before we can interpret the significance of long column length (thick bundles) in type I hair cells.

We used two approaches to examine the effect of adding lateral columns to the ciliary array (FIG. 10). Both the unit bundle and per column approaches suggest that adding lateral columns increases bundle stiffness, and the stiffness increase is greater when the lateral columns are long (FIG. 10, cells b and c). The magnitude of this effect is uncertain, given the different predictions and known limitations of the two approaches. Nevertheless, both approaches suggest that bundles with many, long columns of stereocilia (e.g., cells b, c, and d in FIG. 7) will be stiffer than smaller bundles at the same location on the crista.

ACKNOWLEDGMENTS

We thank Laura DiCaprio for help in collecting the DIC data and preparing FIGURE 1 and Alan Brichta for help in collecting the SEM data.

NOTES AND REFERENCES

A. Only amniotes (mammals, birds, reptiles) possess type I and type II hair cells. Much important information is available about the physiology and adaptation mechanics of type II hair cells in anamniotes (fish, amphibia), especially frog otolithic hair cells,[5–9] but these studies cannot clarify the distinctive functional role of type I receptors.

B. Values calculated by this method reflect the stiffness of the modeled bundle when it first begins to deform. Further deformation produces a realignment of the compliant lateral shaft links, which our current linear model does not simulate. This realignment would increase bundle stiffness, making the values in FIGURE 10A underestimates. Whether living hair bundles exhibit this realignment and stiffness increase is uncertain; experimental results[25,28] suggest that stiffness may be linear over a similar range of deflections.

C. When comparing central with peripheral hair cell morphologies, it is necessary to hold the longitudinal position constant because hair cell structure *also* varies with distance from the wall to the center of the canal. Accordingly, all our central/peripheral comparisons are based on transverse sections through the central zone. In such sections, central type II hair cells occupy the apex of the crista and peripheral type II hair cells occupy the slopes. We omitted any type II hair cells from the planum or torus from these comparisons.

1. MANLEY, G. A. 1990. Peripheral hearing mechanisms in reptiles and birds. Springer-Verlag. New York.

2. ROBERTS, W. M., J. HOWARD & A. J. HUDSPETH. 1988. Hair cells: Transduction, tuning, and transmission in the inner ear. Annu. Rev. Cell Biol. **4:** 63–92.

3. HOWARD, J., W. M. ROBERTS & A. J. HUDSPETH. 1988. Mechanoelectrical transduction by hair cells. Annu. Rev. Biophys. Biophys. Chem. **17:** 99–124.

4. PICKLES, J. O. 1993. A model for the mechanics of the stereocilia bundle on acoustico-lateral hair cells. Hear. Res. **68:** 159–172.

5. BAIRD, R. A. 1994. Comparative transduction mechanisms of hair cells in the bullfrog utriculus. I. Responses to intracellular current. J. Neurophysiol. **71:** 666–684.

6. BAIRD, R. A. 1994. Comparative transduction mechansism of hair cells in the bullfrog utriculus. II. Sensitivity and response dynamics to hair bundle displacement. J. Neuro-physiol. **71:** 685–705.

7. COREY, D. P. & J. A. ASSAD. 1992. Transduction and adaptation in vertebrate hair cells: Correlating structure with function. *In* Sensory Transduction. D. P. Corey & S. D. Roper, Eds.: 325–342. Rockefeller University Press. New York.

8. HUDSPETH, A. J. 1992. Hair-bundle mechanics and a model for mechanoelectrical transduction by hair cells. *In* Sensory Transduction. D. P. Corey & S. D. Roper, Eds.: 358–370. Rockefeller University Press. New York.

9. JACOBS, R. A. & A. J. HUDSPETH. 1990. Ultrastructural correlates of mechanoelectrical transduction in hair cells of the bullfrog's internal ear. Cold Spring Harbor Symp. Quant. Biol. **55:** 547–561.

10. BRICHTA, A. M., D. L. ACUÑA & E. H. PETERSON. 1988. Planar relations of semicircular canals in awake, resting turtles, *Pseudemys scripta*. Brain Behav. Evol. **32:** 236–245.

11. BRICHTA, A. M. & J. M. GOLDBERG. 1996. Afferent and efferent responses from morpho-logical fiber classes in the turtle posterior crista. Ann. N.Y. Acad. Sci. This volume.

12. BRICHTA, A. M. & E. H. PETERSON. 1994. Functional architecture of vestibular primary afferents from the posterior semicircular canal of a turtle, *Pseudemys (Trachemys) scripta elegans*. J. Comp. Neurol. **344:** 481–507.

13. COCHRAN, S. L. & M. J. CORREIA. 1995. Functional support of glutamate as a vestibular hair cell transmitter in an amniote. Brain Res. **670:** 321–325.

14. HUWE, J. A. & E. H. PETERSON. 1995. Differences in the brain stem terminations of large- and small-diameter vestibular primary afferents. J. Neurophysiol. **74:** 1362–1366.

15. JORGENSEN, J. M. 1974. The sensory epithelia of the inner ear of two turtles, *Testudo graeca* L. and *Pseudemys scripta*. Acta Zool. **55:** 289–298.

16. DiCAPRIO, L. L., A. M. BRICHTA & E. H. PETERSON. 1990. Structural and spatial diversity of type I and type II hair cells from the vestibular epithelium of a turtle, *Pseudemys scripta*. Soc. Neurosci. Abstr. **16:** 735.

17. DiCAPRIO, L. L. & E. H. PETERSON. 1992a. Differences in ciliary bundle morphology of type I and type II vestibular hair cells. Soc. Neurosci. Abstr. **18:** 509.

18. DiCAPRIO, L. L. & E. H. PETERSON. 1992b. Differences in hair bundle size of type I and type II ampullary receptors in a turtle, *Pseudemys scripta*. Abstr. Assoc. Res. Otol. **15:** 24.

19. HOUNSGAARD, J. & C. NICHOLSON. 1990. The isolated turtle brain and the physiology of neuronal circuits. *In* Preparations of Vertebrate Central Nervous System *in Vitro*. H. Jahnsen, Ed.: 155–181. John Wiley & Sons. London.

20. KELLY, R. O., R. A. DEKKER & J. G. BLUEMINK. 1973. Ligand-mediated osmium binding: Its application in coating biological specimens for scanning electron microscopy. J. Ultrastruct. Res. **45:** 254–258.

21. TILNEY, L. G., E. H. EGELMAN, D. J. DeROSIER & J. C. SAUNDERS. 1983. Actin filaments, stereocilia, and hair cells of the bird cochlea. II. Packing of actin filaments in the stereocilia and in the cuticular plate and what happens to the organization when the stereocilia are bent. J. Cell Biol. **96:** 822–834.

22. DUNCAN, R. K., J. W. GRANT & E. H. PETERSON. 1993. Finite element analysis of ciliary bundle stiffness. Soc. Neurosci. Abstr. **19:** 1579.

23. DUNCAN, R. K. & J. W. GRANT. 1995. A finite-element model of inner ear hair bundle micromechanics. Submitted.

24. REDDY, J. N. 1993. An Introduction to the Finite Element Method, 2nd edit. McGraw
     Hill. New York.
25. HOWARD, J. & J. F. ASHMORE. 1986. Stiffness of sensory hair bundles in the sacculus of the
     frog. Hear. Res. **23:** 93–104.
26. PETERSON, E. H. Unpublished data.
27. BAGGER-SJÖBÄCK, D. & M. TAKUMIDA. 1988. Geometrical array of vestibular sensory hair
     bundle. Acta Otolaryngol. **106:** 393–403.
28. CRAWFORD, A. C. & R. FETTIPLACE. 1985. The mechanical properties of ciliary bundles of
     turtle cochlear hair cells. J. Physiol. (Lond.) **364:** 359–379.

Ionic Conductances and Hair Cell Tuning in the Turtle Cochlea[a]

J. J. ART[b,c] AND M. B. GOODMAN[d,e]

[b]*Department of Anatomy and Cell Biology*
University of Illinois College of Medicine
Chicago, Illinois 60612

[d]*Committee on Neurobiology*
University of Chicago
Chicago, Illinois 60637

INTRODUCTION

The vertebrate cochlea has evolved to maximize its overall sensitivity, bandwidth, and temporal resolution. In the turtle, sensitivity is optimized in each receptor, or hair cell, by an electrical resonance resulting from a counterbalanced flow of voltage- and time-dependent ionic currents. This electrical resonance can convert small (pA) currents produced by the cell's mechanical transducer into large (> 10 mV), oscillatory receptor potentials. The use of an electrical resonance to maximize sensitivity naturally limits the range of frequencies detected by each cell and compromises temporal resolution. Both problems have been solved by the organization of hair cells and their innervation. For example, the ear detects a wide range of frequencies because it is composed of an array of independent hair cells tuned to different frequencies and arranged tonotopically in the sensory epithelium. Temporal resolution can be restored by synaptic input from efferent nerve fibers which is known to short-circuit the delicate balance of currents. This dampens the inherent resonance and enhances temporal fidelity.[1]

To understand how ionic currents enter into optimization of acoustic sensitivity, bandwidth, and temporal resolution, we examined the response of turtle hair cells *in situ* and *in vitro*. This paper reviews the normal response to sound measured by microelectrode recordings of hair cells in the intact cochlea, focusing on the correspondence between their acoustic and electrical properties. In addition, we discuss whole-cell patch-clamp recordings of cells isolated from known regions of the sensory epithelium. In particular, voltage-clamp recordings were used to characterize ionic currents underlying electrical resonance across the acoustic spectrum and to determine the pharmacology of K^+ currents that dominate the membrane conductance. Currents activated by acetylcholine, the putative efferent neurotransmitter, were also examined.

Our results demonstrate that the range of frequencies is determined by variations in the kinetic properties of two pharmacologically distinct K^+ channel types. At

[a]This work was supported by an A. P. Sloan Foundation fellowship and a National Institutes of Health grant to J.J.A. (DC00454) and a Howard Hughes predoctoral fellowship to M.B.G.

[c]Address correspondence to Jonathan Art, Department of Anatomy & Cell Biology, University of Illinois College of Medicine, 808 South Wood Street, Chicago, IL 60612. E-mail: jart@uic.edu

[e]Current address: Miriam B. Goodman, Institute of Neuroscience, 1254 University of Oregon, Eugene, OR 97403.

frequencies greater than 60 Hz, K^+ current is carried mostly by a large conductance, calcium-activated potassium channel, BK, and for cells tuned to less than 60 Hz these channels are replaced by a purely voltage-activated potassium channel, KV. Throughout the frequency spectrum, these outward currents are balanced against the inward transducer current,[2] a dihydropyridine-sensitive, voltage-gated calcium current,[3] and a K-selective inward rectifier, IR, to generate resonance.[4] We find that the sizes of ionic currents within the ensemble vary systematically with frequency, suggesting that their expression is precisely regulated. Normal hair cell function can also be modified by physiological or experimental alteration of the balance of currents expressed in a cell. These findings are relevant both to our understanding of cochlear function and to the general experimental challenges posed by studying hair cell biophysics.

METHODS

Recording in the Intact Cochlea

Techniques for acoustic stimulation, current injection, and voltage recording of cochlear hair cells in isolated half-head preparations of *Trachemys scripta elegans* were similar to those employed previously.[5] After decapitation, the head was bisected along the midline and the scala tympani exposed by opening the medial aspect of the otic capsule. The preparation was mounted in a Plexiglas chamber gassed with an atmosphere of 95% O_2 and 5% CO_2. The tympanic membrane was sealed to a Beyer DT-48 earphone via an acoustic coupler, and acoustic stimuli were generated by a low-distortion digital oscillator. Sound pressure at the tympanum was monitored with a 0.5-in. microphone through a calibrated probe tube. To produce clicks, the earphone was driven with a 300-μs rectangular pulse and sound was monitored directly with a 0.125-in. microphone.

Glass micropipettes for intracellular recording, filled with 4 M K acetate and 0.1 M KCl, were advanced into the basilar papilla from the scala tympani, and hair cell potentials were measured with respect to a Ag/AgCl electrode in the cervical spinal cord. Electrode resistances were in the range of 200 to 500 MΩ, and the 3 dB bandwidth of the recordings was greater than 1 kHz. Experimental data were stored on FM tape for subsequent analysis.

Tuning curves were constructed from the response to continuous tones swept at constant intensity through the range 20 Hz to 2 kHz. The frequency increased exponentially throughout a 60–90-s sweep. The amplitude of the hair cell response was measured using a digital approximation of two phase-lock amplifiers (see ref. 1). The frequency, F_0, and the quality factor, Q_{3dB}, were measured as described previously.[5] Briefly, F_0 was estimated from the frequency of maximum sensitivity, and Q_{3dB} from the ratio of F_0 and BW_{3dB}, where BW_{3dB} is the width of the tuning curve between the frequencies where the response has fallen to one-half of its maximum power. For the response to acoustic clicks and steps of injected current, F_0 and Q_{3dB} were determined from the measurement of the ringing frequency, F_r, and the rate of decay of the oscillation by: $f_0^2 = f_r^2 + (2\pi\tau)^{-2}$ and $Q_{3dB} = \{(\pi f_r\tau)^2 + 0.25)\}^{1/2}$.

Recording from Solitary Hair Cells

Solitary hair cells were isolated using modifications of a standard procedure.[6] The basilar papilla was dissected out, and the preparation incubated in a low Ca^{2+} saline (100 μM $CaCl_2$) supplemented with 30 μg/mL bacterial protease type XXIV (Sigma P8038). After the tectorial membrane was removed, the epithelium was incubated in either a low Ca^{2+} saline containing 0.5 mg/mL papain, 2.5 mM L-cysteine, and 0.1 mg/mL bovine serum albumin (BSA), or EDTA-buffered saline ($Ca^{2+} \approx 30$ μM, $Mg \approx 5$ mM) containing 200 μg/mL DNase I, type IV. Hair cells were collected while in low Ca^{2+} saline, plated onto glass coverslips, and transferred to the stage of an inverted microscope (Zeiss IM) equipped with Nomarski optics. Cells were superfused with either normal saline or saline supplemented with 0.4 mg/mL BSA. Experiments were performed at 22–24 °C for periods of up to five hours after decapitation.

Cells were exposed to different solutions by means of a pair of six-barreled glass "pan-pipes" (Vitro Dynamics, Rockaway, NJ). Each barrel was perfused from a peristaltic pump, a given barrel selected by means of a remotely controlled miniature solenoid valve (Lee Products, Westbrook, CT). Solution was removed by a U-tube placed at 90° with respect to the pan-pipe arrays. ACh was applied either by superfusion via the U-tube or by high pressure (20–40 PSI) ejection from a small diameter (1–2 μm) pipette placed ~5 μm from the cell. The speed of these methods was determined by measuring the blockade of BK by 1 mM tetraethylammonium (TEA).

Extracellular solutions were based on normal turtle saline composed of (in mM): NaCl, (130); KCl, (4); CaCl$_2$ (2.8); MgCl$_2$ (2.2); HEPES (5); pH adjusted to 7.6 with NaOH. Drugs applied in excess of 1 mM were substituted for an equimolar concentration of NaCl. TEA was obtained as TEA-OH (Aldrich Chemical, Milwaukee, WI) and titrated with HCl to yield a 1 M stock solution. 4-Aminopyridine (4-AP) was diluted from a 30- or 60-mM stock solution prepared daily from solid. After dilution, the pH was adjusted to 7.6 with HCl. Calibrated solutions (1 M) of CaCl$_2$ and MgCl$_2$ were purchased from BDH through their U.S. distributor (Gallard-Schlesinger, Carle Place, NY) and Alfa Chemical (Ward Hill, MA), respectively. Unless indicated, all other reagents were obtained from Sigma Chemical (St. Louis, MO). Osmolarity of extracellular (290 mOsm) and intracellular (270 mOsm) solutions was assayed by freezing-point depression (Advanced Instruments, Natick, MA).

Hair cell membrane current and voltage were recorded using standard whole-cell patch-clamp methods.[7] Pipettes were pulled from soda-glass capillaries and were filled with a solution composed of (in mM): KCl (125); CaCl$_2$ (0.45); MgCl$_2$ (2.8); K$_2$EGTA (5); Na$_2$ATP (2.5); KHEPES (5); pH 7.2. Where indicated, BAPTA was used in place of EGTA. Osmolarity was maintained in solutions containing more than 5 mM BAPTA by reducing the amount of KCl. Membrane current and voltage were recorded with a modified Yale Mark V amplifier.[6] Experiments were recorded with an 8-channel PCM unit (VR-100, Instrutech, Elmont, NY) and analyzed off-line. Unless otherwise indicated, the data were filtered at 3.2 kHz (8-pole Bessel filter) and digitized at up to 24 kHz. All voltages are corrected for liquid junction potentials and errors due to current flow across uncompensated series resistance. Only cells recorded with electrodes having a residual series resistance between 1 and 6 MΩ were included. Leak current was measured from the steady current elicited by small voltage steps (± 5 mV) from a holding potential of -75 mV during superfusion with 5–10 mM Cs^+. All data were analyzed and plotted using Igor Pro 2.0x (WaveMetrics, Lake Oswego, OR).

RESULTS

Response to Acoustic and Electrical Stimuli in the Intact Cochlea

The behavior of hair cells in the intact turtle cochlea is well characterized.[5,8,9] Here, we emphasize the correspondence between the response to acoustic and electrical stimuli. Hair cells produce large, sustained receptor potentials in response to acoustic stimuli at their best or characteristic frequency (CF). An example of this behavior is illustrated in FIGURE 1A, which shows the average response to 220-Hz tone bursts of increasing intensity. For stimuli less than 55 dB_{SPL} (re: 20 μPa), the amplitude of the response is proportional to the stimulus, and once a steady level is achieved, the membrane potential is a faithful sinusoidal copy of the tone. For louder tones (75 dB_{SPL}), two nonlinearities are apparent: the response saturates, increasing by a factor of three for a 10-fold increase in intensity, and the waveform is sharper on the depolarizing phase of each cycle. A very loud sound (95 dB_{SPL}) fully saturates the response at 50 mV_{p-p}, and displays a third nonlinearity, an asymmetry between the amplitude of the depolarizing and hyperpolarizing phases. Because receptor potential amplitude is constant during tone presentations, the response to low-intensity frequency sweeps could be used to characterize hair cell sensitivity across frequency as a tuning curve (see METHODS). Tuning curves show that each cell is sensitive to a relatively narrow range of frequencies (FIG. 1B). The response amplitude increases with frequency, reaches a peak at a frequency that is characteristic for each cell, and declines as the stimulus approaches a high frequency limit (FIG. 1B).

Of the various mechanical and electrical mechanisms that could contribute to tuning in the turtle cochlea, the dominant factor is the electrical behavior of the hair cell.[5,8,9] FIGURE 2 compares the response to acoustic and electrical stimulation of the 488-Hz cell characterized previously (see FIG. 1B). To do this, we used a rapid, acoustic click to provide a stimulus with energy that extends across a wide range of frequencies. The hair cell responded to the click with a prolonged series of lightly damped oscillations in membrane potential. We obtained a second measurement of the cell's characteristic frequency and Q_{3dB} from the frequency of oscillation and its rate of decay (see METHODS), as described previously.[5] Injecting a current step through the recording electrode likewise elicited a series of lightly damped oscillations whose frequency and damping were nearly identical to those seen in the acoustic response. This observation is important for three reasons. First, tuning can be studied without mechanical stimulation of the ciliary bundle because nearly identical responses are obtained with acoustic and electrical stimuli. Second, frequency tuning occurs after transduction of mechanical energy and may, therefore, be preserved in solitary cells isolated from the sensory epithelium. Third, the electrical characterization of hair cells in the intact cochlea can be used to determine whether solitary cells are compromised by the dissociation procedure.

Comparison of Response of Solitary Hair Cells in Current- and Voltage-Clamp

To understand the ionic mechanisms underlying the generation of a highly tuned receptor potential, the response properties of solitary hair cells in current- and voltage-clamp were compared. As for experiments in the intact cochlea, damped oscillations evoked by current injection were used to determine Q_{3dB} and electrical CF or resonant frequency (F_0). Results for a cell isolated from the low-frequency end of the epithelium are shown in FIGURE 3A. The cell was voltage-clamped at its average resting potential, and a small depolarizing step was applied to reproduce the change in membrane potential observed in current clamp (FIG. 3B). A net outward current develops during the course of the step and decays slowly to the resting level upon repolarization. The rate of tail current decay was quantified by fitting the data with a single exponential function with time constant, τ. Previous studies[6,10] have established that F_0 is related to τ at -50 mV according to the function, $F_0 = k\tau^{-1/2}$, where k is an empirical constant. The range of kinetics is illustrated in FIGURE 3C, which shows normalized tail currents recorded in cells isolated from different regions

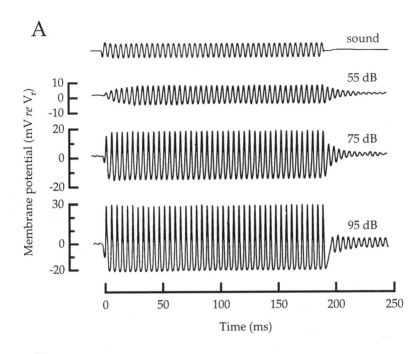

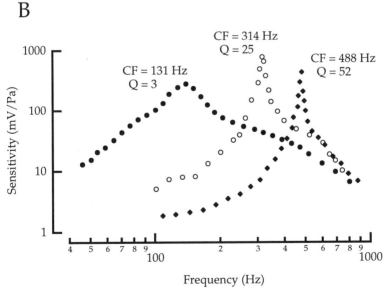

FIGURE 1. Hair cell response to pure tones in the intact cochlea. **(A)** Responses to tone bursts at 55, 75, and 95 dB (*re* 20 μPa) at 220 Hz, the frequency of maximal response (CF). Ordinates are plotted with respect to a mean level of −45 mV and are averages of between 5 and 50 presentations. **(B)** Response of three cells to frequency sweeps between 20 Hz and 2 kHz. The ordinate is the sensitivity of the cell near threshold. Each symbol represents a different cell. The CF and Q_{3dB} for each cell is indicated near the peak of the tuning curve.

of the epithelium. These experiments show that the speed of outward current evoked by depolarization is a major determinant of the frequency of electrical resonance. Because of the correspondence between acoustic and electrical tuning in the intact ear (see FIG. 2), the kinetics of the net current must also determine acoustic CF.

The Extended Current-Voltage Relation

To fully understand the variation in kinetics of the net current, it is necessary to determine the ensemble of currents present in each cell, characterize their voltage- and ionic-sensitivity, and use these results to reconstruct the response in current

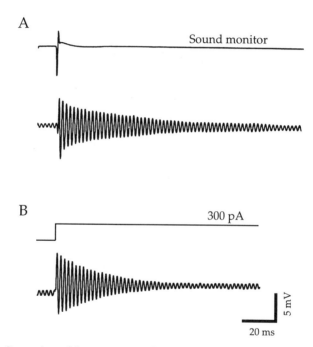

FIGURE 2. Comparison of the response to acoustic and electrical stimuli in the intact cochlea. (A) Voltage response to rarefaction click; the trace is an average of 300 presentations. Oscillation seen before the click is applied reflects spontaneous oscillations generated in the absence of acoustic stimuli. (B) Response to injection of a 300 pA depolarizing current through the recording electrode, an average of 200 presentations. The cell has a mean potential of −58 mV prior to the onset of the current step.

clamp. In this paper we focus on the first two aspects. FIGURE 4 shows representative current-voltage (I-V) relations, which consist of regions of strong inward and outward rectification, separated by a high-impedance region immediately hyperpolarized to the hair cell resting membrane potential. The inset shows membrane current in the 13-Hz cell, which was held near its resting potential of −56 mV, and stepped to a series of depolarizing and hyperpolarizing voltage levels. Whereas current is

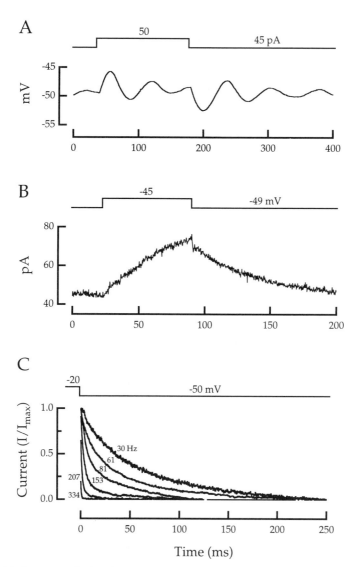

FIGURE 3. Response of a low-frequency solitary hair cell in current and voltage clamp. **(A)** Voltage response to injection of current through the recording electrode. **(B)** Membrane current in the same cell recorded in response to a 4-mV step from −49 mV. **(C)** Normalized tail currents recorded in cells isolated from different regions. Tail currents were recorded at −50 mV following depolarization to −20 mV, and traces were normalized. Each example is either a single trace or the average of two presentations. Frequency was estimated from the time constant of decay as described in the text.

carried by a combination of K^+- and Ca^{2+}-selective ionic currents during a depolarizing step,[11] tail currents are carried almost exclusively by K^+ because they reverse polarity near the K^+ equilibrium potential.[7] An outstanding issue concerns how variations in tail current kinetics are achieved in cells tuned to different frequencies. The variation could be due to modulation of a single type of K^+ channel, or different channel types might be expressed at different frequencies.

Pharmacological Dissection of Potassium Currents across the Frequency Spectrum

A large Ca^{2+}-activated K^+ channel (BK) has been characterized previously in these cells.[12] To discover the degree to which the functional role of this channel is

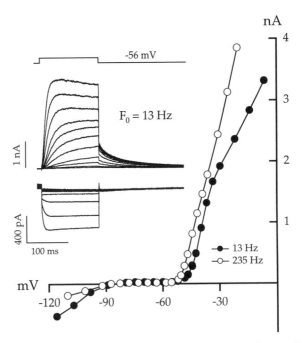

FIGURE 4. Representative net current-voltage curves. The I-V curve shows regions of inward and outward rectification. The inset shows current traces recorded in the 13-Hz cell, held at its resting potential and stepped to a series of voltages between -110 and 0 mV. Resonant frequency of both cells was estimated from the voltage response to a small (<50 pA) current step.

supplemented or replaced by other K^+ channel types as a function of frequency, we measured the sensitivity of potassium current to the broad-spectrum K^+ channel antagonists, TEA and 4-AP. Complete concentration-response relations, testing antagonist concentrations between 10^{-6} and 10^{-3} M were collected from individual hair cells tuned to different frequencies in experiments documented elsewhere.[13] Both TEA and 4-AP inhibit most types of K^+ channel if applied in sufficiently high concentrations. Thus, if single-cell concentration-response relations agree with a single-binding site function, they demonstrate that outward current is carried by a single class of K^+ channels. Initially, we focused on cells tuned to less than ~ 30 Hz and more than ~ 100 Hz. In high-frequency cells, inhibition of outward current was consistent with the presence of a single class of K^+ channels whose apparent affinity for TEA and 4-AP were 0.2 mM and 14 mM, respectively. The apparent affinity for TEA is typical of large conductance, BK channels characterized in other preparations.[14,15] Outward current in low-frequency cells was also carried by a single class of K^+ channels. The apparent affinity constant for TEA (36 mM) was nearly 200-fold lower than in high-frequency cells. This current was very sensitive to 4-AP; half-blocking concentrations lay between 20 and 100 μM. This pharmacological profile is consistent with the presence of a purely voltage-gated K^+ channel, which we call KV. Additional evidence supporting this conclusion comes from a previous study,[3] which showed that the K^+ current in low-frequency cells is unlike the Ca^{2+}-activated K^+ current in high-frequency cells in that it is unaffected by reductions in the external Ca^{2+} concentration.

It is possible to dissect outward current in cells tuned to different frequencies using the apparent affinities of BK and KV for TEA and 4-AP. A complete discussion of the method has been considered elsewhere.[13] The general procedure is illustrated in FIGURE 5. Outward current was activated by depolarization to roughly -40 mV and measured during superfusion with each of five external salines: (1) normal saline, (2) 35 μM 4-AP, (3) 35 μM 4-AP plus 280 μM TEA, (4) 0.8 mM 4-AP plus 280 μM TEA, and (5) 0.8 mM 4-AP plus 6 mM TEA. FIGURE 5A shows the response of a cell tuned to 220 Hz, measured from the speed of deactivation at -50 mV. Potassium current is virtually unchanged during superfusion with 35 μM 4-AP (trace 2), a concentration which would be sufficient to block about half of KV in a low-frequency cell. Addition of 280 μM TEA (trace 3) inhibits slightly more than half of the outward current, suggesting that all of the current in this cell is carried by BK channels. Increasing the 4-AP concentration to 0.8 mM (trace 4) again fails to produce any reduction in current, despite the fact that this concentration is enough to block 95% of KV. By increasing the TEA concentration to 6 mM (trace 5), we block 95% of the BK channels and reveal an inward current, which has been shown previously to be carried by calcium.[6]

Contrast these results with those obtained in a 10-Hz cell (FIG. 5B). In this case, 35 μM 4-AP reduces outward current by half, suggesting that it is carried mostly by KV. Addition of 280 μM TEA to the solution fails to reduce the current further (trace 3). Increasing the 4-AP concentration to 0.8 mM (trace 4) reduces outward current to 5% of its initial amplitude. As expected, no additional reduction occurs with an increase in TEA concentration (trace 5). These results suggest that outward current in cells at the high- and low-frequency ends of the spectrum is carried exclusively by BK and KV, respectively. This pharmacological dissection was used to estimate the sizes of BK and KV expressed by cells isolated from different regions of the sensory epithelium and to determine whether intermediate frequencies express a mixture of the two channel types (see FIG. 6). In all cells, resonant frequency was estimated from the speed of deactivation at -50 mV.

FIGURE 6 shows that the sizes of both KV and BK increase with resonant frequency and that there is very little overlap in the range of frequencies covered by each channel type. In the lower decade, between 6 and 60 Hz, outward current is carried by KV. For cells tuned to frequencies higher than 60 Hz, outward current is carried by increasing numbers of BK channels. A third channel type is expressed by hair cells, an inwardly rectifying current apparent at potentials negative to E_K (see FIG. 4). We have shown in turtle cochlear hair cells that the major inwardly rectifying current, IR, is K^+-selective.[4] Its amplitude was measured from the conductance between -100 and -140 mV and plotted against resonant frequency. As shown in FIGURE 6, IR amplitude declines with F_0 and appears to be present across the entire frequency spectrum. All hair cells also contain a voltage-gated Ca^{2+} current, I_{Ca}, whose size increases with resonant frequency.[3,6]

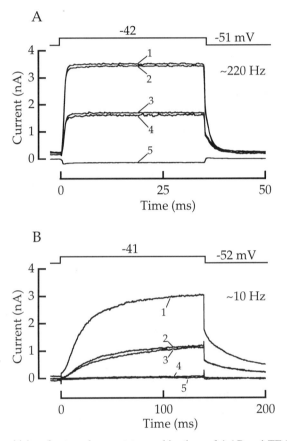

FIGURE 5. Sensitivity of outward current to combinations of 4-AP and TEA. (**A**) Outward current was evoked by a 9-mV step in a 220-Hz cell. Individual traces illustrate the response to superfusion with the following salines: normal (1), 35 μM 4-AP (2), 35 μM 4-AP plus 280 μM TEA (3), 0.8 mM 4-AP plus 280 μM TEA (4), and 0.8 mM 4-AP plus 6 mM TEA (5). (**B**) Outward current evoked by a 11-mV step in a 10-Hz cell exposed to the same series of solutions as in **A**. Resonant frequency of both cells was measured from the time constant of decay as described in the text.

Together, these results suggest that electrical resonance is produced by at least two distinct mechanisms. The first mediates high-frequency resonance and involves primarily BK and I_{Ca}, as demonstrated previously.[6,11] The second operates at low frequencies and involves the interaction of KV, IR, and I_{Ca}. This finding provides a functional role for purely voltage-gated K^+ currents in shaping hair cell receptor

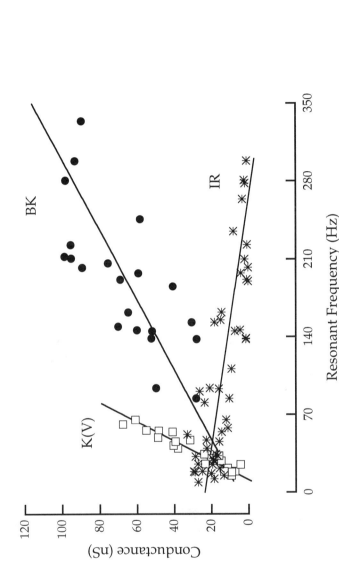

FIGURE 6. Variation in the size of potassium (K) currents with frequency. The total amount of KV (*squares*) and BK (*circles*) expressed by each cell was determined from the measurements of outward current block by TEA and 4-AP. IR size (*stars*) was measured from the conductance between −140 and −100 mV. Straight lines are fits to the data with correlation coefficients of 0.93, 0.83, and −0.79 for KV, BK, and IR, respectively.

potentials. An important role for IR was suggested by its apparent frequency-dependent regulation (FIG. 6) and was confirmed both experimentally[4] and in numerical reconstructions of hair cell resonance.[10] The biophysical properties of the voltage-sensitive ionic currents underlying low-frequency resonance in auditory hair cells may prove relevant to the study of vestibular hair cells. Although a wide variety of ion- and voltage-sensitive ionic channels have been observed in hair cells responsible for detecting linear and angular accelerations as well as substrate vibration,[16–19] their functional roles are only beginning to be understood.

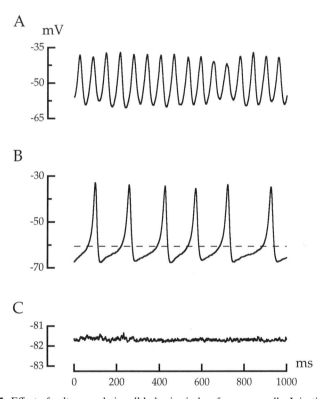

FIGURE 7. Effect of voltage on hair cell behavior in low-frequency cells. Injection of 75 pA depolarized the cell to -50 mV (**A**), and oscillatory potentials reminiscent of the behavior in the intact cochlea are recorded. Injection of 50 pA depolarized the cell to a mean potential of -61 mV (*dashed line* in **B**), and regenerative spiking is observed. The hair cell had a zero-current potential of -82 mV (**C**).

Effects of Voltage and External K⁺ on the Behavior of Low F₀ Hair Cells

In this section, we consider two mechanisms by which tuning is modulated in low-frequency hair cells. Previous studies have examined the voltage-dependence of F_0 and Q_{3dB} and in cells tuned to higher frequencies.[5] FIGURE 7 shows how changes in membrane potential modify resonance in a low-frequency cell. Initially, the cell had a stable zero-current potential of -82 mV, a voltage where the resting impedance of the cell is very high (see FIG. 4). Injecting 50 pA through the recording electrode depolarized the cell to −61 mV, a membrane potential at which regenerative spiking is supported by the interaction of I_{Ca}, IR, and KV. Heuristically, spikes are produced because KV channel activation is relatively sluggish at these potentials and I_{Ca} activates rapidly to produce a regenerative depolarization which is terminated only when sufficient KV channels open to repolarize the cell. When the cell is depolarized further to −50 mV, by injection of 75 pA, the cell produces a faster, sinusoidal oscillatory behavior similar to that observed near the resting potential in the intact cochlea. The shift from spiking to oscillatory behavior is likely to result from voltage-dependent changes in the kinetics of KV and I_{Ca}. With depolarization, KV activates more rapidly and ICa activates more slowly, such that KV is fast enough to counteract the regenerative influx of calcium at −50 mV and reduces the amplitude of the voltage excursions about the mean level.

The behavior of low-frequency hair cells can also be modulated by changes in external K^+. FIGURE 8 shows the effect of an increase in external K^+ from 4 to 10 mM in both voltage- and current-clamp. Comparison of the net current recorded in 4 and 10 mM K^+ (FIG. 8A and B) reveals that the size of the hair cell IR increases, as found for IR in starfish oocytes.[20] In addition, tail currents decrease in proportion to the reduction in driving force for K^+. Surprisingly, this comparison also reveals that outward currents are similar during depolarizing steps and that the steady-state amplitude is essentially unchanged (FIG. 8C). Net current in this voltage range is carried mostly by KV, suggesting that it, like IR, may also be sensitive to external K^+. The maintenance of the steady-state current amplitude in the face of elevating the external K^+ concentration could be explained if the reduced driving force is offset by a compensatory increase in the KV single-channel conductance. It also predicts that in current clamp, modest increases in external K^+ would fail to depolarize low F_0 cells. This second idea was tested in the presence of 25 mM TEA, which was applied to remove any possible contribution of BK to electrical resonance (FIG. 8D). Low-frequency membrane potential oscillations about a mean potential of −50 mV are observed in a solitary cell bathed in 4 mM K^+. Oscillations are silenced by increasing the external K^+ to 10 mM (FIG. 8D, middle trace). The mean membrane potential is relatively unaffected in spite of the fact that the driving force for K^+ is halved at −50 mV.

Ionic Basis of Efferent Control

A third and physiologically important modulation of hair cell resonance is known to occur via activation of the efferent synapse. Hair cells are the target of extensive, largely cholinergic, efferent innervation,[1,21] and, in the intact turtle cochlea, they respond to a train of efferent shocks with a complex postsynaptic potential (PSP) composed of a small, brief depolarization followed by a larger, slower hyperpolarization.[21] The latter component results from an increased permeability to K^+ and reduces the amplitude of the receptor potential. The effect is most acute for tones near the characteristic frequency, so that hair cells under efferent control are broadly tuned and exhibit improved temporal resolution.[1] Evidence for the cholinergic nature of the efferent–hair cell synapse includes the following. First, both components of the PSP are blocked by cholinergic antagonists. Second, superfusion with ACh hyperpolarizes the hair cell and desensitizes the efferent receptor.[21] In this section, we consider ionic currents gated by acetylcholine (ACh) in solitary turtle hair cells.

Superfusion with ACh hyperpolarizes solitary hair cells (FIG. 9A) and evokes

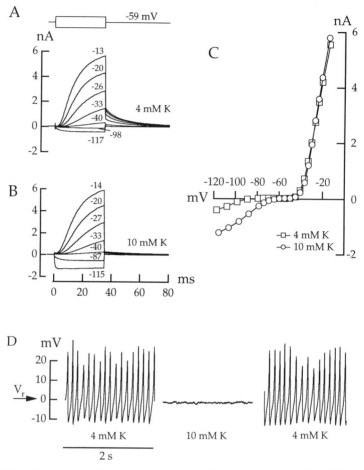

FIGURE 8. Sensitivity of low-frequency cells to changes in external K^+. Voltage-clamp experiments **(A–C)** show that net current is insensitive to modest changes in external K^+. **(A)** Net current in normal ringer (4 mM K^+). The cell was held at -59 mV and subjected to a series of voltage pulses. **(B)** Net current in elevated K^+ saline (10 mM) using the same voltage-clamp protocol. **(C)** Comparison of steady-state I-V in 4 mM K^+ (*squares*) and 10 mM K^+ (*circles*). **(D)** Increasing external K^+ dampens spontaneous oscillations recorded in the presence of 25 mM TEA and has little effect on the average membrane potential (-50 mV). Each trace is a segment of a 10-s record that was used to calculate the average membrane potential in each condition.

both a rapid inward current and a longer-lived outward current (FIG. 9B), indicating that cholinergic receptors are not entirely destroyed by the isolation procedure. However, cells isolated without the use of papain are more likely to exhibit ACh-induced responses. Initially, hair cells were recorded using standard intracellular solutions that preserve electrical resonance. Varying either the capacity or speed of Ca^{2+} buffering in the intracellular solution provides additional evidence to support the idea that ACh-induced events have two separable components. FIGURE

9C shows ACh-induced current in three cells held at a mean potential of −50 mV. In order to facilitate comparison, current was normalized to its peak value in each condition. The ACh-induced current was outward for pipettes containing modest Ca^{2+} buffering (5 mM EGTA). When buffering capacity was increased (65 mM EGTA), the ACh-induced current reversed polarity and was inward. A similar effect was seen observed using BAPTA (5 mM; FIG. 9C, bottom trace) to buffer intracellular Ca^{2+}. These results are consistent with the model proposed for chick hair cells,[22] in which ACh rapidly activates a ligand-gated ion channel that carries sufficient Ca^{2+} to activate a Ca^{2+}-activated potassium current.

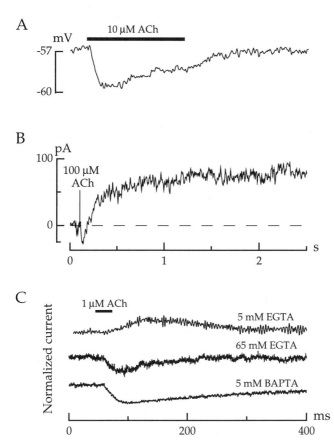

FIGURE 9. Whole-cell recording of ACh-induced currents. **(A)** ACh (10 μM) hyperpolarizes solitary hair cells. Standard pipette solution containing 5 mM EGTA. **(B)** Prolonged bath application (100 μM) evokes a rapid inward current and a longer-lived outward current in another cell voltage-clamped at −52 mV. Membrane current returned to control levels approximately 1 min after ACh superfusion was terminated. Standard pipette solution containing 5 mM EGTA. **(C)** Effect of Ca^{2+} buffering speed and capacity on ACh-induced currents. Normalized membrane current evoked by brief application of ACh (1 μM) in three cells held near −50 mV. Peak values and Ca^{2+} buffers were (top to bottom): +26 pA, 5 mM EGTA; −24 pA, 65 mM EGTA; −230 pA, 5 mM BAPTA.

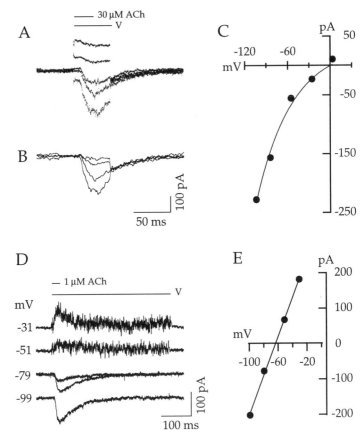

FIGURE 10. Voltage-dependence of ACh-induced currents. **(A)** Membrane current evoked by puffs of ACh (30 μM) applied during depolarizing voltage steps to between −120 and 10 mV. Current evoked by depolarization alone was subtracted from these traces to obtain the ACh-induced current. The pipette contained 30 mM KBAPTA. **(B)** ACh-induced current derived from the traces in **A.** Since the ACh-induced current outlasts the voltage step, its amplitude at the end of the step was used to normalize the response and account for desensitization. Traces were digitally filtered with a high-frequency cut-off of 30 Hz. **(C)** Peak ACh-induced current versus voltage. The smooth line is an exponential function of voltage and yields a reversal potential near 0 mV. **(D)** The total ACh-induced current recorded using 5 mM EGTA in the pipette solution. Puffs of ACh were synchronized to voltage steps from −79 mV. To determine the extent of desensitization, two traces were recorded at −79 mV and used to correct peak current. **(E)** Net ACh-induced current versus voltage derived from the traces in **D.** The straight line was fit to the data and has a slope of 5.6 nS and a reversal potential of −63 mV.

Inasmuch as the two components of ACh-induced response often occur simultaneously, it was necessary to develop a strategy to separate the ionic influx gated by ACh from any subsequent activation of an ionic current gated by elevation of the internal Ca^{2+}. To characterize the voltage dependence of the ligand-gated event, I-V curves were constructed from cells recorded with 30 mM BAPTA in the pipette.

External Ca^{2+} was reduced to 100 μM to further reduce the contribution of a Ca^{2+}-activated conductance to the measured current. The amplitude of inward current activated by puffs of ACh declines with repeated application even when separated by 20-s intervals. We adopted the following strategy to overcome this difficulty. ACh was applied at the same time as steps to the test potentials (FIG. 10A), and each application was bracketed by voltage steps alone (not shown). Since the response to ACh outlasts the voltage step, its amplitude upon repolarization to -84 mV was used to normalize the response. The corrected difference currents are shown in FIGURE 10B, and the peak response was measured from these traces and plotted as a function of voltage (FIG. 10C). The I-V was inwardly rectifying and fit by an exponential function.

The voltage dependence of the total ACh-induced current was determined in the presence of modest Ca^{2+} buffering (5 mM EGTA). Puffs of ACh were synchronized to voltage steps from -79 mV; the difference between this and the current evoked by the step alone is illustrated (FIG. 10D). The increased current noise during depolarizing steps probably results from activation of BK channels, because it was not significantly altered by ACh. The peak ACh-induced current was corrected for the desensitization of the response with repeated application, plotted as a function of membrane potential (FIG. 10E), and fit by a line with a slope of 5.6 nS and a reversal potential of -63 mV. This reversal potential is intermediate between those expected for the physiological charge carriers, Cl^-, K^+, Na^+, and Ca^{2+}, and suggests that the current represents the sum of at least two ionic components. If we assume the net ACh-induced current is carried in part by the ligand-gated current characterized in FIG. 10A–C, then the remaining current is likely to be carried by K^+. The linearity of the I-V in FIG. 10E further suggests that the second component may have only slight outward rectification, and may represent activation of an apamin- and Ca^{2+}-sensitive K^+ channel, SK, recently demonstrated in turtle hair cells.[12,23]

DISCUSSION

Variations in the Mechanism of Electrical Resonance

The existence of multiple strategies for producing electrical resonance across the acoustic spectrum is not entirely unexpected in light of the variety of ionic currents observed in other hair cells.[24] Many previous analyses have relied, in part, on differences in activation, deactivation, and inactivation rates to distinguish between K^+ channel types. However, the smooth variation in kinetics exhibited by cochlear hair cells suggests that either there is a very large number of distinct K^+ channels or that a single-channel type is systematically modified. The pharmacological dissection outlined here indicates that variation in the speed of activation and deactivation of only two classes of K^+ channels, KV and BK, is sufficient to explain tuning in the turtle cochlea. The molecular basis of the kinetic heterogeneity is not understood. It has been suggested that variations in BK kinetics reflect differences in Ca^{2+} accumulation at the inner face of the channel.[25,26] However, measurements of single BK channels isolated from cells tuned to different frequencies demonstrate that the variation in activation and deactivation rates are maintained in the presence of a constant Ca^{2+} concentration.[12] Differences in K^+ channel kinetics might, therefore, result from differential gene expression of a large number of channel isoforms, channels encoded by single genes that have a large number of splice variants, or even editing of single transcripts. Post-translational modifications such as glycosylation and phosphorylation may also contribute to variations in channel kinetics.

The forces that constrain expression of KV to low frequencies and BK to high frequencies are unknown. One possibility is the high impedance needed for sensitivity, produced in part by a delicate balance in the size of inward Ca^{2+} and outward K^+ currents in each cell. The sizes of both currents increase with frequency,[3,6] and the use of a Ca^{2+}-activated K^+ current may be required to ensure that balance is maintained. An alternative determinant of K^+ channel expression is the large conductance of single BK channels. If the small currents in low-frequency cells were carried by BK, approximately 10 channels would be active at rest, and their stochastic behavior would produce significant current noise. Therefore, KV may be better suited to low-frequency resonance as a consequence of its smaller single-channel conductance.[12]

Efferent Modulation of Electrical Resonance

Although temporal resolution is compromised by the use of electrical resonance to maximize sensitivity, it may be restored through efferent activity that is able to transform hair cells into low-pass acoustic filters and improve temporal resolution.[1] Because even single shocks to efferent nerve fibers can dampen electrical resonance, it is possible for the turtle to modulate the degree of tuning over a wide range, trading sensitivity and frequency discrimination for temporal resolution. As yet, it is unknown what behavioral conditions regulate efferent activity and the sensitivity and temporal resolution achieved by the cochlea. We do understand that ACh, one of the putative efferent transmitters, produces a change in the membrane conductance that is sufficient to explain the change in tuning.[1] The results of our preliminary dissection of the ACh-induced current suggest that the efferent–hair cell synaptic potential is generated by at least two currents: an inwardly rectifying, ligand-gated conductance and a voltage-insensitive K^+ conductance. In its main features, our result resembles ACh-induced currents reported in short (outer) hair cells in the chick cochlea.[22]

Is the Modulation by Voltage and External K^+ Relevant to Hair Cell Physiology?

Understanding the behavior of voltage-sensitive conductances used in tuning auditory hair cells to low frequencies may be relevant to the population of vestibular hair cells that contain a similar ensemble of currents. As shown in FIGURE 7, qualitative differences in the electrical behavior are apparent depending on the mean membrane potential. Membrane potential is relatively stable at hyperpolarized levels, but exhibits either spikes or oscillations when depolarized. Injecting < 100 pA is sufficient to depolarize cells by more than 30 mV (FIG. 7). The need to inject a depolarizing current to bring solitary cells to −50 mV, the potential typically recorded in situ, is not unexpected. Depolarizing currents on the order of 50 to 100 pA might be lost during the isolation procedure, because of inadvertent damage to the transduction apparatus and a loss of a fraction of the transducer channels that are on at rest. Of course, other ionic currents may be affected by the dissociation procedure and change the apparent resting potential as well. Thus, the zero-current potential measured in solitary cells may be a poor measure of the resting potential of hair cells in an intact epithelium. For auditory hair cells, an appropriate benchmark has been the membrane potential at which the cells produce the largest acoustic response in the intact cochlea.

Both vestibular and cochlear epithelia are closely packed, providing diffusion barriers at their apical and basal surfaces which may allow the accumulation of K^+ ions. We have shown that a modest increase in extracellular K^+ is sufficient to silence membrane potential oscillations (FIG. 8). This is particularly interesting in light of the additional diffusion barrier produced by calyceal nerve endings in vestibular epithelia. Our results suggest that type I hair cells containing similar currents as low-frequency auditory hair cells may exhibit electrical tuning *in vitro* and resemble a lower resistance, low-pass filter *in situ*. Over the long-term, K^+ in the calyceal synaptic cleft must be removed and may be actively transported into either the hair cell or the calyx. Indeed, the calyx contains a high level of Na^+/K^+-ATPase immunoreactivity.[27] Further experiments testing the response properties of vestibular hair cells *in situ* are required to determine whether K^+ accumulation is important for vestibular function.

ACKNOWLEDGMENTS

We are grateful to R. Fettiplace, A. Crawford, and P. Fuchs who participated in the experiments in the intact cochlea (FIGS. 1 and 2). We would also like to thank T. Denison, H. Denison, and S. Wen for their technical assistance.

REFERENCES

1. ART, J. J., A. C. CRAWFORD, R. FETTIPLACE & P. A. FUCHS. 1985. Efferent modulation of hair cell tuning in the cochlea of the turtle. J. Physiol. **360:** 397–421.
2. COREY, D. P. & A. J. HUDSPETH. 1979. Ionic basis of the receptor potential in a vertebrate hair cell. Nature **281:** 675–677.
3. ART, J. J., R. FETTIPLACE & Y. C. WU. 1993. The effects of low calcium on the voltage-dependent conductances involved in tuning of turtle hair cells. J. Physiol. **470:** 109–126.
4. GOODMAN, M. B. & J. J. ART. 1996. Positive feedback by a potassium-selective inward rectifier enhances tuning in vertebrate hair cells. Biophys. J. In press.
5. CRAWFORD, A. C. & R. FETTIPLACE. 1980. The frequency selectivity of auditory nerve fibres and hair cells in the cochlea of the turtle. J. Physiol. **306:** 79–125.
6. ART, J. J. & R. FETTIPLACE. 1987. Variation of membrane properties in hair cells isolated from the turtle cochlea. J. Physiol. **385:** 207–242.
7. HAMILL, O. P., A. MARTY, E. NEHER, B. SAKMANN & F. J. SIGWORTH. 1981. Improved patch-clamp techniques for high-resolution current recording from cells and cell-free membrane patches. Pflügers Arch. **391:** 85–100.
8. CRAWFORD, A. C. & R. FETTIPLACE. 1981. An electrical tuning mechanism in turtle cochlear hair cells. J. Physiol. **312:** 377–412.
9. CRAWFORD, A. C. & R. FETTIPLACE. 1981. Non-linearities in the response of turtle hair cells. J. Physiol. **315:** 317–338.
10. WU, Y. C., J. J. ART, M. B. GOODMAN & R. FETTIPLACE. 1995. A kinetic description of the calcium-activated potassium channel and its application to electrical tuning of hair cells. Prog. Biophys. Mol. Biol. **63:** 131–158.
11. LEWIS, R. S. & A. J. HUDSPETH. 1983. Voltage- and ion-dependent conductances in solitary vertebrate hair cells. Nature **304:** 538–541.
12. ART, J. J., Y. C. WU & R. FETTIPLACE. 1995. The calcium-activated potassium channels of turtle hair cells. J. Gen. Physiol. **105:** 49–72.
13. GOODMAN, M. B. 1995. A functional analysis of potassium currents in turtle cochlear hair cells. PhD. thesis. University of Chicago. Chicago, IL.
14. YELLEN, G. 1984. Ionic permeation and blockade in Ca^{2+}-activated K^+ channels of bovine chromaffin cells. J. Gen. Physiol. **84:** 157–186.

15. LAGRUTTA, A., K.-Z. SHEN, R. A. NORTH & J. P. ADELMAN. 1994. Functional differences among alternatively spliced variants of Slowpoke, a Drosophila calcium-activated potassium channel. J. Biol. Chem. **269:** 20347–20351.
16. STEINACKER, A. & A. ROMERO. 1991. Characterization of voltage-gated and calcium-activated potassium currents in toadfish saccular hair cells. Brain Res. **556:** 22–32.
17. RENNIE, K. J. & M. J. CORREIA. 1994. Potassium currents in mammalian and avian isolated type I semicircular canal hair cells. J. Neurophysiol. **71:** 317–329.
18. HUDSPETH, A. J. & R. S. LEWIS. 1988. Kinetic analysis of voltage- and ion-dependent conductances in saccular hair cells of the bull-frog, *Rana catesbeiana*. J. Physiol. **400:** 237–274.
19. EATOCK, R. A. & M. J. HUTZLER. 1992. Ionic currents of mammalian vestibular hair cells. Ann. N.Y. Acad. Sci. **656:** 58–74.
20. HAGIWARA, S. & K. TAKAHASHI. 1974. The anomalous rectification and cation selectivity of the membrane of a starfish egg cell. J. Membr. Biol. **18:** 61–80.
21. ART, J. J., R. FETTIPLACE & P. A. FUCHS. 1984. Synaptic hyperpolarization and inhibition of turtle cochlear hair cells. J. Physiol. **356:** 525–550.
22. FUCHS, P. A. & B. W. MURROW. 1992. Cholinergic inhibition of short (outer) hair cells of the chick's cochlea. J. Neurosci. **12:** 800–809.
23. TUCKER, T. & R. FETTIPLACE. 1995. Confocal imaging of calcium microdomains and calcium extrusion in turtle hair cells. Neuron **15:** 1323–1335.
24. FUCHS, P. A. & M. G. EVANS. 1990. Potassium currents in hair cells isolated from the cochlea of the chick. J. Physiol. **429:** 529–551.
25. ROBERTS, W. M., R. A. JACOBS & A. J. HUDSPETH. 1990. Colocalization of ion channels involved in frequency selectivity and synaptic transmission at presynaptic active zones of hair cells. J. Neurosci. **10:** 3664–3684.
26. ROBERTS, W. M. 1994. Localization of calcium signals by a mobile calcium buffer in frog saccular hair cells. J. Neurosci. **14:** 3246–3262.
27. ICHIMIYA, I., J. C. ADAMS & R. S. KIMURA. 1994. Immunolocalization of Na^+, K^+-ATPase, Ca^{2+}-ATPase, calcium-binding proteins, and carbonic anhydrase in the guinea pig inner ear. Acta Otolaryngol. (Stockh.) **114:** 167–176.

Routes of Calcium Entry and Extrusion in Turtle Hair Cells[a]

T. TUCKER, J. J. ART, AND R. FETTIPLACE[b]

Department of Neurophysiology
University of Wisconsin Medical School
Madison, Wisconsin 53706

INTRODUCTION

Cytoplasmic calcium fulfills multiple functions in hair cell transduction.[1,2] It sets the working range of the mechano-electrical transducer channels[3,4] and gates calcium-activated K^+ channels that tune the receptor potentials,[5-9] or mediate efferent inhibition.[10,11] It also triggers exocytosis[12] that will deliver chemical transmitter to the afferent dendrites. Each of these cellular processes is confined to a separate region of the hair cell and is likely to have its own calcium requirements. To permit coordination of the processes, the free calcium in hair cells must be tightly regulated and spatially heterogeneous. The hair cell's voltage-dependent calcium current is both large (up to 0.1 nA/pF) and sustained, being partly activated at the resting potential of -50 mV. The resultant continuous calcium influx presents a substantial burden on the metabolism of the cell, disruption of which may result in saturation of buffers and a rise in free calcium leading to cellular deterioration and death. This may partly account for the hair cell's reputed metabolic vulnerability. It could also explain the sensitivity to aminoglycoside antibiotics, which have been suggested to interfere with metabolism by damaging the mitochondria.[13] The toxic effects of high levels of calcium, acting through disruption of the cytoskeleton, activation of calcium-dependent proteases, and the production of free radicals, have in other neurons been linked to cell death.[14]

To understand how the hair cell copes with such a high calcium metabolism requires knowledge of the sites of entry, the identity and distribution of intracellular calcium buffers, and the mechanism of extrusion. Although a number of previous measurements of calcium in hair cells have been made,[15-18] little is known about the processes that maintain calcium homeostasis and their metabolic cost to the cell. Two previous studies[18,19] have provided evidence for a Na/Ca extrusion mechanism in hair cells. To address these problems we have examined the regulation of intracellular calcium during prolonged calcium loads. The distribution of the ion was followed by real-time confocal imaging of isolated hair cells filled with a fluorescent calcium indicator.

METHODS

Experiments were performed on hair cells isolated from the basilar papilla of the turtle *Trachemys scripta elegans* (for methods see ref. 5). Cells were plated in an

[a]This work was supported by a National Institutes of Health grant DC01362 to R. F. and a training fellowship to T. T. from the Neuroscience Program.

[b]Address correspondence to Robert Fettiplace, 273 Medical Sciences Building, 1300 University Avenue, Madison, WI 53706.

extracellular solution containing (in mM): NaCl, 125; KCl, 4; $CaCl_2$, 5; glucose, 10; NaHEPES, 10, pH 7.6, onto a clean coverslip mounted on the stage of a Zeiss Axiovert 10 microscope. Voltage-dependent calcium currents were recorded using whole-cell patch electrodes filled with a solution of composition (in mM): CsCl, 125; $MgCl_2$, 3; Na_2ATP, 2.5; EGTA, 0.5, 1 or 2; HEPES, 5, neutralized to pH 7.2 with CsOH; the pipette solution also contained 0.1 mM of the hexapotassium salt of Calcium Green 5N (Molecular Probes, Eugene, OR), a low-affinity calcium indicator with an estimated dissociation constant (K_d) of 25 μM. The K_d of Calcium Green 5N in the hair cell was determined by filling cells with solutions containing free calcium buffered at different concentrations with BAPTA or dibromoBAPTA.

Cells were voltage-clamped at a holding potential of −80 mV, and calcium influx was elicited by depolarizing for durations of between 0.1 and 1.5 s at a repetition rate usually of 1/90 s. For most of the experiments described, a 60 mV step to −20 mV, evoking close to a maximal steady-state calcium current, is illustrated. Membrane currents were recorded with a List EPC7 amplifier and stored on a Sony PC-108M DAT recorder at a band width of 20 kHz. Membrane capacitances were read off the dial on the EPC7 after nulling the current transient. Intracellular application of sodium vanadate was achieved by filling the tip of the patch pipette with the control solution and then back-filling the pipette with the blocking agent. This allowed a number of control responses to be acquired prior to diffusion of the blocker into the cell, which took 10 to 15 min. In a separate series of experiments in the absence of intracellular calcium dye, hair cells were stained by extracellular perfusion of 0.5 to 1 μM of the styryl dye FM 1-43 (Molecular Probes), which had been used previously to reveal the recycling of synaptic vesicles.[20] All experiments were performed at a room temperature of about 23 °C.

For fluorescence measurements, hair cells were illuminated with the 488 nm line of a 300-mW argon ion laser and the fluorescence images, obtained through a 515 nm long-pass filter, were collected with an Odyssey real-time laser-scanning confocal microscope (Noran Instruments, Middleton, WI) connected via the bottom TV (Keller) port of the Zeiss optical microscope. Cells were viewed with a 40×/0.75 NA plan-neofluar or a 40×/1.2 NA C-apochromat water-immersion objective, and further magnified with either a 2.5× optivar or the Odyssey's computer-controlled zoom. The thickness of the confocal section could be varied by selecting different detection slit widths. With a 15-μm slit the axial resolution (full width at half-maximum) was about 3.5 μm (plan-neofluar) or 1.5 μm (C-apochromat). The Odyssey generated an RS-170 video-rate signal at 30 interlaced frames per second, and the vertical synchronization pulse of the video signal was employed to trigger the voltage-clamp pulses in order to synchronize their timing with the start of an image. The images were recorded on videocassette using a Sony S-VHS recorder (SVO-9500MD). Subsequent analysis was performed with the MetaMorph software package (Universal Imaging, West Chester, PA) following capture of sequential images into memory of a Pentium computer equipped with a Matrox LC image board. The time course of fluorescence changes in different parts of the cell was measured for regions 1 to 2 μm in diameter using the brightness-over-time function in MetaMorph.

RESULTS

A Novel Calcium-activated Potassium Current

Calcium enters hair cells mainly through voltage-dependent calcium channels, which in a number of species have been shown to be sustained L-type channels that activate at membrane potentials positive to −55 mV.[5,6,21–23] The voltage-dependent calcium current can be isolated using Cs^+ as the major intracellular cation to block the large-conductance calcium-activated K^+ channels involved in the electrical resonance. In turtle hair cells, depolarizing voltage steps to −20 mV evoke a maximal inward current that can be abolished by removal of external calcium or application of 20 μM nifedipine.[24] FIGURE 1A shows examples of the calcium current which activates rapidly on depolarization with a time constant of less than 0.5 ms, and tail currents which turn off equally rapidly on repolarization to −74 mV. The peak amplitude of the calcium current in turtle cochlear hair cells depends on the

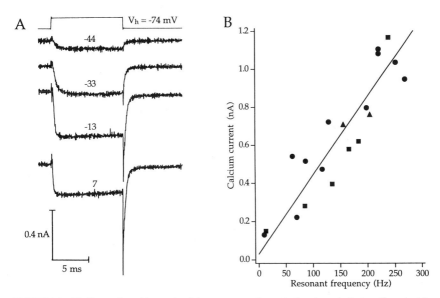

FIGURE 1. (A) Examples of inward calcium currents in an isolated turtle hair cell evoked in response to depolarizing voltage steps from a holding potential of −74 mV to the membrane potential given beside each trace. Note the fast calcium tail currents at the offset of the voltage step. **(B)** Peak amplitude of the calcium currents measured in hair cells tuned to different resonant frequencies. The resonant frequency was determined from the frequency of oscillations in membrane potential in response to a small current step. The calcium current was extracted by blocking the K^+ currents with 25 mM TEA (*triangles*), or replacing external calcium with 5 mM barium (*squares*) or 1 μM calcium (*circles*). Reproduced with modification from reference 24 where the procedures for obtaining the calcium currents are given.

resonant frequency of the cell (FIG. 1B) and hence on the position of the cell along the basilar membrane:[9,24] cells tuned to higher frequencies possess larger calcium currents. When the depolarization lasted for more than a few hundred milliseconds (FIG. 2), the inward current in many cells declined during the step from an initial peak value (ranging between 0.5 and 1.7 nA) and, at the end of the step, on repolarization to −80 mV, an additional slow component of inward tail current appeared. The slow tail current had a complex time course that was a function of the amplitude and duration of the preceding voltage step: generally the longer the step, the larger and slower the tail.

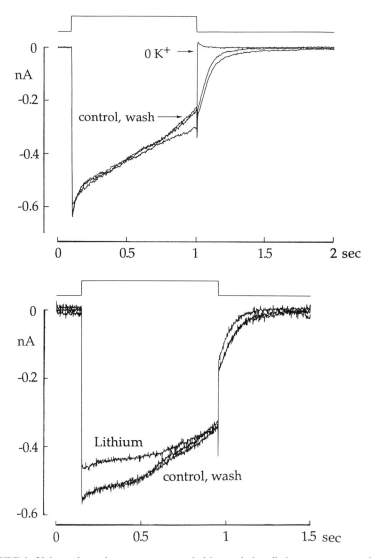

FIGURE 2. Voltage-dependent currents recorded in two hair cells in response to prolonged depolarizations. In both cases, the membrane potential was stepped from -80 mV to -20 mV. The responses consist of a slow calcium-activated current, outward as a Cs^+ current during the pulse and inward as a K^+ current at the end, superimposed on an inward Ca^{2+} current. The slow inward tail current at the end of the pulse was reversibly abolished by removing K^+ from the external solution (*top*), but was virtually unaffected by replacing the Na^+ with Li^+ (*bottom*). Both recordings were made using electrodes filled with a Cs^+-based intracellular solution. The decline in current during the pulse was absent if Cs^+ was replaced by NMG as the main intracellular cation.

Several pieces of evidence[25] indicate that this tail current flows through a second type of calcium-activated K^+ channel: (1) the tail current was abolished by removal of extracellular K^+ (FIG. 2), but was largely unaffected by replacement of Na^+ by Li^+, or substitution of methylsulfate for Cl^- in the extracellular solution; (2) the amplitude of the tail current had a U-shaped voltage dependence that paralleled that of the calcium current and, like the calcium current, it was blocked by 20 μM nifedipine; (3) both the decline in inward current during the voltage step and the tail current were blocked by 0.1 μM apamin; and (4) the sag in current during the voltage step was not seen when N-methyl glucamine (NMG) was used instead of Cs^+ as the intracellular cation. These observations may be explained by assuming that during the depolarization, accumulation of intracellular calcium close to the membrane activates a K^+ channel that is also partially permeable to Cs^+. This K^+ channel is distinct from the large-conductance calcium-activated K^+ channel involved in electrical tuning. Cs^+ flowing out through this channel during the step causes a sag in the inward current, whereas the slow tail current at the end of the pulse is due to K^+ flowing in through the channel. Recordings from membrane patches of turtle hair cells have identified a small-conductance calcium-activated K^+ channel that may underlie these currents.[26] The small-conductance channel is voltage-independent and half-activated by about 2 μM calcium. The tail current provides a useful monitor of the time course of calcium clearance from under the membrane; this time course will depend on the diffusion and buffering of intracellular calcium as well as its rate of extrusion.

Calcium Hotspots

Depolarizing voltage steps, when combined with imaging, elicited an increase in fluorescence around the base of the cell. Under confocal conditions, the fluorescence was seen to be localized to a number of discrete regions (FIG. 3), between one and six such "hotspots" being visible in the basal half of the cell (FIG. 4). In contrast, a much smaller change in fluroescence was found in the rest of the cell, particularly in the vicinity of the hair bundle. For small areas near the centers of the hotspots, the fluorescence intensity increased with time during the depolarization, and then on repolarization it returned to baseline with a time constant of 0.1 s or less; in addition there was a smaller but variable component that decayed with a time constant of 10 s or more (FIG. 5). These hotspots most likely reflect microdomains of intracellular calcium near discrete entry sites. Their presence requires influx of calcium through voltage-dependent channels, which expand during and after the pulse. Evidence in support of this explanation is as follows. First, the peak amplitude of the fluorescence at the end of the voltage step possessed a dependence on membrane potential identical to that of the calcium current. It was maximal near -20 mV, and was indistinguishable from the noise for depolarizations to membrane potentials negative to -50 mV and positive to $+60$ mV. Second, a given hotspot could be reversibly extinguished by local application of a low-calcium solution. In some cases it was possible to achieve sufficient spatial resolution with the pressure application to suppress a given hotspot without affecting neighboring spots. Such a maneuver was associated with a small but rapid decrease in the inward current.

Each fluorescence hotspot expanded throughout the depolarizing pulse from an initial diameter of 1 μm or less. To quantify the growth, a contour at a fixed gray level was drawn around the hotspot in each frame, and the enclosed area calculated. The contour enlarged in sequential frames as the fluorescence intensity increased. Plots of the areal growth versus time were approximately linear and gave slopes ranging

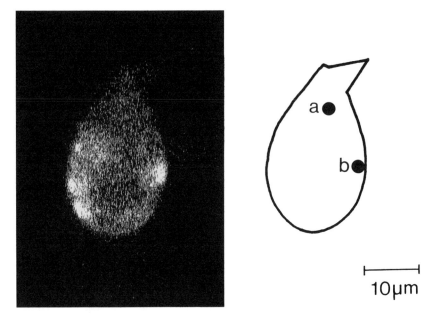

FIGURE 3. Confocal image of a hair cell filled with 100 μM K_6 Calcium Green 5N. Nine frames at the start of a depolarizing pulse to −20 mV have been averaged. Note the four bright regions on the sides of the basolateral membrane, thought to be sites of Ca^{2+} entry. The hair bundle, only faintly stained, is at the top. On the right, superimposed on a drawing of the hair cell, are shown the apical (**a**) and basal (**b**) regions used in constructing the records in FIGURE 5.

from 25 to 108 $\mu m^2 \cdot s^{-1}$. These values are comparable to the range of diffusion coefficients reported for calcium in cytoplasm with the smaller value corresponding to calcium bound to buffer and the larger value tending towards the diffusion of free calcium.[27] The experimental observations are consistent with the idea that calcium is entering through voltage-dependent channels clustered in a few sites on the hair cell base and is diffusing intracellularly away from these sites.

Calcium Extrusion Mechanism

Neurons must expend metabolic energy in extruding calcium ions so as to maintain the cytoplasmic concentration low in the face of a large electrochemical gradient for calcium. Two separate types of calcium-transport mechanism are employed: a Na/Ca exchanger and Ca ATPase (for reviews see refs. 28 and 29). The former mechanism exchanges one Ca^{2+} ion for three Na^+ ions, and utilizes ATP only indirectly, relying primarily on the Na^+ electrochemical gradient that was initially established though a Na/K ATPase. In contrast, the latter mechanism directly hydrolyzes ATP to pump Ca^{2+} ions against their concentration gradient. The Ca ATPase exists as two isoforms,[30] one resident in the plasma membrane and the other in intracellular organelles including the endoplasmic reticulum. These two forms differ structurally and are encoded by separate genes, PMCA for the plasma membrane and SERCA for the endoplasmic reticulum. Both forms of Ca ATPase, like other P-type ATPases, are blocked by low concentrations of the phosphate analogue, vanadate,[31] but the PMCA product is resistant to drugs like thapsigargin and 2,5-di-(*t*-butyl) hydroquinone (BHQ) that are effective blockers of the SERCA pump.[32,33] Some evidence is available to suggest that the SERCA pump is less susceptible to vanadate than the PMCA pump, which in certain cells is half-blocked at submicromolar concentrations.[34]

To test for the presence of a Na/Ca exchanger, external Na+ was replaced by Li+ or NMG, neither of which will support the exchange mechanism. These ionic substitutions had no effect on the time courses of the inward tail current or of calcium removal following a prolonged load. Furthermore, no significant increase in resting calcium-fluorescence occurred during Na+ replacement. However, this maneuver often caused a small but rapidly reversible reduction in the amplitude of the calcium current (FIG. 2). The reason for this reduction in current is presently unknown. The effect of Li+ saline was to reduce the amplitude of the current throughout the voltage range rather than to produce a shift along the voltage axis, which suggests that it might be decreasing the effective single-channel conductance. Although it is difficult to discount completely the contribution of a Na/Ca exchange mechanism to calcium homeostasis in hair cells, much more striking effects were observed on introducing agents that would interfere with a Ca ATPase mechanism.

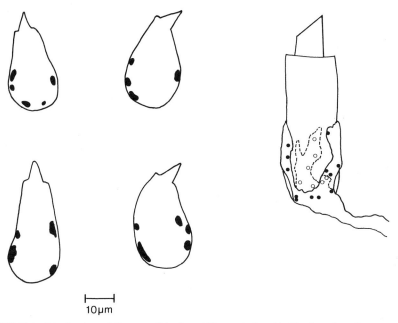

10 µm

FIGURE 4. Distribution of "hotspots" in four different hair cells. The location of spots was obtained by averaging up to nine images during a 300-ms depolarizing voltage pulse and then subtracting the background averaged just prior to the depolarization. The centers of the hotspots are indicated by the filled regions superimposed on the cell outline. On the right is a drawing of the terminal processes of an afferent fiber contacting a hair cell in the turtle basilar papilla; results kindly supplied by Dr. M. G. Sneary. *Circles* indicate the positions of the synaptic dense bodies reconstructed from serial sections; *filled circles* are sites on the near side of the cell, and the *open circles* on the far side. Scale bar applies only to the four cells on the left.

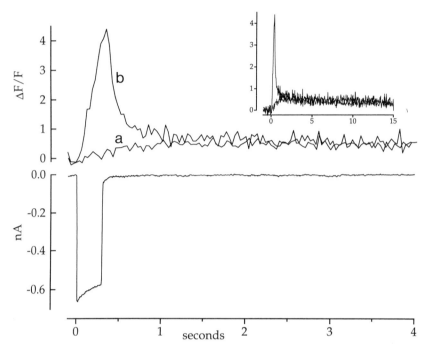

FIGURE 5. Change in fluorescence for the cell of FIGURE 3 in response to a 0.3-s depolarization to −20 mV, starting at time zero. Below is shown the current record and above is the change in fluorescence, ΔF (normalized to the resting fluorescence F) for two 2-μm diameter regions. The larger fluorescence change was taken from a region overlying one of the hotspots, whereas the smaller change was measured at the top of the cell just beneath the hair bundle. The locations of these basal (**b**) and apical (**a**) regions are shown in FIGURE 3. The inset gives the fluorescence change on a slower time scale.

Perfusion of the cytoplasm with 10 μM vanadate invariably lengthened and amplified the inward tail current, and after treatment with 1 mM vanadate, the tail current, after a depolarizing step, often became so prolonged that it did not recover in time for the next stimulus (FIG. 6). At stimulus repetition rates of once every 60 to 90 s, both the tail current and the calcium-fluorescence acquired a staircase appearance suggesting that each calcium load produced an increment in cytoplasmic calcium that was no longer being cleared. A similar sequence of events occurred if the ATP was omitted from the intracellular solution used for filling the electrodes. These observations strongly argue for a central role for a Ca ATPase in the calcium regulation of hair cells.

Additional evidence about the relative roles of plasma membrane and intracellular Ca ATPases in calcium trafficking was derived from use of thapsigargin and BHQ, specific blockers of the endoplasmic reticulum Ca ATPase. When administered extracellularly at concentrations between 10 and 100 μM, BHQ caused an increase in the resting calcium-fluorescence; in addition, after a depolarizing step in BHQ, both the calcium-fluorescence and the inward tail current recovered more slowly. For example, in FIGURE 7, the fast decline in fluorescence at the end of the step was well fit with a time constant of 177 ms in the control, but after BHQ, this time constant lengthened to 433 ms. In some cells a partial recovery was obtained on removal of the BHQ. The effect of BHQ on the hotspots was to make them spread further, and as a consequence, the calcium that entered locally had a wider spatial influence. It should be noted that in no case was BHQ observed to generate the staircase-like behavior seen with high concentrations of vanadate. One explanation would be that some extrusion of calcium persists after uptake into an intracellular compartment has been blocked. The results with these various blockers argue that Ca ATPases in both the plasma and internal membranes make significant contributions to calcium homeostasis in turtle hair cells.

Membrane Recycling

An increase in intracellular calcium in nerve terminals is thought to be the trigger for fusion of synaptic vesicles with the plasma membrane, thus releasing chemical transmitter onto the postsynaptic cell. Such exocytosis must be accompanied by membrane retrieval (endocytosis) in order to preserve a constant area of plasma membrane. Changes in the membrane area, reflecting the processes of exocytosis and endocytosis, may be observed by measurements of membrane capacitance.[35] It

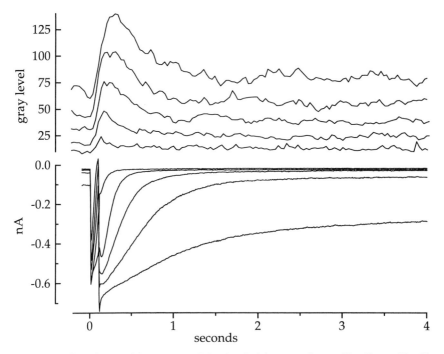

FIGURE 6. Superimposed responses to 0.1-s depolarizing steps from −80 mV to −20 mV, currents shown at the top and fluorescence below. The patch electrode was back-filled with a Cs[+]-based intracellular solution containing 1 mM Na vanadate. The fluorescent response was taken from the rim around the basal pole which included several hotspots. As the vanadate washed in, the decline in current during the pulse became more pronounced, the tail current was more prolonged, and the Ca^{2+} fluorescence increased.

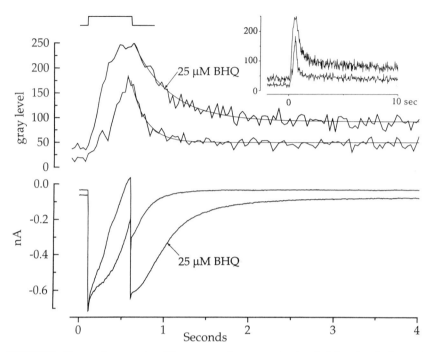

FIGURE 7. Changes in current and fluorescence in response to depolarizing steps before and after external perfusion of 25 μM 2,5-di-(t-butyl) hydroquinone (BHQ) to block the endoplasmic reticulum Ca ATPase. The fluorescence measurements were made from a hotspot; the smooth lines are single-exponential fits to the fast decay in fluorescence with time constants of 177 ms in the control and 433 ms after BHQ.

was evident in many of our experiments that during the prolonged series of depolarizations used to examine the changes in intracellular calcium, there could be substantial changes in the membrane capacitance of the hair cell, which might increase by 10 to 50% over its resting value of about 10 pF. The time course of the capacitance change during depolarization was not examined in any detail though some indication of its calcium dependence was obtained from experiments designed to calibrate the Calcium Green 5N in the cell. In these experiments, hair cells were filled with solutions containing different buffered concentrations of free calcium; the capacitance determined immediately after breakthrough was compared with its final value after equilibration of the intracellular solution. When the calcium was buffered at 18 or 28 μM with 10 mM dibromoBAPTA, no significant long-term change in capacitance was found in six cells, the ratio of final to initial capacitance having a mean value (± SD) of 0.98 ± 0.04. However, when the hair cell was filled with a millimolar concentration of calcium, the ratio of final to initial capacitance in another six cells was 1.39 ± 0.17. These results point to a large membrane turnover that is calcium dependent, but has a relatively low calcium sensitivity.

As an alternative monitor of membrane turnover we have used FM 1-43, a water-soluble styryl dye, which becomes considerably more fluorescent after incorporation into the nonpolar environment of the membrane. It is believed that this dye, when applied in the external solution, inserts into the outer leaflet of the plasma membrane, but because of the presence of two positively charged quaternary nitrogens does not cross the membrane. The course of endocytosis can be then followed by the intracellular accumulation of the dye as the surface membrane is internalized.[20] Brief external application of 0.5 to 1 µM FM 1-43 produced bright fluorescent staining of the plasma membrane and, in particular, highlighted the hair bundle that contains a substantial area of surface membrane. However, after 5 to 10 min of exposure, a significant amount of fluorescence appeared inside the cell. Initially this fluorescence was concentrated in two regions of the hair cell: one just beneath the cuticular plate and the other in the region of the synaptic zone at the basal end of the cell (FIG. 8). Although not shown in FIGURE 8, the staining of the plasma membrane and the bright hair bundle (but not the intracellular staining) could be quickly eliminated by washing with dye-free solution. After continued exposure fluorescence was visible throughout the cell, which indicates a mixing of the two compartments. The results suggest fast and independent recycling of the apical and basal membranes of the hair cell. They are consistent with observations on other polarized epithelial cells, where endocytosis from the apical and basolateral domains

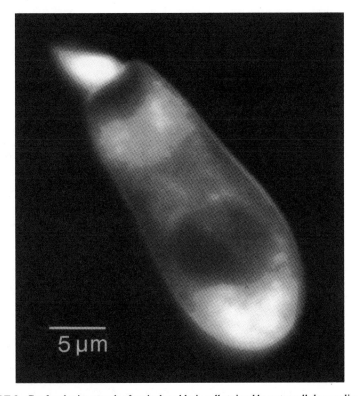

FIGURE 8. Confocal micrograph of an isolated hair cell stained by extracellular application of the impermeant membrane dye 1 µM FM 1-43. Intracellular compartments beneath the dark nucleus and around the cuticular plate were labeled over a period of about 10 min most likely by internalization of the plasma membrane domains at basal and apical poles of the cell. The image was taken while the dye was still present in the external solution so the plasma membrane on the basolateral surface and over the hair bundle is also stained.

of the cell occurs into two distinct early endosomal compartments,[36] which enables the proteins of the two membrane domains to be kept separate.

DISCUSSION

Our confocal imaging experiments with the fluorescent dye Calcium Green 5N have revealed the appearance in hair cells of microdomains of calcium during depolarizations that activate voltage-dependent calcium channels. These observations are consistent with the idea that calcium influx occurs at a small number of sites on the basolateral membrane of the hair cell, and it suggests that the voltage-dependent calcium channels may be arranged in clusters. Such clusters have been previously postulated on the basis of loose-patch recordings[8] and may be localized to the synaptic release sites identified by the presence of presynaptic dense bodies.[37] Hair cells from the turtle's basilar papilla possess between about 17 and 85 such release sites.[38] The larger value was for cells located in the basal membrane area, which would be tuned to higher frequencies[39] and would thus have larger calcium currents (FIG. 1). A correlation between number of release sites and number of calcium channels would be consistent with many of the hair cell's calcium channels being positioned at the active zones.[8] The images revealed far fewer calcium hotspots than release sites even when a series of focal sections were taken throughout the cell. A comparison between the distributions of the hotspots in four cells and the positions of the synaptic release sites for a mid-frequency turtle hair cell is shown in FIGURE 4. The positions of the release sites, characterized by the presence of a synaptic body, and areas of thickened pre- and postsynaptic membrane, were reconstructed from serial electron-micrographic sections.[38] It can be easily imagined that some of these release sites are sufficiently close for their Ca^{2+} domains to fuse during a long depolarization. Therefore, the hotspots visible in the images might correspond to regions where several release sites are close together. Such conglomerations of calcium channels may allow the local intracellular calcium concentration to rise sufficiently high to be detectable in the imaging experiments.

Although the results have stressed the localization of the calcium signals in hotspots around the basal perimeter, it should not be thought that the cytoplasmic free calcium elsewhere in the cell is unaffected by influx via the voltage-dependent calcium channels. Thus, in response to depolarization, there may still be slow attenuated changes in calcium visible even at the top of the cell (see trace a in FIG. 5). Such changes are underemphasized here through use of a calcium dye with low affinity. In the intact inner ear of the turtle, the hair cells will be partially depolarized and thus subject to a continuous calcium influx though the basolateral membrane, which may contribute to the resting calcium concentration in the hair bundle. Physiological changes in resting potential may therefore cause small variations in calcium concentration occurring over a slow time scale of minutes or hours. It is conceivable that these small calcium changes, by affecting the adaptation of the mechano-transduction channels in the hair bundle, could be largely responsible for adjusting the operating range of the transducer.

Our experiments also addressed the mechanism of removal of the calcium entering during depolarization. Both the slow inward tail current, which we argue is an indicator of the calcium concentration at the membrane, and the fluorescence in the hotspots were affected similarly by manipulations that would alter the rate of calcium removal. Although the exact location of the small-conductance calcium-activated K^+ channels responsible for the tail current is unknown, clearly the kinetics of that current and its susceptibility to Ca ATPase blockers paralleled the behavior of the calcium-fluorescence at the hotspots. Both confirm that the major mechanism of extrusion is via a Ca ATPase rather than a Na/Ca exchanger, the most profound effects on calcium regulation being exerted by intracellularly applied vanadate. The slow inward tail current differs from that observed in some other neurons, such as retinal amacrine cells, where it has been attributed to an electrogenic Na/Ca exchange on the basis of its suppression in Li^+ saline.[40] The lack of contribution of a Na/Ca exchanger is unsurprising given that the hair cell does not need a powerful Na/K pumping capacity to handle Na^+ influx during transduction. The hair cell's transducer current is carried by K^+ ions entering from the endolymph, and therefore the requirement for Na^+ extrusion is largely deferred in the cochlea to the Na/K ATPase pumps in the stria vascularis. The main metabolic cost of preserving ionic balance in the hair cell may thus be incurred by calcium pumping and its requirement for ATP.

A hair cell in the intact cochlea of the turtle is normally subject to continual fluctuations in membrane potential,[39] which even in the absence of acoustic stimulation might generate at least 0.1 nA of maintained calcium current flowing into a cell about 2 pl in volume. To balance this load, the cell must possess an extrusion mechanism of comparable potency:[41] this influx of 3×10^8 ion/s would require more than 10^6 Ca ATPase pumps per cell if each were to operate at a maximum capacity of 200 ion/s. A comparable estimate of the number of Ca ATPase pumps required can be arrived at by modeling the experimental time course and distribution of calcium (Tucker *et al.*, unpublished results). If 10^6 calcium pumps were distributed over the hair cell's basolateral membrane, they would be packed at an average density of $1300/\mu m^2$, assuming a membrane area of about 750 μm^2. The surface density would be lower if a proportion of pumps were allocated to an intracellular compartment. Given this degree of calcium pumping, the average ATP utilization can be estimated as at least 0.1 $mmole \cdot l^{-1} \cdot s^{-1}$. The total metabolic cost may be greater than this, particularly in hair cells tuned to the highest frequencies that have the largest calcium currents (FIG. 1), and in cochleas of birds and mammals that have higher body temperatures than the turtle.

With prolonged depolarizations or internal perfusion with a high calcium concentration a significant increase in cell capacitance was found, which may represent fusion of a considerable number of intracellular vesicles with the plasma membrane. Large calcium-dependent changes in capacitance have been previously documented in some detail for saccular hair cells.[12] We obtained supporting evidence for rapid membrane turnover by extracellular perfusion with the dye FM 1-43, which indicated endocytic compartments at both apical and basal poles of the hair cell. Evidence for membrane recycling, especially in the synaptic zone, has also been described using uptake of horseradish peroxidase by mammalian cochlear hair cells.[42] In relating the FM 1-43 fluorescent images to the capacitance measurements, it will be important in future experiments to determine what fraction of the membrane recycling is calcium dependent. It would also be useful to know whether the FM 1-43-labeled intracellular membrane overlaps with the compartment containing the SERCA calcium pumps. Recycling of the synaptic vesicles most likely contributes part or all of the staining at basal pole, but the significance of the endocytic compartment at the apical pole is unclear. It seems unlikely that this compartment reflects migration of stained synaptic vesicles from the basal pole because the apical and basal compartments appeared separate early on in dye perfusion; furthermore, electron-micrographic evidence exists for the presence in turtle hair cells of coated pits and vesicles at the apical membrane beside the hair bundle.[43] Recycling of the apical membrane may be crucial for hair cell function because a prominent sign of an unhealthy or hypoxic turtle hair cell epithelium is the formation of blebs on the apical membrane beside the hair bundle. Such blebs, which can be of a size comparable to the hair bundle, can also be produced by treatment with aminoglycoside antibiotics and other polycations.[44] Ballooning of the apical membrane could result from a promotion of exocytosis by elevated intracellular calcium or to a failure of endocytosis due to lack of the ATP required for removal of the clathrin coats from the internalized endosomes.

ACKNOWLEDGMENTS

We would like to thank Peter Lipton and Michael Wu for helpful discussions. We are grateful to Mike Sneary for allowing us to use data on the distribution of afferent synapses on turtle hair cells.

REFERENCES

1. FETTIPLACE, R. 1992. The role of calcium in hair cell transduction. *In* Sensory Transduction. D. P. Corey & S. D. Roper, Eds. Soc. Gen. Physiol. Ser. **47:** 343–356.
2. LENZI, D. & W. M. ROBERTS. 1994. Calcium signaling in hair cells: Multiple roles in a compact cell. Curr. Opin. Neurobiol. **4:** 496–502.
3. EATOCK, R. A., D. P. COREY & A. J. HUDSPETH. 1987. Adaptation of mechanoelectrical transduction in hair cells of the bullfrog's sacculus. J. Neurosci. **7:** 2821–2836.
4. CRAWFORD, A. C., M. G. EVANS & R. FETTIPLACE. 1989. Activation and adaptation of transducer currents in turtle hair cells. J. Physiol. **419:** 405–434.
5. ART, J. J. & R. FETTIPLACE. 1987. Variation of membrane properties in hair cells isolated from the turtle cochlea. J. Physiol. **385:** 207–242.
6. HUDSPETH, A. J. & R. S. LEWIS. 1988. Kinetic analysis of voltage- and ion-dependent conductances in hair cells of the bullfrog, *Rana catesbeiana*. J. Physiol. **400:** 237–274.
7. FUCHS, P. A., T. NAGAI & M. G. EVANS. 1988. Electrical tuning of hair cells isolated from the chick cochlea. J. Neurosci. **8:** 2460–2467.
8. ROBERTS, W. M., R. A. JACOBS & A. J. HUDSPETH. 1990. Colocalization of ion channels involved in frequency selectivity and synaptic transmission in presynaptic active zones of hair cells. J. Neurosci. **10:** 3664–3684.
9. WU, Y.-C., M. B. GOODMAN, J. J. ART & R. FETTIPLACE. 1995. A kinetic description of the calcium-activated potassium channel and its application to electrical tuning of hair cells. Prog. Biophys. Mol. Biol. **63:** 131–158.
10. SHIGEMOTO, T. & H. OHMORI. 1991. Muscarinic receptor hyperpolarizes cochlear hair cells of chick by activating Ca^{2+}-activated K^+ channels. J. Physiol. **442:** 669–690.
11. FUCHS, P. A. & B. W. MURROW. 1992. Cholinergic inhibition of short (outer) hair cells of the chick's cochlea. J. Neurosci. **12:** 800–809.
12. PARSON, T. D., D. LENZI, W. ALMERS & W. M. ROBERTS. 1994. Calcium-triggered exocytosis and endocytosis in an isolated presynaptic cell: Capacitance measurements in saccular hair cells. Neuron **13:** 875–883.
13. CORTOPASSI, G. & T. HUTCHIN. 1994. A molecular and cellular hypothesis for aminoglycoside-induced deafness. Hear. Res. **78:** 27–30.
14. CHOI, D. W. 1994. Calcium and excitotoxic neuronal injury. Ann. N. Y. Acad. Sci. **747:** 162–171.
15. OHMORI, H. 1988. Mechanical stimulation and fura-2 fluorescence in the hair bundle of dissociated hair cells of the chick. J. Physiol. **399:** 115–137.
16. CHABBERT, C., G. GELEOC, J. LEHOUELLEUR & A. SANS. 1994. Intracellular calcium variations evoked by mechanical stimulation of mammalian isolated vestibular type I hair cells. Pflueg. Arch. Eur. J. Physiol. **427:** 162–168.
17. ASHMORE, J. F. & H. OHMORI. 1990. Control of intracellular calcium by ATP in isolated outer hair cells of the guinea pig cochlea. J. Physiol. **428:** 109–131.
18. IKEDA, K., Y. SAITO, A. NISHIYAMA & T. TAKASAKA. 1992. Na^+-Ca^{2+} exchange in isolated

cochlear outer hair cells of the guinea pig studied by fluorescence image microscopy. Pflueg. Arch. Eur. J. Physiol. **420:** 493–499.

19. MROZ, E. A. & C. LECHENE. 1993. Calcium and magnesium transport by isolated goldfish hair cells. Hear. Res. **70:** 139–145.

20. BETZ, W. J., F. MAO & G. BEWICK. 1992. Activity-dependent staining and destaining of living vertebrate motor nerve terminals. J. Neurosci. **12:** 363–375.

21. OHMORI, H. 1984. Studies of ionic currents in the isolated vestibular hair cell of the chick. J. Physiol. **350:** 561–581.

22. FUCHS, P. A., M. G. EVANS & B. W. MURROW. 1990. Calcium currents in hair cells isolated from the cochlea of the chick. J. Physiol. **429:** 553–568.

23. ZIDANIC, M. & P. A. FUCHS. 1995. Kinetic analysis of barium currents in chick cochlear hair cells. Biophys. J. **68:** 1323–1336.

24. ART, J. J., R. FETTIPLACE & Y-C. WU. 1993. The effects of low-calcium on the voltage-dependent conductances involved in tuning of turtle hair cells. J. Physiol. **470:** 109–126.

25. TUCKER, T. & R. FETTIPLACE. 1994. Calcium regulation in turtle cochlear hair cells. Soc. Neurosci. Abstr. **20:** 968.

26. ART, J. J., Y.-C. WU & R. FETTIPLACE. 1995. The calcium-activated potassium channels of turtle hair cells. J. Gen. Physiol. **105:** 49–72.

27. ALLBRITTON, N. L., T. MEYER & L. STRYER. 1992. Range of messenger action of calcium ion and inositol 1,4,5-trisphosphate. Science **258:** 1812–1815.

28. BLAUSTEIN, M. P., R. DIPOLO & J. P. REEVES. 1991. Sodium-calcium exchange: Proceedings of the second international conference. Ann. N. Y. Acad. Sci. **639.**

29. SCHATZMANN, H. 1989. The calcium pump of the surface membrane and the SR. Annu. Rev. Physiol. **51:** 473–485.

30. GROVER, A. K. & I. KHAN. 1992. Calcium pump isoforms: Diversity, selectivity and plasticity. Cell Calcium **13:** 9–17.

31. PEDERSEN, P. L. & E. CARAFOLI. 1987. Ion motive ATPases. I. Ubiquity, properties and significance for cell function. Trends Biochem. **12:** 146–150.

32. JACKSON, T. R., S. I. PATTERSON, O. THASTRUP & M. R. HANLEY. 1988. A novel tumour promoter, thapsigargin, transiently increases cytoplasmic free Ca^{2+} without generation of inositol phosphates in NG115-401L neuronal cells. Biochem. J. **253:** 81–86.

33. KASS, G. E., S. K. DUDDY, G. A. MOORE & S. ORRENIUS. 1989. 2,5-Di-(tert-butyl)-1-4-benzohydroquinone rapidly elevates cytosolic Ca^{2+} concentration by mobilizing the inositol 1,4,5-trisphosphate-sensitive Ca^{2+} pool. J. Biol. Chem. **264:** 15192–15198.

34. GILL, D. L. & S.-H. CHUEH. 1985. An intracellular $(ATP + Mg^{2+})$-dependent calcium pump within the N1E-115 neuronal cell line. J. Biol. Chem. **260:** 9289–9297.

35. PENNER, R. & E. NEHER. 1989. The patch clamp technique in the study of secretion. Trends Neurosci. **12:** 159–163.

36. MATLIN, K. S. 1992. W(h)ither default? Sorting and polarization in epithelial cells. Curr. Opin. Cell Biol. **4:** 623–628.

37. ISSA, N. P. & A. J. HUDSPETH. 1994. Clustering of Ca^{2+} and Ca^{2+}-activated K^+ channels at fluorescently labeled presynaptic active zones of hair cells. Proc. Natl. Acad. Sci. USA **91:** 7578–7582.

38. SNEARY, M. G. 1988. Auditory receptor of the red-eared turtle. II. Afferent and efferent synapses and innervcation patterns. J. Comp. Neurol. **276:** 588–606.

39. CRAWFORD, A. C. & R. FETTIPLACE. 1980. The frequency-selectivity of auditory nerve fibres and hair cells in the cochlea of the turtle. J. Physiol. **306:** 79–125.

40. GLEASON, G., S. BORGES & M. WILSON. 1995. Electrogenic Na-Ca exchange clears Ca^{2+} loads from retinal amacrine cells in culture. J. Neurosci. **15:** 3612–3621.

41. ROBERTS, W. M., R. A. JACOBS & A. J. HUDSPETH. 1991. The hair cell as a presynaptic terminal. Ann. N.Y. Acad. Sci. **635:** 221–233.

42. SIEGEL, J. H. & W. E. BROWNELL. 1986. Synaptic and Golgi membrane recycling in cochlear hair cells. J. Neurocytol. **15:** 311–328.

43. HACKNEY, C. M., R. FETTIPLACE & D. N. FURNESS. 1993. The functional morphology of stereociliary bundles on turtle cochlear hair cells. Hear. Res. **69:** 163–175.

44. KOTECHA, B. & G. P. RICHARDSON. 1994. Ototoxicity in vitro: Effects of neomycin, gentamycin, amikacin, spectinomycin, neamine, spermine and poly-L-lysine. Hear. Res. **73:** 173–184.

Filtering Properties of Vestibular Hair Cells: An Update[a]

M. J. CORREIA,[b-d] A. J. RICCI,[b] AND K. J. RENNIE[b]

Departments of Otolaryngology[b] and Physiology & Biophysics[c]
University of Texas Medical Branch
Galveston, Texas 77555-1063

At the last of this series of meetings, we[1] summarized the literature and presented results that led us to suggest that, when different, membrane properties such as membrane capacitance, membrane resistance, and ionic conductances in the basolateral membrane of hair cells contribute to different filtering of the hair cell receptor potential. At that time, we discussed hair cells in general (auditory, seismic, and vestibular hair cells). First, we concluded that hair cells of the different specialized senses showed different filtering properties. For example, hair cells in auditory receptors, appear to show a higher quality of electrical resonance around their resting membrane potential than do hair cells of vestibular receptors. Second, we concluded that within the same end organ, hair cells with *different* morphologies and *different* innervation patterns (e.g., inner and outer hair cells of the cochlea and type I and type II hair cells of the vestibular apparatus) have different filtering properties because they have different conductances and passive membrane properties. Finally, we concluded that further study was needed to determine whether hair cells of the same type (with the *same* morphology) but located in different regions of the neuroepithelium of the same receptor had different filtering properties. We pointed out that when differences have been found in the past, cell type (based on shape) always co-varied with location. In the past three years, new studies have been conducted which permit us to speak further about these three conclusions particularly with reference to vestibular hair cells.

DO HAIR CELLS FROM DIFFERENT SPECIALIZED RECEPTORS HAVE DIFFERENT FILTERING PROPERTIES?

The evidence continues to accumulate that the filtering properties of type II hair cells of seismic detectors (the saccule in some species) are different from type II vestibular hair cells (hair cells from the semicircular canals and utricle). Recently, Baird[2] has directly compared the electrical resonant properties of 19 type E hair cells in the frog utricle and 10 unclassified type II hair cells from the frog saccule, a receptor thought to sense substrate-borne vibrations.[3] He recorded receptor potentials using sharp intracellular microelectrodes and observed that saccular hair cells had a higher quality of resonance—an on-ringing response during depolarization

[a]This work was supported in part by NIH grant DC01273. M.J.C. is a NIH NIDCD Claude Pepper investigator; A.J.R. is a NASA research associate; and K.J.R. is a NIH NRSA research fellow.
[d]Address correspondence to correia@mudd.mjclab.utmb.edu or Room 7.102, MRB, UTMB, Galveston, TX 77555.

and an off-ringing response during hyperpolarization—and required smaller depolarization steps to achieve the same quality of resonance as the utricular hair cells.

Although we have not thoroughly tested the complex currents in saccular type II hair cells in pigeon and compared them to those we[4] obtained from the semicircular canals, we[5] have preliminary data suggesting that the complex ionic currents in pigeon gravito-inertial sensing utricular type II hair cells (from the lateral extrastriolar region) are similar to those observed for the rotation sensing semicircular canals. We treated the neuroepithelia of utricles of white king pigeons with papain and processed the tissue as described elsewhere.[6] We vacuumed solitary type II hair cells from the lateral most 200 μm of the macula (the lateral extrastriolar region), and we studied solitary cells using the whole-cell variant of the perforated and ruptured

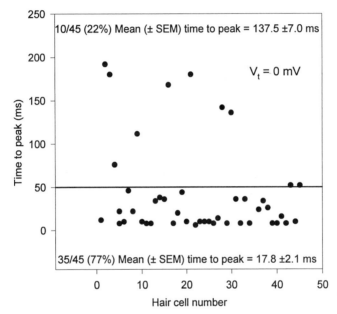

FIGURE 1. A scatter plot of time to peak of complex current for 45 utricular type II hair cells. The horizontal bar is arbitrarily drawn at 50 ms to divide the times into two clusters. The current response was produced using a voltage-clamp protocol previously used for pigeon semicircular canal hair cells.[4] The protocol consists of a hyperpolarizing prepulse (250 ms) to −110 mV from −60 mV followed by a test pulse of 250 ms at 0 mV. The mean time to peak and percentage of cells falling in the two clusters are included in the figure.

patch-clamp technique with the amplifier operating in voltage-clamp mode. The test voltage protocol was a 250-ms conditioning pulse to −110 mV from the zero current potential (V_z) followed by a 250-ms test pulse (V_t) of different peak voltages. FIGURE 1 presents time to peak current for $V_t = 0$ mV. One group of cells (77%) had a fast mean time to peak (17.8 ± 2.1 ms) and showed time-dependent inactivation; a second group of cells (22%) had a much slower mean time to peak (137.5 ± 7.0 ms) and little time-dependent inactivation. Using this same test protocol, we[4] found that 68% of a sample of 19 type II hair cells from the semicircular canals had a fast mean time to peak (~ 6 ms), and 21% had a slower time to peak (~ 55 ms). Using pharmacological methods, we[4] showed that type II hair cells from the semicircular canals containing the former complex current had a dominant A-type potassium (I_A) and a calcium activated potassium $I_{K(Ca)}$ current, whereas the latter complex current was dominated by a delayed rectifier potassium current, which we subsequently labeled I_{KII}.[7]

Type I hair cells in different receptors appear to be *more homogenous* than type II hair cells with respect to their zero current potential, activation, deactivation, slope conductance, and steady-state properties of their ionic currents. We[8] have studied mechanically dissociated type I hair cells from the semicircular canals, utricle, lagena, and saccule of pigeons. Type I hair cells with a neck-to-plate ratio[6] (NPR)

TABLE 1. Measurements from Isolated Pigeon Type I Hair Cells (Group 1)

Measurement (mean ± SEM)	Semicircular Canal	Saccule	Lagena	Utricle
V_z (mV)	-69 ± 1	-67 ± 3	-66 ± 4	-61 ± 2
Slope Conductance (nS)	41 ± 4	35 ± 10	32 ± 4	30 ± 4
Activation A (ms)	11 ± 3	10 ± 1	11 ± 2	10 ± 1
Activation B (ms)	5.0 ± 2.0	1.0 ± 0.2	4.0 ± 1	3.0 ± 1.0
Activation C (ms/mV)	30 ± 4	18 ± 1	28 ± 2	21 ± 2
Deactivation τ_1 (ms)	3.20 ± 0.80	2.40 ± 0.99	5.00 ± 2.00	5.00 ± 2.00
Deactivation τ_2 (ms)	40 ± 8	23 ± 9	35 ± 7	46 ± 11

NOTE: Values for A, B, and C were derived from the equation of a single exponential ($Y = A + B(e^{-x/C})$ fitted to voltage-dependent time constants for each receptor. The time constants were derived by fitting the activation kinetics with a first-order Hodgkin-Huxley equation. The test paradigm consisted of depolarizing the cell to several test potentials (V_t) from a holding potential (V_h); ($V_h = -90$ mV, -80 mV $\leq V_t$ to ≤ 20 mV, in 20-mV increments). Values for τ_1 and τ_2 are deactivation time constants derived from fitting a double exponential function to currents obtained over a voltage pulse range from -80 mV to -120 mV with $V_h = -60$ mV. (Table modified from Ricci *et al.*[8])

< 0.72 and a neck-to-body width ratio[9] (NBR) of < 0.64 comprised this group (designated as group 1), which contains 87% of all type I hair cells that we have studied. Ninety-eight type I hair cells—48 from the semicircular canals, 24 from the utricle, 20 from the lagena, and 6 from the saccule—were studied using the perforated whole-cell patch-clamp technique. No attempt was made to compensate for the small leak current or series resistance. The currents in all cells were reversibly sensitive to 5 mM 4-AP applied to the bath. Some of the measurements shown in TABLE 1 of Ricci *et al.*[8] are presented in TABLE 1. None of the statistics tabulated were statistically significantly different ($p > 0.05$) *across the different receptors.*

DO HAIR CELLS OF THE SAME MORPHOLOGY BUT FROM DIFFERENT REGIONS OF THE SAME RECEPTOR HAVE DIFFERENT FILTERING PROPERTIES?

Little evidence has emerged in the past several years to suggest that hair cells with the *same* morphology but in *different* locations on the neuroepithelium have different conductances. Masetto *et al.*[10] made slices of the frog cristae and recorded primarily from two types of cells (club-shaped and cylindrical) in two different regions of the neuroepithelium (central and peripheral zone) using whole-cell patch-clamp techniques. They found that most cells in the peripheral regions (71% club-shaped) exhibited a transient outward K^+ current (I_A) in conjunction with a slow delayed rectifier outward K^+ conductance (I_K current). However, most cells in the central regions (81% cylindrical) showed little or no I_A, but showed I_k along with an inward rectifier K current (I_{IR}). Cells in both regions showed a rapidly activating, rapidly inactivating Ca^{2+}-dependent outward K^+ current ($I_{K(Ca)}$). The percentages cited above imply that cylindrical and club-shaped cells exist in both the central and peripheral zones. However, apparently cells of the same morphology in different regions do not always have different currents (Masetto, personal communication). Furthermore, Baird[2,11] studied frog hair cells *in vitro* in whole-mount utricles and saccules. He used sharp intracellular electrodes and studied subtypes of utricular type II hair cells identified according to the classification of Lewis and Li.[12] Only type B cells are found throughout the neuroepithelium. Eight type B hair cells, 3 in the medial extrastriolar region and 5 in the lateral or medial striolar regions, were studied, and they "had similar response properties."

DO HAIR CELLS OF DIFFERENT MORPHOLOGY IN THE SAME RECEPTOR HAVE DIFFERENT FILTERING PROPERTIES?

Recent studies[2,10,11,13] continue to show that type II hair cells with different morphology but in the same receptor have different conductances. Holt and Eatock,[13] studied 168 isolated leopard frog saccular hair cells. They observed four currents: an outward calcium-dependent potassium current and three inward currents, a calcium current, and two inward rectifiers, I_{K1} and I_h. The presence of I_{K1} was correlated with morphology and resonance properties. Cells without I_{K1}, which were more spherical than cells with I_{K1}, did not resonate at rest. In contrast, most cells with I_h resonated at rest or required the smallest injected current to resonate.

The comparison of the modulation of receptor potentials of type I and type II vestibular hair cells during current injections provides striking evidence for different filtering properties between vestibular hair cells of different shape and the role played by the major conductances in these cells on the filtering of the receptor potential.

Studies[14-17] of type I hair cells using whole-cell patch-clamp (current-clamp mode) measurements demonstrate a clear difference between the membrane voltage responses of rat, gerbil, and pigeon type I and type II hair cells to current injection. During sinusoidal or pulse current injections, the membrane voltage of gerbil type I hair cells exhibits a low gain, broad frequency response[16] (20% attenuated at 1 kHz, Rennie *et al.*[16]) and no resonance about V_z.[16] These features are caused by a large potassium conductance,[14,15,18-21] which we[7] have called I_{KI}, that is about 50% activated at V_z.[7] When I_{KI} is removed pharmacologically (20 mM TEA in pipette), the resting membrane potential is depolarized ~ 30 mV, the frequency response gain is attenuated $\sim 75\%$ at 1 kHz, and the membrane response to a pulse, changes from a replica of the current pulse injection to a pulse that shows an initial peak followed by a relaxation. Also, I_{KI} can be deactivated by hyperpolarizing the membrane to ~ -90 mV. This deactivation results in approximately a 10-fold decrease in membrane conductance or inversely, approximately a 10-fold increase in membrane resistance.[7]

FIGURE 2 shows the effect of activation and deactivation of I_{KI} on the admittance of the membrane of a pigeon utricular type I hair cell from the striolar region. The recordings were made in voltage clamp using perforated whole-cell patch-clamp techniques. The stimulus (described in detail elsewhere[1,6]) consisted of a pulse

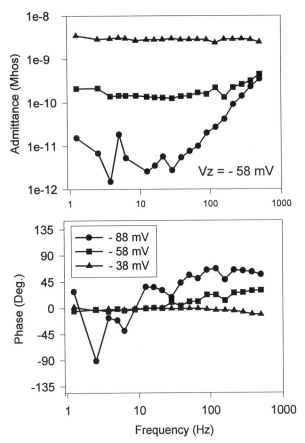

FIGURE 2. A log–log magnitude and log–linear phase plot of membrane admittance of a pigeon utricular type I hair cell. The recordings were made in voltage-clamp mode; the analysis procedure has been described in detail elsewhere.[6] The cell's membrane potential was held at one of three voltage levels (-88, -58, -38 mV), and a sum of 20 sinusoids spanning the frequency range from 1–500 Hz with a waveform amplitude of 6 mV rms was delivered. Note that while the magnitude and phase of the admittance function is relatively flat at $V_z = -58$ mV and -38 mV, at -88 mV, where I_{KI} is mostly deactivated, a trough at ~ 10 Hz is seen, and this trough is accompanied by a phase transition through zero from a lag to a lead. These features are indicative of a resonance. It is not yet clear what conductance, active at this holding potential, contributes to the resonance.

voltage upon which was superimposed a sum of sinusoidal oscillations (20 logarithmically spaced frequencies, 1–500 Hz; with a rms voltage ~ 6 mV). At a holding potential, $V_h = -88$ mV, where I_{KI} is presumably deactivated, the admittance is low and evidence of resonance is present (a trough at ~ 10 Hz in the admittance function and a phase change from phase lag to phase lead). Parenthetically, we have not yet isolated the conductances active at this hyperpolarized membrane potential that contribute to this resonance. At V_z, where I_{KI} is partially activated, the phase is essentially flat and the magnitude component of the admittance is larger in magnitude. Further depolarization of the membrane results in a further increase in admittance magnitude and a flatter phase and magnitude component across frequencies.

Pigeon type I hair cells, like gerbil type I hair cells, show a wide range of input resistances around V_z. Gerbil input resistances[16] around V_z had a mean ($\pm$SD) value of $\sim 21 \pm 14$ MΩ ($n = 25$). Pigeon input resistances for 81 type I hair cells around V_z are presented in FIGURE 3. The mean input resistance is 277 MΩ, an order of magnitude greater than the mean value for the gerbil. The largest input resistances in pigeon are in the range 0.9 to 1.0 GΩ—not that much smaller than the mean described for the pigeon type II hair cells (1.5 $\pm$ 0.3 GΩ^6).

As pointed out elsewhere,[16] if type I hair cells have such a wide range of input resistances *in situ,* then different gains and frequency responses are predicted. The membrane voltage responses of type I hair cells around V_z, with high-input conductances, is determined by the magnitude of the conductance.[16] However, the voltage response of cells with low-input conductances (high-input resistances) appears to be determined primarily by the activation kinetics of the complex current.[17] An analysis leading to this conclusion is presented elsewhere in this volume.[17] Briefly summarized, as current pulses of increasing magnitude are injected into a type I hair cell, the voltage response is first pulsatile (depending on the input resistance of the cell); then as the stimulus magnitude increases, a peak response (still determined by the input resistance of the cell) is followed by a relaxation. The peak response remains a linear function of the cell's input resistance while the steady-state response shows

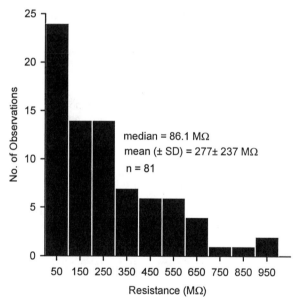

FIGURE 3. A bar histogram of input resistance around $V_h = -60$ mV from 81 pigeon type I hair cells. The range is quite variable (10–1000 MΩ). The mean (277 MΩ) and median (86 MΩ) are presented. If, as suggested in the text and elsewhere,[7,8,16] the input resistance is determined by the amount of activation of I_{KI}, which contributes to the sensitivity, bandwidth, and resting membrane potential of the type I hair cell, then there must be heterogeneity in the filtering properties among type I hair cells in a given receptor.

rectification, the magnitude of which is a function of the recruited conductance. Thus, the linearity of the peak response is determined by the cell's input resistance (established by the steady-state component of the active conductance) and the slow activation of the macro-conductance. The relaxation time constant of the membrane voltage is determined by the activation kinetics of I_{KI}. The shape of this response can be fitted by the resonance equation previously used[6] to characterize avian type II semicircular canal hair cells with a low resonant frequency and a low quality factor (Ricci and Correia, unpublished observations). Because this response is predominately determined by the activation of the major conductance, I_{KI},[8] type I hair cells with higher input resistances will be more sensitive to a narrow band of frequencies than will type II hair cells. The complex currents of type II hair cells are dominated by I_A, I_{KII}, or $I_{K(Ca)}$, each with different activation kinetics and presumably different frequency sensitivities. Therefore, type I hair cells with low-input conductance will operate over a *narrower* but *similar* frequency range in comparison to type II hair cells. It is possible that type I hair cells were added to the neuroepithelium of amniotes to promote sensitivity to the same narrow frequency range.

To further examine the filtering of membrane voltage resulting from intracellular current, particularly that resembling the mechanoelectric transduction current, we injected rectified sine waves into type I and type II hair cells. This method has been used previously by Sugihara and Furukawa[22] in their analysis of "oscillatory" and "spike type" type II hair cells in the goldfish saccule. Responses to rectified sine wave current injections and responses to voltage-clamp and current-clamp pulse protocols are presented for a type II hair cell in FIGURE 4 and a type I hair cell in FIGURE 5.

Test protocols are shown in the upper panels of FIGURE 4A–E. These protocols are described in the figure captions. With the exception of FIGURE 4A and FIGURE 5F, all protocols were current injections. In FIGURES 4A and 5F, values for the voltage protocols are in mV and the current responses are in nA. In the remainder of the panels, current injection values are in nA and the membrane voltage responses are in mV.

The traces in FIGURE 4 were obtained from a pigeon utricular type II hair cell from the medial extrastriolar region. The current response in FIGURE 4A is a fast time–to–peak complex current which shows rapid activation followed by inactivation to a steady-state level. Previously, we[4] showed that this complex current is composed of I_A and I_{KII}, a delayed rectifier unlike the one (I_{KI}) found in type I hair cells. The membrane voltage response to pulse injections is presented in FIGURE 4B. The response to depolarizing current injections is a rapid peak response followed by a rapid relaxation followed by a slower repolarization. Although unproved, but by analogy to the analysis of the voltage response in type I hair cells,[17] the relaxation time constant is probably a function of the whole cell activation kinetics, and the repolarization is a function of the time-dependent inactivation of the transient outward current (I_A). FIGURE 4C–E shows membrane voltage responses to rectified sine wave injections of different frequencies. First, it can be noted that the responses are nonlinear, particularly in comparison with those from type I hair cells shown in FIGURE 5A–E. Second, as previously demonstrated by Sugihara and Furukawa,[22] the ionic conductances and the membrane resistance and capacitance in the utricular type II hair cell, shown in FIGURE 4, cause the membrane potential to become more symmetrical and sine wave-like at a certain frequency, the resonant frequency (cf. FIG. 4C and D). Third, as predicted by Hudspeth,[23] at a frequency of 200 Hz, the membrane properties of the hair cell cause the sinusoidal membrane oscillations to be mathematically integrated and ride about a membrane offset, analogous to temporal summation of postsynaptic potentials.

FIGURE 5F shows the current response of a utricular striolar type I hair cell to the

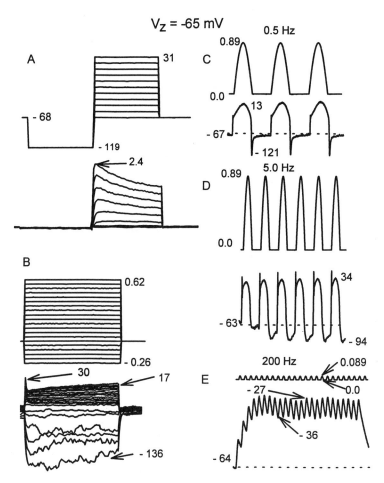

FIGURE 4. Traces obtained from a pigeon utricular type II hair cell located in the medial extrastriolar region. (**A**) Complex currents obtained in voltage-clamp mode. The command voltage protocol was initially $V_h = -70$ mV, then hyperpolarization to -110 mV for 100 ms, then depolarization to a series of test voltages from -70 to $+30$ mV (10 mV increments) for another 100 ms. Numbers in the top trace are actual voltages in mV. The number in the bottom trace is peak current (in nA) at a depolarization of 31 mV. (**B**) Membrane voltage responses to a series of pulses. Current was injected for 200 ms and ranged from -260 pA to 620 pA. (**C–E**) Rectified sine wave current injections of variable frequency. Top trace in each panel is the injected current (in nA), and the bottom trace is the membrane voltage (in mV). Dashed line in C–E represents the resting membrane potential before the current injection.

same voltage pulse protocol as applied to the cell in FIGURE 4A. The larger current (6.9 nA compared to 2.4 nA) at the same voltage (~ 30 mV) is typical of comparisons of the complex ionic currents of type I and type II hair cells. It is interesting to wonder why type I hair cells have such large currents. The membrane voltage responses to current pulses have already been discussed. But, it is interesting to note that the response of the pigeon utricular type I hair cell seen in FIGURE 5G shows

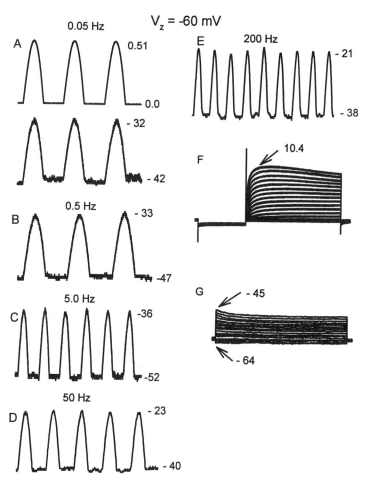

FIGURE 5. Traces obtained from a pigeon utricular type I hair cell located in the striolar region. (**A–E**) Current-clamp responses to rectified sine wave injection. The top trace in panel **A** is the current waveform for the 0.05 Hz injection. In **B–E** the peak current was also 0.51 nA, but the traces are not shown. In the bottom panel of **A** and in traces **B–E,** the membrane voltage (in mV) is shown. (**F**) Voltage-clamp response to a pulse protocol that consisted of hyperpolarizing the membrane to −110 mV for 100 ms and then applying a series of test pulses for 250 ms. The test voltages ranged from −70 mV to 70 mV in 10 mV increments. Peak current (in nA) in response to a 70 mV depolarizing voltage is indicated. (**G**) Current-clamp response to 250 ms current pulse injections. The current amplitude ranged from −0.024 nA to 0.054 nA in 0.005 nA intervals. Maximum and minimum peak membrane voltage in mV is indicated.

little relaxation at higher current injections. Its input resistance around V_z was 128 MΩ. Voltage responses to rectified current injections (zero to peak, 0.51 nA) were obtained at frequencies of 0.05, 0.5, 5.0, 50.0, and 200 Hz. From the traces in FIGURES A–E it can be seen: first, that the responses were exact duplicates of the current injection waveforms; second, that the membrane potential swings varied by only 7 mV over the entire frequency range (indicating little if any resonance); and, third, that no mathematical integration of the membrane potential oscillations occurred at 200 Hz.

It seems clear that the differences in the responses presented for type I and type II hair cells in FIGURES 4 and 5 are a result of different input capacitance, different input resistance, and different complements of ionic conductances. These parameters are summarized in TABLE 2 for pigeon and gerbil based on data from our laboratory.

TABLE 2. Parameters for Solitary Type I and Type II Hair Cells of the Gerbil and Pigeon[a]

Parameter	Animal	Property	Type II Hair Cell	Type I Hair Cell
Zero current potential (V_z)	Gerbil	—	-52.9 ± 11.1 mV, 9[b]	-66.6 ± 9.3 mV, 25[16]
Input resistance (R)	Gerbil	—	0.86 ± 0.27 GΩ, 5[16]	0.021 ± 0.014 GΩ, 25[16]
Input capacitance (C)	Gerbil	—	4.6 ± 1.2 pF, 5[16]	3.4 ± 1.7 pF, 24[16]
Cell time constant (RC)	Gerbil	—	4 ms[16]	0.03–0.4 ms[16]
—	Gerbil	Conductances	?	I_{KI}, $I_{K(Ca)}$[7]
—	Gerbil	Resonance	?	None
—	Gerbil	Bandwidth	?	Roughly flat to 1K Hz
—	Gerbil	Conductance channel blockers	?	I_{KI}—internal TEA (20 mM), external 4-AP (5 mM)[7] $I_{K(Ca)}$—external TEA (50 mM), 100 nM apamin but not 100 nM charybdotoxin[7]
Zero current potential (V_z)	Pigeon	—	-57 ± 11 mV, 15[18]	-70 ± 11 mV, 14[18]
Input resistance (R)	Pigeon	—	1.5 ± 0.8 GΩ, 15[6]	0.27 ± 0.23 GΩ, 81 (see FIG. 3)
Input capacitance (C)	Pigeon	—	12 ± 5 pF, 7[6]	5.5 ± 0.7 pF, 5[7]
Cell time constant (RC)	Pigeon	—	18 ms[6]	1.5 ms
—	Pigeon	Conductances	I_{KII}, $I_{K(Ca)}$, I_A, I_{Ca},[4] I_{IR}[d]	I_{KI}, $I_{K(Ca)}$
—	Pigeon	Resonance	59% of tested cells[6]	None at V_z or $V_h < -70$ mV[c]
—	Pigeon	Bandwidth	?	~flat to 500 Hz @ V_z (see FIG. 2)
—	Pigeon	Conductance channel blockers	I_A—external 4-AP (6 mM)[4] I_{KII}—external TEA (50 mM)[4]	I_{KI}—internal TEA (20 mM)[7] or external 4-AP (5 mM)[7]

[a]Mean ± SD,N. Also included are summaries of conductances and membrane potential properties.
[b]Rennie and Correia, unpublished observations.
[c]Ricci and Correia, unpublished observations.
[d]Masetto and Correia, unpublished observations.

In summary, an accumulating literature suggests that the filtering properties of hair cells involved in seismic detection (e.g., the saccule in some species) are different from hair cells of the utricle and semicircular canals, i.e., those involved in head tilt, translation, and rotation. No studies of hair cells in any of the above-mentioned receptors indicate that location alone or cell body morphology alone or ciliary bundle morphology alone or innervation pattern alone determines the filtering properties of vestibular type II or type I hair cells, because all of these parameters always appear to co-vary. Type II hair cells generally show the same cadre of ionic currents during development[24] across species and across vestibular receptors.[1] The combination of these ionic currents, input capacitance, and input resistance results in a low-quality electrical resonance of the membrane potential in the majority of pigeon semicircular canal type II hair cells,[6] for example, and a temporal summation of injected rectified sine waves at higher frequencies (e.g., 200 Hz) to produce sinusoidal oscillations about a plateau of the membrane potential (FIG. 4E). The low-input conductance around V_z and the more depolarized resting membrane potential found in isolated solitary type II hair cells could suggest that if the relationship of these parameters remain, *in situ,* type II hair cells could be more "sensitive" than type I hair cells. Type I hair cells, when compared to type II hair cells, show a stronger homogeneity in membrane properties (particularly conductances) across receptors.[8] These membrane properties produce in type I hair cells, at least around V_z, different filtering properties when compared to those of type II hair cells. Type I hair cells show little if any electrical membrane resonance around V_z. Type I hair cells can faithfully pass injected sinusoidal current up to around 1 kHz. And the high-input conductance of isolated type I hair cells causes smaller membrane potential swings than for comparable current injections into type II hair cells. These properties result from I_{KI}, the dominant current in type I hair cells. This current, partially activated at V_z, in isolated type I hair cells, sets a more negative resting membrane potential, a greater conductance at V_z, a decreased sensitivity around V_z, and an increased frequency response. Finally, although the input resistance of type I hair cells is a continuum, those cells with an input resistance above 100 MΩ show special filtering properties that may explain their addition to the neuroepithelium in amniotes. These properties discussed in this and another paper in this volume[17] suggest that *all* type I hair cells with an input resistance above a certain value (e.g., 100 MΩ) would behave identically and enhance membrane potential responses in the same narrow frequency range. These properties are derived from the input resistance of the cell as well as the activation kinetics and steady-state properties of the dominant current in type I hair cells, I_{KI}.

REFERENCES

1. CORREIA, M. J. 1992. Filtering properties of hair cells. Ann. N.Y. Acad. Sci. **656:** 49–57.
2. BAIRD, R. A. 1994. Comparative transduction mechanisms of hair cells in the bullfrog utriculus. I. Responses to intracellular current. J. Neurophysiol. **71(2):** 666–684.
3. KOYAMA, H., E. R. LEWIS, E. L. LEVERENZ & R. A. BAIRD. 1982. Acute seismic sensitivity in the bullfrog ear. Brain Res. **250:** 168–172.
4. LANG, D. G. & M. J. CORREIA. 1989. Studies of solitary semicircular canal hair cells in the adult pigeon. II. Voltage-dependent ionic conductances. J. Neurophysiol. **62(4):** 935–945.
5. CORREIA, M. J., A. J. RICCI & K. J. RENNIE. 1994. Characteristics of basolateral ionic currents in type I and type II hair cells dissociated from the pigeon. ARO Abstr. **509:** 128.
6. CORREIA, M. J., B. N. CHRISTENSEN, L. E. MOORE & D. G. LANG. 1989. Studies of solitary

semicircular canal hair cells in the adult pigeon. I. Frequency- and time-domain analysis of active and passive membrane properties. J. Neurophysiol. **62:** 924–934.

7. RENNIE, K. J. & M. J. CORREIA. 1994. Potassium currents in mammalian and avian isolated type I semicircular canal hair cells. J. Neurophysiol. **71(1):** 317–329.

8. RICCI, A. J., K. J. RENNIE & M. J. CORREIA. 1996. Electrophysiologic comparison of avian vestibular type I hair cells. Pflügers Arch. In press.

9. RICCI, A. J., K. J. RENNIE, G. A. KEVETTER & M. J. CORREIA. 1996. Morphologic identification of vestibular type I and type II hair cells in the pigeon and gerbil. J. Neurosci. Methods. Submitted.

10. MASETTO, S., G. RUSSO & I. PRIGIONI. 1994. Differential expression of potassium currents by hair cells in thin slices of frog crista ampullaris. J. Neurophysiol. **72(1):** 443–455.

11. BAIRD, R. A. 1994. Comparative transduction mechanisms of hair cells in the bullfrog utriculus. II. Sensitivity and response dynamics to hair bundle displacement. J. Neurophysiol. **71(2):** 685–705.

12. LEWIS, E. R. & C. W. LI. 1975. Hair cell types and distributions in the otolithic and auditory organs of the bullfrog. Brain Res. **83:** 35–50.

13. HOLT, J. R. & R. A. EATOCK. 1995. Inwardly rectifying currents of saccular hair cells from the leopard frog. J. Neurophysiol. **73(4):** 1484–1502.

14. EATOCK, R. A. & M. J. HUTZLER. 1992. Ionic currents of mammalian vestibular hair cells. Ann. N.Y. Acad. Sci. **656:** 58–74.

15. EATOCK, R. A., W.-Y. CHEN & M. SAEKI. 1994. Potassium currents in mammalian vestibular hair cells. Sens. Syst. **8(3–4):** 21–28.

16. RENNIE, K. J., A. J. RICCI & M. J. CORREIA. 1996. Electrical filtering in gerbil isolated type I semicircular canal hair cells. J. Neurophysiol. In press.

17. RICCI, A. J., K. J. RENNIE & M. J. CORREIA. 1996. A delayed rectifier conductance shapes the voltage response of type I hair cells. Ann. N. Y. Acad. Sci. This volume.

18. CORREIA, M. J. & D. G. LANG. 1990. An electrophysiological comparison of solitary type I and type II vestibular hair cells. Neurosci. Lett. **116:** 106–111.

19. RENNIE, K. J. & J. F. ASHMORE. 1991. Ionic currents in isolated vestibular hair cells from the guinea pig crista ampullaris. Hear. Res. **51:** 279–292.

20. GRIGUER, C., A. SANS & J. LEHOUELLEUR. 1993. Non-typical K^+-current in cesium-loaded guinea pig type I vestibular hair cell. Pflügers Arch. **422:** 407–409.

21. LAPEYRE, P. N. M., P. H. KOLSTON & J. F. ASHMORE. 1993. GABA$_B$-mediated modulation of ionic conductances in type I hair cells from guinea pig semicircular canals. Brain Res. **609:** 269–276.

22. SUGIHARA, I. & T. FURUKAWA. 1989. Morphological and functional aspects of two different types of hair cells in goldfish sacculus. J. Neurophysiol. **62:** 1330–1343.

23. HUDSPETH, A. J. 1983. Transduction and tuning by vertebrate hair cells. Trends Neurosci. **6(9):** 366–369.

24. SOKOLOWSKI, B. H. A., L. M. STAHL & P. A. FUCHS. 1993. Morphological and physiological development of vestibular hair cells in the organ-cultured otocyst of the chick. Dev. Biol. **155:** 134–146.

Ionic Current Contribution to Signal Processing by Toadfish Semicircular Canal Hair Cells[a]

A. STEINACKER[b]

Institute of Neurobiology
University of Puerto Rico Medical Sciences Campus
201 Blvd. del Valle
San Juan, Puerto Rico 00901

INTRODUCTION

The vertebrate vestibular semicircular canal system provides neural information in response to angular acceleration of the head to supply the necessary sensory signal for compensatory eye, head, and body movements. The sensory hair cells mediating this process are located across the crista of the canal with their hair bundles (multiple stereocilia and a single kinocilium) inserted into an overlaying gelatinous cupula. Movement of this hair cell bundle in its "on" direction results in a transduction current across the apical surface of the hair cell. The transduction current interacts with the ionic currents of the hair cell's basolateral surface to control transmitter release from the basal surface of the hair cell. To date, the outward ionic currents characterized in the basal surface of vestibular hair cells have been potassium currents.[1–10] Earlier experiments from isolated toadfish horizontal semicircular canal (HSCC) hair cells using whole-cell patch-clamp recording showed that both the species and kinetics of the potassium currents varied from cell to cell,[4,8] indicating that individual hair cells may be extracting different information from the sensory signal. The data below provide more quantitative information on the kinetics and pharmacological sensitivity of these HSCC hair cell basolateral potassium currents. In conjunction with the peripheral mechanics and afferent fiber properties,[11–15] this work using the toadfish HSCC as a model system may lead to an understanding of the process by which the peripheral vestibular canal system provides the necessary signal of angular acceleration to the central nervous system.

METHODS

HSCCs were removed from anesthetized, paralyzed toadfish (MS222, 50 mg/L sea water and Pancuronium, 40 μg/kg intramuscularly; Sigma, St. Louis, MO). The crista was divided before enzyme treatment into central and peripheral regions, as previously defined by Boyle *et al.*[13] The tissue was treated for 10 min in Sigma type A collagenase at 0.25 mg/mL (Sigma) in normal Ringer followed by a 20-min exposure to 0.5 mg/mL papain (Fluka Biochemicals, Switzerland) combined with 0.5 mg/mL trypsin inhibitor (Sigma) in calcium-free Ringer. Hair cells were maintained at 12 °C

---

[a] Much of this work was supported by NSF 9120497 and NIMH MH 48190 and was done at the Marine Biological Laboratory, Woods Hole, Massachusetts.
[b] E-mail: Toni@wums.wustl.edu

in a microscope dish perfused with teleost Ringer (in mM: NaCl 165, KCl 5, CaCl$_2$ 4, MgCl$_2$ 1, Hepes 10 adjusted to pH 7.2 with NaOH).

Quartz glass patch pipettes were filled with (in mM): KCl 165, CaCl$_2$ 0.1, MgCl$_2$ 1.5, Hepes K$^+$ salt 5, EGTA 10, and K$^+$ ATP 2.5. Using an Axoclamp B or D amplifier (Axon Instruments, Foster City, CA), a giga seal was made and pipette capacitance compensated. Following patch rupture to whole-cell voltage-clamp mode, series resistance and capacity were adjusted manually using the transient from a -20 mV pulse from a -60 mV holding potential, the holding potential used for all experiments here. Any remaining transient response to this -20 mV pulse was recorded at intervals throughout the experiment using pClamp to calculate residual series resistance and capacity from the time constant of decay and area of the transient. All command pulses were repeated with 5-s intervals to prevent inactivation of the currents during the trial.

Data acquisition and digitization were done using the Digidata interface (Axon Instruments) or a Labmaster interface (Scientific Solutions, Solon, OH). Data were filtered at 5 kHz and digitized on line at 10–50 kHz, depending upon the command protocol used. PClamp (V 6.0, Axon Instruments) was used to run the experiments and for data analysis. Ionic current activation time was measured as the 10–90% rise time. Rise time and current/voltage relationships were measured using peak current values. Quality factor (Q) and resonant frequency were calculated as given by Art and Fettiplace[16]: $Q = [(\pi * F_o \tau_o)^2 + \frac{1}{4}]^{1/2}$, where τ_0 is the time constant of decay of the membrane potential oscillation following current onset. The data below were taken from 52 hair cells selected for stable recording values from a larger pool of cells. Because recording time using patch-clamp methodology is often limited, two basic but optimal voltage command protocols and two pharmacological blocking agents were used to selectively define the current.

RESULTS

Resonance in Horizontal Semicircular Canal Hair Cells

In current-clamp recordings from the isolated HSCC hair cells, the membrane potential response to 100 pA current commands was assessed from several holding potentials set by manually varied holding currents (FIG. 1). As with saccular hair cells,[17] the HSCC hair cell resonance showed the highest Q values at holding potentials between -45 and -55 mV. The frequency having the highest Q value was used as the resonant frequency of that cell. At 12 °C, the resonant frequencies for HSCC hair cells ranged from 44 Hz to 360 Hz ($n = 7$). In several cells, it was possible to change from current clamp to voltage clamp to record the ionic current composition in cells from which resonance had been recorded. This current could be completely and rapidly blocked by TEA (2–20 mM) (FIG. 2). This same cell was subjected to a voltage protocol designed to reveal inactivation and to separate possible inactivating and non-inactivating currents (FIG. 3A). This consisted of a series of 1-s, 20-mV incremental voltage prepulses from -120 mV to $+20$ mV followed by a test pulse to $+40$ mV (FIG. 3). A class of cells showed no inactivating current in response to this voltage protocol (FIG. 3A). Based on the lack of inactivation in the outward current and the high sensitivity to the potassium current blocker TEA (FIG. 2), the current in these high Q resonant hair cells has been tentatively designated IKCa, and this current appears to be the only outward current in these hair cells. Only a small minority of the cells (approx. 10% of recorded cells)

A

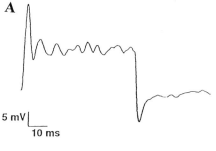

5 mV |
        10 ms

B

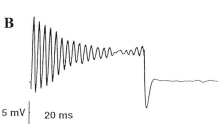

5 mV | 20 ms

FIGURE 1. In current-clamp mode, hair cells of the horizontal semicircular canal are capable of high-frequency, high Q resonance in response to a 100 pA command. Frequency (RF) and quality factor (Q) are shown to the right. These hair cells are of the class in FIGURE 2 and FIGURE 3A, which show no inactivating current.

showed no decrease in current with time or voltage in response to the above voltage protocol.

Two Outward Currents as Defined by Voltage and Pharmacological Protocols

In the majority of HSCC hair cells, the outward current showed partial inactivation in response to positive voltage command steps suggesting the presence of at least two components to the current. The outward current in response to the test pulse of +40 mV following a negative prepulse of −120 mV was a rapidly activating, inactivating, and deactivating outward current. Following the more positive prepulses, the response to the test pulse progressively lost the inactivating component until, at a prepulse voltage near −40 mV, the current in response to the test pulse had only a non-inactivating current. Subtraction of the test pulse current preceded by a −40 mV prepulse (depending upon the prepulse voltage necessary for complete inactivation) from the test pulse response preceded by a −120 mV prepulse, was used to separate the inactivating from the non-inactivating current (FIG. 4). Based solely on inactivation, this class of cells expressed at least two components in the outward current. When measured by tail current analysis, the outward current in both classes of cells shows a reversal potential close to the calculated K^+ equilibrium potential (−88 mV). When the response to the test pulse of +40 mV was plotted against prepulse voltages as the percentage of maximal test pulse response, normalized to 1, the inactivating current in this cell was 50% inactivated at −53 mV and fully inactivated following the prepulse of −40 mV. This response to the test pulse following different prepulse values is shown on an expanded time scale in FIGURE 4B and C. There, and in FIGURES 5–7 below, the rise time of the inactivating current is considerably faster than that of the non-inactivating component.

In some HSCC hair cells, all or most of the outward current appears to be an inactivating current. However, an additional calcium-dependent, non-inactivating current can be demonstrated by increasing the external calcium level from 4 mM to 10 mM (FIG. 5). Under these conditions, this additional current does not inactivate, and its rise time is slower than that of the inactivating current. That this is not a current from which inactivation has been removed by the increased calcium is shown by the slowing of the rise time of the additional current. Since inactivation can slow rise time by removing some channels from activity during the process of inactivation, a decrease in current activation time would be expected. The opposite effect is actually seen; current activation time slows (FIG. 5C). This lack of effect of increased calcium on inactivation has also been shown using Shaker potassium currents.[18]

To pharmacologically separate the inactivating and non-inactivating currents described above, two potassium current blockers (4-AP and TEA) were used whose concentration range and specificity for potassium channels in hair cells are well established.[5,16,17,19,20] In a cell that had shown a rapidly inactivating and a non-inactivating current in response to the prepulse, test pulse protocol described above, a rapid and complete block of the inactivating component of the HSCC hair cell current was produced by 1 mM 4-AP (FIG. 6B). An additional voltage protocol was used here, which consisted of +10 mV incrementing steps from −60 mV to +20 mV in order to assess the current/voltage relationship and activation time of the two current components. Using this protocol, 1 mM 4-AP left untouched a non-inactivating outward current while blocking completely the inactivating current

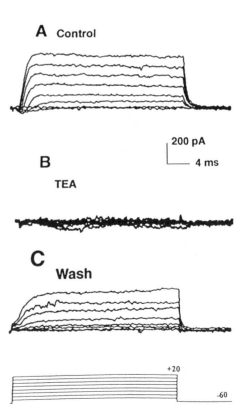

A Control

200 pA

4 ms

B

TEA

C

Wash

+20

-60

FIGURE 2. In some hair cells, the total ionic current of the hair cell can be reversibly blocked by low concentrations of TEA. These cells show no inactivation of outward current. See also FIGURE 3A.

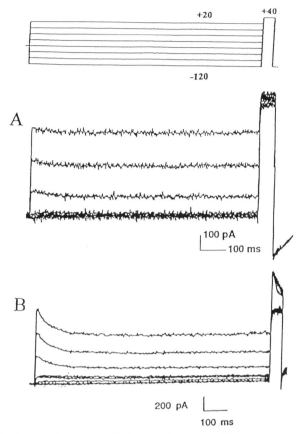

FIGURE 3. Total outward current profile in two cells showing different current composition in response to a protocol designed to reveal inactivation. Cell **A** has only a non-inactivating current in response to all test pulses; cell **B** expresses at least two outward currents, an inactivating and a non-inactivating component.

(FIG. 6). Again, it is readily apparent that the activation time of the 4-AP-sensitive current is faster than the 4-AP-insensitive current.

In some cells that showed an inactivating and non-inactivating current in response to the prepulse test pulse protocol, the cell was held long enough to separate two different current components in the same cell using two different blocking agents with Ringer wash between applications (FIG. 7). In FIGURE 7A, total outward current shows a small inactivating component. Application of 20 mM TEA left a residual current that showed a rapid inactivation (FIG. 7B). TEA was then removed by washing with control Ringer. When the current returned to control levels, the cell was exposed to 1 mM 4-AP. This blocked the inactivating current, leaving the non-inactivating component (FIG. 7C). In FIGURE 7 (plot to right), data taken from the use of TEA to separate the currents have been used to plot the current activation time (measured as the 10–90% rise time to peak current level). The activation of the TEA-sensitive, 4-AP-insensitive current was again slower than that of the TEA-insensitive, 4-AP-sensitive current. The same subtraction protocols and the data from 4-AP application yield the same results; that is, the TEA-insensitive, 4-AP-sensitive current activates more rapidly than 4-AP-insensitive, TEA-sensitive current.

Delayed Rectifier

The delayed rectifier (IK), so prominent in toadfish saccular hair cells,[17,20,21] was not seen in HSCC hair cells when the same voltage and pharmacological protocols

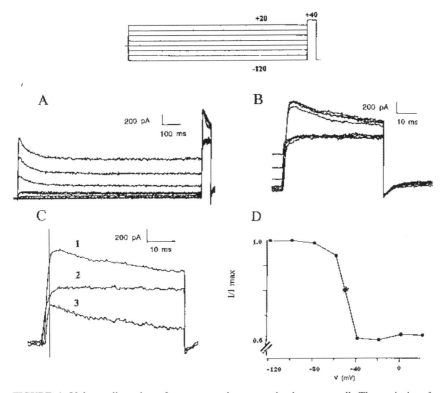

FIGURE 4. Voltage dissection of two outward currents in the same cell. The majority of horizontal semicircular canal hair cells show both an inactivating and a non-inactivating current (**A, B**). Data in **B** is the response to the 40 mV test pulse seen in **A**, plotted on a faster time base. **C** shows (on a yet faster time scale) the isolation of inactivating and non-inactivating components by subtraction. Trace 1 is the test pulse response following a −120 mV prepulse which contains both inactivating and non-inactivating currents; trace 2 is the response following the −40 mV prepulse from which the inactivating current has been removed by the positive holding potential. The subtraction of the non-inactivating current (2) from the total outward current (1) isolates the inactivating current (3). When the response to the test pulse following different voltage prepulses is plotted as the percentage of the maximum current, the voltage dependence of inactivation is revealed. The process of inactivation begins between −100 and −80 mV and is complete at −40 mV. The voltage for half inactivation is −53 mV (asterisk in **D**).

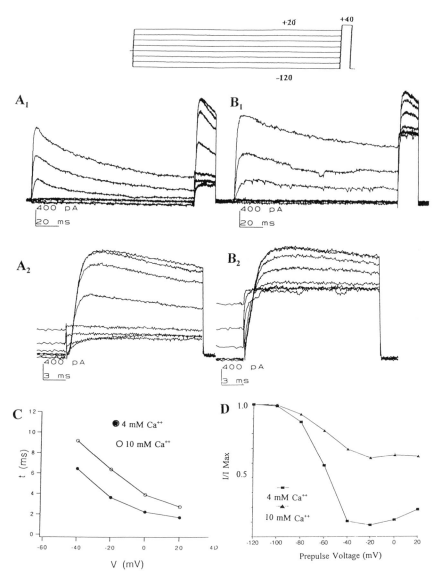

FIGURE 5. Some hair cells have no apparent non-inactivating current (**A**) in response to the voltage protocol consisting of variable voltage prepulses and a test pulse (shown above). However, increase of the calcium level in the bath (from 4 mM in **A** to 10 mM in **B**) reveals the presence of a non-inactivating current in the cell. In A_2 and B_2 are plotted the response to the test pulses on a faster time scale. When the 10–90% rise time of the prepulse current is plotted against prepulse voltage (**C**), the current evoked by the additional calcium in the bath (IKCa) shows a slower rise time than current from the same cell in control levels of calcium (4 mM). In **D**, the current in response to the test pulse at the two calcium levels is plotted as the current vs. maximum current (normalized) against prepulse voltage. Although little additional current is evoked at more negative prepulse voltages, perhaps due to the failure of hair-cell calcium channels to open at negative prepulse values (4, 16, 18), at more positive prepulse values, the additional current is seen in both the response to positive prepulses (arrows) and in the following response to the test pulses.

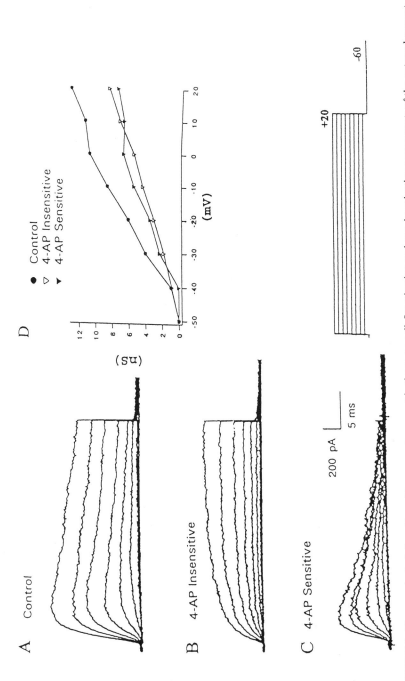

FIGURE 6. Pharmacological dissection of two currents present in the same cell. Inactivating and non-inactivating components of the outward current have a differential sensitivity to 4-AP (1 mM). (**A**) Control response to the voltage command protocol above. (**B**) Current remaining after exposure to 1 mM 4-AP. Subtraction of the 4-AP insensitive component (**B**) from total outward current (**A**) reveals the 4-AP sensitive current (**C**). (**D**) Plot of conductance vs. voltage for the three currents plotted in **A**, **B**, and **C**.

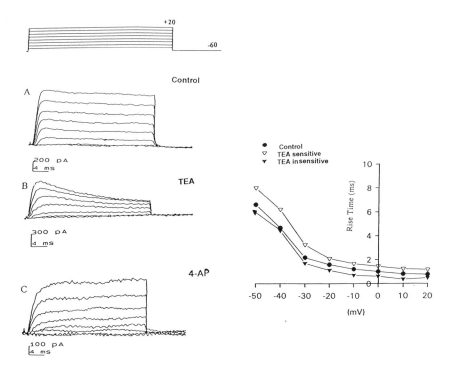

FIGURE 7. Inactivating and non-inactivating components of the outward current in the same cell have a different sensitivity to TEA and 4-AP applied sequentially. In **A,** the total outward current in response to the voltage command protocol shown above the current recording suggests the presence of an inactivating and a non-inactivating current in the cell. The cell was then exposed to 20 mM TEA and the same voltage protocol repeated, revealing an inactivating current **(B).** TEA was removed by Ringer wash and 4-AP (1 mM) applied **(C),** revealing the 4-AP insensitive non-inactivating current. When the rise time of the outward current (measured as the 10–90% rise time) is plotted against the command voltage, the TEA-insensitive current has a faster activation time than the TEA-sensitive current. This is an invariant finding in hair cells in which both currents are found together. When 4-AP is used as the blocking agent, the 4-AP-sensitive current shows the faster activation time.

were used as were used to define IK in saccular hair cells. In the toadfish saccular hair cells, insensitivity to TEA (2–25 mM), external calcium, and cadmium (0.5 mM) distinguished IK from IKCa. The slow inactivation process of IK distinguishes IK from the rapidly inactivating IA. However, in the cells of the HSCC, IK could not be unequivocally identified by any of the above means.

Inward Rectifier

Although no voltage command protocol was used to specifically explore the properties of the inward rectifier, its presence is revealed by the negative prepulses of the prepulse, test pulse protocol. This current was never seen in the "IKCa only" class of hair cells. (This had also been true for this class of hair cells in the toadfish saccule.) When the inward rectifier was found in the HSCC hair cells, it was always found in cells originating in the center of the crista.

Properties of the Hair Cell Bundle

The properties of the hair cell bundle differ between fish species and within end-organs of the same fish.[22,23] The hair cell bundle (stereocilia and kinocilium) of toadfish HSCC cells is considerably longer than that of the saccular hair cells of the same animal. The HSCC hair bundles with kinocilia exceeding 100 μm are shown in FIGURE 8. An equivalent light micrograph of the toadfish saccule is not available for comparison but the necessary information can be obtained from scanning electron micrographs of toadfish saccular hair cell bundles (A. Steinacker, unpublished data). The longest saccular hair cell bundles are found as a single border of cells at the outer edge of the macula and do not exceed 12 μm.[24]

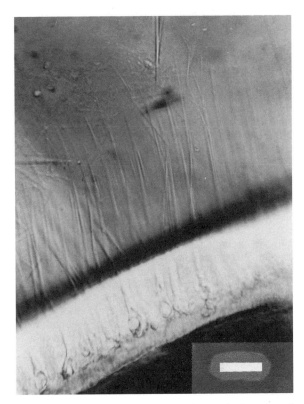

FIGURE 8. An optical slice of the horizontal semicircular canal crista taken through a section of the canal with intact crista and cupula using a 40× water immersion lens with Nomarski optics shows the relationship between hair cell soma and hair bundle length. Calibration bar equals 20 μm.

DISCUSSION

Unlike many animals where the semicircular canals are embedded in a dense temporal bone, the toadfish crista are virtually suspended in the cerebral spinal fluid, allowing easy access to the hair cells and afferent fibers. An additional advantage of the toadfish is that the toadfish has only type II hair cells. The toadfish belongs to the anamniotes—that is, it has not evolved the extraembryonic membrane containing the fetus and the amniotic fluid. Another characteristic of amniotes is the type I hair cell[25] and, perhaps more importantly, the evolution of the neck, around which the head may make rapid movements, independent of the body. Thus, the more simple HSCC of the toadfish, *Opsanus tau,* has many advantages for the study of sensory coding of angular acceleration.

On the basis of their ionic currents, two clear and separate classes of toadfish HSCC hair cells can be defined. As in the toadfish saccule,[20] a small subset of cells appears to express only one potassium current, and this current displayed the characteristics of an IKCa. This class of cells is notable for the complete absence of an inward rectifying current component in both saccule and crista. No regional (central vs. peripheral) distribution of the IKCa-only cell type was found. It is also in this class of IKCa-only cells that high Q, high-frequency resonance was found. The same was true for the cells in the toadfish saccule; the cells with IA did not show resonance.[17]

In the majority of the HSCC cells, two current components are seen in the total outward current. One current is a calcium[8] and TEA-sensitive, 4-AP-insensitive, non-inactivating current (IKCa), and the other a TEA-insensitive, 4-AP-sensitive, rapidly inactivating current (IA).[9] When this latter class of cells originated from the center of the crista, they were sometimes found with the inward rectifying potassium current. The same class of cells arising from the periphery of the crista did not express an inward rectifier. This regional distribution of the inward rectifier was also found in hair cells from the frog crista.[10]

In cells with IKCa-only, an inward current is visible as a small negative glitch preceding the outward current (FIG. 2A) and following TEA block of outward current (FIG. 2B). This is presumed to be a calcium current because, with possible exceptions,[26,27] the only inward current described in hair cells is carried by calcium. This class of cells appears to be similar to that described in the auditory system of the turtle[16] and the frog.[19] The IKCa in the resonating IKCa-only hair cells may differ from the IKCa found in combination with IA. In guinea-pig outer hair cells, two classes of IKCa, one of low conductance (SK) and another of high conductance (BK), were described.[28] In goldfish saccular hair cells, a range of unitary IKCa conductances, activation and deactivation times, and calcium sensitivities have been described.[29] More recently, separate classes of calcium-activated potassium channels that differ in their sensitivity to calcium and in their kinetics were described in the turtle auditory hair cells.[30] Further experiments are needed that are designed specifically to explore the properties of IKCa in HSCC hair cells to differentiate possible classes.

The interaction of IKCa and ICa kinetics and magnitude has been proposed as the source of the resonant frequency whose putative function is to sharpen the characteristic frequency of the cell. In these auditory end-organs, an inverse relationship exists between the hair cell bundle lengths and resonant or characteristic frequency;[16,31] this inverse relationship is not seen in the HSCC hair cells whose long hair cell bundles are paired with fast current kinetics and high resonant frequencies. The toadfish HSCC hair cell data can be compared with those from the saccule (the auditory end-organ) of this same animal taken using similar experimental methods but at 22 °C. On the basis of current thinking in the field, it would be expected that current kinetics of the saccule would be faster than those from the canal because the frequency range of toadfish hearing extends to 600 Hz,[32] whereas the natural frequency of HSCC stimulation via toadfish head movement is slower than 1 Hz. Endolymph deflection of the hair cell bundle would be at the frequency of the natural stimulation.

To compare resonant frequency or current kinetics taken from canal cells at 12 °C with those of toadfish saccular hair cells taken at 22 °C,[17,21] a Q_{10} of 2 was used. An experimentally measured Q_{10} of 1.8 has been reported for frog saccular resonance.[33] Using a Q_{10} of 2 results in a frequency range for HSCC hair cells of 88 Hz to 720 Hz compared to resonance values of 107 Hz to 175 Hz for the saccule. The range of resonant frequencies is in agreement with the ionic current kinetics in both end-organs. These discrepancies suggest that resonating HSCC cells must be specialized for processing a stimulus attribute other than frequency of endolymph movement resulting from head movement.

The same is true for the coexistence of fast current kinetics and long hair cell bundles coupled to low-frequency head movements. An alternative approach to the current feedforward concept of resonance is to have the membrane potential resonance feedback to tune the stiffness of the hair cell bundle to optimally extract a necessary attribute of the stimulus. In that case, an interaction between membrane potential resonant frequency and the mechanical frequency of the hair cell bundle is implied. Two options that would explain the linking of long hair bundles, fast current kinetics, and high resonant frequencies could be considered. The first is that long hair bundles are more capable of signal amplification because, for a given stimulus, the deflection at the hair bundle tip is greater the longer the hair bundle. Second, membrane potential resonance may make it possible to more accurately track low-frequency head and hair bundle movements with a high sampling rate in order to best preserve the head acceleration signal. A high-frequency update of stereocilia stiffness may be the end result of membrane potential resonance because both compliance and adaptation of the hair bundle are calcium and voltage sensitive. Such a feedback is implied in the description of active hair bundle movements and the membrane potential oscillations in the turtle auditory hair cells.[34]

Does the Coexistence of IKCa and IA Permit a Hair Cell to Switch Operating Modes depending on the Properties of the Stimulus?

Because the IA activates before IKCa over most of its operational range, IA will be the first outward current to respond to stimuli, and the response would be optimal for high-frequency low-amplitude events. Activation of this current may produce a short-lived delay in depolarization in response to the sensory stimulus and result in initial inhibition of transmitter release. This inhibition may be overridden by a maintained transduction or low-frequency slowly rising events that would remove IA by inactivation. In response to higher-amplitude low-frequency transduction currents, IKCa will be recruited by both the positive voltage and calcium entry, conditions favorable to removal of IA. The presence of these two currents with different kinetic properties and overlapping temporal and voltage ranges suggests that a hair cell may have two operating modes and be capable of switching between these modes in response to the transduction current and/or efferent transmitters. If the IKCa of IKCa-only hair cells differs from that of the IKCa found with IA, there would be three distinct operational modes in the hair cells of the crista.

ACKNOWLEDGMENTS

The author wishes to thank Dr. Stephen M. Highstein for the photograph of the HSCC hair cells in FIGURE 8 and Dr. Philip Bayly for helpful discussions.

REFERENCES

1. OHMORI, H. 1984. Studies of ionic currents in the isolated vestibular hair cell of the chick. J. Physiol. **350:** 561–581.
2. HOUSLEY, G. D., C. H. NORRIS & P. S. GUTH. 1989. Electrophysiological properties and morphology of hair cells isolated from the semicircular canal of the frog. Hear. Res. **38:** 259–276.
3. LANG, D. G. & M. J. CORREIA. 1989. Studies of solitary semicircular canal hair cells in the adult pigeon. II. Voltage-dependent ionic conductances. J. Neurophysiol. **62:** 935–945.
4. STEINACKER, A., J. MONTERRUBIA, R. PEREZ & S. M. HIGHSTEIN. 1992. Potassium current composition and kinetics in toadfish semicircular hair cells. Biol. Bull. **183:** 346–347.
5. NORRIS, C. H., A. J. RICCI, G. D. HOUSLEY & P. S. GUTH. 1992. The inactivating potassium currents of hair cells isolated from the crista ampullaris of the frog. J. Neurophysiol. **68:** 1642–1653.
6. GRIGUER, C., C. J. KROS, A. SANS & J. LOHOUELLEUR. 1993. Potassium currents in type II vestibular hair cells isolated from the guinea pig crista ampullaris. Pflügers Arch. **425:** 344–352.
7. RENNIE, K. J. & M. J. CORREIA. 1994. Potassium currents in mammalian and avian isolated type I semicircular canal hair cells. J. Neurophysiol. **71:** 317–329.
8. STEINACKER, A. & D. C. ZUAZAGA. 1994. Calcium and voltage sensitivity of potassium current activation in toadfish semicircular canal hair cells. Biol. Bull. **187:** 267–268.
9. STEINACKER, A., J. MONTERRUBIO, R. PEREZ, A. F. MENSINGER & A. MARIN. Outward currents of toadfish, *Opsanus tau*, semicircular canal hair cells: Electrophysiological and pharmacological characterization. Submitted.
10. MASETTO, S., G. RUSSO & I. PRIGIONI. 1994. Differential expression of potassium currents by hair cells in thin slices of frog crista ampullaris. J. Neurophysiol. **72:** 443–455.
11. RABBITT, R. D., R. BOYLE & S. M. HIGHSTEIN. 1995. Mechanical indentation of the vestibular labyrinth and its relationship to head rotation in the toadfish, *Opsanus tau*. J. Neurophysiol. **73:** 2237–2260.
12. RABBITT, R. D., R. BOYLE & S. M. HIGHSTEIN. 1994. Sensory transduction of head velocity and acceleration in the toadfish horizontal semicircular canal. J. Neurophysiol. **72:** 1041–1048.
13. BOYLE, R., J. P. CAREY & S. M. HIGHSTEIN. 1991. Morphological correlates of response dynamics and efferent stimulation in horizontal semicircular canal afferents of the toadfish, *Opsanus tau*. J. Neurophysiol. **66:** 1504–1521.
14. BOYLE, R. & S. M. HIGHSTEIN. 1990. Resting discharge and response dynamics of horizontal semicircular canal afferents in the toadfish, *Opsanus tau*. J. Neurosci. **10:** 1557–1569.
15. HIGHSTEIN, S. M., R. D. RABBITT & R. BOYLE. 1996. Determinants of semicircular canal afferent response dynamics in the toadfish, *Opsanus tau*. J. Neurophysiol. **75:** 565–596.
16. ART, J. J. & R. FETTIPLACE. 1987. Variation of membrane properties in hair cells isolated from the turtle cochlea. J. Physiol. **38:** 207–242.
17. STEINACKER, A. & A. ROMERO. 1992. Resonance and voltage gated potassium conductance in the toadfish saccular hair cells. Brain Res. **574:** 229–236.
18. LOPEZ-BARNEO, J., T. HOSHI, S. H. HEINEMANN & R. W. ALDRICH. 1993. Effects of external cations and mutations in the pore region on C-type inactivation of *Shaker* potassium channels. Recept. Channels **1:** 61–71.
19. HUDSPETH, A. J. & R. S. LEWIS. 1988. Kinetic analysis of voltage- and ion-dependent conductances in saccular hair cells of the bull-frog, *Rana catesbeina*. J. Physiol. **400:** 237–274.

20. STEINACKER, A. & A. ROMERO. 1991. Characterization of voltage gated and calcium activated potassium currents in saccular hair cells. Brain Res. **556:** 22–32.
21. STEINACKER, A. & L. PEREZ. 1992. Sensory coding in the saccule: Patch clamp study of ionic currents in isolated cells. Ann. N. Y. Acad. Sci. **656:** 27–48.
22. POPPER, A. N. 1977. A scanning electron microscopic study of the sacculus and lagena in the ears of fifteen species of teleost fishes. J. Morphol. **153:** 397–417.
23. PLATT, C. 1977. Hair cell distribution and orientation in goldfish otolith organs. J. Comp. Neurol. **172:** 283–298.
24. STEINACKER, A., D. MENTON & A. ROMERO. 1990. Toadfish saccular hair cell bundle has a preferred orientation in the otolithic membrane. Hear. Res. **48:** 145–149.
25. WERSALL, J. 1956. Studies on the structure and innervation of the sensory epithelium of the cristae ampullares in the guinea pig. A light and electron microscopic investigation. Acta Oto-Laryngol. Suppl. **126:** 1–85.
26. FUCHS, P. A. & M. G. EVANS. 1988. Voltage oscillations and ionic conductances in hair cells isolated from the alligator cochlea. J. Comp. Physiol. A **164:** 151–163.
27. WITT, C. M., H.-Y. HU, W. E. BROWNELL & D. BERTRAND. 1994. Physiologically silent sodium channels in mammalian outer hair cells. J. Neurophysiol. **72:** 1037–1040.
28. ASHMORE, J. F. & R. W. MEECH. 1986. Ionic basis of membrane potential in outer hair cells of guinea pig cochlea. Nature **322:** 368–371.
29. SUGIHARA, I. 1994. Calcium-activated potassium channels in goldfish hair cells. J. Physiol. **476:** 373–390.
30. ART, J. J., R. FETTIPLACE & Y.-C. WU. 1995. The calcium activated potassium channels of turtle hair cells. J. Gen. Physiol. **105:** 49–72.
31. CRAWFORD, A. C. & R. FETTIPLACE. 1981. An electrical tuning mechanism in turtle cochlear hair cells. J. Physiol. **312:** 377–412.
32. FISH, J. F. & G. C. OFFUTT. 1972. Hearing thresholds from toadfish *Opsanus tau* measured in the laboratory and field. J. Acoust. Soc. Am. **51:** 1318–1321.
33. SMOTHERMAN, M. S. & P. M. NARINS. 1995. Temperature dependence of resonant frequency in frog saccular hair cells. Soc. Neurosci. **21:** 397.
34. CRAWFORD, A. C. & R. FETTIPLACE. 1985. The mechanical properties of ciliary bundles of turtle cochlear hair cells. J. Physiol. **36:** 359–379.

Synaptic Organization of the Crista Ampullaris in Vertebrates[a]

ANNA LYSAKOWSKI[b]

Department of Anatomy and Cell Biology
University of Illinois College of Medicine
808 South Wood Street
Chicago, Illinois 60612

INTRODUCTION

In ongoing investigations of the vestibular sensory epithelium of two species, chinchilla and squirrel monkey,[1,2] certain general features of synaptic organization have become apparent. These have included regional variations in cytoarchitecture, in afferent innervation per hair cell, and in synaptology. A comparative overview of some of these synaptic features in vertebrates will be presented in this paper. These data are suggestive that more quantitative comparisons in a future study will be useful.

Previously, we have reported on the synaptic organization of the crista ampullaris in the chinchilla and squirrel monkey. One motivation for this previous ultrastructural work was earlier studies demonstrating that morphological and physiological properties varied regionally within the vestibular sensory epithelium.[3–5] In morphophysiological studies in mammals, three classes of afferents were demonstrated. (1) Calyx afferents, consisting of large chalice-shaped endings, were restricted to the central zone of the crista, had irregular spontaneous discharge patterns, and were less sensitive to head rotations compared to irregularly discharging dimorphic afferents. (2) Bouton afferents, consisting of solely bouton terminals, were restricted to the peripheral zone, had regular spontaneous discharge patterns, and were relatively insensitive to head rotations. (3) Dimorphic afferents, consisting of both calyceal and bouton terminals, were distributed throughout the crista and had spontaneous discharge patterns and response dynamics that varied depending upon their location within the sensory epithelium. Other investigators working with species lacking calyceal afferent terminals and thus type I hair cells, such as the guitarfish,[6] bullfrog,[7,8] and toadfish,[9,10] have shown comparable differences in the physiological properties of vestibular primary afferents. In the present work, we have chosen to report on ultrastructural observations made in the cristae of different species in several different vertebrate classes. The notion is that the properties of individual hair cells or the organization of the sensory epithelium help to determine the physiological properties.

The crista has been chosen because its organization is somewhat simpler than that of the macular end organs. From a survey of the material and the literature, one sees that there are similar regional variations in the macular end organs, with the striolar region equivalent to the central zone and the extrastriolar region equivalent to the peripheral zone. The cristae in different vertebrate classes exhibit many

[a]This work was supported by grants DC-02521 and DC-02290 and the University of Illinois Campus Research Board.
[b]E-mail: aLysakow@uic.edu

similar features: regional differences in the sizes and shapes of hair cells, in the numbers of afferent boutons per type II hair cell, and in the thickness of individual stereocilia and calyces.

METHODS

Samples were taken from cristae of species in diverse taxonomic classes, including skate, bullfrog, turtle, pigeon, zebra finch, mouse, rat, guinea pig, chinchilla, and rhesus monkey. In each case, animals were perfused transcardially with heparinized saline (pH 7.4), and then with a trialdehyde fixative consisting of 3% paraformalde-hyde, 2% glutaraldehyde, and 1% acrolein in a buffer, either 0.08 M sodium cacodylate buffer or 0.1 M phosphate buffer (for mammals) or a Ringer's solution (for submammalian species). End organs were dissected in buffer, postfixed with a solution of 1% OsO_4 in 0.08 M sodium cacodylate, rinsed with buffer, stained *en bloc* with 1% uranyl acetate, dehydrated in a series of graded alcohols, and embedded in Araldite. Serial semithin (2 μm) sections were cut with a glass knife and mounted on slides. Ultrathin sections were cut with a diamond knife (Delaware) and mounted on Formvar-coated single-slot grids. Grids were examined in a JEOL 100CX electron microscope.

RESULTS

Skate

The little skate, *Raja erinacea,* is an elasmobranch, or cartilaginous fish. One striking cytoarchitectural feature, observable even at the light microscopic level (FIG. 1A), is that fish vestibular end organs have no calyceal endings. The implication is that fish have only one type of hair cell, type II hair cells. In our observations of the crista ampullaris of the skate, we noted two types of hair cells. Both types are present in the central zone. One type is wider, with thicker stereocilia and cuticular plates, and contacts fewer afferent (about 2–4 per section for a total of about 6–12 per hair cell;[c] see TABLE 1) and efferent boutons than the other type. The other type has thinner stereocilia and cuticular plates and thus is similar to peripheral hair cells (see below). Within the central zone, most myelinated fibers lose their myelin just before entering the sensory epithelium. However, some fibers lose their myelin at a distance (10–15 μm) from the epithelium and then branch. Less commonly, other fibers keep their myelin for a short distance (≈ 2 μm) into the epithelium. One unanswered question remains: Are the hair cells innervated by thick fibers the same as those with thick stereocilia?

Hair cells in the peripheral zone are long and narrow with thinner stereocilia and cuticular plates than those in the central zone. Immature hair cells (indicated by

---

[c]From our previous serial section studies in which several whole hair cells were reconstructed, we learned that we can extrapolate from the number of bouton profiles present in a single ultrathin section to the total number present on an entire reconstructed hair cell. The total number was approximately three times the number present on a single ultrathin section. We have assumed a similar multiplicative factor for the other species in this study. For the purposes of this study and throughout the remainder of the paper, extrapolations are made instead of presenting quantitative data. Entries based upon such extrapolations are noted in TABLE 1 with an asterisk.

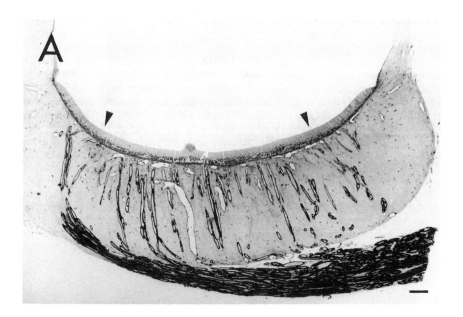

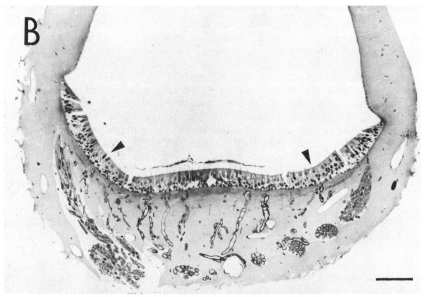

FIGURE 1. Longitudinal sections: (**A**) Skate horizontal crista and (**B**) bullfrog posterior crista. Central zone is the area between the arrowheads. Scale bar represents 100 μm.

short, thin stereocilia and a relatively undifferentiated cytoplasm) are also present, although mostly at the external margin of the peripheral zone. Hair cells with thinner stereocilia had more boutons in the peripheral zone (about 20 per hair cell) than in the central zone (about 6 per hair cell). Some features did not differ by region. Synaptic ribbons[d] were all spherical regardless of region (FIG. 5A and B, see TABLE 1). Efferent boutons did not appear to differ by region in number or type. They mostly terminated as C (cisternal)-synapses upon hair cells. Occasionally, however, efferent boutons terminated as postsynaptic densities (PSDs) onto afferent fibers. The efferent boutons had smaller mitochondria than afferent boutons, and their synaptic vesicles were smaller (FIG. 2A) compared to mammalian efferent synaptic vesicles (FIG. 2B), similar to the microvesicles observed in the toadfish by Sans and Highstein.[11] Typical dense core vesicles were also present within efferent boutons in the skate.

Other studies have suggested the possibility of different hair cell types in the fish. Recent studies from Popper's laboratory have described the heterogeneity of sensory hair cells in the fish utricle. Studies by Chang et al.[12] in the oscar (*Astronotus ocellatus*), a cichlid fish, and by Saidel et al.[13] in the goldfish, a cyprinid fish, describe striolar- and extrastriolar-type hair cells. Striolar or central hair cells have well-defined perinuclear cisternae located just below the nucleus, large perinuclear mitochondria, and small, clustered synaptic bodies. Striolar hair cells have an average of 15 synaptic ribbons per hair cell with 7.5 afferent boutons per hair cell and 4.3 efferent boutons per hair cell. Extrastriolar hair cells lack the perinuclear cisternae and contain large, individually dispersed synaptic bodies. Extrastriolar or peripheral hair cells have an average of 4.3 synaptic ribbons per hair cell with 1.7 afferent boutons per hair cell and 0.1 efferent boutons per hair cell. The authors suggest that striolar hair cells closely resemble amniote type I hair cells and extrastriolar hair cells resemble amniote type II hair cells. Not discussed explicitly in their paper, but an interesting question nonetheless, is whether all striolar hair cells were "striolar-type" or whether some extrastriolar hair cells were mixed in. Further confirmation for the idea of structural diversity in fish crista is seen in the recent work of Lanford and Popper[14] in the goldfish crista in which they described single enlarged afferent terminals that envelop the basolateral portion of several hair cells. Unfortunately, there is no mention of whether these enlarged terminals are found exclusively in the central zone or are present throughout the sensory epithelium.

Earlier work by Wegner[15] in the lagena of an anabantid fish (*Colisa labiosa*), and by Jensen[16] in the saccular and lagenar macular end organs of the herring (*Clupea harengus*), had similarly described two types of hair cells, one centrally located in an area that Wegner called region A (after Werner), and the other in the periphery, in an area termed region B. Based upon serial reconstructions of eight hair cells, Wegner determined that central hair cells were wide and short, with variations in mitochondria from small to large, with an average of 25 ribbons per hair cell with 11 per afferent bouton, 1.5 efferent boutons per hair cell, and thick fibers with large bowl-shaped endings. Jensen also described the innervation of the central area by large-diameter fibers (5–14 μm, ≈ 10% of total) and the presence of large T- or star-shaped nerve endings in the central zone. Jensen compared the latter to the giant candelabra nerve endings found in the cristae of cyclostomes such as the

---

[d]For simplicity, we use the term "synaptic ribbons," rather than "synaptic bodies," to mean all synaptic contacts that hair cells make with afferent processes. Sometimes these are in the shape of elongated bars, or "ribbons"; at other times they are in the shape of spheres, barrels, plates, etc.

TABLE 1. Comparative Overview of Synaptic Innervation of the Vestibular End Organs in Vertebrates

SPECIES Zones[a]	Cytoarchitecture HCs	Fiber Diameters (μm)	Stereocilia/ Cuticular Plate	Synaptic Ribbons OF[b]	Shapes, etc.	n/HC	Efferents Characteristics[c]	n/HC	Afferent Boutons per HC[d]	Other Features
FISHES										
Skate crista (*Raja erinacea*, present study)										
Central	Wide, long	0–20	Thick and thin	NA	All spheres	ND	C-synapses, microvesicles	ND	6–12*	Occas. myel. fibers in epith.
Peripheral	Narrow long Immature HCs	0–11	Thin	NA	All spheres	ND	Smaller mitochondria	ND	12–20*	No myel. fibers in epith.
Oscar utricle (*Astronotus ocellatus*, Chang et al.[12])										
Central	Wide, short Perinuclear cisternae	ND	ND	NA	All spheres, clusters	15	C-synapses, microvesicles	4.3	7.5	Myel. fibers in epith.
Peripheral	Narrow, low	ND	ND	NA	All spheres	4.3	No C-synapses	0.1	1.7	No myel. fibers in epith.
Anabatid lagena (*Colisa labiosa*, Wegner[15])										
Central	Wide, short	5–14[f]	ND	NA	All spheres, clusters	25	C-synapses	1.5	1–4	Myel. fibers in epith.
Peripheral	Narrow, long	>2[f]	ND	NA	ND	4	No C-synapses	0.0	1–3	No myel. fibers in epith.
Toadfish crista and utricle (*Opsanus tau*, Sans and Highstein;[11] Boyle et al.[10])										
Central		3–12	ND	NA	ND	ND	C-synapses, microvesicles PSDs	Many[e]	ND	Some microvesicles darken with cacodylate buffer
Peripheral		3–9	ND	NA	ND	ND		Many[e]	ND	
AMPHIBIANS										
Bullfrog crista and utricle (*Rana catesbiana*, present study)										
Central	Wide	0–18[g]	Thick and thin	NA	Large spheres	ND	C-synapses only	ND	15*	No myel. fibers in epith.
Peripheral	Narrow	0–11[g]	Thin	NA	All spheres	ND	No PSDs	ND	30*	No myel. fibers in epith. Liposomes in HCs thruout
REPTILES										
Turtle crista (*Pseudemys scripta*, present study)										
Central	Wide	0–7[h]	Thick (I)–thin (II)	yes	Large spheres, clusters	ND	C-synapses (II), PSDs (I)	ND	5–10*	Occas. myel. fibers in epith.
Peripheral	Narrow	0–3[h]	Thin (II)	no	All spheres	ND	Smaller mitochondria	ND	20–25*	No myel. fibers in epith.
Lizard crista (*Calotes versicolor*, Schessel et al.[25])										
Central	Wide	1–11	ND	no	Spheres	ND	C-synapses (II), PSDs (I)	ND	ND	Occas. myel. fibers in epith.
Peripheral	Narrow	1–5	ND	no	Spheres	ND	Smaller mitochondria	ND	ND	No myel. fibers in epith.

(continued)

TABLE 1. (Continued)

SPECIES Zones[a]	Cytoarchitecture			Synaptic Ribbons			Efferents		Afferent Boutons per HC[d]	Other Features
	HCs	Fiber Diameters (μm)	Stereocilia/Cuticular Plate	OF[b]	Shapes, etc.	n/HC	Characteristics[c]	n/HC		
BIRDS										
Finch crista (*Tupaia guttata*, present study)										
Central	Wide and short	ND	Thick (I)–thin (II)	yes	Spheres, plates, clusters	ND	C-synapses (II), PSDs (I)	ND	10*	No myel. fibers in epith.
Peripheral	Narrow and long Immature HCs	ND	Thin (II)	no	Spheres	ND	Smaller mitochondria	ND	18*	No myel. fibers in epith.
Pigeon crista (*Columba livia*, Correia *et al.*[28])										
Central	Wide and short	ND	Thick (I)–thin (II)	yes[e]	Spheres	ND	C-synapses (II), PSDs (I)	ND	ND	Myelination pattern ND
Peripheral	Narrow and long	ND	Thin (II)	ND	Spheres	ND	Smaller mitochondria	ND	ND	Myelination pattern ND
MAMMALS										
Rodent cristae and utricle (*Chinchillas, guinea pigs, rats and mice,* Lysakowski and Goldberg[i] present study)										
Central	Wide and short	0–7[i]	Thick (I)–thin (II)	yes	Spheres, bars, clusters	10	C-synapses (II), PSDs (I)	3–4	5–10	No myel. fibers in epith.
Peripheral	Narrow and long	0–6[i]	Thin (I and II)	no	Spheres, bars	20	Smaller mitochondria	3–4	25	No myel. fibers in epith.
Primate crista (*Saimiri and Rhesus,* Lysakowski and Goldberg[2] present study)										
Central	Wide and short	0–8[i]	Thick (I)–thin (II)	yes	Spheres, bars	10	C-synapses (II), PSDs (I)	2–4	11	No myel. fibers in epith.
Peripheral	Narrow and long	0–7[i]	Thin (I and II)	no	Spheres, bars	25	Smaller mitochondria	1–10	40	No myel. fibers in epith.

[a] Central zone refers to central (crista ampullaris) and striolar (otolith organ) regions. Peripheral refers to peripheral (crista ampullaris) and extrastriolar (otolith organ) regions.

[b] OF refers to synaptic ribbons in type II hair cells that synapse on the outer face of calyces surrounding type I hair cells.

[c] Characteristics for efferent boutons apply to all regions except in the case of *Astronotus* and *Colisa,* in which central and peripheral differences are noted.

[d] Afferent boutons per hair cell refers to type II hair cells in amniote species and to as-yet-undefined subtypes in anamniote species. In some cases (indicated by an asterisk), the numbers have been extrapolated from single section observations, by multiplying the number of boutons observed in a single section by three. Based upon previous serial section reconstruction studies, this appears to be a valid approximation.

[e] No regional distinctions given.

ND, not determined. Data on fiber diameters taken from *Jensen*[16]; *Honrubia et al.*[8]; *Brichta and Peterson*[45]; and *Lysakowski and Goldberg* (unpublished data). Those measured in the present study are unmyelinated axons diameters. HC, hair cell; PSD, postsynaptic density; myel., myelinated; epith., epithelium.

NA, not applicable; ND, not determined.

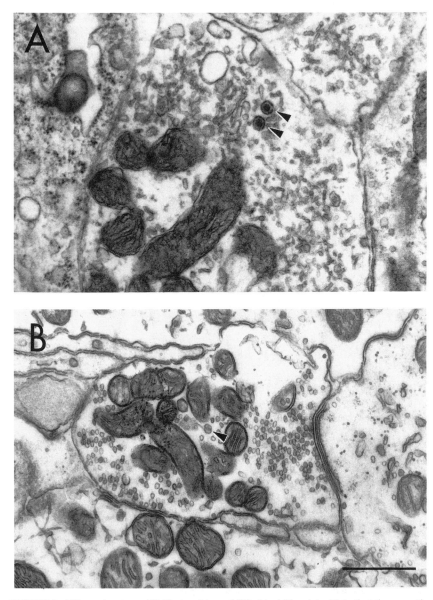

FIGURE 2. Efferent boutons: (**A**) Skate crista and (**B**) chinchilla crista. Note that the synaptic vesicles in the skate efferent are small ("microvesicles") compared to those in the chinchilla. Note also the dense-cored vesicles (*arrowheads*). Scale bar represents 0.5 μm.

lamprey,[17] and suggested that they might be forerunners of the calyceal endings of amniotes.

Based upon five serially reconstructed hair cells, Wegner found that peripheral hair cells were thin and long, with an average of 4 ribbons per hair cell, 1.5 ribbons per afferent bouton, and no efferent boutons per hair cell. Jensen reported that the peripheral area was innervated by small diameter fibers (2 μm or less, ≈50%). A transitional area innervated by intermediate-sized fibers (3–4 μm) was found between the other two regions.

Thus, morphological evidence exists that fish have two types of hair cells in the crista, even though they lack calyceal endings. One of these hair cell types is distributed throughout the sensory epithelium whereas the other is confined to the central zone.

Bullfrog

The bullfrog, *Rana catesbiana,* has no calyceal afferents and so, by definition, has only type II hair cells (FIG. 1B). In the crista ampullaris of the bullfrog, we noted again that these type II hair cells fall into two classes. Central hair cells are wider than peripheral hair cells. Hair cell length does not appear to vary significantly between the two regions. Central hair cells can possess either thick or thin stereocilia. Those with thick stereocilia contain larger, darker mitochondria. Central hair cells are innervated by thick fibers (up to 15 μm, unmyelinated axon diameter) that retain their myelin almost to the basement membrane. Peripheral hair cells possess long, thin stereocilia and are contacted by more boutons (about 30 per hair cell, see TABLE 1) than are central hair cells (about 15 per hair cell). In the periphery, thin fibers (about 3 μm in diameter) lose their myelin or become very thinly myelinated at distances of up to 20 μm away from the sensory epithelium. In sections through the entire length of the crista and the utriculus, only cisternal-type efferent synapses were observed; no PSD-type efferent synapses were observed. All synaptic ribbons observed were spherical in shape, regardless of region. Central ribbons were so large as to be visible at the light microscopic level under oil immersion (FIG. 5C and H) whereas peripheral ribbons were somewhat smaller (FIG. 5D).

Lewis and Li[18] described several hair cell types (A–G) based upon hair bundle composition. Based on microelectrode and morphological studies of hair cell properties in different regions of the bullfrog utriculus, Baird[19] noted four subtypes of hair cells. These hair cell subtypes were B (most common, thin stereocilia, confined to the extrastriola), C (thin stereocilia, striolar), E (bulbed kinocilium, thicker stereocilia, striolar), and F (thicker stereocilia, striolar). Morphologically, two of these subtypes, B and C, appear to be equivalent in regional distribution to type II hair cells in amniotes and to have response properties similar to those of regularly discharging afferents, whereas the other two types, E and F, are analogous to type I hair cells in amniotes with current and gain response properties similar to high-gain irregular afferents. Large club-like or claw-like endings[7,20] innervate the E cells, reminiscent of calyx endings in the amniote vertebrates. Physiologically, thick fibers with irregular discharge are characteristic of the central region of the crista.[7,8]

Flock and Orman[21] observed that in the bullfrog crista, the thickness (and therefore presumably the stiffness) of the stereocilia correlated to the response of the hair cell. Hair bundles with thick stereocilia, found mainly in the central zone, returned quickly (phasically) following displacement, while hair bundles with thin stereocilia, found throughout the crista, returned slowly (tonically) following displacement of their hair bundle. Baird and Lewis[7] found that the afferent response dynamics correlated with variations in the "length of the kinocilium relative to that of the stereocilia," suggesting that "kinociliary morphology ... determines the response dynamics of the receptor and, ultimately, the afferent discharge." Myers and Lewis[22] corroborated these findings and added further evidence for a direct correlation with the afferent innervation pattern. Thus, both studies found that the hair bundle responses corresponded to the response of afferents in the study by Honrubia et al.[8] Geisler et al.[23] showed the fiber diameter distribution to be similar to that of the mammal with the exception that they found fewer small-diameter fibers than in the mammal.

Turtle

The red-eared turtle, *Pseudemys scripta,* has type I hair cells restricted to two zones in the vertical cristae, one in the hemicrista on either side of a central eminentia (or septum) cruciatum (composed of supporting cells, the so-called torus), whereas type II hair cells are found throughout the crista (FIG. 3A). The horizontal crista consists of a single hemicrista. Both transverse sections through the central zone and longitudinal sections along the apex of the crista were examined. The former were used to examine the periphery near the base of the crista, and the latter to examine the peripheral zones near the planum and the torus. Central hair cells, both type I and type II, were wider than peripheral hair cells, which were type II hair cells. Type I hair cells, concentrated in the central zone, had stereocilia and cuticular plates that were thicker than type II hair cells anywhere in the sensory epithelium. Central type II hair cells were contacted by fewer, but larger, afferent boutons (about 5–10 per hair cell) than were peripheral type II hair cells (about 20–25 per hair cell). Postsynaptic density-type efferent synapses were observed on the afferent processes and on calyces surrounding type I hair cells, and cisternal-type (C-synapse) efferent synapses were observed on type II hair cells throughout the sensory epithelium (see TABLE 1). Efferent boutons of both types were particularly common and large in the central zone. Synaptic ribbons making contact with the outer face of calyceal afferents were common in the central zone. Our qualitative assessment was that synaptic ribbons were more common in type I hair cells contained within complex calyces and that these were often found in pairs. Synaptic ribbons were spherical in shape. No elongated ribbon synapses were observed. Central ribbons, as in the frog, were so large as to be visible at the light microscopic level under oil immersion (FIG. 5E); peripheral ribbons were smaller (FIG. 5F and G). One reciprocal synapse was observed. Some myelinated fibers were seen penetrating the sensory epithelium, but such fibers were restricted to the central zone.

Previous studies by Jorgenson on the ultrastructure of the turtle labyrinth[24] described thicker afferent fibers innervating the central zones of the two hemicristae and the striola of the macular end organs. He also described the segregation of type I hair cells into the central regions of the two hemicristae. Schessel et al.[25] corroborated the findings concerning fiber diameters in the lizard (*C. versicolor*). Furthermore, these authors added that they found no synaptic ribbons on the outer surface of calyces surrounding type I hair cells in 19 serially reconstructed calyx units. It was unclear, however, whether this was also true of calyces in dimorphic units, present in smaller proportions (17%) in the lizard than calyx units (78%). Such synaptic ribbons were first described in mammals by Engström et al.[26] and Ross et al.[27] They were found to be common in the central zone in both chinchillas and squirrel monkeys[1,2] and in turtles (present study) and have been observed contacting physiologically-characterized serially-reconstructed calyx units in the chinchilla (Lysakowski, unpublished observations). Of the species that have calyces and that were directly examined or reviewed for this paper, the lizard appears to be unusual in this lack of

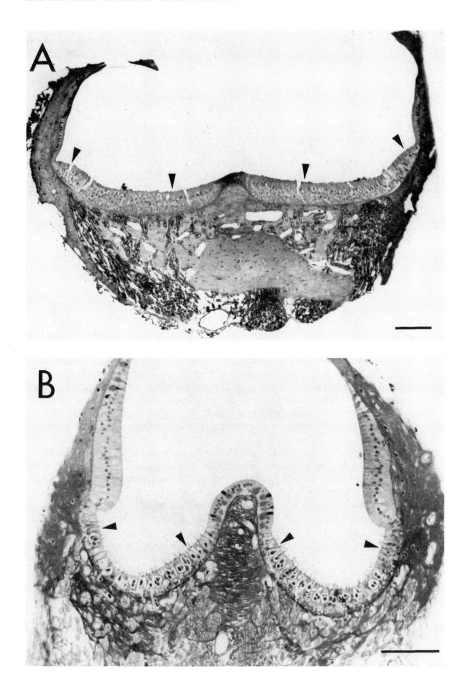

FIGURE 3. Longitudinal sections: (**A**) Turtle posterior crista and (**B**) zebra finch superior crista. Central zone is the area between the arrowheads in each hemicrista. Scale bar represents 100 μm.

outer-face ribbons (see TABLE 1). The lizard also has myelinated fibers extending into the sensory epithelium, similar to the turtle, but in the lizard they penetrate both the central and intermediate zones, rather than being restricted to the central zone as in the turtle.

Zebra Finch

The zebra finch, *Taeniopygia guttata,* has a sensory epithelium similar to the pigeon and the turtle, in that there is a central zone containing predominantly type I hair cells and a concentric peripheral zone that contains only type II hair cells (FIG. 3B). These are contained within each hemicrista. Immature hair cells, characterized by short thin stereocilia and a relatively undifferentiated cytoplasm, were occasionally observed in the periphery. The vertical cristae have an extensive septum cruciatum and type II hair cells that extend onto the planum semilunatum. The horizontal crista actually consists of a single hemicrista, sloped to an angle approaching 45°. The peripheral zone near the septum cruciatum differs slightly from that near the planum semilunatum; that is, although both contain exclusively type II hair cells, the hair cells near the planum are longer and thinner and in possession of much longer, thinner stereocilia than those near the septum cruciatum. There were more afferent boutons per type II hair cell in the peripheral zone (about 18 per hair cell) than in the central zone (about 10 per hair cell).

In terms of synaptic innervation, synaptic ribbons were common in type I hair cells, and outer-face ribbons were common between central type II hair cells and the outer face of calyces surrounding type I hair cells (FIG. 5L). Most synaptic ribbons were small spheres (FIG. 5I–L), and they frequently occurred in clusters, particularly in the central zone (FIG. 5I). In one instance, however, a large elongated plate-like ribbon was observed (not shown) in a central type II hair cell synapsing on the outer surface of a complex calyx containing five type I hair cells visible in a single section. Efferent boutons were observed making synaptic contacts of the appropriate type on both the outer surface of calyces surrounding type I hair cells and on type II hair cells.

A previous ultrastructural study on the crista ampullaris in pigeons done in Correia's laboratory[28] has noted the unusually large numbers of type I hair cells found in single complex calyces (71.7% of all calyces are complex (multiple) and contain 2–12 type I hair cells each). This study also provided some details about synaptic innervation, namely, that synaptic ribbons are spherical, efferents come in two varieties, outer-face calyx ribbons are present (although regional location is not noted, a central location is assumed in TABLE 1), and calyceal invaginations are present. Estimates of the numbers of synaptic ribbons, efferent boutons or afferent boutons per hair cell were not determined. Examination of their published micrographs reveals that stereocilia do vary in thickness between type I and type II hair cells, at least in the central zone, and that type I hair cells bulge at their apical surfaces as they do in other species.

Mouse

The albino mouse, *Mus musculus,* has a sensory epithelium similar to other rodents (FIG. 4A), for example, the rat,[25] guinea pig (Lysakowski, unpublished observations), gerbil (Fernández, personal communication), and chinchilla.[1,29,30] Type I and type II hair cells are evenly distributed throughout the epithelium. The

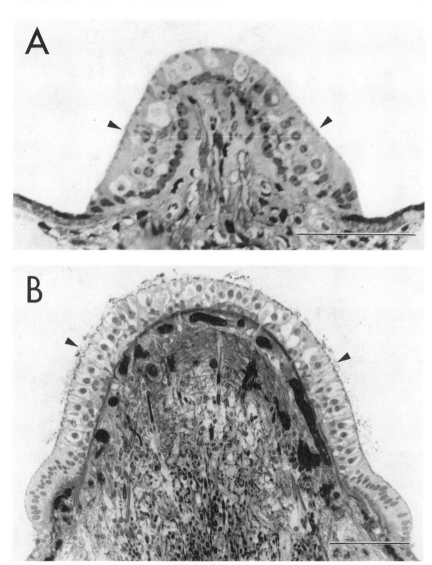

FIGURE 4. Transverse sections: **(A)** Mouse horizontal crista and **(B)** macaque superior crista. Central zone is the area between the arrowheads. Scale bar represents 100 μm.

apical surfaces of type I hair cells bulge compared to type II hair cells. A septum cruciatum exists in the vertical semicircular canals in the mouse, rat, and gerbil, but not in the chinchilla. The number of afferent boutons per type II hair cell in the central zone of the mouse crista is about 5–10, whereas the number in the periphery is about 20–25. Efferent innervation is similar to other rodents with about three efferent boutons per hair cell. As in the chinchilla, synaptic ribbons in type I hair cells in mice are typically small and spherical (FIG. 5M), although occasionally elongated

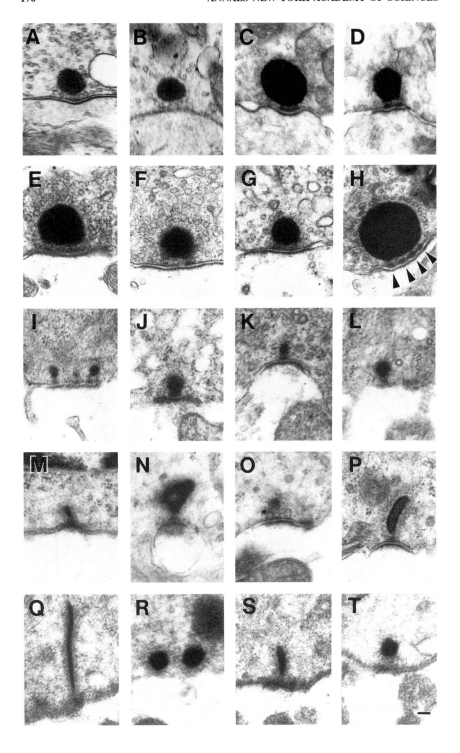

ribbons are found (FIG. 5P). Ribbons in type II hair cells are more variable, ranging from small spheres or bars, to large hollow ribbons (FIG. 5N), especially in the central region as compared to the peripheral region. Outer-face ribbons were also common in the central zone (FIG. 5O), as noted before.[1,2]

Rhesus Monkey

The rhesus monkey, *Macaca mulatta*, has a sensory epithelium (FIG. 4B) similar to the other primate that we and others have previously studied, the squirrel monkey.[2,26] The ratio of type I hair cells to type II hair cells is comparable to those we obtained in the squirrel monkey (3:1 compared to 1:1 in rodents[30,31]). As might be expected with fewer type II hair cells in the sensory epithelium, the number of calyx units in monkeys is three times higher than in rodents, while the number of bouton units is less than half.[31] There were fewer afferent boutons per type II hair cell (and slightly more efferent boutons) in the central zone (≈ 15 per hair cell) than in the peripheral zone (≈ 24 per hair cell), similar to our results in the squirrel monkey. With far fewer type II hair cells in the monkey, particularly in the central zone, the implication for synaptic innervation is that far fewer outer-face synaptic ribbons are found; indeed, none were observed in our samples of macaque crista, almost assuring that the calyx units found there receive input exclusively from type I hair cells. Synaptic ribbons in type I hair cell ribbons were either elongated (FIG. 5Q and S) or spherical (FIG. 5T), whereas type II hair cell ribbons showed variations in size and

←—————————————————————————————

FIGURE 5. Synaptic ribbons taken from different regions and hair cell types in several vertebrates. In each case, the hair cell type and region are given. (**A**) Central zone of the skate crista. (**B**) Peripheral zone of the skate crista. (**C**) Central zone of the bullfrog crista. (**D**) Peripheral zone of the bullfrog crista. (**E**) Type I hair cell contained within a complex calyx in the central zone of the turtle crista. (**F**) Type II hair cell in the peripheral (torus or septum cruciatum) zone of the turtle crista. (**G**) Type II hair cell in the peripheral (planum) zone of the turtle crista. (**H**) Striola of the bullfrog sacculus. Note the four presynaptic specializations (*arrowheads*) present between the spherical ribbon and the presynaptic membrane. These are also present in **C**, but not as clearly as shown here. (**I**) Type I hair cell contained within a complex calyx in the central zone of the zebra finch crista. Note triplet of synaptic ribbons; the middle one is not fully in this plane of section. Clusters of synaptic ribbons such as this were common in the central zone of the finch crista. (**J**) Type II hair cell in the peripheral (septum cruciatum) zone of the zebra finch crista. (**K**) Type II hair cell in the peripheral (planum) zone of the zebra finch crista. (**L**) Type II hair cell making synaptic contact with the outer surface of the calyx surrounding a type I hair cell in the central zone of the zebra finch crista. (**M**) Type I hair cell in the central zone of the mouse crista. (**N**) Type II hair cell in the central zone of the mouse crista. Central core of this ribbon is less electron dense than the rim. Such "hollow" or "barrel-shaped" ribbons were commonly found in the central zone (13% of total central ribbons in the chinchilla) in our previous ultrastructural studies. (**O**) Type II hair cell making synaptic contact with the outer surface of the calyx surrounding a type I hair cell in the central zone of the mouse crista. (**P**) Type I hair cell in the medial extrastriola of the mouse utriculus. Note elongated shape of ribbon. (**Q**) Type I hair cell contained in a complex calyx in the central zone of the macaque crista. Note elongated shape of ribbon. Both elongated and spherical ribbons were observed in type I hair cells in the macaque. (**R**) Type II hair cell in the central zone of the macaque crista. Note pair of synaptic ribbons. Multiple ribbons were more common in the central zone of all amniote species examined. (**S**) Elongated ribbon found in a type I hair cell in the peripheral zone of the macaque crista. (**T**) Spherical ribbon found in a type II hair cell in the peripheral zone of the macaque crista. Scale bar for all panels in this figure represents 0.1 μm.

shape, i.e., they were more often multiple and larger in the central zone (FIG. 5R) compared to the peripheral zone (not shown).

DISCUSSION

Regional variations in morphology and physiology in the crista ampullaris have been well documented now in several different species (fish;[10] turtle, Brichta and Goldberg, this volume; chinchilla;[3] and squirrel monkey[5]) and appear to be a general feature of vestibular sensory processing in vertebrates. Elements proposed to be responsible for these regional differences range from hair cell characteristics (such as hair cell size, hair bundle composition, and membrane ionic channel distribution) to afferent characteristics (such as myelination pattern, terminal morphology, and membrane ionic channel distribution). Efferent effects may even influence regional response dynamics. Recent work from Peracchio's laboratory (Purcell and Perachio, this volume) has demonstrated a differential distribution of efferents within different regions of the end organ based upon the projection pattern from the efferent nucleus in the brain stem.

The properties of hair cells that appear to be conserved through vertebrate phylogeny include characteristics of the hair bundle, cytoplasmic composition, and membrane ionic channel composition. Previous studies have described the use of individual characteristics of stereocilia[32] (such as diameter and length) and hair bundle size[33] as criteria to distinguish between type I and type II hair cells. Such criteria have proven extremely useful and have been extended to other species in the present study, such that it is possible to distinguish different hair cell types in species in which there are no calyceal afferents. Previous studies have also used stereociliary differences and other criteria to distinguish different hair cell types in anamniotes (fish[12] and frogs[7,18,19,21]). Studies of vestibular hair cell response properties have demonstrated in some cases that many of the response properties of hair cells mirror those of the afferents they supply.[7,19,21,22] Recent patch-clamp studies in several amniote species have determined that type I and type II hair cells have distinctive potassium ion channels (e.g., turtle, Brichta, Eatock, and Goldberg, personal communication; pigeons;[34] guinea pigs;[35] rats;[36] mouse, Rüsch and Eatock, this volume). Future patch-clamp studies may show that ionic currents in anamniote hair cells also correlate with differing morphological types of hair cells.

Properties of afferents that are conserved through phylogeny are spontaneous discharge patterns, certain sinusoidal response dynamics (phase and gain), regional fiber diameter distribution, and myelination patterns. One group of central fibers is thick and myelinated right up to the basement membrane or even a short distance into the sensory epithelium. These myelinated fibers have been demonstrated in amniotes to be calyx units, as morphophysiological,[25] ultrastructural ("M" fibers of Ross et al.[27]), and HRP- and immunolabeled afferent[32] studies have shown. A second group of central fibers is composed of medium to thick fibers that lose their myelin at some short distance from the epithelium. These are dimorphic fibers (or "M/U" fibers, according to Ross and colleagues), based upon evidence from the same studies. Thinner fibers in the periphery that lose their myelin at some distance from the epithelium can be either dimorphic or bouton fibers. No clear means of distinguishing dimorphic or bouton fiber types on purely morphological grounds exists yet. Thus, in mammals[3,5] and reptiles,[25] we can correlate calyx units or M fibers with relatively low-gain irregularly discharging afferent and dimorphic units or M/U fibers with high-gain irregularly discharging afferents. Because we have the same two morphological types (myelinated and unmyelinated fibers) in anamniotes (fish and frogs) and we have studies showing similar physiological classes,[6–8,10] it seems likely, but remains to be verified that the correlation also holds in anamniotes.

Specific efferent effects upon vestibular afferents do not appear to be conserved throughout phylogeny. Efferent effects upon afferents have been found to be either purely excitatory, as in the monkey,[37] or have been mixed (excitatory and/or inhibitory), as in the toadfish[10] (also, Highstein, personal communication), frog[38,39] and turtle (Brichta and Goldberg, this volume), where both effects (increases and decreases in afferent discharge rate) have been observed. One possibility to explain such effects is that one of the effects is postsynaptic (PSD-type, on the afferent) and the other is presynaptic (cisternal-type, on the hair cell). We might then expect to find only one type of efferent contact in mammals and both types of efferent contact in toadfish and turtles. This, however, does not appear to be the case in mammals. Conversely, frogs have both types of efferent effects and yet have no direct efferent-afferent contacts (demonstrated by both physiological studies in which efferent stimulation did not evoke direct EPSPs or IPSPs in afferents[39] and the present ultrastructural results in which no PSDs were observed). On the other hand, turtles have both effects (in fact, the two effects, excitation and inhibition, are regionally segregated; see Brichta and Goldberg, this volume), yet the two types of efferent contacts are not regionally segregated.

Another possibility to explain the differing efferent effects is that there are different types of cholinergic receptors. Several recent preliminary studies have presented evidence for this. Some studies have shown different nicotinic receptor subunits in different regions of the epithelium in light microscopic *in situ* hybridization experiments. Alpha-9 subunits have been found on hair cells (indicating a presynaptic, or hair cell, location for cholinergic effects) in both the cochlear[40] and the vestibular[41] sensory epithelium, whereas α-7 subunits have been found on type I cochlear ganglion cells[42] and α-4[43] and α-4–7[41] subunits have been found on vestibular ganglion cells (indicating a postsynaptic, or afferent, location for cholinergic effects). In addition, muscarinic receptor subtypes M1, M2, and M5 have been identified from recent molecular biological studies[44] as being present in human vestibular sensory ganglia and in end-organ tissue (thought to be consistent with a localization in type II hair cells). Such studies indicate that presynaptic and postsynaptic cholinergic effects can be explained by both ligand-gated (presumably inhibitory, such as a regular nicotinic receptor coupled to a potassium channel, or the more unusual α-9 receptor subtypes) and metabotropic (presumably excitatory, such as muscarinic) receptor mechanisms.

Whatever the calyx is doing—and an interesting theoretical discussion of its purpose is presented by Goldberg (this volume)—its sole purpose is not to enable anatomists to distinguish type I hair cells from type II hair cells. We are confident that these will be defined eventually by other means, presumably morphological, biochemical, and patch-clamp studies. Phylogenetically, the calyx had forerunners in the candelabra and giant club-like endings of anamniotes. It emerged in restricted zones of the vestibular sensory epithelium in reptiles, became a very elaborate structure in birds where it can enclose many hair cells at once, and finally became dispersed throughout the epithelium in mammals. One key to its function may come from this regional distribution.

ACKNOWLEDGMENTS

The technical assistance of Steven Price and Victoria Johnson is greatly appreciated. The author is also grateful to the Electron Microscopic Facility of the Research

Resources Center of the University of Illinois at Chicago for providing equipment and assistance to conduct this study.

REFERENCES

1. LYSAKOWSKI, A. & J. M. GOLDBERG. 1989. Regional variations in the synaptic organization of the chinchilla cristae. Soc. Neurosci. Abstr. **15:** 502.
2. LYSAKOWSKI, A. & J. M. GOLDBERG. 1993. Regional variations in the synaptic organization of the squirrel monkey cristae. Soc. Neurosci. Abstr. **19:** 1578.
3. BAIRD, R. A., G. DESMADRYL, C. FERNÁNDEZ & J. M. GOLDBERG. 1988. The vestibular nerve of the chinchilla. II. Relation between afferent response properties and peripheral innervation patterns in the semicircular canals. J. Neurophysiol. **60:** 182–203.
4. GOLDBERG, J. M., G. DESMADRYL, R. A. BAIRD & C. FERNÁNDEZ. 1990. The vestibular nerve of the chinchilla. V. Relation between afferent discharge properties and peripheral innervation patterns in the utricular macula. J. Neurophysiol. **63:** 791–804.
5. LYSAKOWSKI, A., L. B. MINOR, C. FERNÁNDEZ & J. M. GOLDBERG. 1995. Physiological identification of morphologically distinct afferent classes innervating the cristae ampullares of the squirrel monkey. J. Neurophysiol. **73:** 1270–1281.
6. O'LEARY, D. P. & R. F. DUNN. 1976. Analysis of afferent responses from isolated semicircular canal of the guitarfish using rotational acceleration white-noise inptus. I. Correlation of response dynamics with receptor innervation. J. Neurophysiol. **39:** 631–644.
7. BAIRD, R. A. & E. R. LEWIS. 1986. Correspondences between afferent innervation patterns and response dynamics in the bullfrog utricle and lagena. Brain Res. **369:** 48–64.
8. HONRUBIA, V., L. F. HOFFMAN, S. SITKO & I. R. SCHWARTZ. 1989. Anatomic and physiological correlates in bullfrog vestibular nerve. J. Neurophysiol. **61:** 688–701.
9. BOYLE, R. & S. M. HIGHSTEIN. 1990. Resting discharge and response dynamics of horizontal semicircular canal afferents of the toadfish, *Opsanus tau.* J. Neurosci. **10:** 1557–1569.
10. BOYLE, R., J. P. CAREY & S. M. HIGHSTEIN. 1991. Morphological correlates of response dynamics and efferent stimulation in horizontal semicircular canal afferents of the toadfish, *Opsanus tau.* J. Neurophysiol. **66:** 1504–1521.
11. SANS, A. & S. M. HIGHSTEIN. 1984. New ultrastructural features in the vestibular labyrinth of the toadfish, *Opsanus tau.* Brain Res. **308:** 191–195.
12. CHANG, J. S. Y., A. N. POPPER & W. M. SAIDEL. 1992. Heterogeneity of sensory hair cells in a fish ear. J. Comp. Neurol. **324:** 621–640.
13. SAIDEL, W. M., P. J. LANFORD, H. Y. WAN & A. N. POPPER. 1995. Hair cell heterogeneity in the goldfish saccule. Brain Behav. Evol. **46:** 362–370.
14. LANFORD, P. J. & A. N. POPPER. 1996. A novel afferent terminal structure in the crista ampullaris of the goldfish, *Carassius auratus.* J. Comp. Neurol. **366:** 572–579.
15. WEGNER, N. 1982. A qualitative and quantitative study of a sensory epithelium in the inner ear of a fish (*Colisa labiosa;* Anabantidae). Acta Zool. **63:** 133–146.
16. JENSEN, J. C. 1984. On the polarization and innervation of the pars inferior sensory epithelia of the herring labyrinth. Acta Zool. **65:** 61–74.
17. LOWENSTEIN, O., M. P. OSBORNE & R. A. THORNHILL. 1968. The anatomy and ultrastructure of the labyrinth of the lamprey (*Lampetra fluviatilis*). Proc. R. Soc. Lond. B **170:** 113–134.
18. LEWIS, E. R. & C. W. LI. 1975. Hair cell types and distributions in the otolithic and auditory organs of the bullfrog. Brain Res. **83:** 35–50.
19. BAIRD, R. A. 1992. Morphological and electrophysiological properties of hair cells in the bullfrog utriculus. Ann. N.Y. Acad. Sci. **656:** 12–26.
20. BAIRD, R. A. & N. R. SCHUFF. 1992. Peripheral innervation patterns of vestibular nerve afferents in the bullfrog utriculus. J. Comp. Neurol. **342:** 279–298.
21. FLOCK, Å. & A. ORMAN. 1983. Micromechanical properties of sensory hairs on receptor cells of the inner ear. Hear. Res. **211:** 249–260.

22. MYERS, S. F. & E. R. LEWIS. 1990. Hair cell tufts and afferent innervation of the bullfrog crista ampullaris. Brain Res. **534:** 15–24.
23. GEISLER, C. D., W. A. VAN BERGEIJK & L. S. FRISHKOPF. 1964. The inner ear of the bullfrog. J. Morphol. **114:** 43–58.
24. JORGENSON, J. M. 1974. The sensory epithelium of the inner ear of two turtles, *Testudo graeca L.* and *Pseudemys scripta* (Schoepff). Acta Zool. **55:** 289–298.
25. SCHESSEL, D. A., R. GINZBURG & S. M. HIGHSTEIN. 1991. Morphophysiology of synaptic transmission between type I hair cells and vestibular primary afferents. An intracellular study employing horseradish peroxidase in the lizard, *Calotes versicolor.* Brain Res. **544:** 1–16.
26. ENGSTRÖM, H., H. B. BERGSTRÖM & H. W. ADES. 1972. Macula utriculi and macula sacculi in the squirrel monkey. Acta Otolaryngol. Suppl. **301:** 75–126.
27. ROSS, M. D., C. M. ROGERS & K. M. DONOVAN. 1985. Innervation patterns in rat saccular macula. Acta Otolaryngol. **102:** 75–86.
28. CORREIA, M. J., D. G. LANG & A. R. EDEN. 1985. A light and transmission electron microscope study of the neural processes within the pigeon anterior semicircular canal neuroepithelium. *In* Contemporary Sensory Neurobiology. Prog. Clin. Biol. Res. **176:** 247–262.
29. GOLDBERG, J. M., A. LYSAKOWSKI & C. FERNÁNDEZ. 1990. Morphophysiological and ultrastructural studies in the mammalian cristae ampullares. Hear. Res. **49:** 89–102.
30. GOLDBERG, J. M., A. LYSAKOWSKI & C. FERNÁNDEZ. 1992. Structure and function of vestibular nerve fibers in the chinchilla and squirrel monkey. Ann. N.Y. Acad. Sci. **656:** 92–107.
31. FERNÁNDEZ, C., A. LYSAKOWSKI & J. M. GOLDBERG. 1995. Hair cell counts and afferent innervation patterns in the cristae ampullares of the squirrel monkey. J. Neurophysiol. **73:** 1253–1269.
32. LYSAKOWSKI, A. 1992. Possible morphological features to distinguish calyx vs. dimorphic type I vestibular hair cells in the chinchilla cristae. Soc. Neurosci. Abstr. **18:** 1400.
33. DICAPRIO, L. L. & E. H. PETERSON. 1992. Differences in ciliary bundle morphology of type I and type II vestibular hair cells. Soc. Neurosci. Abstr. **18:** 509.
34. CORREIA, M. J. & D. G. LANG. 1990. An electrophysiological comparison of solitary type I and type II vestibular hair cells. Neurosci. Lett. **116:** 106–111.
35. RENNIE, K. J. & J. F. ASHMORE. 1991. Ionic currents in isolated vestibular hair cells from the guinea pig crista ampullaris. Hear. Res. **51:** 279–291.
36. EATOCK, R. A., W.-Y. CHEN & M. SAEKI. 1994. Potassium currents in mammalian vestibular hair cells. Sens. Syst. **8:** 21–28.
37. GOLDBERG, J. M. & C. FERNÁNDEZ. 1980. Efferent vestibular system in the squirrel monkey: Anatomical location and influence on afferent activity. J. Neurophysiol. **43:** 986–1025.
38. BERNARD, C., S. L. COCHRAN & W. PRECHT. 1985. Presynaptic actions of cholinergic agents upon the hair cell–afferent fiber synapse in the vestibular labyrinth of the frog. Brain Res. **338:** 225–236.
39. ROSSI, M. L. & M. MARTINI. 1991. Efferent control of posterior canal afferent receptor discharge in the frog labyrinth. Brain Res. **555:** 123–134.
40. ELGOYEN, A. B., D. S. JOHNSON, J. BOULTER, D. E. VETTER & S. HEINEMANN. 1994. α9: An acetylcholine receptor with novel pharmacological properties expressed in rat cochlear hair cells. Cell **79:** 705–715.
41. HEIL, H., D. DRESCHER, A. ELGOYEN & B. J. MORLEY. 1995. nACHR subunits in the peripheral vestibular system. The Molecular Biology of Hearing and Deafness Meeting, Bethesda, MD. Abstr.: 119.
42. LI, H.-S., H. HEIL, H. K. HAPPE, J. LINDSTROM, R. J. WENTHOLD & B. J. MORLEY. 1995. Expressions of nicotinic cholinergic subunits in rat cochlea. The Molecular Biology of Hearing and Deafness Meeting, Bethesda, MD. Abstr.: 118.
43. WACKYM, P., P. POPPER, I. LOPEZ, A. ISHIYAMA & P. E. MICEVYCH. 1995. Expression of alpha 4 and beta 2 nicotinic acetylcholine receptor subunit mRNA and localization of alpha-bungarotoxin binding proteins in the rat vestibular periphery. Cell Biol. Intl. **19:** 291–300.

44. WACKYM, P., C. T. CHEN, R. M. PETTIS & A. ISHIYAMA. 1995. Selective amplification and sequencing of muscarinic acetylcholine receptor cDNAs from the human vestibular periphery. The Molecular Biology of Hearing and Deafness Meeting, Bethesda, MD. Abstr.: 81.

45. BRICHTA, A. M. & E. H. PETERSON. 1994. Functional architecture of vestibular primary afferents from the posterior semicircular canal of a turtle, *Pseudemys (Trachemys) scripta elegans.* J. Comp. Neurol. **344:** 481–507.

Afferent and Efferent Responses from Morphological Fiber Classes in the Turtle Posterior Crista[a]

ALAN M. BRICHTA[b,c] AND JAY M. GOLDBERG[d]

[b]*Department of Surgery—Otolaryngology-Head & Neck Surgery*
[d]*Department of Pharmacological and Physiological Sciences*
University of Chicago
Chicago, Illinois 60637

INTRODUCTION

It is well established that vestibular-nerve afferents differ in their terminal morphology.[1,2] In the last 10 years intra-axonal labeling has allowed us to relate the peripheral terminations of afferents with their physiological properties. Fish and frogs have type II hair cells innervated by bouton fibers.[3] The afferents in these animals have diverse physiological properties that are related to their longitudinal position in the crista, as well as to their branching patterns.[4–6] In mammals, type I and type II hair cells are found throughout the neuroepithelium,[3] and there are three kinds of afferent fibers.[7,8] Calyx units innervate type I hair cells in the central zone, and bouton units supply type II hair cells in the peripheral zone. Dimorphic units supply all parts of the neuroepithelium and provide a mixed innervation to both kinds of hair cells. Calyx and bouton fibers each have relatively homogeneous physiological properties, whereas those of dimorphic units show a considerable variation related to the zone of the neuroepithelium they innervate.[9,10]

The present study extends the analysis to the posterior crista of the turtle. We became interested in the turtle posterior crista because in some ways it shares features with the end organs of mammals and in other ways it resembles the end organs of anamniotes (fish and amphibians). Like mammals, there are type I hair cells[11,12] innervated by calyx and dimorphic fibers.[12] At the same time, the turtle crista has a longitudinally arranged peripheral zone containing only type II hair cells innervated by bouton fibers,[11,12] with the branching patterns of the latter[12] resembling those seen in fish[5] and frogs.[6] One purpose of the present study was to compare the discharge properties of calyx-bearing and bouton afferents in the turtle. That the two kinds of fibers might differ in their physiology was suggested by their distribution within the turtle crista. As in other reptiles and birds,[11] type I hair cells and calyx-bearing afferents are confined to a central zone, whereas type II hair cells and bouton afferents are concentrated in a peripheral zone. It was hoped that any difference between calyx-bearing and bouton afferents might provide clues as to the distinctive contributions made by type I and type II hair cells. In addition, we were interested in comparing the functional organization of the crista in a reptile with that found in other vertebrate groups. A second purpose concerned the responses to

[a]This work was supported by NIDCD grants DC 02058 and 00110.

[c]Address correspondence to Dr. Alan M. Brichta, Department of Surgery—Otolaryngology-Head & Neck Surgery, University of Chicago Hospitals and Clinics, 5841 S. Ellis Avenue, Chicago, IL 60637. E-mail: bric@midway.uchicago.edu

183

electrical activation of efferent pathways. In fish and mammals, efferent effects are exclusively excitatory.[13,14] In contrast, both excitatory and inhibitory responses have been observed in frogs[15] and possibly in birds.[16] In preliminary studies, we found excitatory and inhibitory efferent responses in turtles as well.[17] The issue addressed here was whether the two kinds of efferent actions are targeted to distinctive groups of afferents differing in their responses to head rotation and possibly in their locations within the neuroepithelium.

To study these problems, we adapted the half-head preparation of the turtle previously developed to study the physiology of the basilar papilla.[18]

PHYSIOLOGICAL CHARACTERISTICS

The preparation was placed on a rotating device, and extracellular recordings were made from the posterior branch of the vestibular nerve. Afferents innervating the posterior crista were characterized by their background discharge rate, discharge regularity, and rotational responses.

Background rates varied from 0–55 spikes/s with a mean ($\pm$SD) of 19 ± 13 spikes/s. Discharge regularity was quantified by cv*, a coefficient of variation appropriate to a mean interspike interval of 50 ms. The cv*s ranged from 0.1 (regularly discharging) to 0.9 (irregularly discharging). Responses to sinusoidal head rotations were characterized by their gains and phases. Data are shown for two afferents (FIG. 1A and B). Unit 1 is regularly discharging and has relatively low rotational gains. Unit 2 is irregularly discharging and has higher gains. The two units also differ in their response dynamics. Gain and phase curves of unit 1 resemble those of the torsion-pendulum model: gains are constant above 0.1 Hz, and responses are nearly in phase with head velocity in the same frequency range. In contrast, the gains of unit 2 continue to increase with frequency, and phase leads $> 45°$ are seen at 0.3 Hz.

To characterize the response dynamics of individual units, the ratio of their gains at 0.1 and 1.0 Hz is plotted against the phase lead at 0.3 Hz (FIG. 1C). A gain ratio of 1 and a phase of 0° imply that the unit encodes head velocity (V), whereas a gain ratio of 10 and a 90° phase would be consistent with acceleration encoding (A). The points for most units fall between these two limits.

FIGURE 2 shows the rotational gains and phases for 0.3-Hz sinusoidal head rotations obtained from a large population of extracellularly recorded turtle afferents. Data are plotted against cv*. For many of the units (○), gains and phases increase with cv*. As is particularly evident in the phase plot (FIG. 2B), these units appear to fall into two clusters, one with small phases encoding near head velocity and the other with larger phases encoding nearer head acceleration. In addition, there are irregular units with relatively low gains and phases (●).

Intra-axonal labeling techniques were used to identify the several groups of units.

INTRA-AXONAL LABELING STUDIES

The turtle crista is divided into two triangular-shaped hemicristae (FIG. 3A), which meet at a raised elevation or torus. Each hemicrista has a central zone surrounded by a peripheral zone, the latter extending from the torus to the planum. The central zone is innervated by bouton, calyx, and dimorphic fibers, whereas the peripheral zone only has bouton fibers.[12] Fifty-four posterior crista afferents were

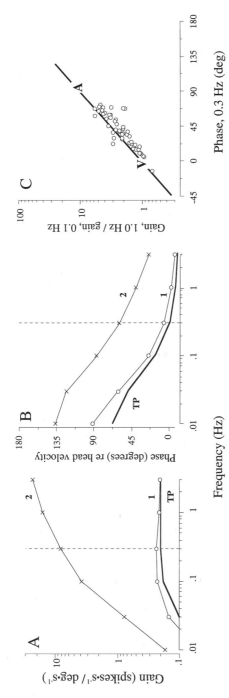

FIGURE 1. Responses of turtle posterior-crista afferents to sinusoidal head rotations in a frequency range from 0.01 to 3 Hz. Individual afferents are characterized by their gains in spikes · s⁻¹/deg · s⁻¹ (**A**) and phase leads re head velocity in degrees (**B**). Unit 1 is regularly discharging; its gain and phase curves parallel those expected of a torsion pendulum function with a first-order time constant of 3 s (TP). Unit 2 is more irregularly discharging and has larger gains and phases. Dotted lines indicate the frequency (0.3 Hz) that provided maximum separation between individual units. (**C**) The ratio of gains at 0.1 and 1.0 Hz are plotted versus the phase lead at 0.3 Hz for several units. Letters indicate the relation between the two variables if a unit encoded head velocity (V) or head acceleration (A).

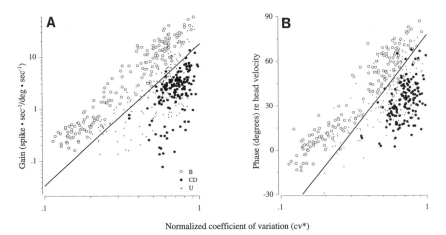

FIGURE 2. Relation between discharge regularity (cv*) and the gain (**A**) and phase (**B**) of extracellularly recorded units responding to 0.3 Hz sinusoidal head rotations. There is a general trend for gains and phases to increase with cv*. Based on a discriminant analysis of intra-axonally labeled units, a line has been drawn in each graph to separate extracellularly recorded units into B, CD, and U classes (see text). With few exceptions, B (bouton) units are above the line, and CD (calyx-bearing) units below it.

first physiologically characterized and then intra-axonally labeled with biocytin. Physiological testing was confined to 0.3-Hz sinusoidal head rotations, a frequency at which there was a clear separation in the gains and phases of units belonging to different morphological classes.

Three examples are shown in Fig. 3b–d, one from each morphological group. Labeled bouton units were found throughout the crista and were similar in appearance whether they supplied the central zone or the peripheral zone near the torus or near the planum; most of them had over 80 bouton endings (Fig. 3b). As expected, calyx and dimorphic units were only found in the central zone. Calyx units possessed both simple and complex endings. The example illustrated had a complex ending enclosing five hair cells (Fig. 3c). Dimorphic units, in addition to their calyx endings, had boutons. There were usually a small number of the latter endings, which were located on relatively short branches (Fig. 3d).

Calyx and dimorphic units were found to be irregularly discharging, whereas bouton units could be regular or irregular. Because calyx and dimorphic units had similar discharge properties, we combined them into a single calyx-bearing (CD) class. They had lower gains and phases than did irregularly discharging bouton (B) units. CD units were divided into CD-low and CD-high groups based on whether their background rates were less or greater than 5 spikes/s. Of the two groups, CD-low units had lower gains and lower phases and were located nearer the planum. A striking relation was found between the longitudinal position of B units and their physiological properties. This was so even though terminal branching patterns and numbers of endings were similar for units at different locations. B units found near the planum were regularly discharging and had relatively low gains and phases, whereas those found near the torus combined an irregular discharge with high gains and phases. Only a few labeled bouton units innervated the central zone. In their physiological properties, they resembled peripheral bouton units located at the same longitudinal position in the crista.

To summarize, CD units are irregularly discharging and have lower gains and phases than do irregularly discharging B units. CD units with low background rates have especially low rotational gains. The discharge properties of B units are correlated with their longitudinal position, but not with their terminal morphology.

DISCRIMINANT ANALYSIS

The physiology of CD and B units are distinctive, raising the possibility that the morphological class of an extracellularly recorded unit could be deduced solely from its physiological properties. This would facilitate the analysis for several reasons. First, in our hands, only one labeled unit can be unambiguously identified in a single preparation. Second, although it is relatively easy to impale most units, it remains difficult to maintain intracellular contact for the long periods required to complete some physiological protocols. Third, the labeling of units with thin axons is still a challenge. We now describe a statistical procedure that has allowed us to infer the morphological class of extracellular units.

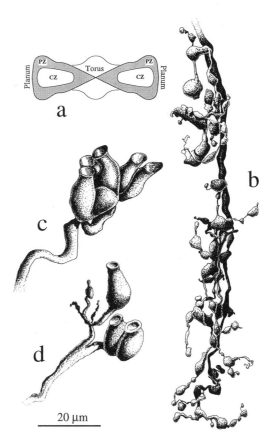

FIGURE 3. (a) A map of the turtle posterior crista showing the two triangular-shaped hemicristae. The bases of these hemicristae are near the canal wall (planum), and their apices join at the middle of the canal (torus). Each hemicrista can be separated into two regions: a central zone (CZ) surrounded by a peripheral zone (PZ). Reconstructions of intra-axonally labeled units; a bouton (b), calyx (c), and dimorphic (d) units.

20 μm

Discriminant analysis, a multivariate statistical procedure, was applied to our intra-axonally labeled sample. For each labeled unit, we calculated a single score, $D = a_1x_1 + a_2x_2 + a_3x_3$, where $x_1 = \log_{10}(cv^*)$, $x_2 = \log_{10}(gain)$, and $x_3 = $ phase. The coefficients ($a_1 < 0$, $a_2 > 0$, $a_3 > 0$) were chosen to maximize the difference between $\overline{D}_{CD}$ and $\overline{D}_B$, the mean scores for CD and B units. From the signs of the coefficients, $\overline{D}_{CD} < \overline{D}_B$. With one exception among the 54 labeled units, all of the CD scores were lower than the lowest B score. The analysis was used to define a boundary separating the two populations. The probability of assigning a new unit to the wrong category was estimated to be $p = 0.056$. To make the probability of misassignment, $p < 0.01$, we included an unassigned (U) category. Two boundaries, D_{UPPER} and D_{LOWER}, were calculated. A unit was assigned to the B class if its score was greater than D_{UPPER}; to the U class if the score fell between D_{UPPER} and D_{LOWER}; and to the CD class if the score was less than D_{LOWER}.

The discriminant analysis is illustrated for our extracellular sample in FIGURE 2. Separate symbols denote units assigned to the two morphological categories. Of the 554 units in the extracellular sample, 223 (40%) were B units, 226 (41%) were CD units, and 105 (19%) were unassigned. The CD units are distinctive in being irregular units with relatively low gains and phases. Stated an equivalent way, CD units are more irregular than are B units with similar gains and phases. As was the case for the intracellular sample, CD-high units have considerably larger gains than do CD-low units (FIG. 4); mean values ($\pm$ SD) for 0.3-Hz sinusoids are 3.6 ± 2.5 and 0.7 ± 0.5 spikes·s^{-1}/deg·s^{-1}. There appear to be two groups of B units: one with regular discharge, low gains and small phases; the other with irregular discharge, high gains and large phases. B units will be referred to as bouton-velocity (B-vel) or bouton-acceleration (B-acc) if their phases at 0.3 Hz are $< 45°$ and $> 45°$, respectively. Our intra-axonal labeling results imply that B-vel units are located near the planum; the B-acc units, near the torus.

RATE-INTENSITY RELATIONS

We compared the relation between response and stimulus intensity for extracellularly recorded B-vel, B-acc, CD-high, and CD-low units. Rate-intensity plots were obtained in response to 2-s ramps of angular velocity with final values ranging from < 1 to > 500 deg/s. The situation illustrates the advantage of the discriminant classification as applied to extracellular units. The physiological protocol was relatively lengthy. More importantly, it would have been difficult to hold impaled units during the larger accelerations.

FIGURE 5 presents rate-intensity curves for the four groups. The data were obtained from the last 0.5 s of the 2-s velocity ramp. For each group, the points are the mean response rates (r) for several units plotted against the average head velocity during the sampling interval (x); the curves are fits of the mean rates by the empirical function, $r = b_1 atan[(x - b_2)/b_3]$. The maximum rate is given by $\pi b_1/2$; the low-intensity or linear gain by b_1/b_3; and the threshold by b_2. The b_3 is a scale factor indicating the linear stimulus range, i.e., the intensity range over which the response is close to a linear function of stimulus intensity. (When $x - b_2 = b_3$, the expected response deviates from linearity by 21.5%.) Except for some CD-low units, thresholds were zero.

B-vel units encode over a wide range of head velocities ($b_3 = 94 \pm 8$ deg/s). By contrast, B-acc units linearly encode only very low intensities ($b_3 = 3.8 \pm 0.3$ deg/s) and become saturated for head velocities > 20 deg/s. CD-high units have a linear stimulus range similar to that of B-vel units ($b_3 = 81 \pm 10$ spike/s), and CD-low units have an even broader range ($b_3 = 215 \pm 39$ deg/s). CD units reach considerably higher maximum response rates than do B units; the maximum values have the following means $\pm$ SD (in spikes/s): B-vel (72 ± 3), B-acc (59 ± 1), CD-high (192 ± 11), and CD-low (189 ± 19).

EFFERENT ACTIVATION

We recorded the response of afferents to electrical stimulation of efferent fibers. A bipolar stimulating electrode was placed on the nerve bundles running between the anterior and posterior rami of the vestibular nerve. All of the efferent fibers

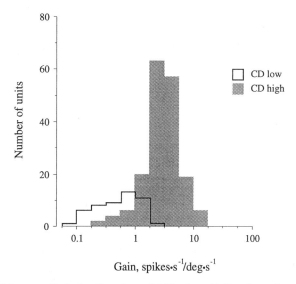

FIGURE 4. Histograms displaying the gains to 0.3-Hz sinusoidal head rotations of two groups of extracellularly recorded calyx-bearing (CD) units. CD-low units had background rates < 5 spikes/s, whereas CD-high units had comparable rates ≥ 5 spikes/s. Units were assigned to the CD class based on their discriminant scores.

destined for the posterior crista travel in these bundles, but none of the afferents to the posterior crista do so.[19] Once again, extracellularly recorded units were used, and their morphological class was inferred from their discriminant scores.

Responses to brief shock trains are shown in FIGURE 6A–D. Responses outlasted stimulation by 1 s or more. Units were either excited (FIG. 6A and B), inhibited (FIG. 6C) or showed a mixed response consisting of an initial inhibition followed by an excitation (FIG. 6D). The delayed excitation seen in mixed responses is not merely a postinhibitory rebound. This can be seen in FIGURE 6E, taken from the same unit as illustrated in FIGURE 6D. By lowering the shock rate and prolonging the shock train, the two response components could be separated in time with the large poststimulus excitation now being preceded by several seconds of weak excitation. The type of efferent response shown by a unit was unaffected by variations in shock intensity, shock rate or shock-train duration.

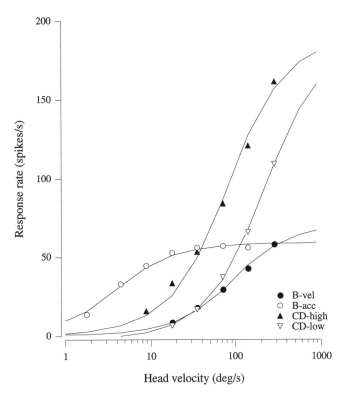

FIGURE 5. Rate-intensity functions for four groups of extracellularly recorded units. Data were collected during the last 0.5 s of a 2-s head-velocity ramp. For each group, the points are the mean response rates (actual rate minus background rate) for several units plotted against the average stimulus velocity during the collection interval. Curves are fits to the mean points by an empirical formula (see text). Units were assigned to the calyx-bearing (CD) or bouton (B) categories based on their discriminant scores. B units were called B-vel (velocity) or B-acc (acceleration) depending on whether the phase of their response to 0.3-Hz sinusoidal head rotations was less or greater than 45°. CD units were called high-rate (CD-high) or low-rate (CD-low) depending on whether their background rate was less or greater than 5 spikes/s. Number of units: B-vel (8), B-acc (8), CD-high (12), and CD-low (13).

Excited units were of the CD (FIG. 6A) and B-vel (FIG. 6B) varieties, with the former units having much larger responses. Almost all of the inhibited units were of the B-acc type. Most of the units showing mixed responses were B-acc units (FIG. 6D) or CD units (not shown). Combining the efferent data with our labeling results leads to the conclusion that the efferent actions are regionally organized. In the peripheral zone, inhibitory or mixed effects are found near the torus, whereas excitation predominates near the planum. The principal action in the central zone is excitation. Although most CD units are excited by efferent activation, some show a mixed response. Whether the latter units are calyx or dimorphic units can only be clarified by labeling studies. Many CD-low units were silent at rest, and most of these remained silent during efferent stimulation.

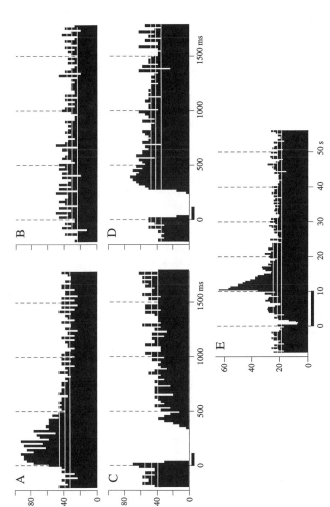

FIGURE 6. Responses of four extracellularly recorded afferents (**A–D**) when efferent fibers were electrically stimulated. (**A**) A CD-high unit shows an excitatory response > 40 spikes/s. (**B**) A B-vel unit shows a smaller excitatory response of ≈5 spikes/s. (**C**) A B-acc unit is inhibited. (**D**) A B-acc unit shows a mixed response consisting of an initial inhibition followed by an excitation. Stimulus, indicated by bar below lower histograms, was 20 shocks at 200/s. Each histogram is based on 26 stimulation trials interleaved with the same number of control trials. Bins are 20 ms. The horizontal lines show the mean rate ± SD based on the control trials. (**E**) The same B-acc unit as in **D** was stimulated with 1000 shocks, 100/s. The initial inhibition was transient, giving way to a weak excitation lasting for the remainder of the shock train. There is still a large poststimulus excitation even though it was preceded by several seconds of excitation. For the classification of extracellularly recorded units, see legend to FIGURE 5.

COMPARISON WITH OTHER SPECIES

Bouton units in the turtle show a diversity of response characteristics related to their longitudinal position in the crista. In some respects, the spatial organization of the bouton fibers resembles that seen in fish and frogs, which only have type II hair cells. In the latter animals, as in turtles, so-called B-vel units are located near the planum, while B-acc units are found near the middle of the organ.[5,6] Differences in efferent responses exist across species. In fish, both B-vel and B-acc units are excited by efferent activation.[13] In contrast, efferent actions in the turtle include an excitation of B-vel units and an inhibition or a mixed inhibition-excitation of B-acc units. Both efferent excitation and efferent inhibition have been seen in the frog,[15] although the excited and inhibited units have not been characterized in terms of their rotational responses or their locations in the crista.

We now turn to CD units, which in turtles are only found in a central zone. It is profitable to compare the central zones in turtles and in mammals because they both have calyx and dimorphic fibers innervating type I hair cells. As calyx and dimorphic units in the turtle have similar discharge properties, they have been included in a single CD class. Their discharge is irregular, they have modest phase leads of 20–45°, and they can give large excitatory responses to efferent activation. Gains are considerably higher for CD-high than for CD-low units. Central calyx-bearing afferents in mammals resemble turtle CD units in their discharge regularity, phase, and efferent responses.[9,10] In addition, two groups of mammalian units can be distinguished on the basis of their gains. In mammals, however, the two groups differ in their morphology, but not in their background discharge; the high-gain afferents are dimorphs and the low-gain afferents are calyx units.

The comparison between turtles and mammals can be extended to the rest of the crista. Unlike the situation in turtles, type I hair cells are distributed throughout the mammalian neuroepithelium, as are dimorphic, but not calyx units.[7,8] The discharge properties of dimorphic units are related to their epithelial location with those located in the central zone being more irregularly discharging and having higher gains and phases than those innervating the peripheral zone.[9,10] Bouton units are only found in the peripheral zone of mammals.[7,8] They resemble peripheral dimorphs in their discharge properties,[9,10] and both categories of fibers are similar to the B-vel units of turtles. The resemblance includes efferent excitatory responses smaller in size than those of centrally located CD units. One clear difference is that mammals do not have any units approaching the high gains and large phase leads of B-acc units.

We can summarize the comparative data as follows. In anamniotes, the crista is longitudinally arranged with afferent fibers near the planum, differing in their morphology and physiology from those near the center of the organ. As is the case in other reptiles and birds, the turtle hemicrista has a peripheral zone containing only type II hair cells and a central zone containing both type I and type II hair cells. The turtle peripheral zone has a longitudinal organization similar to that seen in the entire crista of anamniotes. In some respects, CD units in the turtle central zone resemble central dimorphs and calyx units in mammals. The structural organization of the mammalian crista is unusual in at least three ways. First, type I and type II hair cells are found throughout the neuroepithelium. Second, morphological and physiological gradients are concentrically, rather than longitudinally, organized. This is especially clear in the peripheral zone, which rings the entire circumference of the crista. Peripheral units have similar morphology and physiology whether they are located near the planum or near the middle of the organ. Third, one class of afferents, corresponding to the B-acc units of turtles, is not present in mammals.

COMPARISON OF CALYX-BEARING AND BOUTON AFFERENTS

Type I and type II hair cells are likely to play distinctive roles in vestibular processing, and these should be reflected in the discharge properties of the afferents innervating them. Previous work in mammals has not been particularly successful in defining differences between calyx-bearing and bouton afferents.[9,10] One difficulty has been that B units in mammals have thin axons and are not easily impaled and labeled.[9] Furthermore, bouton afferents make up only 10–20% of the fibers in the mammalian vestibular nerve.[7,8] A comparison between B and CD units has proved easier in the turtle crista. Relatively large samples of the two kinds of units have been physiologically characterized and labeled. Their physiology is sufficiently distinctive that we can assign extracellularly recorded units to either the B or CD categories based solely on a combination of their discharge properties. As reflected by the discriminant analysis, CD units are more irregularly discharging than B units with the same gain and phase.

Although the discriminant score has proved useful descriptively, its functional interpretation is obscure. In particular, CD units are not distinctive in any of the individual properties making up the score. Two other discharge properties are more easily interpreted. First, CD units have maximum response rates that are three times larger than those of B units. The increased response range can potentially increase the low-intensity gain and the linear stimulus range (FIG. 5). As is described by Goldberg (this volume),[20] the extended response range might be explained by a postsynaptic depolarization of calyx endings by intercellular potassium accumulation. The other candidate property concerns excitatory efferent responses, which are considerably larger in CD-high than in B-vel units. Two observations suggest that large efferent responses may not be a distinctive feature of CD units. First, many CD-low units in turtles are unaffected by efferent activation. Second, dimorphic units located in the peripheral zone of mammals have small efferent responses[14] even though they are known to receive a postsynaptic efferent innervation.[21] On this basis, it can be suggested that the one property distinguishing CD units is their expanded response range. A critical test of this idea would be to compare the rate-intensity functions of B and CD units in mammals.

A FUNCTIONAL INTERPRETATION

The posterior crista of the turtle is a remarkable organ capable of encoding with high sensitivity both small head movements (< 10 deg/s) and large head movements (> 100 deg/s). Separate classes of units may be used in monitoring the two kinds of head movements. B-acc units are well suited to encoding the small head perturbations involved in postural control, whereas B-vel and CD units might be better at monitoring head motion during locomotion and other voluntary motor acts. Among the CD units, those with low background rates have especially large linear stimulus ranges, extending above 200 deg/s.

The efferent system exerts a mixed action in the posterior crista that is regionally organized. B-acc afferents are inhibited, whereas B-vel and CD afferents are excited. It has been suggested that lateral-line efferents are activated in anticipation of movement.[22,23] Were vestibular efferents to respond similarly, they could switch the organ from a "postural" mode to a "volitional" mode by inhibiting units that would be saturated by large head movements and activating units having large dynamic ranges.

REFERENCES

1. LORENTE DE NÓ, R. 1926. Etudes sur l'anatomie et la physiologie du labyrinthe de l'orielle et du VIIIe nerf. Deuxième partie. Quelques données au sujet de l'anatomie dans organes sensoriels du labyrinthe. Trab. Lab. Invest. Biol. Univ. Madrid **24:** 53–153.
2. POLJAK, S. 1927. Über die Nervenendigungen in den vestibularen Sinnesendstellen bei den Säugetieren. Z. Anat. Entwicklungsgesch. **84:** 131–144.
3. WERSÄLL, J. & D. BAGGER-SJÖBÄCK. 1974. Morphology of the vestibular sense organ. In Handbook of Sensory Physiology. Vol. 6. Vestibular System. Part 1. Basic Mechanisms. H. H. Kornhuber, Ed.: 123–170. Springer-Verlag. Berlin.
4. O'LEARY, D. P., R. F. DUNN & V. HONRUBIA. 1976. Analysis of afferent responses from isolated semicircular canal of the guitarfish using rotational acceleration white noise inputs. I. Correlations of response dynamics with receptor innervation. J. Neurophysiol. **39:** 631–644.
5. BOYLE, R., J. P. CAREY & S. M. HIGHSTEIN. 1991. Morphological correlates of response dynamics and efferent stimulation in horizontal semicircular canal afferents of the toadfish, *Opsanus tau.* J. Neurophysiol. **66(5):** 1504–1521.
6. HONRUBIA, V., L. F. HOFFMAN, S. SITKO & I. R. SCHWARTZ. 1989. Anatomic and physiological correlates in bullfrog vestibular nerve. J. Neurophysiol. **61(4):** 688–701.
7. FERNÁNDEZ, C., R. A. BAIRD & J. M. GOLDBERG. 1988. The vestibular nerve of the chinchilla. I. Peripheral innervation patterns in the horizontal and superior semicircular canals. J. Neurophysiol. **60:** 167–203.
8. FERNÁNDEZ, C., A. LYSAKOWSKI & J. M. GOLDBERG. 1995. Hair-cell counts and afferent innervation patterns in the cristae ampullares of the squirrel monkey with a comparison to the chinchilla. J. Neurophysiol. **73:** 1253–1269.
9. BAIRD, R. A., G. DESMADRYL, C. FERNÁNDEZ & J. M. GOLDBERG. 1988. The vestibular nerve of the chinchilla. II. Relation between afferent response properties and peripheral innervation patterns in the semicircular canals. J. Neurophysiol. **60:** 182–203.
10. LYSAKOWSKI, A., L. B. MINOR, C. FERNÁNDEZ & J. M. GOLDBERG. 1995. Physiological identification of morphologically distinct afferent classes innervating the cristae ampullares of the squirrel monkey. J. Neurophysiol. **73:** 1270–1281.
11. JØRGENSEN, J. M. 1974. The sensory epithelia of the inner ear of two turtles, *Testudo graeca* and *Pseudemys scripta.* Acta Zool. **55:** 289–298.
12. BRICHTA, A. M. & E. H. PETERSON. 1994. Functional architecture of vestibular primary afferents from the posterior semicircular canal of a turtle, *Pseudemys (Trachemys) scripta.* J. Comp. Neurol. **344:** 481–507.
13. BOYLE, R. & S. M. HIGHSTEIN. 1990. Efferent vestibular system in the toadfish: Action upon horizontal semicircular canal afferents. J. Neurosci. **10(5):** 1570–1582.
14. GOLDBERG, J. M. & C. FERNÁNDEZ. 1980. Efferent vestibular system in the squirrel monkey: Anatomical location and influence on afferent activity. J. Neurophysiol. **43:** 986–1025.
15. ROSSI, M. L., M. MARTINI, B. PELUCCHI & R. FESCE. 1994. Quantal nature of synaptic transmission at the cytoneural junction in the frog labyrinth. J. Physiol. (Lond.) **478(1):** 17–35.
16. DICKMAN, J. D. & M. J. CORREIA. 1993. Bilateral communication between vestibular labyrinths in pigeons. Neuroscience **57(4):** 1097–1108.
17. BRICHTA, A. M. & J. M. GOLDBERG. 1992. Afferent and efferent response properties of morphologically identified fibers from the posterior semicircular canal of the turtle. Soc. Neurosci. Abstr. **18:** 510.
18. CRAWFORD, A. C. & R. FETTIPLACE. 1980. The frequency selectivity of auditory nerve fibres and hair cells in the cochlea of the turtle. J. Physiol. (Lond.) **306:** 79–125.

19. FAYYAZUDDIN, A., A. M. BRICHTA & J. J. ART. 1991. Organization of eighth nerve efferents in the turtle, *Pseudemys scripta.* Soc. Neurosci. Abstr. **17:** 312.
20. GOLDBERG, J. M. 1995. Transmission between the type I hair cell and its calyx ending. Ann. N.Y. Acad. Sci. This volume.
21. GOLDBERG, J. M., A. LYSAKOWSKI & C. FERNÁNDEZ. 1990. Morphophysiological and ultrastructural studies in the mammalian cristae ampullares. Hear. Res. **49:** 89–102.
22. RUSSELL, I. J. & B. L. ROBERTS. 1972. Inhibition of spontaneous lateral line activity by efferent nerve stimulation. J. Exp. Biol. **57:** 77–82.
23. TRICAS, T. C. & S. M. HIGHSTEIN. 1990. Visually mediated inhibition of lateral line primary afferent activity by the octavolateralis efferent system during predation in the free-swimming toadfish, *Opsanus tau.* Exp. Brain Res. **83(1):** 233–236.

Evidence of a Sensory Processing Unit in the Mammalian Macula

THOMAS C. CHIMENTO[a] AND MURIEL D. ROSS

NASA Ames Research Center
Life Sciences Biocomputation Center, MS 239-11
Moffett Field, California 94035-1000

INTRODUCTION

Mammalian vestibular maculae are sensory end organs that are responsive to linear acceleration. Primary afferent endings in the maculae have a unique morphology (FIG. 1). Large terminal calyces wrap around the bodies of type I hair cells. Synaptic input to the calyx from a type I hair cell occurs largely at the base of the hair cell. Type II hair cells, which synapse with the outer membrane of calyces and with the heads of afferent processes, provide additional input to the primary afferents.

Emanating from the neuron branch and calyx are projections we call processes. The processes are similar in some ways to the spines found on pyramidal cell dendrites.[1,2] Like spines, vestibular afferent processes consist of a stem and a bulbous head. However, most processes are larger than dendritic spines and they lack a spine apparatus. Ultrastructural research and three-dimensional (3-D) reconstructions reveal a wide range of synaptic connections on macular receptor cells and primary afferents, and a complex connectivity between the neural elements. Most processes are postsynaptic to ribbon synapses in the type II cells, that is, the processes are afferent endings. Other processes contain numerous vesicles and on morphological grounds are efferent (FIG. 1). They make horizontal connections to adjacent type II hair cells where they end opposite subsynaptic cisterns (c synapses),[3,4] or terminate as asymmetric synapses on calyces and other neuron branches. Finally, some processes contain both pre- and postsynaptic elements, defining them as recurrent (also known as reciprocal). Current physiological techniques are not capable of exploring the functions of processes. This makes compartmental modeling appealing as a method to investigate the effects of morphology on voltage spread within single primary vestibular afferents.

Compartmental modeling has been used (1) to determine whether large dendritic trees can be collapsed into simpler equivalent cylinder representations,[5-9] (2) to examine depolarization within single cells,[10-12] (3) to confirm the quality of electrophysiological recordings,[13] and (4) to study the connections between two or more cells.[14] Although many of the original models explored passive flow of current in dendrites and dendritic spines,[15-18] later simulations included active channels.[1,19]

In this report we describe results of computer simulations based on compartmental models that address the following issues: (1) the relative synaptic contribution to afferent output when stem dimension is varied, (2) synaptic summation, and (3) the properties of efferent processes. A primary goal was to determine whether employing the accuracy of ultrastructural morphometry in compartmental models of neural electrodynamics affects action potential (AP) generation and peak latency (henceforth referred to simply as latency), or peak depolarization magnitude (henceforth

---

[a] E-mail: chimento@biocomp.arc.nasa.gov

referred to as depolarization magnitude or depolarization) at the spike initiation zone (SIZ). We used data from serial sections and from 3-D reconstructions to build our neuron models, and we examined the consequences of systematically varying membrane resistivity and synaptic conductance. By comparing this large parametric series of simulations to published electrophysiology, we could estimate the most likely values for membrane resistivity and synaptic conductance. These values were then applied to simulations of whole primary afferents.

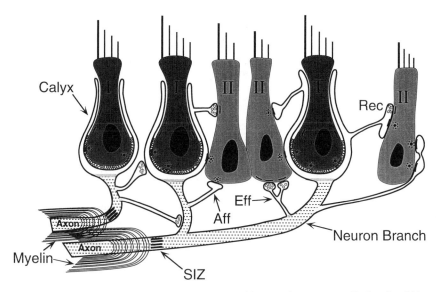

FIGURE 1. Schematic representation of the principal innervation patterns of hair cells within the utricular macula of the rat. Type I and type II hair cells are the sensory receptor cells. The calyx wraps around the bodies of type I hair cells. An unmyelinated neuron branch begins at the base of each calyx (*shaded areas*). When there is more than one neuron branch, the branches connect distal to the first heminode. The heminode is the assumed site of the spike initiation zone (SIZ). Processes contribute to the afferent (Aff) input by receiving synaptic transmission from type II hair cells. Processes may provide efferent (Eff) output to type II hair cells or neuron branches through presynaptic contacts. The type II hair cell on the far right displays a recurrent (Rec) synapse. Presynaptic vesicles and a postsynaptic thickening are found together in a single process head. This diagram does not include all the possible connections found in the macula. For example, this diagram does not include efferent endings described as originating from the central nervous system.

METHODS

Histology

Rat utricular maculae were fixed by rapid immersion and perfusion with 2.5% glutaraldehyde + 0.5% paraformaldehyde in 0.1 M Millonig phosphate buffer at pH 7.4. All tissues were postfixed for 1 h in 1.0% osmium tetroxide in Millonig phosphate buffer and dehydrated in steps from 30% to 70% ethanol. Samples were then microdissected to obtain maculae free of temporal bone, dehydration was completed, and the tissues were embedded in Spurr resin. Following sectioning at 1 μm to reach the area of choice, ultrathin sections (~ 0.15 μm) were cut on a Reichart ultramicrotome. Sections were mounted on slot grids previously coated with Formvar, then stained with 4% uranyl acetate and 2% lead citrate.

Electron Microscopy and Reconstructions

Electron micrograph mosaics of serial sections were used to produce 3-D images of vestibular primary afferent endings. Each reconstruction was made using 300–600 serial sections. Every third or fifth section was photographed at 3000× and micrographs were printed at 4500× for the mosaics. Selected afferent terminals and all hair cells contacting them were traced onto acetate sheets. The tracings were digitized into a PC and reassembled as filled slice reconstructions.[20,21] Data were transferred to a Silicon Graphics IRIS 4D/210 VGX graphics workstation for 3-D reconstruction using software developed in our laboratory.

Simulations

The compartmental modeling program NEURON,[22,23] which uses one-dimensional (1-D) cable "sections" to analyze voltage changes, was used for the simulations. Each section is composed of a user-specified number of cylindrical isopotential compartments. The sections can be connected to construct an arbitrary branched cable. Membrane properties, such as resistivity, capacitance, reversal potential, and the presence of Hodgkin-Huxley membrane mechanisms, can be specified for any section.

The number of compartments used in a simulation was derived empirically by increasing compartments until a finer spatial mesh did not markedly affect the results of the computation. The number of compartments was then doubled for the simulations. All process sections were modeled using 30 compartments, and the neuron branch was modeled with 100 compartments. When an entire afferent ending was simulated, each neuron branch and each calyx were modeled with 10 compartments. Axons were constructed with 10-compartment internodal regions and a 1-compartment node of Ranvier.

All the local electrical properties used here, such as cytoplasmic resistivity and the widely accepted value of $1 \mu F/cm^2$ for specific membrane capacitance (C_m) are taken from the literature.[1,5,9,10,13,24–28] For all simulations, the axial (cytoplasmic) resistivity (R_i) was 100 Ωcm, and resting membrane potential was set at −65 mV. Simulations were run with membrane resistivity (R_m) of 5000, 20,000 or 50,000 Ωcm². The calyces, processes, and neuron branches were all modeled as passive structures. To simulate the SIZ and nodes of Ranvier, we multiplied the maximum sodium, potassium, and leakage conductances in the Hodgkin-Huxley equations by 100 and adjusted the rate function to 15 °C. These parameters produced simulated APs that approximated the duration and amplitude of mammalian responses. To model the insulating property of the myelinated axon, the specific membrane resistivity along internodal regions was increased to 1 MΩcm².

A synapse, modeled as a time-varying conductance, was located on the distal end of each process or near the base of a calyx. The time course of the conductance for all simulations was modeled as a standard α-function, with a time to peak of 0.25 ms, a maximum synaptic conductance (g_{syn}) of 0.1, 1, or 5 nS, and an absolute reversal potential of 0 mV.

Simulated voltage was recorded at two sites on the isolated neuron branch, at one end of the neuron branch, and at the distal end of efferent processes (a presynaptic site in the head). In simulations of an entire primary afferent, measurements at the SIZ replaced recordings at the end of the neuron branch.

Calyx Model

Calyx endings pose a unique problem for compartmental modeling. Their structure can be described as a two-membrane, planar surface wrapped around the type I hair cell(s). This morphology is difficult to convert to a form that can be analyzed with 1-D cable equations. Our solution was to approximate the calyx as a cylinder within a cylinder, each cylinder representing one cell membrane. The lengths of the cylinders were measured from each reconstructed calyx. The area of the annulus produced by the two cylinders was used to define a single cylinder of equivalent cross-sectional area for use in the simulations (FIG. 2). The reasoning was

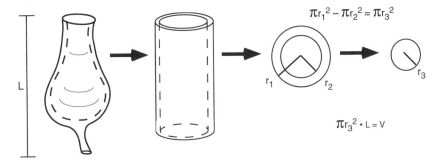

$$\pi r_1^2 - \pi r_2^2 = \pi r_3^2$$

$$\pi r_3^2 * L = V$$

FIGURE 2. Procedure for converting a calyx into an equivalent cylinder for entry into NEURON. First the calyx is approximated by a cylindrical annulus. The radius of the inner (r_2) and outer (r_1) membranes is determined from measurements of 3-D reconstructions of calyces. The "cylinder-within-a-cylinder" provides a close approximation of the total surface area and volume measured from the original calyx. The two radii are used to produce a single cylinder with a cross-sectional area equivalent to the annulus. The radius of this equivalent cylinder (r_3) is entered into the model along with the measured length of the original calyx. The membrane capacitance (C_m) of the calyx is increased to 2 μF/cm^2 and the membrane resistivity (R_m) decreased to 2500 Ωcm^2 to compensate for the near halving of the total membrane surface area.

that this produced a good set of approximations for the length of the calyx, the volume of cytoplasm, and the cross-sectional area of the calyx. Therefore, the resistance to current flow along the length of the equivalent cylinder calyx approximated the resistance of the calyx.

The one parameter of the equivalent cylinder approximation of the calyx that was not accurate was the total surface area, which was less than that of the original calyces largely because the calyx has inner and outer membranes. To account for this discrepancy, the specific membrane capacitance was increased to 2 μF/cm^2, and the membrane resistivity was decreased to 2500 Ωcm^2. These changes in the calyceal membrane made the total capacitance, resistance, and time constant (τ) of the equivalent cylinder representation of the calyx closely approximate the values in the original calyx.

RESULTS

Simulations of a Process on a Neuron Branch

Effects of Stem Dimension on Voltage

We systematically examined the effects of length and diameter by varying the diameter of the stem while keeping all other parameters constant, and then by varying just the length of the stem while holding the diameter constant. Using this methodology we investigated a 6 × 6 matrix of possible stem sizes (FIG. 3). The lengths and diameters of the processes examined extended slightly beyond those measured in our sample of serial section electron micrographs because of the relatively small number of the longer and thinner processes that have been accurately measured. Two membrane parameters were varied: membrane resistivity and peak synaptic conductance. Selecting these two parameters is difficult because of the range of values that have been measured experimentally. Membrane resistivity was set at 5000, 20,000 and 50,000 Ωcm^2 and synaptic conductance at 5, 1, and 0.1 nS. All permutations of these parameters were tested. For the following simulations, voltages were recorded at the end of the neuron branch.

Three sets of simulations are shown (FIG. 3A–F). The top row displays the magnitude of depolarization from rest (-65 mV), and the bottom row is the latency. Membrane resistivity was 5000 Ωcm^2 for all cases. Synaptic conductance was 5 nS for A and B, 1 nS for C and D, and 0.1 nS for E and F. The smaller dark region in 3C is the overlap between the stem dimensions of spines in the cerebellum[29] and vestibular afferent processes. The larger lined region is the overlap between stem dimensions of hippocampal CA1 spines[29] and vestibular afferent processes. The spine dimensions also extended off the matrix, because some spines are both thinner and shorter than any of the stems observed in the macula.

The results demonstrate that a large range in magnitude of depolarization can exist at the end of the neuron branch when the length and diameter of the stem are varied (FIG. 3A). The range of voltage values across matrix A is 15.7 mV (from 16.8 mV to 1.1 mV). Voltage increases are mostly restricted to the longest processes (16 μm) and occur when the diameter increases from 0.05 to 0.4 μm. When synaptic conductance is 1 nS, the voltage range is reduced to 3.1 mV. Therefore, there can be a sizable difference in depolarization across the range of stem dimensions commonly found in the utricular macula depending on the values selected for membrane resistivity.

When membrane resistivity was varied (not shown), virtually no change in the range of depolarization was observed with any of the three synaptic conductances tested.

Effects of Stem Dimension on Latency

A gradual increase in latency occurred as stem diameter was varied from short and wide to long and thin. In general, increasing stem length increases latency and, conversely, increasing stem diameter decreases latency (FIG. 3B). Latency varied from 1.66 to 2.68 ms. This 1-ms range is sufficient to modify the temporal summation of simultaneous synaptic input.

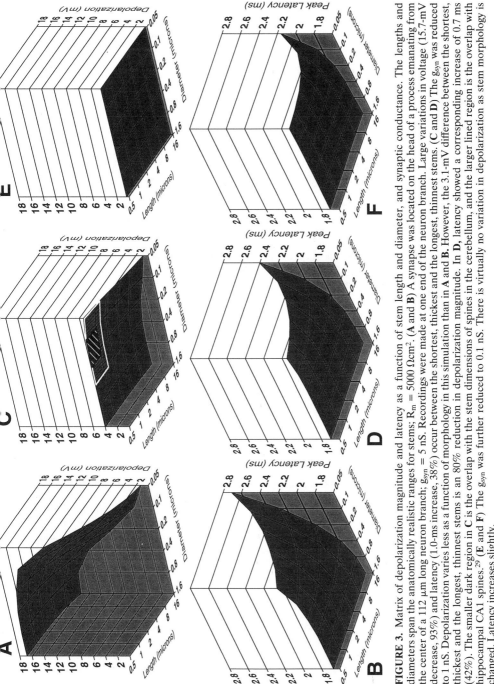

FIGURE 3. Matrix of depolarization magnitude and latency as a function of stem length and diameter, and synaptic conductance. The lengths and diameters span the anatomically realistic ranges for stems; R_m = 5000 Ωcm². (**A** and **B**) A synapse was located on the head of a process emanating from the center of a 112 μm long neuron branch; g_{syn} = 5 nS. Recordings were made at one end of the neuron branch. Large variations in voltage (15.7-mV decrease, 93%) and latency (1.0-ms increase, 38%) occur between the shortest, thickest and the longest, thinnest stems. (**C** and **D**) The g_{syn} was reduced to 1 nS. Depolarization varies less as a function of morphology in this simulation than in **A** and **B**. However, the 3.1-mV difference between the shortest, thickest and the longest, thinnest stems is an 80% reduction in depolarization magnitude. In **D**, latency showed a corresponding increase of 0.7 ms (42%). The smaller dark region in **C** is the overlap with the stem dimensions of spines in the cerebellum, and the larger lined region is the overlap with hippocampal CA1 spines.[29] (**E** and **F**) The g_{syn} was further reduced to 0.1 nS. There is virtually no variation in depolarization as stem morphology is changed. Latency increases slightly.

Simulation of Efferent Processes

Effects of Stem Morphology on Voltage and Latency at the Distal End of an Efferent Process

Many of the processes on a primary afferent make presynaptic connections with adjacent type II hair cells, calyces, and neuron branches. These processes are arranged in a manner that would permit them to function analogously to interneurons, but with only one synaptic delay. Just as local interneurons provide for communication within their territory, so would efferent processes communicate calyx or neuron branch activity to nearby type II hair cells, calyces, and neuron branches. This output could affect type II hair cell activity, which would influence the output of vestibular afferents. Therefore, for network modeling it is necessary to determine those factors that affect the magnitude of depolarization reaching presynaptic release sites in efferent processes.

A single 5-nS synapse on the neuron branch was activated to provide the current source. Depolarization magnitude (FIG. 4A) and latency (FIG. 4B) at the presynaptic site (head) of an efferent process are virtually unaffected by process morphology. There is a maximum increase of 0.43 ms and 0.2 mV between the shortest, large-diameter stem (0.5×1.6 μm) and the longest, thinnest stem (16×0.05 μm). Varying the membrane resistivity and synaptic conductance, as was done in previous simulations, simply shifted the matrix results up or down (not shown).

Simulations of Primary Afferents with Passive Spike Initiation Zone

Once we understood the effects of process morphology on depolarization using an isolated neuron branch, we expanded the simulations by using morphology from actual primary afferent endings. We selected four afferents for simulation (FIG. 5). Their dimensions were measured from 3-D reconstructions. Two identical processes were placed on each primary afferent, one on the calyx most distal to the SIZ (arrows, FIG. 5) and one on the neuron branch nearest the SIZ (arrowheads, FIG. 5).

How would the choice of membrane resistivity and synaptic conductance affect these results? Simulations were conducted using afferent A from FIGURE 6. In FIGURE 6 the synaptic conductance was held at 5 nS while the membrane resistivity was varied. Under these conditions depolarization varies less than 1 mV. However, increasing the membrane resistivity also increases the time constant of the membrane, and, therefore, the membrane remains depolarized longer.

The membrane resistivity was held constant at 50,000 Ωcm^2 while the synaptic conductance was varied from 5 to 0.1 nS. Under these conditions, a large drop in depolarization of the membrane occurred (FIG. 7). The magnitude of depolarization declined nearly 75% between 5 and 1 nS. At 0.1 nS the cells were barely depolarized. However, the difference in excitatory postsynaptic potential (EPSP) magnitude remained proportional across the four afferents as the synaptic conductance was decreased.

The previous results demonstrate that synaptic conductance affects the size of the EPSP, whereas membrane resistivity primarily affects the rate of return to the resting membrane potential. How could these results guide the selection of parameters for a whole cell simulation? Would particular values be critical, or could the values vary with little effect on the result? To explore these questions we selected one primary afferent (FIG. 5D) and placed a total of four afferent processes on its calyces and neuron branches. One synapse was placed on each afferent process head and 10

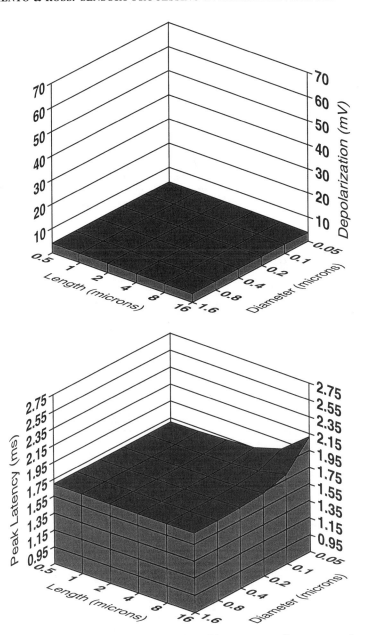

FIGURE 4. Matrix of depolarization magnitude and latency at an efferent process head as a function of stem length and diameter. (**A** and **B**) A synapse was activated at a proximal site on the primary afferent, and recordings were made at the head. All other parameters are the same as in FIGURE 3B. With a proximal depolarization source, voltage and latency vary little at the distal end of an efferent process for the range of stem dimensions tested. When membrane resistivity and synaptic conductance were varied, the only change observed was a slight shift of the entire surface along the Z axis (not shown).

synapses were placed near the base of each calyx. The total of 44 synapses and their distribution are representative of the population observed in mammalian end organs. We used this afferent (FIG. 8) for a number of simulations described below.

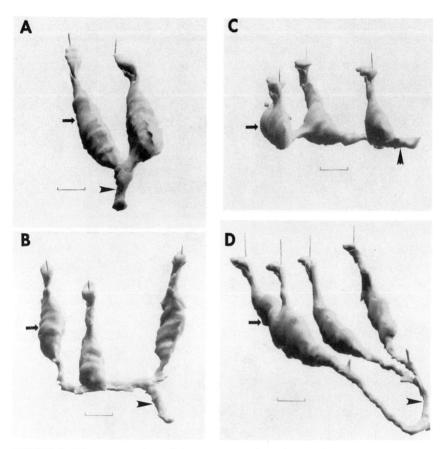

FIGURE 5. 3-D reconstructions of four representative primary afferents. Arrow on each reconstruction indicates the location of a process added to the model of a calyx. Arrowhead indicates the location of a process added to the model of a neuron branch. These processes were not part of the original reconstructions but were placed at commonly observed sites to study systematically the effects of process location on depolarization magnitude at the SIZ. Scale bar is 10 μm.

Summation of Synaptic Inputs

Our previous simulations examined the effects of process location on depolarization magnitude at the SIZ. In those simulations, identical processes with identical synapses were placed at various locations on the afferent terminal. However, synapses along the inner membrane of the calyx from type I hair cells and along the outer membrane from the type II hair cells are more numerous sources of synaptic input to the afferent. Synapses on calyces were assessed by the next set of simulations

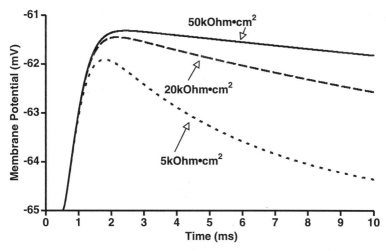

FIGURE 6. Effects on excitatory postsynaptic potential magnitude when R_m is changed from 50,000 Ωcm^2 to 5000 Ωcm^2 while keeping g_{syn} constant at 5 nS. Simulations were conducted using afferent A from FIGURE 6. Depolarization is reduced by slightly more than 0.5 mV. However, the greatest effect is on the decay rate of the membrane potential. This is a consequence of decreasing the time constant of the membrane, thereby allowing the membrane to discharge more quickly.

using the representative afferent described above. In one case, active membrane was placed at the SIZ and at the nodes of Ranvier. Internodal regions were modeled as high-resistance regions of membrane (1 MΩcm^2).

For the simulation shown in FIGURE 9, membrane resistivity was 5000 Ωcm^2 and

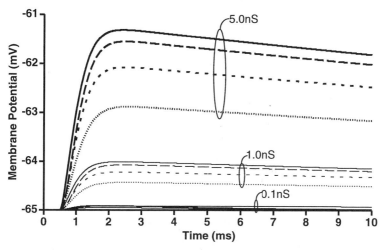

FIGURE 7. Excitatory postsynaptic potential (EPSP) magnitude as g_{syn} is varied from 5 nS to 0.1 nS. Simulations were conducted using afferent A from FIGURE 6. R_m was set at 50,000 Ωcm^2 to prevent traces from overlapping. The EPSP magnitude remains proportional across the four afferents as synaptic conductance is decreased.

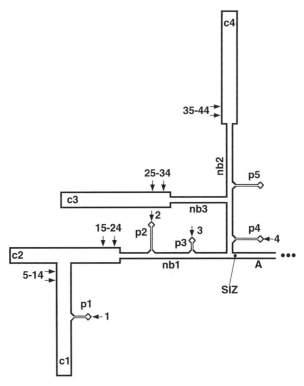

FIGURE 8. Schematic representation of the reconstructed afferent in FIGURE 6D. This diagram illustrates the general structure used in the simulation. A, axon; SIZ, heminode; nb1–nb3, three neuron branches; c1–c4, four equivalent cylinder calyces; and p1–p5, five processes. The numbered, small arrows on the calyces and process heads are the 44 synaptic inputs to the afferent, 10 on each calyx and one on each process. In all simulations calyces and neuron branches are divided into 10 compartments, and processes are divided into four sections of 30 compartments each. The axon is composed of a one-compartment heminode connected to a 30-μm, 10-compartment internode, followed by a 3-μm, one-compartment node, a 1000-μm, 10-compartment internode, and a final 3-μm, one-compartment node. Nodes have active (Hodgkin-Huxley-like) membranes.

synaptic conductance was 1 nS. In the first simulation, the 44 synapses were activated one at a time and the individual results summed. In the second simulation, all 44 synapses were activated simultaneously. In this case, peak depolarization was approximately 14% less than the sum of the individual synaptic responses, demonstrating that synaptic currents did not sum linearly.

Simulations of Primary Afferents with Active Spike Initiation Zone

FIGURE 9 illustrates the results of adding active membrane to the first heminode (the SIZ) and to nodes along the axon. Synapses were activated individually and their responses summed. In this case, peak depolarization is reduced and the rate of repolarization is more rapid. An afterhyperpolarization similar to that observed following an AP is displayed, even though depolarization is subthreshold. These results demonstrate that simulation of subthreshold depolarizations on an afferent with only passive properties yields different values from simulations that include active membrane at the SIZ.

DISCUSSION

Selection of Simulation Parameter Values

Values for synaptic conductance and membrane resistivity are not easily selected for compartmental simulations because results suggested by *in vitro* and *in vivo* electrophysiological studies vary widely. We hoped to narrow the choices by examining the consequences of varying parameters across a range of reasonable values. Indirect methods of selecting the particular parameters are necessary because direct measurements of membrane resistivity and synaptic conductance are not available for vestibular primary afferents. One such indirect method is to use EPSP amplitude. EPSPs measured in primary afferents in the vestibular system of frogs,[30] lizards,[31] and toads,[32] and in the auditory system of goldfish[33] provide values between 0.5 and 1.0 mV. Our findings suggest that a 1.0 nS synaptic conductance is most appropriate for use in vestibular afferent simulations because 1.0 nS produces an appropriate

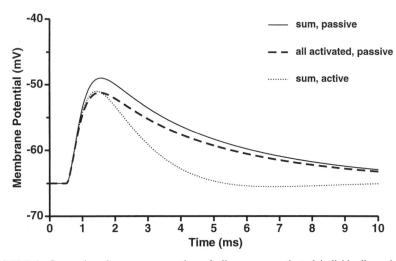

FIGURE 9. Comparison between summation of all synapses activated individually and all synapses activated simultaneously. This simulation used the afferent shown in FIGURE 10. R_m = 5000 Ωcm^2, g_{syn} = 1 nS. The solid line is produced by the sum of 44 synapses activated individually on a passive afferent ending, and the heavy-dashed line by the simultaneous activation of the same 44 synapses. The difference between these two traces demonstrates that summation of simultaneously activated synapses is nonlinear. The dotted line is the sum of 44 individually activated synaptic inputs with active nodes on the axon. Addition of Hodgkin-Huxley active sites to the nodes produces an intermediate amplitude response that repolarizes more quickly than either of the previous responses. Also, there is a clear afterhyperpolarization not seen in the other two traces.

amplitude EPSP (see FIG. 7). Altering membrane resistivity did not change the EPSP amplitude enough to provide a basis for choosing between the values tested. However, EPSP duration was closest to that obtained experimentally when the membrane resistivity was 5000 Ωcm^2 (FIG. 6). Including an active SIZ in the simulation (FIG. 9) brought the EPSP duration even closer to measured values.

Effects of Stem Dimension

Our first set of simulations was a systematic analysis of simplified processes with biologically appropriate stem lengths and diameters. If processes are viewed as electronic devices, the voltage drop across the stem of both afferent and efferent processes is controlled by impedance matching. There are two impedance matching problems: head to stem, and stem to neuron branch. In afferent processes, the head to stem impedance matching is a consequence of the ratio g_{syn}/g_{stem} (the conductance of the synapse divided by the conductance of the stem). The net effect of a synapse on depolarization of the neuron branch (or calyx) is determined by the ratio of the conductance loading provided by the neuron branch (or calyx) to the conductance of the stem. If g_{syn} is large and g_{stem} is small (i.e., the diameter of the stem is small), the process can act as a fixed voltage source,[12] but only if the conductance of the neuron branch (or calyx) is small. On the other hand, if the conductance of the neuron branch is large compared with the stem, then the stem cannot transfer sufficient current to depolarize the neuron branch—that is, there is an impedance mismatch. Under these conditions, impedance mismatch decreased the magnitude of depolarization more than 60 mV (see also ref. 14 and FIG. 2).

Current flow in the opposite direction (antidromically) produces a different result. Because of the relatively small diameter of the process stems, they have a high input impedance compared with the neuron branch or calyx from which they emanate. Just as the high input impedance of an oscilloscope allows it to accurately reflect the voltage of some system, the high input impedance of the stems allows the processes to accurately reflect the magnitude of depolarization within calyces and neuron branches. Thus, processes act as voltage followers. This result agrees with findings obtained in models of dendrites and dendritic spines by Shepherd and Brayton.[14]

Including Active Membrane

The addition of active (Hodgkin-Huxley) channels at the SIZ reduces the amplitude and duration of subthreshold depolarizations. Active channels serve to increase the temporal dynamics of the system by more rapidly returning the cell to resting potential. For a series of subthreshold responses, the contributions of individual synapses to depolarization of the afferent would be significantly less than estimated from simulations of passive neurons, especially if the synapses are not simultaneously activated. In contrast to most neuronal models that have the SIZ far removed from the sites of synaptic input, many of the terminal endings in the vestibular periphery are electrically close to the SIZ and all are in continuity with it. Continuity with the active membrane for spike generation requires inclusion of this active zone in simulations of synapses, even though the synapses may be located in a passive region of the cell.

Influences of Distal Spread of the Action Potential

Vestibular afferent neurons are bipolar cells structurally capable of bidirectional conductance of APs initiated along the axon. On histochemical grounds, the SIZ of nerve fibers with long unmyelinated neuron branches is likely located at the first heminode.[34,35] No cell body separates the SIZ from the terminal endings. Therefore, the typical cellular conditions that might produce attenuation of the depolarizing effects of an AP on the most distal calyx processes are not present. Dendrites on classical neurons in the central nervous system tend to be much longer and more branched than macular endings, electrically isolating the distal tips of the dendrite from the SIZ.

The primary purpose of the AP is to transmit depolarization rapidly along the axon toward the central nervous system. A secondary consequence of the AP is a large, rapid, synchronous spread of depolarization distally into the primary afferent ending. With minimal delay, all the calyces on an afferent that has fired will be isopotential. Likewise, all the neuron branches, process stems, and process heads will be nearly isopotential. Simultaneous with the AP, sufficient depolarization to release transmitter from the efferent endings will arrive at the efferent heads (i.e., greater than 20 mV depolarization).

Moreover, as the distal spread of depolarization approaches zero mV, synaptic input to the afferent will be altered, thereby changing the discharge characteristics of the nerve fiber. When the depolarization at the head exceeds the reversal potential of the synaptic channels (0 mV), the electromotive driving force at the synapse will change from inward to outward, shunting current out of the cell. Therefore, when the cell is depolarized by the distal spread of the AP, the inward synaptic current will first slow and then reverse when the local potential is above 0 mV. In some afferents, no inward flow of ions will pass through the synapse beginning 0.3 ms after onset of AP, and this effect will last for nearly 0.4 ms. Any postsynaptic channels that open will provide the afferent ending with a more rapid return to resting, not further depolarization. Therefore, during an AP, the electromotive driving force acting at a synapse would modulate the flow of current through the synaptic channel, acting as an "excitatory self-inhibition." This modulation could have consequences for the rate and regularity of repetitive firing of the primary afferent.

Possible Roles of Efferent Processes

Our results indicate that all efferent processes emanating from a single primary afferent, regardless of process morphology, receive synchronous depolarization sufficient to provide a unified output to adjacent cells in the macula. The consequences of activating the efferent processes depend on whether they form excitatory or inhibitory synapses. The neurotransmitter at these efferent processes is currently unknown.

A common inhibitory neurotransmitter in the central nervous system is γ-amino-butyric acid (GABA). GABA has been localized to the vestibular end organ in hair cells and primary afferents,[36–40] but is differentially localized according to the species examined. Nonmammalian species contain GABAergic elements within the hair cells whereas mammals tend to contain GABA in afferent fibers (guinea pig) or efferent fibers (squirrel monkey). In the rat, only the upper parts of the calyces in the sensory epithelia showed evidence of GABA.[39]

The presence of GABA suggests that some synapses in the macula are inhibitory. A large percentage of the processes intrinsic to the macula are vesiculated and presynaptic to adjacent type II hair cells and other primary afferents.[41] A possible function for the unusual arrangement of these endings is lateral inhibition, such as the center/surround organization in the retina. However, if these peripheral endings are GABAergic and the central terminations of the afferents in the vestibular nucleus are excitatory (as they most likely are), we are left with a single neuron producing two different neurotransmitters with opposite actions. The co-localization of the excitatory and inhibitory neurotransmitters glutamate and GABA, although uncommon, has been found in hippocampal mossy fibers,[42] the basal forebrain magnocellular complex of the rat and monkey,[43] the striatal projection neurons in the rat,[44] and the bipolar cells of the tiger salamander retina.[45]

SUMMARY

We cut serial sections through the medial part of the rat vestibular macula for transmission electron microscopic (TEM) examination, computer-assisted 3-D reconstruction, and compartmental modeling. The ultrastructural research showed that many primary vestibular neurons have an unmyelinated segment, often branched, that extends between the heminode (putative site of the spike initiation zone) and the expanded terminal(s) (calyx, calyces). These segments, termed the neuron branches, and the calyces frequently have spine-like processes of various dimensions with bouton endings that morphologically are afferent, efferent, or reciprocal to other macular neural elements. The major questions posed by this study were whether small details of morphology, such as the size and location of neuronal processes or synapses, could influence the output of a vestibular afferent, and whether a knowledge of morphological details could guide the selection of values for simulation parameters. The conclusions from our simulations are (1) values of 5.0 kΩcm^2 for membrane resistivity and 1.0 nS for synaptic conductance yield simulations that best match published physiological results; (2) process morphology has little effect on orthodromic spread of depolarization from the head (bouton) to the spike initiation zone (SIZ); (3) process morphology has no effect on antidromic spread of depolarization to the process head; (4) synapses do not sum linearly; (5) synapses are electrically close to the SIZ; and (6) all whole-cell simulations should be run with an active SIZ.

REFERENCES

1. SEGEV, I. & W. RALL. 1988. Computational study of an excitable dendritic spine. J. Neurophysiol. **60(2):** 499–522.
2. WILSON, C. 1992. Nonlinear synaptic integration in neostriatal spiny neurons. *In* Analysis and Modeling of Neural Systems 2: 393–405. Kluwer Academic Publishers. Norwell, MA.
3. CONRADI, S. 1969. Ultrastructure and distribution of neuronal and glial elements on the motoneuron surface in the lumbosacral spinal cord of the adult cat. Acta Physiol. Scand. Suppl. **332:** 5–48.
4. MCLAUGHLIN, B. J. 1972. The fine structure of neurons and synapses in the motor nuclei of the cat spinal cord. J. Comp. Neurol. **144:** 429–460.
5. DURAND, D., P. L. CARLEN, N. GUREVICH, A. HO & H. KUNOV. 1983. Electrotonic parameters of rat dentate granule cells measured using short current pulses and HRP staining. J. Neurophysiol. **50(5):** 1080–1097.
6. JACK, J. J. B. & S. J. REDMAN. 1971. An electrical description of the motoneuron and its application to the analysis of synaptic potentials. J. Physiol. **215:** 321–352.

7. RALL, W. 1962. Theory of physiological properties of dendrites. Ann. N.Y. Acad. Sci. **96:** 1071–1092.

8. RALL, W. 1984. Dendritic neuron theory and dendrodendritic synapses in a simple cortical system. Handbook of Physiology: 552–565. American Physiological Society. Bethesda, MD.

9. ROSE, P. K. & S. J. VANNER. 1988. Differences in somatic and dendritic specific membrane resistivity of spinal motoneurons: An electrophysiological study of neck and shoulder motoneurons in the cat. J. Neurophysiol. **60(1):** 149–165.

10. BROWN, T. H., D. H. PERKEL, J. C. NORRIS & J. H. PEACOCK. 1981. Electrotonic structure and specific membrane properties of mouse dorsal root ganglion neurons. J. Neurophysiol. **45(1):** 1–15.

11. COLEMAN, P. A. & R. F. MILLER.1989. Measurement of passive membrane parameters with whole-cell recording from neurons in the intact amphibian retina. J. Neurophysiol. **61(1):** 218–230.

12. KOCH, C., A. ZADOR & T. H. BROWN. 1992. Dendritic spines: Convergence of theory and experiment. Science **256:** 973–974.

13. HESTRIN, S., R. A. NICOLL, D. J. PERKEL & P. SAH. 1990. Analysis of excitatory synaptic action in pyramidal cells using whole-cell recording from rat hippocampal slices. J. Physiol. **422:** 203–225.

14. SHEPHERD, G. M. & R. K. BRAYTON. 1979. Computer simulation of a dendrodendritic synaptic circuit for self- and lateral-inhibition in the olfactory bulb. Brain Res. **175:** 377–382.

15. RALL, W. 1967. Distinguishing theoretical synaptic potentials computed for different soma-dendritic distributions of synaptic input. J. Neurophysiol. **30:** 1138–1168.

16. RALL, W. 1969a. Distributions of potential in cylindrical coordinates and time constants for a membrane cylinder. Biophys. J. **9:** 1509–1541.

17. RALL, W. 1969b. Time constants and electrotonic length of membrane cylinders and neurons. Biophys. J. **9:** 1483–1508.

18. RALL, W. & G. M. SHEPHERD. 1968. Theoretical reconstruction of field potentials and dendrodendritic synaptic interactions in olfactory bulb. J. Neurophysiol. **31:** 884–915.

19. SHEPHERD, G. M., R. K. BRAYTON, J. P. MILLER, I. SEGEV, J. RINZEL & W. RALL. 1985. Signal enhancement in distal cortical dendrites by means of interactions between active dendritic spines. Proc. Natl. Acad. Sci. USA **82:** 2192–2195.

20. KINNAMON, J. C., S. J. YOUNG & T. J. SHERMAN. 1986. 3DEd, Recon. and Show. Laboratory for High Voltage Electron Microscopy. University of Colorado, Boulder, CO.

21. YOUNG, S. J., S. M. ROYER, P. M. GROVES & J. C. KINNAMON. 1987. Three-dimensional reconstructions from serial micrographs using the IBM PC. J. Electron Microsc. Tech. **6:** 207–217.

22. HINES, M. 1989. A program for simulation of nerve equations with branching geometries. Int. J. Bio-Med. Comput. **24:** 55–68.

23. HINES, M. 1991. Neuron and Hoc Interpreter. Neurobiology Department, Duke University Medical Center. Durham, NC.

24. JOHNSTON, D. & T. H. BROWN. 1983. Interpretation of voltage-clamp measurements in hippocampal neurons. J. Neurophysiol. **50(2):** 464–483.

25. RAJAN, R. & B. M. JAHNSTONE. 1988. Biaural acoustic stimulation exercises protective effects at the cochlea that mimic the effects of electrical stimulation of an auditory efferent pathway. Brain Res. **459:** 241–255.

26. CHERUBINI, E., R. A. NORTH & J. T. WILLIAMS. 1988. Synaptic potentials in rat locus coeruleus neurons. J. Physiol. **406:** 431–442.

27. RANDALL, A. D., J. G. SCHOFIELD & G. L. COLLINGRIDGE. 1990. Whole cell patch clamp recordings of an NMDA receptor mediated synaptic current in rat hippocampal slices. Neurosci. Lett. **114:** 191–196.

28. YAMAGUCHI, K. & H. OHMORI. 1990. Voltage-gated and chemically gated ionic channels in the cultured cochlear ganglion neurone of the chick. J. Physiol. **420:** 185–206.

29. HARRIS, D. & J. K. STEVENS. 1989. Dendritic spines of CA1 pyramidal cells in the rat

hippocampus: Serial electron microscopy with reference to their biophysical characteristics. J. Neurosci. **9:** 2982–2997.

30. ROSSI, M. L., P. VALLI & C. CASELLA. 1977. Post-synaptic potentials recorded from afferent nerve fibres of the posterior semicircular canal in the frog. Brain Res. **135:** 67–75.
31. SCHESSEL, D. A., R. GINZBERG & S. M. HIGHSTEIN. 1991. Morphophysiology of synaptic transmission between type I hair cells and vestibular primary afferents. An intracellular study employing horseradish peroxidase in the lizard, Calotes versicolar. Brain Res. **544:** 1–16.
32. SUGAI, T., M. SUGITANI & H. OOYAMA. 1991. Effects of activation of the divergent efferent fibers on the spontaneous activity of vestibular afferent fibers in the toad. Jpn. J. Physiol. **41:** 217–232.
33. FURUKAWA, T., Y. HAYASHIDA & S. MATSUURA. 1978. Quantal analysis of the size of excitatory post-synaptic potentials at synapses between hair cells and afferent nerve fibres in goldfish. J. Physiol. **276:** 211–226.
34. SAIDEL, W. M. 1988. Variations of trigger zones in vestibular afferent fibers of fish. Neurosci. Lett. **84:** 161–166.
35. ROSS, M. D., L. CUTLER, D. DOSHAY, R. CHENG & A. NADDAF. 1991. A new theory of macular organization based on computer-assisted 3-D reconstruction, Monte Carlo simulation and symbolic modeling of vestibular maculas. Acta Otolaryngol. (Stockh.) Suppl. **481:** 11–14.
36. USAMI, S.-I., M. IGARASHI & G. C. THOMPSON. 1987a. GABA-like immunoreactivity in the chick vestibular end organs. Brain Res. **418:** 383–387.
37. USAMI, S.-I., M. IGARASHI & G. C. THOMPSON. 1987b. GABA-like immunoreactivity in the squirrel monkey vestibular end organs. Brain Res. **417:** 367–370.
38. USAMI, S.-I., J. HOZAWA, M. TAZAWA, M. IGARASHI, G. THOMPSON, J.-Y. WU & R. J. WENTHOLD. 1989. Immunocytochemical study of the GABA system in chicken vestibular endorgans and the vestibular ganglion. Brain Res. **503:** 214–218.
39. YLIKOSKI, J., U. PIRVOLA, O. HAPPOLA, P. PANULA & I. VIRTANEN. 1989. Immunohistochemical demonstration of neuroactive substances in the inner ear of rat and guinea pig. Acta Otolaryngol. **107:** 417–423.
40. DIDIER, A., J. DUPONT & Y. CAZALS. 1990. GABA immunoreactivity of calyceal nerve endings in the vestibular system of the guinea pig. Cell Tissue Res. **260:** 415–419.
41. ROSS, M. D., C. M. ROGERS & K. M. DONOVAN. 1986. Innervation patterns in rat saccular macula: A structural basis for complex sensory processing. Acta Otolaryngol. **102:** 75–86.
42. SANDLER, R. & A. D. SMITH. 1991. Coexistence of GABA and glutamate in mossy fiber terminals of the primate hippocampus: An ultrastructural study. J. Comp. Neurol. **303:** 177–192.
43. MARIN, L. J., C. D. BLACKSTONE, A. I. LEVY, R. L. HUGANIR & D. L. PRICE. 1993. Cellular localization of AMPA glutamate receptors within the basal forebrain magnocellular complex of rat and monkey. J. Neurosci. **13:** 2249–2263.
44. WHITE, L. E., H. D. HODGES, K. M. CARNES, J. L. PRICE & J. M. DUBINSKY. 1994. Colocalization of excitatory and inhibitory neurotransmitter markers in striatal projection neurons in the rat. J. Comp. Neurol. **339:** 328–340.
45. YANG, C. Y. & S. YAZULLA. 1994. Glutamate-, GABA-, and GAD-immunoreactivities co-localize in bipolar cells of tiger salamander retina. Visual Neurosci. **11:** 1193–1203.

Determinants of Semicircular Canal Afferent Response Dynamics in Fish[a]

R. D. RABBITT,[b,c,f] S. M. HIGHSTEIN,[d,f] AND R. BOYLE[e,f]

[b]Department of Bioengineering
University of Utah
2480 Merrill Engineering Building
Salt Lake City, Utah 84112

[d]Department of Otolaryngology
Washington University School of Medicine
4566 Scott Avenue, Box 8115
St. Louis, Missouri 63110

[e]Department of Otolaryngology/Head-Neck Surgery & Physiology
Oregon Health Sciences University
Portland Oregon 97201

[f]Marine Biological Laboratory
Woods Hole, Massachusetts 02543

INTRODUCTION

The vestibular semicircular canals sense angular head movements and generate first-order neural signals that are transmitted to the brain stem via the VIIIth cranial nerve. These signals are combined centrally with other sensory inputs for the purpose of controlling motion and motor outputs. The vestibular inputs in particular are essential to the proper function of key motor systems, including the vestibulospinal and vestibulo-ocular reflex arcs which serve to control head/body stability and posture, and the motion of the eyes, respectively. Angular motion sensation by the semicircular canals relies upon angular head accelerations to induce macromechanical response of the endolymphatic fluid, micromechanical cupular and stereociliary-bundle motion, nanomechanical gating of hair cell transduction channels, ion movement through excitable basolateral membrane surfaces, presynaptic processes leading to neurotransmitter release, and postsynaptic processes leading to afferent spike trains. The overall input-output behavior of this cascade is experimentally determined by recording the responses of individual afferents to various waveforms of head motion. Although this input-output relationship is relatively well documented, the specific contribution of each segment in the cascade in shaping the neural response is a subject of ongoing research. Present results contribute to this effort by parsing the overall process into two parts: (1) mechanical and (2) post-transduction current (PTC).

First-order semicircular canal neurons exhibit several nonlinearities that influence their response dynamics. In addition to the nonlinearities of conditional spike generation, the most prominent is a frequency-dependent saturating nonlinearity, which appears to be due primarily to hair cell/afferent biophysics.[1–10] The saturating

[a]This work was supported by the National Institute of Deafness and Other Communications Disorders grant DC-01837.
[c]Corresponding author. E-mail: rabbitt@biomech.bioen.utah.edu

nonlinearities are most important only at high levels of stimulation, such that for each afferent there is a stimulus level below which the response is essentially linear. Existence of a low-level linear regime is in contrast to the physiology of the auditory system where a sensitivity-enhancing nonlinearity becomes dominant at low levels near the threshold of hearing.[11,12] This nonlinearity is in addition to a second, saturating nonlinearity that is analogous to that present in canal afferents. For the semicircular canals, the level at which the saturating nonlinearity begins to be significant varies between individual afferents and species. In some cases the linear range can be predicted reasonably well from the afferent response type or from the afferent/synaptic morphology.[1,13–16] In numerous previous studies the relative importance of nonlinearities is quantified using Fourier methods and reported in the form of harmonic distortion. Although harmonic distortion is informative, numerical values are highly sensitive to the degree of phase-locking in afferent responses and hence is not a direct measure of input-output linearity. Rather than using harmonic distortion to indicate nonlinearity, present results employ the fundamental definition that requires input-output relations to obey the superposition principle.[17] In using this definition the input is defined as the stimulus and the output is defined as the constrained first-harmonic afferent response (see METHODS). A response is classified as nonlinear if the input-output relation violates the basic definition of linearity. In this study, stimuli were maintained at low levels in order to restrict responses to the effective linear regime. This allowed for the use of linear transfer functions in interpreting the results and in separating the subprocesses involved in the sensation of angular head motion.

For sinusoidal head oscillations in the physiological frequency range, the response of most semicircular canal afferents is frequency modulated (FM). More precisely, the instantaneous spike frequency elicited during harmonic head oscillations contains a first-harmonic component that modulates with an amplitude and phase determined by a frequency-dependent function of the stimulus. (See METHODS for a definition of the first-harmonic relevant to cut-off neural responses.) Within the linear range these first-harmonic neural responses can be written as transfer functions from head velocity (or head acceleration) to the afferent response. In all species studied to date, ranging from fish to primates, transfer functions show that individual canal afferents encode primarily angular head velocity, angular head acceleration or a combination of the two.[1,7,15,18–31] In our experimental model, the oyster toadfish *Opsanus tau*, some horizontal canal (HC) afferents modulate their instantaneous firing rate with an amplitude and phase reflecting the angular velocity of sinusoidal head motion, whereas others within the same animal reflect the angular acceleration.[1] The entire population of approximately 300 HC afferents define a continuous distribution of response sensitivities falling primarily between these two extremes. Exactly how this interafferent diversity is generated has not yet been determined.

Previous work provides evidence of diversity at each stage leading to individual neural responses. On a macroscopic scale, contributions from the following three parts of the overall process can be inferred from the literature: (1) synaptic mechanisms and afferent dynamics, (2) hair cell biophysics, and (3) spatiotemporal mechanical activation of hair cells. In some species, correlations have been established between the afferent response dynamics and resting discharge statistics,[18,32–35] but the same measure does not hold universally across species nor does it hold across all hair cell/afferent morphological types.[1,15,35] Because the stochastic properties of resting discharge are determined primarily by synaptic and afferent dynamics,[35,37–41] the existence of such correlates suggests that afferent response dynamics are partially determined by these mechanisms. Correlations between response dynamics and/or resting discharge statistics have also been established with respect to the topological organization of neuronal projections into crista.[13,15,21,36,42–45] These correlates suggest that the mechanical activation of hair cells differs across various regions of the crista and/or that PTC processing exhibits spatial organization within the crista. Some evidence also exists that the kinetics of hair cell basolateral currents may vary systematically with spatial location in the crista.[46–48] Direct measurements of stereociliary bundle displacement during physiological stimulation in the semicircular canal are unavailable to provide the spatiotemporal distribution of mechanical activation of hair cells. Nevertheless, low-frequency or quasi-static measurement of cupula displacement,[49–51] inhomogeneous structure of the cupula,[52,53] diversity of stereocilia deflection and cupular interaction,[53,54] and theoretical studies,[55,56] all indicate that spatial diversity in the mechanical activation of hair cells probably does exist. Taken together these findings support the hypothesis that interafferent diversity present in the population of semicircular canal afferents is due to contributions from both the canal mechanics and PTC mechanisms.

Results presented here illustrate the extent to which mechanical and PTC mechanisms contribute separately to individual HC afferent responses in the toadfish. This separation was achieved by recording individual afferent responses during mechanical stimulation, which excites hair cells by modulation of stereocilia displacements, and during electrical stimulation, which excites hair cells by modulation of the apical-face Nernst-Plank potential. Mechanical indentation of the HC limb was used to mimic sinusoidal head rotation and to eliminate the need to rotate the fish.[57–61] In the same preparation, current passing and voltage measuring electrodes were placed in the endolymphatic space of the anterior canal (AC) to modulate the voltage of the endolymph relative to the intracellular hair cell and the extracellular basolateral voltages. For individual afferents, both the electrical and mechanical stimuli employ the same PTC biophysics and morphological pathway. In effect, the electrical stimulus bypasses the mechanics such that differences between the afferent responses for the electrical and mechanical stimuli can be used to extract the mechanical component of the overall signal processing.[62] Results provide evidence of the extent to which individual afferent responses are predetermined by mechanical events leading to the gating of hair cell transduction channels, and also the extent to which they are further modified by PTC mechanisms.

METHODS

Methods have been previously described by Boyle and Highstein[1] (e.g., afferent recordings and analysis), Highstein *et al.*[62] (e.g.: endolymphatic polarization), and Rabbitt *et al.*[60] (e.g.: mechanical indentation). Briefly, adult toadfish, *Opsanus tau*, of either sex (ca. 500 g) were supplied by the Marine Biological Laboratory, lightly anesthetized by immersion in MS222 (3-aminobenzoic acid ethyl ester; Sigma, St. Louis, MO), and partially immobilized by an intramuscular injection of pancuronium bromide (Pavulon, 0.05 mg/kg; Sigma). Fish were then secured in a Lexan tank filled with fresh seawater and mounted on a vibration isolation table. The vestibular labyrinth and afferent nerves were exposed with a dorsal craniotomy as illustrated in FIG 1. The cerebrospinal fluid space was filled with a fluorocarbon (FC-75, 3-M).

Mechanical stimuli were delivered by sinusoidal indentation of the horizontal canal.[57] A piezoelectric actuator (Burleigh PZL-060 or -100) was placed on the long-and-slender limb of the horizontal canal (FIG. 1, point HCI). Linear motion of the piezoelectric drive was measured using a linear variable differential transformer (LVDT, Schaevitz DC-E 050). This will subsequently be referred to as *mechanical* stimulation or *indentation*. Care was taken to insure that the flat surface of the indenter (1.2 mm diam. glass rod) was flush with the labyrinth and preloaded as described in Rabbitt *et al.*[60] The piezoelectric actuator was driven by a function generator (Tektronics AFG602) and a high-voltage amplifier (TrigTek 207A) to generate sinusoidal mechanical indentation of the horizontal canal limb from 0.02 to 40 Hz.

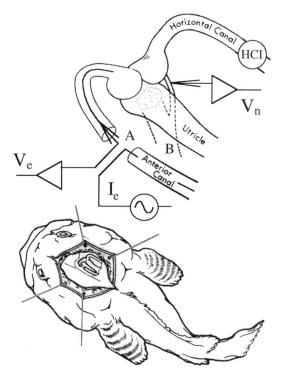

FIGURE 1. Experimental setup. The anterior canal was divided at the dorsal extreme (A) for access to the endolymphatic space. Polarization was achieved using sinusoidal current injection (I_e) into the posterior section of the anterior canal (Ag/AgCl electrode), and the resulting polarization voltage was measured using an endolymph-filled glass electrode within the anterior canal ampulla (V_e). Horizontal canal indentation (HCI) was applied to the lateral limb to mimic sinusoidal head rotation in the horizontal plane. Extracellular and/or intra-axonal neural responses were measured (V_n) in the horizontal canal branch of the VIIIth cranial nerve (B), and discriminated spike times were recorded for both the electrical and mechanical stimuli from ~ 0.02 to 30 Hz.

The AC was carefully divided at about one-third of the distance between the AC ampulla and common crus (FIG. 1, point A), and the free ends were electrically isolated in air above the fluorocarbon-filled cranial space. For electrical polarization, a Ag/AgCl wire was placed into the distal limb of the AC to serve as the current passing electrode, and a 100 μm internal tip diameter endolymphatic voltage recording pipette (V_e, FIG. 1), filled with endolymph taken from a donor fish, was placed in the proximal end and lowered into the AC ampulla. Current (I_e, FIG. 1) was injected into the endolymph using a current source (WPI, A395), with command current provided by a function generator (Tektronix, AFG5102), via the chlorided wire. Fluctuations in the endolymphatic voltage (V_e) were measured relative to a common muscle reference ground. This is henceforth referred to as *endolymphatic polarization* or *electrical* stimulation.

Extracellular or intraaxonal afferent responses were recorded from the horizontal canal nerve (V_n, FIG. 1), amplified, threshold discriminated, and converted to impulse times. Afferent spike times and stimulus triggers were recorded to a resolution of 80 µs. Calibrated indenter displacement (amplified LVDT voltage), endolymphatic polarization voltage, and current injection were amplified to span the 12-bit range of the A/D converter (Cambridge Electronic Design 1401plus, Apple Macintosh interface) and digitized at a rate of ~0.4 ms.

Waveform averaging, synchronized to the stimulus, was applied to determine the first-harmonic amplitude and phase of the mechanical indentation and the polarization voltage. For sinusoidal stimuli, this method yields equivalent results as obtained by discrete Fourier transform (DFT) or least-squares. The first-harmonic amplitude and phase of afferent responses were determined from 100 bin/cycle phase histograms synchronized to the same stimulus trigger. Because the afferent responses are often cut off and result in some empty bins, a constrained least-squares (CLS) procedure was applied for the neural responses rather than a DFT (as employed for waveforms). In this, empty bins were ignored and the DC level was restricted to be $\geq$ 0 (i.e., the zero[th] harmonic is associated with background firing rate and was required to be $\geq$ 0 in the fit). For afferent responses containing $\geq$ 50% empty bins (which commonly occurs at stimulus frequencies $\geq$ ~20 Hz), Gaussian distributions were fitted to the phase histograms. For the Gaussian fits, the peak value defines the amplitude of the afferent response and the mean determines the phase. The amplitude and phase obtained by these methods shall henceforth be referred to as the *first-harmonic* (note the difference between the present usage of the term first-harmonic and the standard Fourier definition). We define here the *afferent response dynamics* as the frequency-dependent gain and phase determined by dividing the complex number representation of the first-harmonic afferent amplitude and phase by the complex number representation of the corresponding stimulus at each frequency.

The procedure noted above can be applied to compute the first-harmonic afferent gain and phase regardless of whether the afferent responds linearly or not. It is only in the interpretation of results that linearity becomes important. In the present work we define the "effective linear regime" with respect to the constrained first-harmonic responses as computed using the procedure described above. Following the standard definition, this requires the amplitude of the first-harmonic response (output) to grow linearly with the amplitude of the stimulus (input) and also requires the superposition principle to apply for multiple inputs. This is a restricted definition that does not directly address distortion products. Even with this definition, at high stimulus levels and at high frequencies, afferent responses begin to deviate from the linear regime. For all afferents included in results, multiple levels were tested in order to insure that stimuli were in the effective linear regime at 2 Hz.

RESULTS

Mechanical Stimuli

Mechanical indentation of the HC canal limb was used to mimic head rotation. For the purpose of illustration, the firing patterns of two afferents from the same fish are shown in FIGURE 2 in response to ± 3 µm mechanical indentation of the HC limb at 1 Hz. Raw spikes (mV; A_2, B_2) and corresponding, instantaneous spike frequencies (imp/s; A_1, B_1) are shown along with the mechanical stimulus (μm; C). The LG afferent (B_1, B_2) responds in phase with positive indentation (compression of the canal) with a gain of ~ 4 (spike/s per μm), and the HG afferent (A_1, A_2) responds

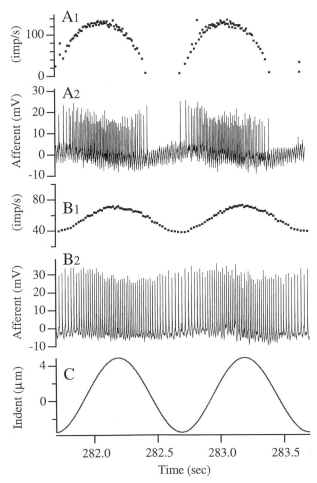

FIGURE 2. Response to mechanical indentation. Raw spikes (mV; A_2 and B_2) and externally discriminated impulses (imps/s; A_1 and B_1) are shown for two horizontal canal afferents from a single fish in response to 1 Hz mechanical indentation (μm; C). The top afferent is classified as high-gain and the lower afferent is classified as low-gain. The same afferents can be excited using endolymphatic polarization or rotation of the head to elicit similar responses.

with a phase lead of ~ 38 deg and gain of ~ 27 (spike/s per μm). These responses can be reproduced in the same afferents by rotating the animal[60] or by applying appropriate endolymphyatic polarization.[62] As discussed below, this correspondence is because all three stimuli employ the same hair cell/synaptic machinery and differ primarily in the activation of hair cell transduction currents.

Endolymphatic Polarization

Steps or waveforms of current were delivered via an Ag/AgCl electrode positioned in the posterior limb of the AC (I_e, FIG. 1) and generated isopotential voltage modulations of the 3-canal endolymphatic space. This voltage was continuously monitored using an endolymph-filled glass electrode placed within the AC ampulla (V_e, FIG. 1). Almost all of the injected current flowed to muscle ground through a relatively low impedance that drops from a constant value of ~ 1100 Ω below 0.02 Hz to a constant value of ~ 200 Ω above 2 Hz. This impedance primarily reflects leakage of the labyrinthine membrane wall, and was not measurably influenced either by sequentially severing and isolating the canal and otolithic nerves, or by connecting an active voltage follower to force the various nerve insertions at the end organs to reference ground.[62] Regardless of the action of the voltage follower, positive steps of current increased the endolymphatic voltage and increased the corresponding firing rate of individual afferents, whereas negative steps of current decreased the endolymphatic voltage and decreased or silenced afferent firing rates. For current steps applied at increasing levels there is an irreducible delay of ~ 0.7 ms from the onset of endolymphatic voltage to afferent spike initiation consistent with the delay reported during mechanical stimuli.[60,62] This delay, shown in FIGURE 3 for one neuron, exceeds that attributed to spike propagation along the neuron to the recording site, and is believed to primarily reflect the chemical nature of synaptic transmission.[63,64] The fact that the delay is the same for both mechanical and electrical stimuli provides evidence that endolymphatic polarization acts presynaptically and, further, that it acts via the same pathway as physiological stimuli, at least in the toadfish.

Additional evidence of the presynaptic action of endolymphatic polarization is provided by applying sinusoidal stimuli. In seven afferents tested, the gain and phase during electrical stimulation were unaffected by actively forcing the extracellular nerve bundle to ground; hence, neural modulation is not due to direct excitation of the afferents. Also, the response dynamics elicited by endolymphatic polarization are distinct from those obtained for modulated current injection via a bridge circuit into axons of the same afferent nerves. The polarization responses are also distinct from those obtained for mechanical stimuli. Inasmuch as neural responses persist even when the extracellular space surrounding the basolateral surfaces of sensory hair cells is maintained near the reference ground, the site of action of endolymphatic polarization is deduced to be at the apical face. The excitatory action of endolymphatic polarization is therefore consistent with simple modulation of the Nernst-Plank potential at the apical face of sensory hair cells, and with the associated modulation of ion transport through the hair cell transduction channels.[62]

As noted previously, injecting DC current into the endolymphatic space causes an increased average firing rate of individual semicircular canal afferents. The average discharge rate increases in an approximately linear fashion with increasing transepithelial voltage and passes through zero near $V_e = -50$ mV. In relating this value to the membrane potential it is important to note that the intracellular hair cell voltage (isopotential V_i) can be measured relative to the apical-membrane surface or the basolateral-membrane surface, which yield two distinct membrane potentials. The data are consistent with the view that the apical-face membrane potential is approximately -50 mV at rest (i.e., when $V_e = 0$)—a figure that is consistent with the membrane potential reported to yield robust mechanically induced receptor

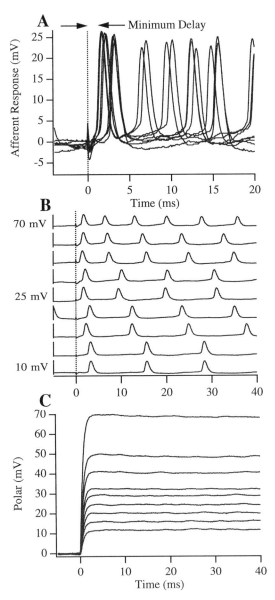

FIGURE 3. Electrical recruitment of spikes. Square pulses of current were delivered to the endolymph at increasing levels to produce the endolymph voltages shown in **C.** As the voltage is increased, spikes (**A** and **B**) are recruited at shorter and shorter latencies until an irreducible delay of approximately 0.7 ms is reached.

potential modulation in isolated saccular hair cells.[4] Superimposing sinusoidally varying potentials on top of the DC polarization shows that, unlike the average firing rate, the gain and phase of afferent responses are relatively unaffected by the DC polarization level (for stimuli -30 mV $< V_e < +30$ mV[62]). This is illustrated in the form of phase histograms for an example afferent in FIGURE 4A–C for DC polarizations of $V_e = +9$, -5, and -29 mV, respectively. The afferent response is shown using the scale on the left (histograms; imp/s per mV) and the electrical stimulus is shown using the scale on the right (solid sinusoidal lines; mV). Dotted lines show the sinusoidal first-harmonic CLS fit of the bin-histogram afferent response. It is

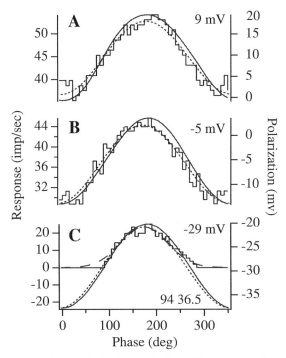

FIGURE 4. Influence of DC polarization level. Phase histograms and corresponding first-harmonic fits (*short dashed lines*) show the neural response to endolymphatic polarization (*solid curve*) for DC potentials of $+9$ (**A**), -5 (**B**), and -29 (**C**) mV. The average firing of afferents is increased for positive polarization and decreased for negative polarization. In **C** (-29 mV) the afferent response is partially cut off. Even though the background rate changes, the gain and phase in response to sinusoidal polarization are insensitive to the DC potential in the range $\sim \pm35$ mV from the rest (referenced to 0 mV endolymph).

important to note that as the DC polarization level becomes more negative the average firing rate decreases until the afferent becomes silent, but the gain and phase relative to the stimulus modulation remain nearly constant. This is precisely what would be expected if endolymphatic polarization acts only to modulate the Nernst-Plank potential driving ions through the partially open transduction channels.

Nature of the Afferent Response

The stimulus-dependent firing of individual afferents for endolymphatic polarization exhibits characteristics similar to those observed for head rotation[1] or mechanical indentation[60] in the same species. At low frequencies of sinusoidal polarization, individual afferent fibers exhibit sinusoidal modulation of instantaneous firing frequency (FM mode of response). At high frequencies of simulation, individual spikes become locked to a specific phase relative to the stimulus and fire in a stochastic fashion every n^{th} cycle of the stimulus (PL, phase-locked mode of response, $n = 1, 2, 3...$). This is illustrated in FIGURE 5 where endolymphatic polarization responses of a single afferent are shown from top to bottom for stimulation at 1, 6, 12, 20, and 35 Hz (solid lines indicate the polarization stimulus). Responses at 1 and 6 Hz are of the FM type, whereas the response shown in the bottom panel at 35 Hz is of the PL type. Sinusoidal curves fit the low-frequency afferent responses quite well (short dashed lines at 1 and 6 Hz), whereas Gaussian curves are more appropriate at high frequencies (dashed line at 35 Hz). In contrast to the multimode transition present at 12 and 20 Hz for this afferent, some other afferents show a smooth transition from the FM to PL mode and are easily fit over the entire frequency range using the CLS sinusoids at low frequencies and Gaussian curves at high frequencies. For these afferents the gain and phase obtained using the Gaussian fit match those obtained using the CLS method when $\sim 50\%$ of the histogram bins are empty (see FIG. 4C for an example of this). In general it is appropriate to use Gaussian fits for responses with $> 50\%$ empty bins and CLS sinusoids for responses with $\leq 50\%$ empty bins. At the low- and high-frequency extremes where FM or PL responses dominate, the appropriate gain and phase are easily identifiable by the amplitude and phase of the sinusoid (low frequencies) or Gaussian curves (high frequencies). At intermediate frequencies, for a majority of neurons, neither a single Gaussian nor a single sinusoid is satisfactory. For the neuron illustrated in FIGURE 5 at 12 Hz three peaks are present in the phase histogram, and the response here could be viewed as three separate Gaussian amplitudes locked at three distinct phases. As the frequency is further increased to 20 Hz, one of the three peaks attenuates to zero amplitude, and we are left with two Gaussian-shaped peaks appearing at relative phases P_1 and P_2. The sinusoidal fit shown at 20 Hz does not reproduce the amplitude or phase of either peak. Further increasing the frequency to 35 Hz results in a single Gaussian peak occurring at $P_1 \sim 90$ deg phase advanced from the stimulus. This peak is identified with the left-most peak occurring at 20 Hz and with the center peak occurring at 12 Hz. Note that the average firing rate (determined by the area under the curve divided by 360 deg) fluctuates according to the phase-locked frequency, but in general is relatively constant in comparison to the peak instantaneous rate. At even higher frequencies the afferent maintains a single Gaussian PL response, but begins to fire every cycle, and later, every n^{th} cycle. For sufficiently high frequencies of mechanical indentation or endolymphatic polarization the phase begins to roll off as determined, in part, by synaptic and afferent delay.[60,62]

Electrical versus Mechanical Stimuli

To compare the response dynamics induced by mechanical stimuli to those induced by endolymphatic polarization the gain and phase of individual afferent responses were determined as a function of frequency (i.e., transfer functions) for both electrical and mechanical stimuli. As detailed in METHODS, afferent responses were time averaged using 100 bin/cycle histograms, and first-harmonic sinusoids

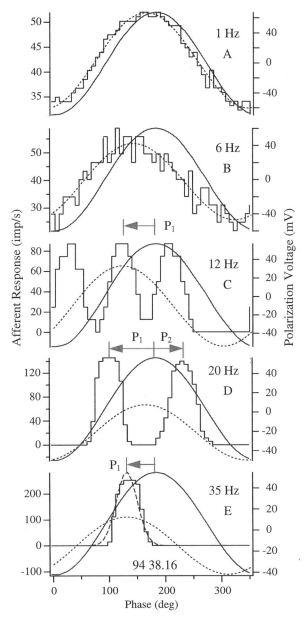

FIGURE 5. Frequency modulation and phase locking. Phase histograms of a single afferent are shown for sinusoidal endolymphatic polarization (*solid lines*) from 1 to 35 Hz. At low-stimulus frequencies (< ~10 Hz) all semicircular canal afferents are frequency modulated (FM) and at high-stimulus frequencies are phase locked (PL; > ~30 Hz for this afferent). In the middle frequency range (~10 to 30 Hz) responding afferents undergo a transition from the FM to the PL regime. Phase histograms of the neural response in the FM regime are fit well by sinusoids (*short dashed lines*), whereas phase histograms in the PL regime are fit well by Gaussian distributions (*dashed line; 35 Hz*).

were fitted using the CLS method. For the purpose of the present comparison, afferent responses having $\geq$ 50% empty bins were classified as PL and Gaussian fits were used to define the amplitude and phase; all other responses were classified as FM and fit with CLS sinusoids. Results provided in FIGURES 6–10 pertain to response dynamics determined in this way. Slightly different curves are obtained at stimulation above $\sim$ 12 Hz if CLS sinusoidal fits are used exclusively, but this

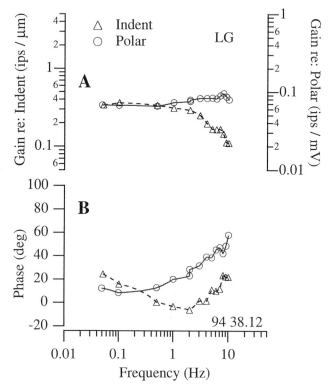

FIGURE 6. Low-gain (LG) afferent. Response dynamics of a single LG afferent are shown for endolymphatic polarization (*continuous* ○) and mechanical indentation (*dashed* △). Symbols denote the gain (**A**) and phase (**B**) as determined by fitting the neural phase histograms (see METHODS). Gains provide the afferent modulation above the DC rate in impulses per second (ips) per unit stimulus amplitude (mV or μm). Phases (**B**) denote the peak response relative to the stimuli such that positive values denote a neural phase lead.

approach does not accurately reflect the amplitude of the PL-type responses captured by the Gaussian fits. In comparing afferent responses for electrical and mechanical stimuli, either approach is valid because the data analysis method influences both mechanical and electrical results in precisely the same way.

By stimulating with multiple inputs at various levels, we were able to determine straightforwardly the linearity of the responses. Each afferent was tested for linearity at 2 Hz, and stimuli were subsequently maintained at low levels well within the linear regime. The linear amplitude range (e.g., μm indentation) determined at 2 Hz extends to the lowest physiological frequencies but does not extend unconditionally to high frequencies. In general, the linear regime is maintained for afferents responding in the FM mode but is compromised for highly PL responses. For PL responses the variance of the Gaussian phase histogram decreases as the amplitude increases, but this accommodation rapidly saturates. This frequency dependence complicates interpretation of results $>$ ~ 14 Hz where a majority of the afferents tested show some degree of phase locking. In order to construct Bode plots up to 40 Hz, both electrical and mechanical stimuli were maintained at a constant level across the entire frequency band tested. Changing the level within the linear regime (established at 2 Hz) does not influence the Bode plots at low frequencies but does have an impact at higher frequencies. For this reason the same level was used for both the electrical and mechanical stimuli yielding nearly equal afferent responses. Typically the level was set at $\sim 50\%$ of that associated with the initiation of the saturating nonlinearity at 2 Hz. Levels of electrical and mechanical stimuli were both adjusted to achieve the same level of afferent response when applied independently at 2 Hz. When applied simultaneously these balanced stimuli cause constructive interference (doubling the response generated by one stimulus) or destructive interference (canceling the afferent response) depending upon their relative phases.[60,62] This approach facilitates comparison of the mechanically and electrically induced response dynamics by insuring nearly linear responses in the low-frequency range and minimizing differences in the nonlinearities induced by the two different stimuli in the high-frequency range.

As noted in the INTRODUCTION, individual semicircular canal afferents exhibit a relatively wide range of response dynamics that together define a population encoding various components of head movement. Previous studies in the toadfish have divided the population into three groups according to the sensitivity during head rotation.[1] For this species an indenter displacement of $\pm$ 1 μm mimics a head velocity $\sim$ ± 4 deg/s (for stimuli $\sim$ < 2 Hz and indenter location shown in FIG. 1), and hence the equivalent (HG, LG, A) groups can be formed using afferent responses to mechanical indentation rather than to head rotation.[60] Results are shown according to these groups identified during mechanical stimuli.

FIGURE 6 shows the response dynamics of a single afferent to endolymphatic polarization and mechanical indentation. Gains (imp/s per μm and imp/s per mV) are shown in the upper panel (**A**) and the corresponding phases are in the lower panel (**B**). Based on the head-velocity-sensitive (indenter-displacement-sensitive) phase and flat gain recorded during mechanical stimulation at 2 Hz, this afferent falls within the LG group. Differences between the curves for electrical and mechanical stimuli are significant. The magnitude of the response to endolymphatic polarization is insensitive to frequency (0.05–10 Hz), whereas the response to mechanical indentation declines markedly above 2 Hz. Correspondingly, the phase during electrical stimulation exceeds that present during mechanical stimulation above 0.2 Hz. Below 0.2 Hz the phase lead present during the mechanical stimulation exceeds that present during electrical stimulation.

The response dynamics for a single afferent falling within the HG group are shown in FIGURE 7. For afferents in this group the gains elicited by electrical and mechanical stimuli show very similar frequency dependencies over the entire range tested. The phase, however, is more advanced during mechanical indentation both at low frequencies ($\sim$ < 0.2 Hz) and again at high frequencies ($\sim$ > 10 Hz). Error bars at 2 Hz, approximately equal to the symbol size, indicate one standard deviation calculated on the basis of $\geq$ 10 repeated tests at stimulus levels spanning the linear range. The small size of the error bars reflects both high linearity (see METHODS) and repeatability.

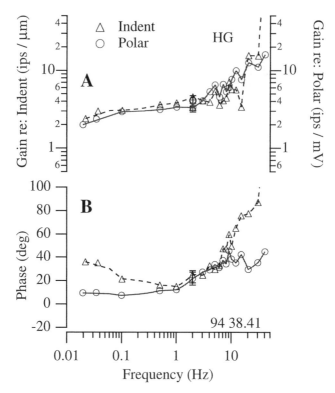

FIGURE 7. High-gain (HG) afferent. Same notation as in FIGURE 6, but for a different afferent falling within the HG group from the same fish. Error bars appearing at 2 Hz show ±1 SD in the results for > 10 repeated tests of the same afferent at various stimulus levels.

For comparison, the response dynamics of a single afferent falling within the A group are shown in FIGURE 8 (cf. FIGS. 6 and 7 recorded from different HC afferents within the same fish). It is significant to note that the phase during mechanical indentation is more advanced than that during electrical stimulation across the entire frequency range tested. Also, the slope of the gain in response to the mechanical stimuli is steeper than the slope in response to electrical stimuli (note that the left and right gain axes both span two orders of magnitude). Differences in the phase and slope of the gain are significant.

FIGURE 9 summarizes the response dynamics of 35 afferents tested for mechanical stimulation. Afferents were divided into groups (LG, HG, A) according to their responses to mechanical stimulation[1,60] and plotted in the form of gain and phase. Transfer functions averaged for each group are summarized in FIGURE 9A and B, and scatter plots for all individual afferents tested are provided in FIGURE 9C and D. Error bars shown on the summary curves (FIG. 9A and B) reflect interafferent variability within each group (1 SD). The scatter plots illustrate that the population of afferent responses form a continuum with gains spanning more than two orders of magnitude and phases spanning more than 120 deg. There is very little overlap between the three groups, particularly with respect to phase, which is the key determinant in classifying the afferents. For mechanical stimuli the LG group responds in phase with head velocity (indenter displacement) at 2 Hz and has a relatively low and flat gain. In contrast, the A group responds nearly in phase with head acceleration (indenter velocity) and shows a gain that increases markedly with frequency of the mechanical stimulus. The phase of the HG group during mechanical stimulation falls between these two extremes.

FIGURE 10 summarizes the results for the same 35 afferents tested during endolymphatic polarization (same notation as FIG. 9). Differences distinguishing the LG, HG, and A groups during mechanical stimulation simply do not hold for the same afferents stimulated by electrical polarization of the endolymph. The phases during electrical stimulation exhibit only small deviations for all three groups, and in the middle frequency range are statistically equivalent (FIG. 10B). Because the response to endolymphatic polarization reflects PTC mechanisms and bypasses the mechanics, we conclude that differences leading to interafferent diversity in phase primarily reflect the mechanics (up to and including activation of the transduction channel). Differences in gain between LG, HG, and A groups during electrical stimulation are primarily a shift in the magnitude of the entire curve without a change in slope (FIG. 10A and C). This is in contrast to results obtained during mechanical stimulation where A group afferents show an increasing gain with

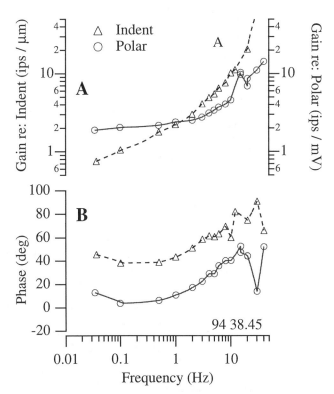

FIGURE 8. Acceleration (A) afferent. Same notation as in FIGURE 6, but for a different afferent falling within the A group from the same fish.

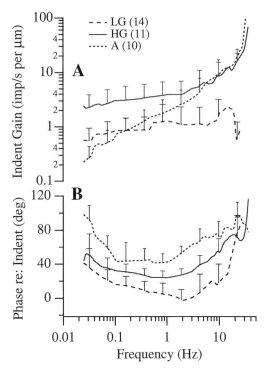

FIGURE 9. Summary of mechanical responses. For the purpose of discussion, afferents are grouped according to gain and phase to mechanical indentation as described in METHODS. Average results are shown (**A** and **B**) along with data for individual afferents (**C** and **D**). Curves denote group averages for 14 low-gain afferents (LG, *dashed*), 11 high-gain afferents (HG, *solid*), and 10 acceleration-sensitive afferents (**A**, *short dashed*). Error bars show standard deviations associated with interafferent variability within each group and hence span the region between the average curves. The slope of the gain for the A group, the level of the gain for the HG group, and the level of the phase for all three groups are notable (portions replotted from Highstein *et al.*[62]).

frequency and LG afferents do not (cf. FIG. 9A and C). Hence, interafferent diversity in the magnitude of the gain is influenced partially by diversity in PTC processing, but the frequency dependence is not; interafferent diversity in the frequency dependence appears to be a result of the mechanics leading to the transduction currents.

FIGURE 11 summarizes results for all 35 afferents for both electrical and mechanical stimuli. The number of cells at each frequency is shown in A, the gains are shown in B, and the phases in C. Solid curves show the population average for endolymphatic polarization, and dashed curves show the population average for mechanical indentation. The error bars denote 1 SD and reflect interafferent variability within the population. When averaged across the population, a remarkable agreement is found between the frequency dependence of the gain for both the mechanical and electrical stimuli (B). Based on this we conclude that the high-frequency (0.2–10 Hz) gain and phase enhancements present in the population

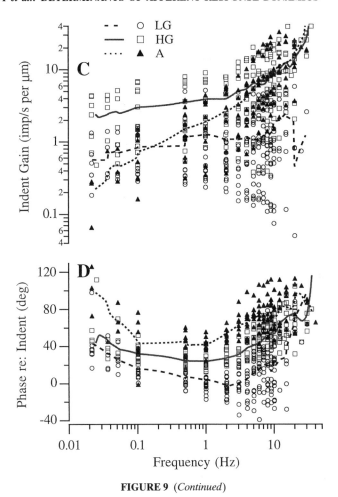

FIGURE 9 (*Continued*)

average primarily reflect hair cell/afferent (PTC) processing. As previously noted, this agreement holds for the population average but does not extend to individual afferents (FIGS. 6–10) nor to the LG, HG, and A groups (FIGS. 9 and 10). The phase, when averaged across the population, shows a marked increase during mechanical indentation at low frequencies ($\sim <0.2$ Hz) that is absent during endolymphatic polarization. This phase lead during mechanical stimuli is consistent with attenuation of the mechanical activation of hair cells due to mechanical stiffness and/or mechanical adaptation of the transduction current. There is approximately a 15 deg phase advance at low frequencies of endolymphatic polarization, which indicates that afferent adaptation is relatively small in comparison to mechanical effects. Another deviation in phase is observed at high-stimulus frequencies (>10 Hz) where phase lead during mechanical stimulation exceeds that present during electrical polarization, but interpretation of these high-frequency data is complicated by the transition from FM to PL responses.

DISCUSSION

It is significant that individual afferent responses elicited by the electrical and mechanical stimuli show different frequency dependencies (FIGS. 6–11). Consider, for example, the LG afferent shown in FIGURE 6. The response to endolymphatic polarization has a flat gain, whereas the response to mechanical indentation attenuates above ~0.8 Hz. Also, the phase during mechanical stimulation lags during electrical polarization over the same frequency range. These differences are statistically significant. All individual afferents tested show differences between responses to mechanical and electrical stimuli. We argue below that the difference is primarily due to the mechanics, which is bypassed during the electrical stimulus. We begin with a brief discussion of the action of each stimulus in modulating the hair cell transduction currents, followed by a discussion of the specific results.

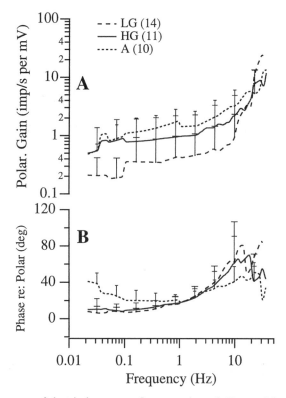

FIGURE 10. Summary of electrical responses. Same notation as in FIGURE 9, but in response to sinusoidal endolymphatic polarization. Individual afferents and average curves are for the identical groups of neurons as shown in FIGURE 9. In comparison to the mechanical responses, the phases are much more uniform between afferent groups, and the gains vary primarily in amplitude and not in slope or frequency dependence (portions replotted from Highstein et al.[62]).

Mechanically Modulated Transduction Currents

The technique of compressing the long-and-slender duct to excite the canal was first used by Ewald in 1892 (see ref.[65]), and was subsequently refined by Dickman *et al.*[57-59] to allow for various waveforms of stimuli to be accurately applied. For the toadfish ±1 μm sinusoidal HC indentation generates the equivalent afferent responses as ±4 deg/s head velocity for sinusoidal stimuli below 2 Hz, and this correspondence is explained on the basis of canal macromechanics. However, at higher frequencies (> 2 Hz) the correspondence is less direct because the amplitude and phase of indentation must be modified as a function of frequency to reproduce the rotational stimuli.[60] Because indentation does not require movement of the

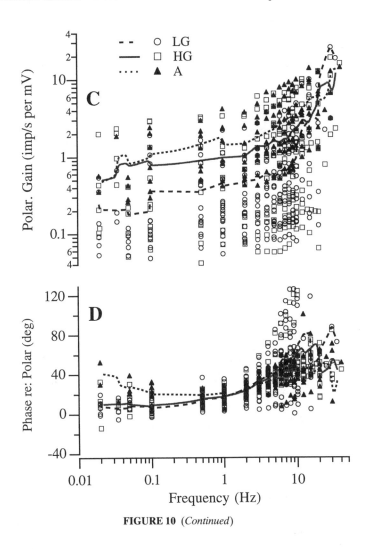

FIGURE 10 (*Continued*)

animal in space, it facilitates experiments requiring numerous probes and manipulators, and hence was selected as the mechanical stimulus for the present study.

Macromechanical stimuli, such as mechanical indentation or head rotation, modulate hair cell transduction currents by inducing endolymph flow, cupular displacement, micromechanical stereociliary bundle displacements, and corresponding nanomechanical gating of ion channels. The mechano-sensitive gating of hair cell

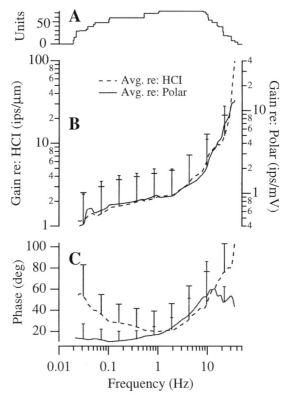

FIGURE 11. Average electrical and mechanical responses. Averaging over the population of afferents (**A**) shows that the average gains (**B**) for endolymphatic polarization and mechanical indentation are remarkably similar, which is not the case for individual afferents or subgroups of afferents (cf. FIGS. 6–10). The average phase advance (**C**) during mechanical stimulation exceeds that due to endolymphatic polarization below ~0.2 Hz, confirming the existence of a mechanical lower-corner frequency. In the range from 1 to 10 Hz the electrical and mechanical responses are remarkably similar. Error bars show 1 SD and reflect interafferent variability in responses at each frequency (replotted from Highstein *et al.*[62]).

transduction channels can be described in terms of the channel open probability P, which is a function of bundle displacement x and time t.[4,6,66–72] For a large number of channels the open probability determines the fraction of channels open, and thus modulates the Nernst-Planck–driven flow of salient ions, K^+ and Ca^{2+}, through the channels into the hair cell. Since the open probability is approximately 13% at rest, a significant fraction of the maximum transduction current is continuously flowing even at rest. During mechanical indentation the open probability is modulated to induce intracellular hair cell voltage modulations on the order of 300 $\mu V/\mu m$.[62] For the Bode results, low stimulus levels were employed so the receptor potential modulations are small relative to the hair cell resting potential, and the Nernst-Plank potential is approximately constant during mechanical stimulation. As a result, the open probability and corresponding current flow changes in a nearly linear fashion with small magnitude mechanical displacements of stereociliary bundles. This coupled sequence of events is reflected in hair cell receptor potentials recorded at low stimulus levels[4,62] and, ultimately, in semicircular canal neural responses (FIGS. 2–11; also see ref. 1). In summary, low-level mechanical stimuli act to modulate the open probability of hair cell transduction channels without significantly influencing the Nernst-Plank potential acting across the apical surface.

Electrically Modulated Transduction Currents

In contrast to the mechanical stimuli, endolymphatic polarization acts to modulate the electrochemical gradient without significantly influencing the open probability. In the toadfish the apical tight junctions between hair cells and supporting cells form an electrical barrier with an impedance much higher than the impedance between the extracellular basolateral space and ground.[41,62] Because of this, endolymphatic polarization drives the transduction current via modulation of the apical-face Nernst-Plank potential without significantly influencing the basolateral voltage. This is evidenced, in part, by the transsynaptic nature of the electrical stimulus. Upon delivering increasing steps of endolymphatic polarization voltage, action potentials are recruited with an irreducible delay of ~ 0.7 ms (FIG. 2). The delay is interpreted as being due to the chemical nature of synaptic transmission,[41,63,64,73–76] thus indicating that the electrical stimulus acts presynaptically. The delay obtained using electrical polarization is, in fact, the same as that obtained from high-frequency phase-shifts of the neural response using mechanical stimulation in this species.[60] Additional evidence that the extracellular basolateral space is in good continuity with ground was obtained by noting that the response of individual afferents to endolymphatic polarization is not influenced by actively grounding or electrically isolating the extracellular neural space.[62] Endolymphatic polarization is distinct from galvanic stimulation where voltage modulations influence firing of afferent nerves directly without synaptic delay.[37,77,78] Based on these observations, we conclude that polarization of the endolymph causes modulation of the Nernst-Plank potential acting across the apical face of hair cells, and this in turn leads to modulation of the hair cell transduction current.

The high impedance of the apical surface is not expected to extend indefinitely for increasing frequencies because of the high-pass character of hair cell and supporting-cell membranes. We have validated, by direct measurement, that the cutoff frequency associated with longitudinal flow of current through viable PC-12 cells deformed into a cylindrical geometry (~ 8 $\mu m \times 20 \mu m$) is approximately 10 MHz—a value very similar to that observed in other cells.[79,80] The cutoff frequency is primarily determined by the cell membrane, but can be perturbed somewhat by changes in the relatively low impedance of the cytoplasm. Although there is no direct evidence to suggest that the apical surface of hair cells has a significantly lower cutoff frequency, it is presumed that the stereociliary bundles will introduce some additional capacitance which has not yet been directly measured. If this capacitive leakage were to play a role in the present experiments, the bundle/channel geometry would need to reduce the effective membrane capacitance by about one million, which would probably not be the case. Results presented by Dallos and Evans[81] for cochlear outer hair cells indicate that a capacitive voltage divider may influence the response at frequencies as low as ~ 300 Hz. This implies that the effective capacitance of hair cell membranes may be considerably lower than would be expected from a simple lipid bilayer. Even if this does apply to semicircular canal hair cells in the toadfish, the cutoff frequency is still well above the range of the present experiments. Therefore, in the interpretation of the results, we ignore frequency-dependent capacitive leakage into hair cells and/or into the basolateral extracellular space.

It has been shown previously that polarization of the endolymph induces motility of semicircular canal hair cell stereocilia.[82] How this may relate to responses during mechanical stimuli is not yet known. The important question in comparing afferent responses is whether any motility that may be induced by endolymphatic polarization is the same as that induced by mechanical stimulation. If the motility were driven by intracellular voltage modulation, then it would be identical for the two stimuli. This follows because the two stimuli are easily balanced at each frequency to produce equivalent afferent responses, which implies that they also produce equivalent neurotransmitter release and associated intracellular conditions including voltage modulation. Events associated with the intracellular voltage are equivalent for the two stimuli, and, hence, motility driven by an intracellular signal does not influence interpretation of the present results. What must be addressed, therefore, is the possibility of an extracellular voltage signal inducing motility. This extracellular voltage modulation is present during endolymphatic polarization but absent during mechanical stimulation. The endolymph voltage was routinely recorded during mechanical indentation, and it does not exhibit stimulus-dependent fluctuations above the noise level (10 μV). Therefore, under mechanical stimulation the endolymph voltage is essentially constant and is not expected to be involved in significant electromechanical feedback. It remains possible that modulation of the endolymph voltage induces nonphysiological motility of hair bundles, but evidence provided by Rüsch and Thurm[82] indicates that this effect is relatively small. Differences between afferent responses to mechanical and electrical stimuli reported here are substantial and often differ in gain by more than an order of magnitude and differ in phase by more than 45 deg, which cannot be accounted for by stereociliary motility. In interpreting the present results, we therefore assume that any motility linked to the endolymph voltage is negligible, and that motility linked to the intracellular voltage is equivalent for the two stimulus types and thus is included in these results as a PTC mechanism.

In summary, evidence is consistent with the view that low-level endolymphatic polarization modulates the apical-face Nernst-Plank potential without significantly influencing the open probability of hair cell transduction channels. Endolymphatic polarization directly drives the transduction current and bypasses the mechanics normally interposed between the external stimulus (head motion or canal indentation) and the resulting motion of hair cell stereocilia. Therefore, afferent response dynamics reported for endolymphatic polarization reflect PTC mechanisms in the absence of mechanical processing.

Combining the electrical and mechanical stimuli causes transport of ions through the nonselective transduction channels in analogy to current flow in a simple electrical circuit where the voltage driving each ion is derived from the Nernst-Planck potential and the conductance is proportional to the open probability.[62,68,83,84] Hence, to good approximation for small stimuli, the identical transduction current can be obtained by modulating the Nernst-Planck potential for a fixed open probability (endolymphatic polarization) or by modulating the open probability for a fixed Nernst-Plank potential (mechanical indentation). This is precisely what was done in the present work.

Role of PTC Processing in Determining Afferent Response Dynamics

Individual afferent responses recorded during sinusoidal electrical polarization of the endolymph reflect signal processing that takes place in the chain of events between the transduction currents in the hair cell and the spike initiation zone in the afferent. Afferent responses summarized in FIGURE 11 clearly show that PTC mechanisms are responsible for the high-frequency (1–10 Hz) gain and phase enhancements observed across the population during both electrical and mechanical stimulation. Hence, hair cell/afferent dynamics introduce a rate-of-change component that is not present, on average, in the mechanics. This processing is universal across all afferents tested in *Opsanus,* and shows relatively little variability between individual cells, as can be seen by comparing responses of individual or groups of afferents during electrical stimulation. The specific biophysical source of the rate-of-change component is not yet known, but presumably is related to synaptic dynamics[85] and/or hair cell conductances.[86] In sharp contrast to responses recorded during mechanical stimulation, the phases of all three groups during electrical stimulation are identical at 2 Hz ($\sim 20°$) and do not show any significant differences in frequency dependence (FIG. 10B). The frequency dependence of the gain is also uniform for LG, HG, and A groups, with nearly identical absolute values for the HG and A groups (FIG. 10A). The clear differences in gain and phase between these groups during mechanical stimulation simply do not appear during endolymphatic polarization (cf. FIGS. 9 and 10). Endolymph polarization as a stimulus does not reveal the diversity of response dynamics seen using rotational and mechanical stimuli. Individual afferents cannot be identified as belonging to the LG, HG, or A group based on responses to endolymphatic polarization alone. Thus, interafferent variability reflected by the LG, HG, and A groups is primarily a result of canal mechanics and not PTC mechanisms. The only clear interafferent difference in response to endolymphatic polarization is a frequency-independent amplitude and some additional high-frequency gain enhancement in a limited number of afferents. Although PTC mechanisms play a significant role in determining high-frequency gain and phase enhancements seen across the entire afferent population and in the absolute level of the gain, PTC mechanisms do not appear to contribute as significantly to diversity in phase.

These findings imply that PTC signal processing is relatively uniform across the LG, HG, and A groups in the toadfish. The extent to which these groups differ in response to electrical polarization is primarily a frequency-independent sensitivity—not a frequency dependence of the gain or phase. Hence, correlates between the afferent groups and the morphology of dendritic arborizations in this species[13] probably do not reflect differences in PTC processing, but rather reflect diversity in the topology of micromechanical activation of hair cells. If this extends to other species, one would hypothesize that established correlates between spatial location on the crista and neural response dynamics may primarily reflect spatial diversity in the mechanical activation of hair cells.[15,21,42,44,45] In addition, results are consistent with the view that systematic variations in hair cell basolateral currents across regions of the crista[46–48] may be involved in modifying afferent-specific sensitivity (FIG. 10A).

Role of Mechanics in Determining Afferent Response Dynamics

In comparing average responses of the present afferent population for electrical and mechanical stimuli, it is clear that canal mechanics is responsible for a vast majority of the low-frequency (<0.2 Hz) phase enhancement seen in all afferents. Data show that the average phase during mechanical indentation at 0.02 Hz is ~60 deg advanced, but the average phase during endolymphatic polarization is less than 20 deg advanced at all frequencies below 1 Hz. The corresponding gains are shown using logarithmic scales, and, as expected, the small change in gain that would be predicted by theory to accompany the 40 deg mechanical phase difference is not discernible in the average data. The residual low-frequency phase advance present during electrical polarization may be due to afferent adaptation, which has been identified using galvanic stimulation.[37,77,78]

Above 12 Hz the average phase during mechanical stimulation leads the average phase during electrical stimulation. Although interpretation is complicated by PL neural responses, this difference in phase may be partially due to the distinction between the average cupula displacement and the local displacement at the surface of the sensory epithelium, as suggested by theoretical analysis of the unsteady endolymph-cupula interaction. Theoretical results provided in FIGURE 12 illustrate this effect for a simple axisymmetric model of the cupula/ampulla.[56] At low frequencies the angular deflection of the model cupula at its connection to the crista reflects the average displacement of the cupula and moves in phase with average endolymph flow. This is not the case at higher frequencies where unsteady, multidimensional, fluid flow causes both the phase and gain of the deflection at the surface of the crista to differ from the average deflection. A difference is also found between points located near the surface of the crista and points located a small distance in from the surface. Although unsteady profiles have not yet been measured in the semicircular canals, similar displacement profiles are known to exist in other sinusoidally driven flows having similar physical characteristics and associated nondimensional groups.[87] Viscous coupling of the stereociliary bundles with the cupula is also expected to contribute to the high-frequency response. Although presently available experimental data and mathematical models are not adequate to draw firm conclusions, the limited evidence is consistent with the hypothesis that multidimensional unsteady mechanics is responsible for at least part of the diversity in response dynamics present during mechanical stimulation but missing during electrical stimulation.

The most striking differences between afferent response dynamics to endolymphatic polarization and mechanical indentation appear in results for individual afferents and for the LG, HG, and A groups (three examples are shown in FIGS. 6–8; also see ref. 62). The same interafferent variability present during mechanical indentation does not exist during endolymphatic polarization (cf. FIGS. 9 and 10). It is particularly interesting that the gain of the A group shows a steep slope and crosses the LG and HG curves during mechanical indentation, but the same group is not so distinguished during electrical stimulation. Also, significant phase differences are found between the various groups during mechanical stimulation that are not present during electrical stimulation. We attribute these differences to canal mechanics.

The influence of canal mechanics is quantified in FIGURE 13 where the data are replotted to eliminate PTC processing. This is achieved by dividing the average mechanically induced transfer functions in FIGURE 9 by the electrical counterparts in FIGURE 10. Results are shown for each afferent group. It is the difference between these curves that is the primary contributor to interafferent diversity characterized by the LG, HG, and A groups. It is interesting that when all three curves are averaged together, we obtain a single curve almost identical to the HG curve. Thus, HG afferents reflect the population average and might be considered the group to which LG and A groups should be compared. The solid HG curve in FIGURE 12 is also representative of the average mechanical response ascertained by this method. All afferents exhibit phase leads and gain decreases (e.g., angular head velocity) at low frequencies attributed to canal mechanics.[88] Although previous theoretical efforts capture the average trend at low frequencies[55] and some additional detail at high frequencies,[56] it appears that these models do not yet contain adequate geometrical and constitutive descriptions to predict the mechanical activation of hair cells

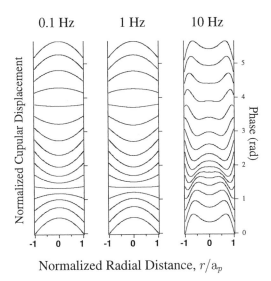

FIGURE 12. Displaced shape of the cupula predicted by a simple axisymmetric model of HC canal dynamics. In this model the cupula is treated as a circular membrane spanning the ampullary cross section. Distance from the center of the ampulla is shown as the radial distance normalized to the radius. Solid curves are the predicted displaced shapes of the cupula, greatly amplified for visualization, at various times in relation to the stimulus as denoted by the phase on the right axis. Note the predicted displacement of the cupula and its dependence on frequency (replotted from Damiano and Rabbitt[56]).

innervated by individual afferent fibers reflected in FIGURE 13. The most substantial differences between afferents belonging to the various groups appear at stimulus frequencies $> \sim 0.2$ Hz where differences in both phase and gain are present. These differences may be related to the topology of mechanical activation of hair cells. Above 10 Hz all three groups show increasing phase advance in the mechanics that is inconsistent with torsion-pendulum type models. As noted above, these high-frequency effects may be related, in part, to viscous coupling of stereociliary bundles to cupula and multidimensional fluid/cupula mechanics in the ampulla.

In summary, the LG group of afferents innervate hair cells that are mechanically activated with a phase lag at high frequencies (1–10 Hz). They also show decreasing mechanical gain at high frequencies. In contrast, PTC processing shows an increased gain and phase in the same frequency range. Results imply that the LG group of afferents effectively encode angular head velocity during physiological movement by offsetting high-frequency mechanical attenuation and phase lag with PTC amplifica-tion and phase lead. The A group is perhaps the most distinguished in that the mechanical gain activating these cells increases almost linearly with frequency and the mechanical phase is advanced by 30–40 deg over the entire range tested (FIG. 10A and B). Results imply that this mechanical effect adds constructively with high-frequency phase and gain enhancements caused by PTC processing so that A

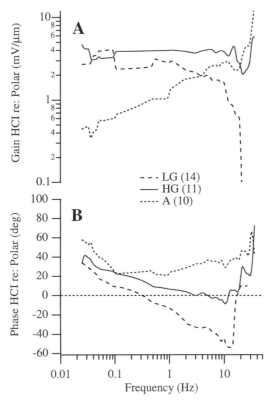

FIGURE 13. Mechanical response dynamics. Curves show the result of dividing the afferent response dynamics for mechanical stimuli by that for electrical stimuli for each afferent group. This calculation should remove post-transduction-current effects and leave only mechanical transfer functions. Results indicate that various afferents receive differing mechanical inputs that are the primary determinant of the LG, HG, and A groups (replotted from Highstein et al.[62]).

group afferents effectively encode angular head acceleration during physiological movement. The HG group falls between the LG and A extremes. Results imply that the mechanics activating HG afferents reflects angular head velocity such that the high-frequency phase and gain enhancements in these afferents is due primarily to PTC mechanisms.

In addition to linking canal mechanics with the LG, HG, and A groups, present results show that the increases in phase and gain present in the population average from 1 to 10 Hz are due to hair cell/afferent processing (PTC mechanisms). There is a remarkable agreement between the population average obtained for endolymphatic polarization and that obtained for mechanical indentation in the 1–10 Hz range (FIG. 11). This provides further evidence that mechanical effects add to some afferent responses and subtract from others, but overall do not contribute to the population average in the 1–10 Hz range. Action in this range is the domain of the hair cell/afferent complex. Outside of this range, mechanical effects influence the population average and also introduce additional interafferent variability as discussed above.

SUMMARY

Present results separate the relative contributions of semicircular canal biomechanics from hair cell/afferent biophysics in determining the amplitude and phase of afferent responses to sinusoidal motion of the head. Separation was achieved by combining electrical polarization of the endolymph with mechanical indentation of the canal limb to modulate the instantaneous firing rate of horizontal semicircular canal afferents. The electrical stimulus drives hair cell transduction currents via modulation of the Nernst-Planck potential, whereas the mechanical stimulus mimics head rotation and modulates the open probability of the transduction channels. Responses for electrical polarization therefore reflect post-transduction-current (PTC) mechanisms, and responses for mechanical stimulation include the additional influence of canal mechanics. Linear transfer functions defining individual afferent response dynamics were obtained for low levels of each stimuli and are reported in Bode form providing gain (spikes/s per μm or mV) and phase (deg re: peak stim) over the frequency range from 0.02 to 40 Hz. Combined results for electrical and mechanical stimuli distinguish the component of sensory signal processing carried out by canal mechanics from that carried out by the hair cell/afferent complexes. Individual afferents were categorized according to their response to the mechanical stimuli as low-gain velocity (LG), high-gain velocity (HG) or acceleration (A) sensitive, groups as originally defined by Boyle and Highstein[1] to describe interafferent diversity present within the population. In contrast to the results for mechanical stimuli, all afferent groups exhibit nearly equal increases in gain and phase for increasing frequencies of electrical stimulation. Comparison of individual afferent responses for the two stimuli leads to the conclusion that the LG, HG, and A groups are distinguished primarily by diversity in the mechanical activation of associated hair cells and not by PTC mechanisms. Even though PTC processing does not contribute significantly to determining these groups, it is the primary determinant underlying high-frequency gain and phase enhancements observed in the population average. Comparison of mechanical and electrical responses also reveals the mechanical lower-corner responsible for phase enhancements and gain decreases in all afferents at low frequencies of mechanical stimulation (<0.05 Hz). Results imply that LG afferents encode angular head velocity by canceling a phase lag and gain attenuation due to the mechanics with a phase lead and gain enhancement due to PTC mechanisms above ~0.2 Hz. In contrast, A group afferents encode angular head acceleration by combining high-frequency phase leads and gain enhancements present in both the mechanics and PTC mechanisms across the physiological frequency spectrum. HG afferents fall between these two extremes, and, other than the influence of the mechanical lower-corner, their response primarily reflects PTC processing.

REFERENCES

1. BOYLE, R. & S. M. HIGHSTEIN. 1990. Resting discharge and response dynamics of horizontal semicircular canal afferents of the toadfish, *Opsanus tau.* J. Neurosci. **10:** 1557–1569.
2. FERNÁNDEZ, C. & J. M. GOLDBERG. 1971. Physiology of peripheral neurons innervating the semicircular canals of the squirrel monkey. II. Response to sinusoidal stimulation and dynamics of peripheral vestibular system. J. Neurophysiol. **34:** 661–676.
3. O'LEARY, D. P. & C. WALL III. 1979. Analysis of nonlinear afferent response properties from the guitarfish semicircular canal. Adv. Oto-Rhino-Laryngol. **25:** 66–73.
4. HUDSPETH, A. J. & D. P. COREY. 1977. Sensitivity, polarity, and conductance change in the response of vertebrate hair cells to controlled mechanical stimuli. Proc. Natl. Acad. Sci. USA **74:** 2407–2411.
5. HUDSPETH, A. J. 1982. Extracellular current flow and the site of transduction by vertebrate hair cells. J. Neurosci. **2:** 1–10.
6. HUDSPETH, A. J. 1985. The cellular basis of hearing: The biophysics of hair cells. Science **230:** 745–752.
7. SEGAL, B. N. & J. S. OUTERBRIDGE. 1982a. Vestibular (semicircular canal) primary neurons in the bullfrog: Nonlinearity of individual and population response to rotation. J. Neurophysiol. **47:** 545–562.
8. SEGAL, B. N. & J. S. OUTERBRIDGE. 1982b. A nonlinear model of semicircular canal primary afferents in bullfrog. J. Neurophysiol. **47:** 563–578.
9. GAUMOND, R. P., C. E. MOLNAR & D. O. KIM. 1982. Stimulus and recovery dependence of cat cochlear nerve fiber spike discharge probability. J. Neurophysiol. **48:** 856–873.
10. JARAMILLO, F., V. S. MARKIN & A. J. HUDSPETH. 1993. Auditory illusions and the single hair cell. Nature **364:** 527–529.
11. RHODE, W. S. 1971. Observations of the vibration of the basilar membrane in squirrel monkeys using the Mössbauer technique. J. Acoust. Soc. Am. **49:** 1218–1231.
12. BROWNELL, W. E., C. R. BADER, D. BERTRAND & Y. DE RIBAUPIERRE. 1985. Evoked mechanical responses of isolated cochlear outer hair cells. Science **227:** 194–196.
13. BOYLE, R., J. P. CAREY & S. M. HIGHSTEIN. 1991. Morphological correlates of response dynamics and efferent stimulation in horizontal semicircular canal afferents of the toadfish, *Opsanus tau.* J. Neurophysiol. **66:** 1504–1521.
14. BRICHTA, A. M. & E. H. PETERSON. 1994. Functional architecture of vestibular primary afferents from the posterior semicircular canal of a turtle, Pseudemys (Trachemys) scripta elegans. J. Comp. Neurol. **334:** 481–507.
15. BRICHTA, A. M. & J. M. GOLDBERG. 1994. Afferent and efferent responses from morphologically identified fibers from the posterior semicircular canal of the turtle. Soc. Neurosci. Abstr. **18:** 510.
16. BRICHTA, A. M. & J. M. GOLDBERG. 1996. Afferent and efferent responses from morphological fiber classes in the turtle posterior crista. Ann. N.Y. Acad. Sci. This volume.
17. BOYCE, W. E. & R. C. DIPRIMA. 1970. Introduction to Differential Equations. John Wiley & Sons. New York.
18. FERNÁNDEZ, C. & J. M. GOLDBERG. 1971. Physiology of peripheral neurons innervating semicircular canals of the squirrel monkey. II. Response to sinusoidal stimulation and dynamics of peripheral vestibular system. J. Neurophysiol. **34:** 661–675.
19. PRECHT, W., R. LLINAS & M. CLARKE. 1971. Physiological responses of frog vestibular fibers to horizontal angular rotation. Exp. Brain Res. **13:** 378–407.
20. BLANKS, R. H. I., M. S. ESTES & C. H. MARKHAM. 1975. Physiologic characteristics of vestibular first-order canal neurons in the cat. II. Response to angular acceleration. J. Neurophysiol. **38:** 1250–1268.
21. O'LEARY, D. P., R. F. DUNN & V. HONRUBIA. 1976b. Analysis of afferent responses from isolated semicircular canal of the guitarfish using rotational acceleration white-noise inputs. II. Estimation of linear system parameters and gain and phase spectra. J. Neurophysiol. **39:** 645–659.
22. ANDERSON, J. H., R. H. I. BLANKS & W. PRECHT. 1978. Response characteristics of

semicircular canal and otolith system in the cat. I. Dynamic responses of primary vestibular fibers. Exp. Brain Res. **32:** 491–507.

23. HARTMANN, R. & R. KLINKE. 1980. Discharge properties of afferent fibers of the goldfish semicircular canal with high frequency stimulation. Pfluegers Arch. **388:** 111–121.

24. ANASTASIO, T. J., M. J. CORREIA & A. A. PERACHIO. 1985. Spontaneous and driven responses of semicircular canal primary afferents in the unanesthetized pigeon. J. Neurophysiol. **54:** 335–347.

25. ESTES, M. S., R. H. I. BLANKS & C. H. MARKHAM. 1975. Physiologic characteristics of vestibular first-order neurons in the cat. I. Response plane determination and resting discharge characteristics. J. Neurophysiol. **38:** 1239–1249.

26. LANDOLT, J. P. & M. J. CORREIA. 1980. Neurodynamic response analysis of anterior semicircular canal afferents in the pigeon. J. Neurophysiol. **43:** 1746–1762.

27. SCHNEIDER, L. W. & D. J. ANDERSON. 1976. Transfer characteristics of first and second order lateral canal vestibular neurons in gerbil. Brain Res. **112:** 61–76.

28. SHIMAZU, H. & W. PRECHT. 1965. Tonic and kinetic responses of cat's vestibular neurons to horizontal angular accelerations. J. Neurophysiol. **28:** 991–1013.

29. LOWENSTEIN, O. & A. SAND. 1940. The mechanism of the semi-circular canals: A study of responses of single fiber preparations to angular accelerations and to rotation at constant speed. Proc. R. Soc. Lond. B Biol. Sci. **129:** 256–275.

30. CORREIA, M. J., J. P. LANDOLT, M. D. NI, A. R. EDEN & J. L. RAE. 1981. A species comparison of linear and nonlinear transfer characteristics of primary afferents innervating the semicircular canal. *In* The Vestibular System: Function and Morphology. T. Gualtierotti, Ed.: 280–316. Springer-Verlag. New York.

31. RABBITT, R. D., R. BOYLE & S. M. HIGHSTEIN. 1994. Sensory transduction of head velocity and acceleration in the toadfish horizontal semicircular canal. J. Neurophysiol. **72:** 1041–1048.

32. GOLDBERG, J. M. & C. FERNÁNDEZ. 1971a. Physiology of peripheral neurons innervating semicircular canals of the squirrel monkey. I. Resting discharge and response to constant angular accelerations. J. Neurophysiol. **34:** 635–660.

33. GOLDBERG, J. M. & C. FERNÁNDEZ. 1971b. Physiology of peripheral neurons innervating semicircular canals of the squirrel monkey. III. Variations among units in their discharge properties. J. Neurophysiol. **34:** 676–685.

34. HONRUBIA, V., L. F. HOFFMAN, S. SITKO & I. R. SCHWARTZ. 1989. Anatomic and physiological correlates in bullfrog vestibular nerve. J. Neurophysiol. **61:** 688–701.

35. GOLDBERG, J. M., A. LYSAKOWSKI & C. FERNÁNDEZ. 1992. Structure and function of vestibular nerve fibers in the chinchilla and squirrel monkey. Ann. N.Y. Acad. Sci. **656:** 93–107.

36. GOLDBERG, J. M. 1991. The vestibular end organs: Morphological and physiological diversity of afferents. Curr. Opin. Neurobiol. **1:** 229–236.

37. GOLDBERG, J. M., C. E. SMITH & C. FERNÁNDEZ. 1984. Relation between discharge regularity and responses to externally applied galvanic currents in vestibular nerve afferents of the squirrel monkey. J. Neurophysiol. **51:** 1236–1256.

38. SMITH, C. E. & J. M. GOLDBERG. 1986. A stochastic afterhyperpolarization model of repetitive activity in vestibular afferents. Biol. Cybern. **54:** 41–51.

39. MILLER, M. I. & J. WANG. 1993. A new stochastic model for auditory-nerve discharge. J. Acoust. Soc. Am. **94(4):** 2093–2107.

40. KERNELL, D. 1968. The repetitive impulse discharge of a simple neurone model compared to that of spinal motoneurones. Brains Res. **11:** 685–687.

41. HIGHSTEIN, S. M. & A. L. POLITOFF. 1978. Relation of interspike baseline activity to the spontaneous discharges of primary afferent from the labyrinth of the toadfish, *Opsanus tau*. Brain Res. **150:** 182–187.

42. O'LEARY, D. P., R. F. DUNN & V. HONRUBIA. 1974. Functional and anatomical correlations of afferent responses from the isolated semicircular canal. Nature **251:** 225–227.

43. O'LEARY, D. P., R. F. DUNN & V. HONRUBIA. 1976a. Analysis of afferent responses from isolated semicircular canal of the guitarfish using rotational acceleration white-noise inputs. I. Correlation of response dynamics with receptor innervation. J. Neurophysiol. **39:** 631–644.

44. BAIRD, R. A., G. DESMADRYL, C. FERNÁNDEZ & J. M. GOLDBERG. 1988. The vestibular nerve of the chinchilla. II. Relation between afferent response properties and peripheral innervation patterns in the semicircular canals. J. Neurophysiol. 60: 182–203.
45. SCHESSEL, D. A., R. GINZBERG & S. M. HIGHSTEIN. 1991. Morphophysiology of synaptic transmission between type I hair cells and vestibular primary afferents. An intracellular study employing horseradish peroxidase in the lizard, Calotes versicolor. Brain Res. 544: 1–16.
46. MASETTO, S. G. RUSSO & I. PRIGIONI. 1994. Differential expression of potassium currents by hair cells in thin slices of frog crista ampullaris. J. Neurophysiol. 72: 443–455.
47. STEINACKER, A., R. MONTERRUBIO, R. PEREZ & S. M. HIGHSTEIN. 1992. Potassium current composition and kinetics in toadfish semicircular canal hair cells. Biol. Bull. 183: 346–347.
48. STEINACKER, A. 1996. Ionic current contribution to signal processing by vestibular hair cells. Ann. N. Y. Acad. Sci. This volume.
49. MCLAREN, J. W. & D. E. HILLMAN. 1979. Displacement of the semicircular canal cupula during sinusoidal rotation. Neuroscience 4: 2001–2008.
50. HILLMAN, D. E. & J. W. MCLAREN. 1979. Displacement configuration of semicircular canal cupulae. Neuroscience 4: 1989–2000.
51. OMAN, C. M., L. S. FRISHKOPF & M. H. GOLDSTEIN. 1979. Cupula motion in the semicircular canal of the skate (Raja erinacea). Acta Otolaryngol. 87: 528–538.
52. HILLMAN, D. E. 1974. Cupular structure and its receptor relationship. Brain Behav. Evol. 10: 52–68.
53. RÜSCH, A. & U. THURM. 1989. Cupula displacement, hair bundle deflection, and physiological responses in the transparent semicircular canal of young eel. Pflügers Arch. 413: 533–545.
54. BELANGER, L. F. 1961. Observations on the intimate structure and composition of the chick labyrinth. Anat. Rec. 139: 5–45.
55. OMAN, C. M., E. N. MARCUS & I. S. CURTHOYS. 1987. The influence of semicircular canal morphology on endolymph flow dynamics. Acta Otolaryngol. 103: 1–13.
56. DAMIANO, E. R. & R. D. RABBITT. 1996. A singular perturbation model of fluid dynamics in the vestibular semicircular canal and ampulla. J. Fluid Mech. 307: 333–372.
57. DICKMAN, J. D., P. A. REDER & M. J. CORREIA. 1988. A method for controlled mechanical stimulation of single semicircular canals. J. Neurosci. Methods 25: 111–119.
58. DICKMAN, J. D. & M. J. CORREIA. 1989a. Responses of pigeon horizontal semicircular canal afferent fibers. I. Step, trapezoid, and low-frequency sinusoid mechanical and rotational stimulation. J. Neurophysiol. 62: 1090–1101.
59. DICKMAN, J. D. & M. J. CORREIA. 1989b. Responses of pigeon horizontal semicircular canal afferent fibers. II. High-frequency mechanical stimulation. J. Neurophysiol. 62: 1102–1112.
60. RABBITT, R. D., R. BOYLE & S. M. HIGHSTEIN. 1995. Mechanical indentation of the vestibular labyrinth and its relationship to head rotation in the toadfish, Opsanus tau. J. Neurophysiol. 73: 2237–2260.
61. BOYLE, R. & S. M. HIGHSTEIN. 1991. Responses of horizontal semicircular canal afferents to rotatory and mechanical stimulation. Biol. Bull. 181: 319.
62. HIGHSTEIN, S. M., R. D. RABBITT & R. BOYLE. 1996. Determinants of semicircular canal afferent response dynamics in the toadfish, Opsanus tau. J. Neurophysiol. 75(2): 575–596.
63. CLUSIN, W. T. & M. V. L. BENNETT. 1977a. Calcium-activated conductance in skate electroreceptors. Current clamp experiments. J. Gen. Physiol. 69: 121–143.
64. CLUSIN, W. T. & M. V. L. BENNETT. 1977b. Calcium-activated conductance in skate electroreceptors. Voltage clamp experiments. J. Gen. Physiol. 69: 145–182.
65. CAMIS, M. 1930. The Physiology of the Vestibular Apparatus. Clarendon Press. Oxford, UK.
66. COREY, D. P. & A. J. HUDSPETH. 1979. Ionic basis of the receptor potential in vertebrate hair cells. Nature 281: 675–677.
67. COREY, D. P. & A. J. HUDSPETH. 1983b. Kinetics of the receptor current in bullfrog saccular hair cells. J. Neurosci. 5: 962–976.

68. COREY, D. P. & A. J. HUDSPETH. 1983a. Analysis of the microphonic potential of the bullfrog's sacculus. J. Neurosci. **3:** 942–961.
69. CRAWFORD, A. C., M. G. EVANS & R. FETTIPLACE. 1991. The actions of calcium on the mechano-electrical transducer current of turtle hair cells. J. Physiol. **434:** 369–398.
70. ASSAD, J. A. & D. P. COREY. 1992. An active motor model for adaptation by vertebrate hair cells. J. Neurosci. **12:** 3291–3309.
71. EATOCK, R. A., D. P. COREY & A. J. HUDSPETH. 1987. Adaptation of mechanoelectrical transduction in hair cells of the bullfrog's sacculus. J. Neurosci. **7:** 2821–2836.
72. OHMORI, H. 1987. Gating properties of the mechano-electrical transducer channel in the dissociated vestibular hair cell of the chick. J. Physiol. (Lond.) **387:** 589–609.
73. ROTH, A. 1968. Electroreception in the catfish, *Amiurus nebulosus*. Z. V. Gl. Physiol. **61:** 196–202.
74. ROTH, A. 1978. Further indications of a chemical synapse in the electroreceptors of the catfish. J. Comp. Physiol. **126:** 147–150.
75. TEETER, J. H. & M. V. L. BENNETT. 1981. Synaptic transmission in the ampullary electroreceptor of the transparent catfish, *Kryptopterus*. J. Comp. Physiol. **142:** 371–377.
76. OBARA, S. 1976. Mechanisms of electroreception in ampullae of lorenzini of the marine catfish, *Plotosus*. *In* Electrophysiology of Nerve, Synapse, and Muscle. J. P. Ruben, D. P. Purpura, M. V. L. Bennett & E. R. Kandel, Eds.: 129–147. Raven Press. New York.
77. LOWENSTEIN, O. 1955. The effect of galvanic polarization on the impulse discharge from nerve endings in the isoloated labyrinth of the thornback ray (Raja clavata). J. Physiol. (Lond.) **127:** 104–117.
78. GOLDBERG, J. M., C. FERNÁNDEZ & C. E. SMITH. 1982. Responses of vestibular-nerve afferents in the squirrel monkey to externally applied galvanic currents. Brain Res. **252:** 156–160.
79. BORDI, F., C. CAMETTI & A. DIBIASIO. 1990. Determination of cell membrane passive electrical properties using frequency domain dielectric spectroscopy technique. A new approach. Biochim. Biophys. Acta **1028:** 201–204.
80. BAO, J-Z., C. C. DAVIS & R. E. SCHMUKLER. 1992. Frequency domain impedance measurements of erythrocytes. Constant phase angle impedance characteristics and a phase transition. Biophys. J. **61:** 1427–1434.
81. DALLOS, P. & B. N. EVANS. 1995. High-frequency motility of outer hair cells and the cochlear amplifier. Science **267:** 2006–2009.
82. RÜSCH, A. & U. THURM. 1990. Spontaneous and electrically induced movements of ampullary kinocilia and stereovilli. Hear. Res. **48:** 247–264.
83. GOLDMAN, D. E. 1943. Potential, impedance, and rectification in membranes. J. Gen. Physiol. **27:** 37–60.
84. HODGKIN, A. L. & B. KATZ. 1949. The effect of sodium ions on the electrical activity of the giant axon of the squid. J. Physiol. (Lond.) **108:** 37–77.
85. SILVER, R. B., M. SUGIMORI, E. J. LANG & R. LLINÀS. 1994. Time resolved imaging of Ca²⁺-dependent aequorin luminescence of microdomains and QEDs in synaptic preterminals. Biol. Bull. **187:** 293–299.
86. ART, J. J., R. FETTIPLACE & Y. C. WU. 1993. The effects of low calcium on the voltage-dependent conductances involved in tuning of turtle hair cells. J. Physiol. **470:** 109–126.
87. FUNG, Y. C. 1993. Biomechanics: Motion, Flow, Stress, and Growth. Springer-Verlag, New York.
88. STEINHAUSEN, W. 1933. Über die beobachtungen der Cupula in der Bognegangsampullen des Labyrinthes des libenden Hecths. Pflügers Arch. **232:** 500–512.

Responses of Identified Vestibulospinal Neurons to Voluntary Eye and Head Movements in the Squirrel Monkey[a]

R. BOYLE,[b,c] TIM BELTON,[d] AND ROBERT A. McCREA[d]

[b]Departments of Otolaryngology/Head-Neck Surgery and Physiology
Neuro-Sensory Research Center
Oregon Health Sciences University
3181 S.W. Sam Jackson Park Road
Portland, Oregon 97201

[d]Department of Pharmacological and Physiological Sciences
University of Chicago
947 East 58th Street
Chicago, Illinois 60637

INTRODUCTION

The simplest vestibulocollic reflex (VCR) pathways are three-neuron arcs interconnecting vestibular-nerve afferents, secondary vestibulospinal neurons, and cervical motoneurons.[1,2] The middle link of the VCR is routed through both the medial (MVST) and lateral (LVST) vestibulospinal tracts.[3] Another possible link of the VCR is made by vestibulo-ocular-collic neurons, which have dual destinations: one to the cervical spinal cord via the descending medial longitudinal fasciculus (MLF), like MVST axons, and the other to the oculomotor nuclei via the ascending MLF.[4–7] In addition to direct VCR pathways, there are indirect vestibulo-reticulo-spinal pathways.[3]

The response of secondary vestibular neurons to an externally applied movement of the head is in the form of a firing rate modulation that encodes the angular velocity of the movement, and reflects in large part the input "head velocity in space" signal carried by the semicircular canal afferents. In addition to the head velocity signal, the majority of vestibular neurons carry a more processed signal that includes eye position or eye velocity, or both.[8–11] Many of these latter cells have been identified as the middle link of the vestibulo-ocular reflex (VOR) and possibly the VCR.[12–17]

To understand the control signals used by the central vestibular pathways in the generation of reflex head stabilization, such as the VCR, and the maintenance of head posture, it is essential to record directly from identified vestibulospinal neurons projecting to the cervical spinal segments in the alert animal. The present report provides two key features of primate vestibulospinal neurons recently determined in separate experiments. To identify the secondary vestibulospinal neuron, electrical pulses were applied to (1) wires implanted into the ventromedial funiculi at C_1 to antidromically excite the vestibulospinal neuron, and (2) middle ear electrodes to determine the same neuron's orthodromic relationship to the VIIIth nerve. The first

[a]This research was supported in part by grant P60 DC02072 from the National Institutes of Health, U.S. Public Health Service.

[c]Corresponding author. E-mail: boyler@ohsu.edu

244

series of experiments were preformed in the alert squirrel monkey prepared for chronic single-unit and eye movement recordings in the head restrained condition to determine the eye movement signal content, if any, carried by identified secondary vestibulospinal neurons. The results show that many secondary vestibulospinal neurons do indeed carry a more integrated signal that includes both the position and the movement of the eyes in orbit, and that these eye movement-related signals interact constructively and destructively with the head velocity signal to provide a variable input to the neck spinal circuits. The second series of experiments were designed to determine the head movement signal content carried by the same class of secondary vestibulospinal neurons during the actual execution of the VCR and during self-generated, or active, rapid head movements. To accomplish this experiment a head unrestrained (or "head free") paradigm was used. In this condition the animal could make head movements about the vertical axis of ± 45° and about the interaural axis of about ± 10°. Isolation of single units was not compromised, even for velocities of active head movements up to 400°/s. Although the data set is still small in this series of experiments, the results are noteworthy: (1) Vestibulospinal neurons do not encode the actual head velocity in space during self-generated head movements, and (2) they encode the velocity of *externally applied* head movements not only as the animal is performing the VCR, but also when the animal is executing rapid, orienting head movements.

METHODS

Squirrel monkeys, *Saimiri sciureus,* were prepared under gas or barbiturate anesthesia for chronic eye movement and extracellular unit recordings from the brain stem. All surgical and experimental procedures were conducted according to the National Institutes of Health Guide for the Care and Use of Laboratory Animals. A stainless steel bolt was fixed to the occipital bone using dental acrylic for head restraint, a chamber was positioned over a hole made in the cranium to allow electrode penetrations in the left brain stem, and a coil was attached to the sclera of one or both eyes using fine sutures to measure the horizontal and vertical eye position using the magnetic search coil technique. Bilaterally, the middle ear space was exposed by a retroauricular approach. One Teflon-coated silver wire (250 μm in diameter, bared 1 mm from the tip and coated with $AgCl_2$) was inserted into a hole made in the promontory (cathode), and another wire bared 3–4 mm from the tip was placed in the middle ear space (anode) for electrical stimulation of the VIIIth nerve to identify the neuron's orthodromic relationship to the ipsilateral vestibular nerve. The posterior arch of the atlas was exposed through a 2-cm skin incision and muscle retraction, and 75-μm platinum wires were inserted through a small hole in the dura rostral to the atlas into the ventromedial funiculi on both sides of the midline; in some cases another wire was also inserted into the left ventrolateral funiculus. To electrically activate vestibulospinal axons positive and negative constant current pulses of 100-μs duration at 1 pulse/s were applied in a bipolar fashion between the wires, and the current intensity was carefully monitored in each recording session to ensure that the pulses did not evoke even the slightest behavioral response of the animal; vestibulospinal axons are typically activated between 200 and 650 μA. Thresholds of antidromic activation using stimulus current of opposite polarity were carefully measured for several vestibulospinal cells; the separation in current amplitudes to activate the cells was between 15 and 40 μA. These values are not sufficient to provide a reliable measure of the laterality of activated axons, particularly in an alert animal in which the cell's level of excitability is constantly changing. Cells exhibiting an evoked potential at a constant latency down to near-threshold current amplitudes and a collision between the potential and a spontaneously occurring or VIIIth nerve-induced spike were used as criteria for antidromicity. FIGURE 1 shows the orthodromic (A) and antidromic (B) identification of a secondary vestibulospinal neuron.

During experiments, the monkey sat upright in a primate chair either (1) with its head held stationary by fixing the skull bolt to the chair and pitched 15° nose-down to

A

n. VIIIth Orthodromic Ressponse

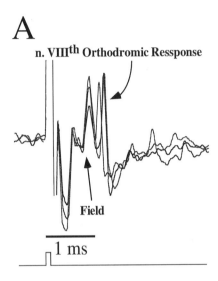

Field

1 ms

B

C₁ Antidromic Response

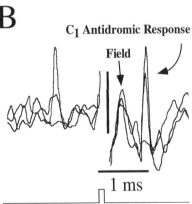

Field

1 ms

FIGURE 1. Identification of a secondary vestibulospinal neuron. **(A)** Orthodromic responses to electrical stimulation of the ipsilateral VIIIth nerve at three stimulus intensities. Minimum latency was 1.05 ms. **(B)** Antidromic responses to electrical stimulation of the ventromedial funiculus at C_1 having a fixed latency of 0.8 ms and the collision of the evoked potential with a spontaneously occurring spike.

position the horizontal semicircular canals in the plane of rotation or (2) with the skull bolt attached by a mini-universal joint and Delrin rod to a double-bearing (Barden) mounting that permitted head movements about the vertical axis (yaw) of ± 45° and about the interaural axis (pitch) of about ± 5°; a separate coil was mounted to the head to measure the horizontal and vertical displacements of the head with respect to the shoulder. The primate chair was mounted atop a turntable that delivered angular acceleration about the vertical axis with velocity profiles generated by either a programmable function generator or digitally at 500 Hz by computer. Single-unit recordings were made using insulated tungsten microelectrodes introduced into the brain stem through a 22-gauge guide tube. Extracellular action potentials were conventionally amplified, filtered, converted into idealized TTL pulses using a spike amplitude discrimination circuit, and digitized, together with the voltage signals of the scleral and head coils, the chair, and the optokinetic and target stimuli, using digital I/O and ADC circuits (Cambridge Electronic Design, CED 1401Plus) interfaced to an 80486 computer. The cell's discharge was examined during (1) spontaneous rapid eye movements and during fixation of presented visual targets, (2) applied yaw rotation in dark and light with the head held stationary and during episodes as the animal suppressed reflex eye movements by fixating a head-referenced visual target, (3) optokinetic stimulation, (4) ocular pursuit of a sinusoidally moving visual target, and (5) in the head unrestrained experiments, as the animal made self-generated head movements in dark and light and in conjunction with an applied yaw rotation of the chair.

Data were transferred to a Macintosh platform and quantitatively analyzed off-line using routines written for the Igor (WaveMetrics) package. Each cell's best eye position vector was calculated using multiple regression analysis by measuring its horizontal and vertical eye position sensitivity during selected episodes of steady fixation > 100 ms in length at a minimum of 60 ms from a rapid eye movement for > 50 fixations. To calculate the cell's sensitivity to pursuit eye movements, the eye position records were differentiated, desaccaded, and averaged with the firing rate, to construct cycle histograms and sine waves that were matched to the responses using a least-squares algorithm. The cell's response (gain in impulses/second per degree/second, or imp/s per °/s, and phase in ° re:ipsilateral chair velocity) to applied whole-body rotation was estimated by using Fourier analysis and by constructing cycle histograms and least-squares fitting of a sine wave at the stimulus frequency. In the head unrestrained experiments each cell's best head position vector with respect to space (equal to head position with respect to shoulder when the chair was stationary) was calculated from selected periods of steady head fixations using multiple regression analysis similar to that used to measure the cell's eye position sensitivity. Multiple regression analysis also was made on the cell's firing rate and the horizontal and vertical head position, velocity (differentiated from head position), and acceleration (double differentiated from head position) during periods of 30–600 s of spontaneous head movements made in dark and in light. Head velocity with respect to space during applied chair rotation was calculated by adding the head velocity signal and the chair velocity, using the convention of rightward and upward head movements as positive values and leftward and downward head movements as negative values. Gaze velocity was calculated by adding the head velocity re:space and the eye velocity re:head following the same convention of direction values. During applied chair rotation the animal either made fast, self-generated head movements or made compensatory slow head movements that characterize the vestibulocollic reflex. To estimate the cell's sensitivity to the fast (voluntary) and slow (reflex) head movements, selected periods of the record were identified in which compensatory head movements were made (the cell's firing rate was not displayed during this procedure). An idealized sine wave of the stimulus frequency was created and inverted, and its amplitude was adjusted manually to best fit the head velocity record; the amplitude of the idealized wave was typically 0.1–0.2 of the stimulus velocity (equals the maximum gain of the vestibulocollic reflex). Head velocity values falling within an amplitude window of the idealized wave were labeled, with the cell's firing rate and the calculated head velocity re:space, as slow epochs; head velocity values outside the window were labeled, with the corresponding firing rate and the calculated head velocity re:space, as fast epochs. Linear regression analyses were then made on the cell's firing rate with respect to head velocity re:space for the two epochs.

RESULTS

Classification of Neurons

Neurons were extracellularly recorded from the left vestibular nuclei and neighboring regions. They were classified as secondary vestibular nuclei neurons based on the latency of the orthodromically evoked action potential of < 1.3 ms, that is, monosynaptic, following electrical stimulation of the ipsilateral VIIIth nerve (see FIG. 1A); cells having an evoked response at > 1.3 ms were classified as nonsecondary vestibular nuclei neurons. Cells unresponsive to electrical stimulation of the VIIIth nerve will not be presented in this report. Secondary and nonsecondary vestibular neurons were further identified as vestibulospinal cells on the basis of the evoked antidromic action potential following electrical stimulation of the spinal cord at C_1 (see FIG. 1B); the spinal-projecting cells reported here were presumed medial vestibulospinal tract cells having axons traveling in the ventromedial funiculi based on threshold testing between sets of implanted wires in some animals or the absence of an ipsilateral ventrolateral funicular wire in the others.

Eye Movement-related Firing Behavior of Vestibulospinal Neurons

Secondary Vestibulospinal Neurons

All secondary vestibulospinal neurons in this report displayed a type I response to applied chair rotation with the animal's head held stationary, characterized by an increase in firing rate during ipsilateral (leftward) rotation and a decrease in firing rate in the opposite sense ($n = 12$). FIGURE 2A and B shows the responses of one neuron to applied chair rotation. The cell was typed as an ipsilateral eye and head velocity cell (iEHV after Scudder and Fuchs[16]); iEHV firing behavior represented 58% of the sample population of secondary vestibulospinal neurons (7 of 12 cells). Compare the response modulations over the time period of 2–6 s in FIGURE 2A, labeled VOR, and those over the time period of 0–6 s in FIGURE 2B, labeled VOR Suppress(ion). During the performance of the VOR (gain ∼ 0.8), the cell's response was characterized by having a sensitivity of 0.7 imp/s per °/s and the peak of modulation led peak ipsilateral chair velocity by 36°. During voluntary VOR suppression (VOR gain < 0.15), the response sensitivity increased to 1.2 imp/s per °/s (20° phase lead). For the 7 iEHV secondary vestibulospinal neurons a 54% increase in the response sensitivity during execution of the VOR was observed when the animal voluntarily suppressed the reflex eye movements (0.52 ± 0.23 vs. 0.8 ± 0.36 imp/s per °/s of chair velocity).

FIGURE 2C shows the firing behavior of the same iEHV cell during ocular pursuit of a moving visual target made with the head stationary. The modulation of the cell's firing rate was closely in phase with ipsilateral movements of the visual stimulus and the eyes, and had a sensitivity of 0.8 imp/s per °/s of horizontal eye velocity (19° phase lead). The average eye velocity sensitivity of the 7 iEHV cells was 1 imp/s per °/s (±0.48 SD), and indicates that on average iEHV vestibulospinal neuron has a larger eye velocity sensitivity than that to an applied vestibular stimulus. Three of the 7 iEHV cells also had a static eye position sensitivity for ipsilateral fixations, average 0.44 ± 2.5 imp/s per °; the neuron in FIGURE 2 had no significant eye position sensitivity.

Of the remaining five secondary vestibulospinal neurons, four were typed as "pure" vestibular having firing rates unrelated to the movement and position of the

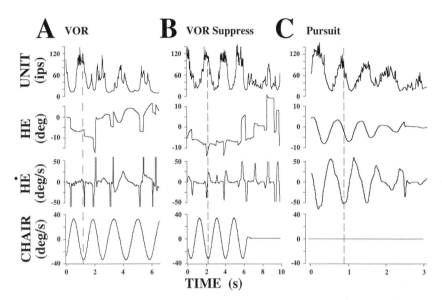

FIGURE 2. Eye movement-related firing rate modulation of a secondary medial vestibulospinal tract neuron recorded in the left vestibular nuclei; latency of antidromic activation from C_1 was 0.75 ms, and the cell was orthodromically activated from the ipsilateral VIIIth nerve at a minimum latency of 1.0 ms. Traces from top to bottom in each panel are instantaneous firing rate in imp/s, horizontal eye position in degrees, horizontal eye velocity in °/s, and the chair velocity in °/s. Right eye and chair movements are up, left movements are down; this convention is used, when required, in the remaining figures. Neuron typed as an ipsilateral eye and head velocity response in the head-restrained paradigm. Dashed vertical lines in **A** and **B** mark peak ipsilateral chair velocity, and in **C** the line is aligned with peak ipsilateral eye velocity. (**A** and **B**) Responses to ipsilateral chair velocity; note the increase in response modulation when the eye movements were reduced. (**C**) Firing rate modulated to the velocity of ipsilaterally directed pursuit eye movements.

eyes in orbit, and one cell had a sensitivity to contralateral eye position. None of the secondary vestibulospinal neurons in this study had a firing rate that was significantly influenced, either in the way of a cessation or pause or in a burst in discharge, by fast phases of the VOR or optokinetic nystagmus or during saccadic eye movements. It should be mentioned that electromyographic recordings were not taken from dorsal neck muscles, so it is uncertain whether or not the animal attempted at any time to move its head during the recording sessions.

Nonsecondary Vestibulospinal Neurons

All 10 nonsecondary vestibulospinal neurons displayed a type II response to applied chair rotation with the animal's head held stationary, characterized by an increase in firing rate during contralateral (rightward) rotation and a decrease in firing rate in the opposite sense. Eight cells were typed as "pure" vestibular, one had a sensitivity to both contralaterally directed eye and applied head velocity (contralateral eye-head velocity, or cEHV after Scudder and Fuchs[16]), and one had an ipsilateral eye position sensitivity that could significantly alter, and even occlude, the firing rate modulation evoked by chair rotation (see FIG. 2 of Boyle[19]). None of the nonsecondary vestibulospinal neurons had a firing rate that was significantly influenced by rapid eye movements made in any direction.

Head Movement-related Firing Behavior of Vestibulospinal Neurons

In one monkey 38 vestibular neurons were recorded during periods of time when the animal could voluntarily make rapid, orienting head movements and reflex head movements made in response to externally applied perturbations. Of this sample, seven were identified as secondary MVST neurons. All seven neurons displayed a type I response to yaw rotation in the head restrained paradigm. Regression analysis techniques were used to determine whether or not the firing rate of the neuron was correlated with the acceleration, velocity or position of spontaneous and evoked eye movements, with head position re:shoulder or with gaze position. Interestingly, no significant correlations were found in this sample of secondary vestibulospinal neurons, and thus they were typed as "pure" vestibular cells. The results of these cells are qualitatively similar, and will be represented by the responses of one secondary MVST neuron provided in FIGURES 3–8.

Head-Restrained Paradigm

FIGURE 3 shows the averaged firing rate of a secondary vestibulospinal neuron (lower histogram) to a 1-Hz yaw rotation (dashed line, "Chair") in the *head-restrained* paradigm. The velocity trace labeled "Head re:Shoulder" (solid and thinner line), representing the differentiated head position signal detected by the head coil, is given in this and the subsequent figures. Typically in the head-fixed condition, the head position is not measured. However, in our head-restrained paradigm the animal can still make with forced effort a head movement of up to about 50°/s. In the figure 42 cycles of rotation were selected where the head velocity re:shoulder was close to 0°/s. The velocity trace labeled "Head re:Space" (solid and thicker line), representing the sum of the chair velocity and the head velocity re:shoulder, is also given and closely corresponds to the applied chair velocity. The averaged response to applied chair rotation was characterized as having a sensitivity of 1.4 imp/s per °/s, reaching its peak at 11° before peak leftward or ipsilateral chair velocity.

Head-Free Paradigm

Lack of correlation between cell discharge and head velocity during self-generated head movements. In the *head-free* paradigm the animal made self-generated head movements that reached velocities up to 350–400°/s; however, the majority of head movements were made in the range of 20 to 50°/s. FIGURE 4 shows the firing rate of the neuron (darkened histograms) during a portion of a 5-min record in which the animal made self-generated horizontal eye (solid and thinner line) and head (solid and thicker line) movements in the head-free paradigm; the sum of eye in head and head on shoulder, or horizontal gaze velocity (dashed trace), is also given. Also provided in the figure is the predicted response of the neuron (striped line, open histograms) superimposed on the actual firing rate. The predicted response is based on the assumption that the cell's firing rate is entirely dependent on its head velocity re:space input, and was calculated by the cell's response to the applied chair rotation as presented in FIGURE 3. As seen by the raw records and the predicted response in

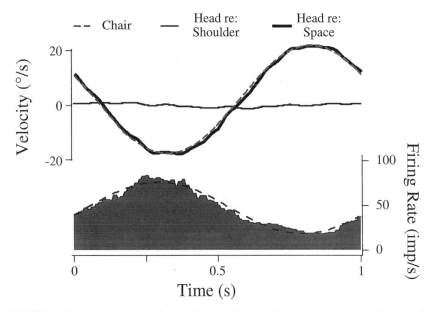

FIGURE 3. Response of a secondary medial vestibulospinal tract neuron recorded in the left vestibular nuclei to a 1-Hz applied chair rotation in the head-restrained paradigm averaged over 42 cycles of rotation; cell was orthodromically excited from the ipsilateral VIIIth nerve at a latency of 1.0 ms and antidromically activated from C_1 at a latency of 0.6 ms. Upper traces are velocity records of horizontal chair (*dashed line*) and head on shoulder (*thin line*), and their sum or head in space (*thick line*); lower plot is the cell's response in the form of a rate histogram and a sine fit to the response. The response was characterized by a sensitivity of 1.4 imp/s per °/s and a phase of +11° with respect to peak ipsilateral chair velocity.

this figure, no clear relationship is apparent between the cell's firing rate and the self-generated horizontal head movements. The relationship between the cell's firing rate and the self-generated head movements is quantitatively analyzed in FIGURE 5, which plots the cell's firing rate (crosses) as a function of head velocity re:shoulder or space (mean 0 ± 30°/s SD). Note the scatter of the firing rate. Linear regression analysis (not shown) indicated no significant relationship existed between the cell's firing rate and the head velocity occurring during active head movements, examined either over the entire record (slope, −0.1; r = −0.1) or over selected ranges of head velocity. The dashed line is the expected response (slope, −1.44) based on the

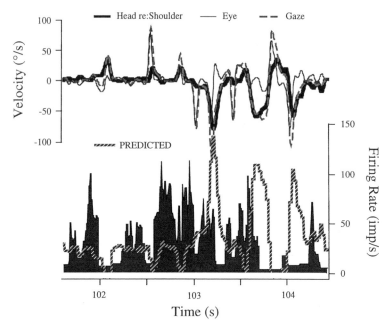

FIGURE 4. Firing rate during self-generated horizontal head movements. Same neuron as in previous figure. Upper traces are the velocity records of horizontal eye (*thin line*) and head (*thick line*) and their sum or gaze (*dashed line*). No obvious relationship is apparent between the firing rate of the medial vestibulospinal tract neuron and eye or head movement in the head-free paradigm.

response of the same cell to applied chair rotation in the head restrained paradigm as shown in FIGURE 3. Interestingly, when the animal held its head quite stabile (head movements less than 10°/s), the cell's "background" firing rate exhibited its widest variation, from silence to 180 imp/s.

Response to applied chair rotation. To determine whether the cell continued to encode an externally applied change in head position in the head-free paradigm, cycles of applied chair rotation were delivered. In this condition the animal could either respond to the applied stimulation by eliciting the vestibulocollic reflex, a compensatory response with head movements made in the opposite direction to the applied stimulus, or generate exploratory, or other orienting head movements. FIGURE 6 shows the raw records of the cell's firing rate during a 1-Hz applied chair rotation. The head movement record is divided into two epochs, together with the corresponding firing rate, to illustrate the mode of analysis we used to evaluate the cell's firing rate as a function of head velocity. One epoch is termed "slow" (striped, lighter trace) and represents in this instance head movements made within a window of an ideal sine wave that modeled the vestibulocollic reflex (mean $-0.5 \pm 5°$/s). The other epoch is termed "rapid" (solid, thicker trace) and represents rapid head movements (mean $1.3 \pm 52°$/s). Striped and solid histograms correspond to the slow and rapid epochs of head velocity, respectively. Discontinuities between the two head velocity traces represent head movements that fell outside both windows (thin line not included in the legend; firing rate during these periods is represented by open histograms). During the beginning and end portions of the record in FIGURE 6, the animal is holding its head relatively stabile and the head velocity in space (dashed trace) approximates that of the applied chair velocity (solid, light line). Over the middle portion of the record the animal began to make a compensatory head movement (at about 49.5 s), which is terminated by a rapid, contralaterally directed head movement followed by a rapid, ipsilaterally directed head movement (from about 50 to 50.5 s). Note that the cell's discharge continued to follow the profile of the chair velocity, even during the execution of a rapid, ipsilaterally directed head movement made close to the peak of the applied stimulus.

FIGURE 7 plots the cell's averaged firing rate and the averaged chair, head re:shoulder and head re:space velocity traces for the two separate epochs of head

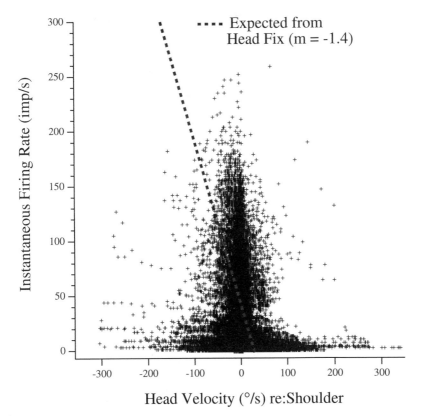

Head Velocity (°/s) re:Shoulder

FIGURE 5. Firing rate as a function of head velocity during self-generated head movements. Same neuron as in previous figure. No external stimulus was applied and thus head velocity on shoulder equals head velocity in space. The cell's firing rate was sorted by the amplitude of leftward (negative values) and rightward (positive values) head movements over a 180-s period. The *expected* fit of slope -1.4 is drawn to represent the cell's response to applied chair rotation derived from the response shown in FIGURE 3. The linear regression fit (not included in figure) revealed that no significant relationship exists between the cell's firing rate and the velocity of voluntary head movements (slope, -0.1; $r = -0.1$).

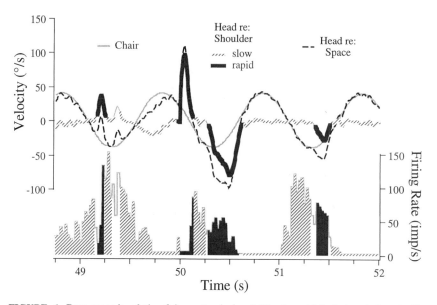

FIGURE 6. Raw records of the firing rate during 1-Hz sinusoidal chair rotation in the head-free paradigm. Same neuron as in previous figure. The head velocity record is divided into two epochs, a slow (*striped line*) and a rapid (*thick, solid line*) one (see text for explanation), to illustrate the execution of the vestibulocollic reflex and the periods of rapid head movements. The cell's firing rate, given in the rate histograms, is shaded to correspond to the two epochs of head movement. The head re:space (*dashed line*) is the sum of the chair and the undivided head velocity.

velocity, the slow in A and the rapid in B; 162 cycles of rotation at 1 Hz were averaged for each plot. A dashed, vertical line marks the peak ipsilateral chair velocity in both plots. In A, the head re:shoulder trace (striped trace) reveals the low-amplitude compensatory vestibulocollic reflex (head velocity/chair velocity, or gain = 0.11). During these periods of the record, the cell maintained a response sensitivity to applied chair rotation (1.1 imp/s per °/s and a phase lead of 9°) comparable to its response in the head restrained paradigm (see FIG. 3). In B, a reduced but present modulation related to the applied chair rotation is still observed during epochs when the animal made rapid head movements (sensitivity of 0.4 imp/s per °/s and a phase lead of 2°). Note that in this particular epoch of the trial the averaged peak ipsilateral head velocity re:space actually exceeded that in A ($-55°$/s vs. $-34°$/s, or 1.38 vs. 0.89 with respect to chair velocity). Thus, although the cell's firing rate was independent of head velocity for self-generated head movements, the applied head velocity was still monitored by the cell.

Response to forced head turning. During applied chair rotation in the head-restrained paradigm, the head velocity on shoulder signal is usually zero, and thus the head velocity in space is equal to the applied chair rotation. In the head-free paradigm, the head velocity on shoulder and the head velocity in space are one and the same in the absence of an external stimulus. In an attempt to produce an external force that mimics the high-velocity, rapid head movements made by the animal itself, and also to indirectly assess the influence of neck proprioceptive signals in shaping the outflow of the vestibulospinal neuron, the animal's head was manually turned.

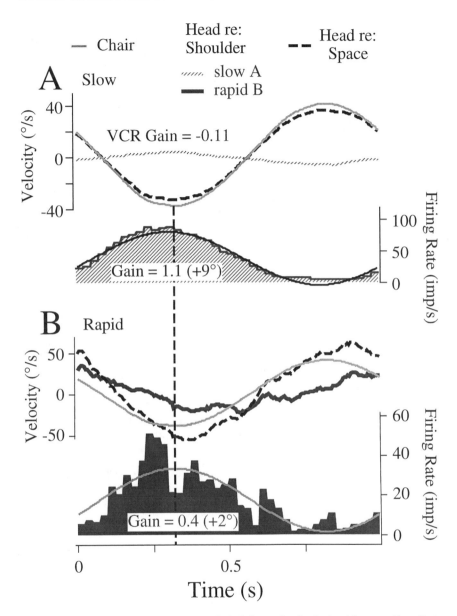

FIGURE 7. Averaged cell responses to applied chair rotation in the head-free paradigm. Same neuron as in FIGURE 6; head velocity recorded was divided into slow (**A**) and rapid (**B**) epochs of head movement as shown in previous figure. During slow epochs of head movement presented in **A**, the vestibulocollic reflex is counterrotating the head at a gain of about 0.1; as a result, the head velocity in space is corresponding reduced by nearly 10%. The cell's response during the execution of the vestibulocollic reflex is nearly identical to that for the same chair rotation in the head-restrained paradigm (from Fig. 3). Note in **B** that, whereas the cell's firing rate was not correlated to the velocity of voluntary head movements (see Figs. 4 and 5), the cell continued to respond, although at a reduced sensitivity, to the applied chair rotation during the performance of active, rapid head movements. Also note that rapid head movements were on average made in the same direction as the chair rotation.

This stimulus thus applied a high-velocity, rapid head movement on the shoulders. The results are presented in FIGURE 8. The cell's firing rate, the horizontal eye velocity (thin trace), and the head velocity re:shoulder (thick trace) signals are shown over about a 4-s period; cycles of forced head turning approached 4 Hz, ± 90°/s. The response to forced head turning (gain −1.1) is comparable to that obtained both during the execution of the vestibulocollic reflex in the head free paradigm (−1.1 imp/s per °/s; FIG. 7A) and during applied rotation in the head restrained paradigm (−1.4 imp/s per °/s; FIG. 3).

DISCUSSION

The most striking finding of the present study is that the firing rate output of a *second-order* vestibular neuron, recorded in the brain stem and shown to receive a direct, short-latency synaptic input from the VIIIth cranial nerve afferents, is dynamically modified by the behavioral context in which the movement is made. Externally applied head perturbations or repetitive passive movements of the whole body are faithfully encoded by the neuron; self-generated, active movements of the head are not. The central vestibular representation of movement is thus dynamically controlled by volition, beginning even at the initial stages of central processing of the afferent sensory signals. This finding is even more remarkable because the output pathway of the second-order vestibular neuron was identified and shown to belong to the vestibulospinal pathway controlling reflex head and neck stabilization and posture.

Vestibulospinal neurons were antidromically identified by using electrical pulses applied to wires implanted into the ventromedial funiculi in the region of the MLF on both sides at C_1. The MLF is the principal conduit through which the vestibulospinal axons belonging to the MVST follow to reach their targets in the cervical segments of the spinal cord.[18] The MVST descends bilaterally. Our techniques used for electrical activation of axons were suited to the nature of the experiment, but could not allow a determination of laterality of the axon (see METHODS). Therefore, our sample of cells belong to crossed or uncrossed or both populations of vestibulospinal axons. In addition, some vestibulospinal axons join the MLF more caudal to our electrode placement site,[19] and others may course in and out of the MLF along their trajectory through the caudal brain stem and spinal cord.[20] Thus, even if the electrodes were ideally positioned in the MLF, some MVST neurons might have escaped identification. With respect to electrode placement and the current amplitude applied to the wires, several empirical observations in the course of this and related studies support the assumption that the reported neurons do indeed belong to the MVST. In animals not reported here, wires were implanted into the lateral and ventral funiculi in an attempt to electrically activate lateral vestibulospinal tract neurons. Using comparable electrical stimulation parameters as applied in the present study, neurons located in the dorsal lateral vestibular (Deiters') nucleus were routinely antidromically activated. In those experiments iEHV cells (example shown in FIG. 2) and type I "vestibular only" neurons having a sensitivity of response to yaw rotation > 0.5 imp/s per °/s (examples shown in FIGS. 3–8) were not antidromically activated. Based on anatomical markings and depth of recording, the present sample of cells were recorded more ventral and medial to dorsal Deiters' nucleus, namely, in an area that includes the ventral lateral, lateral medial, and rostral descending vestibular nuclei. These regions of the vestibular nuclei have been shown using degeneration techniques[21] and intracellular recording and labeling techniques[22,19] to contain MVST cells. Further, neurons located in dorsal lateral

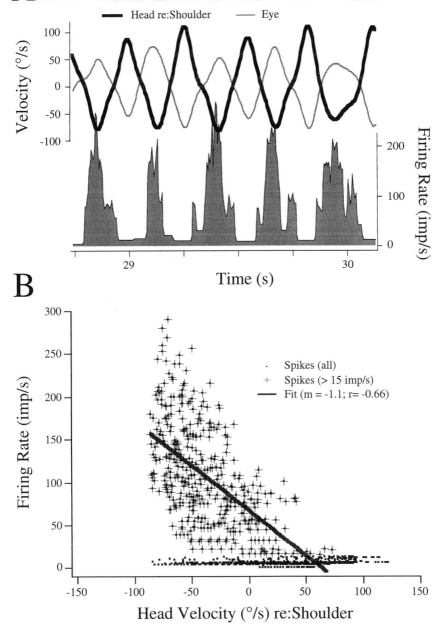

FIGURE 8. Response of the medial vestibulospinal tract (MVST) cell to forced head turning. Same neuron as in FIGURES 3–7. To elicit an externally applied head velocity on shoulder input that approximates that made by the animal itself during voluntary head turning, the animal's head was manually turned ($< \pm 15°$ peak displacement). The cell's response was equivalent to that obtained for the head-restrained paradigm (see FIG. 3) and to the modulation present during the slow epochs (vestibulocollic reflex) of head movement in the head-free paradigm (FIG. 7A). Although indirect, this result indicates that head on shoulder rotation alone may not significantly contribute to the uncoupling of the secondary vestibulospinal neuron's firing rate to head velocity in space during self-generated head movements. One hypothesis is that an efference copy of an intended head movement opens a gate that passes the neck reafference signal to remove the self-generated component of head movement on the MVST neuron.

vestibular nucleus were never antidromically activated in the present study. Consequently, we will refer to the present sample of vestibulospinal neurons as MVST cells.

This study reveals several important new findings on MVST cells. Identified secondary and nonsecondary MVST neurons can carry an eye movement-related signal when the head is stationary. The electromyographic activity of some cat dorsal neck muscles reflects horizontal deviation of the eye in orbit.[23] It is likely that these eye position signals to cervical motoneurons arrive not only via reticulospinal,[24-26] but also MVST cells.[14,17] Although none of the 29 MVST cells recorded in 3 animals had a firing rate that was directly correlated with saccades or the rapid phases of vestibular nystagmus, we cannot outrightly exclude saccade-related neurons from the population of MVST cells until a larger sample is collected under different experimental conditions, including changes in the placement of the stimulating electrodes, in more experiments.

If we assume that the recorded MVST cells participate in the generation of the VCR, then their output to the cervical cell groups controlling neck excitation contains a processed signal that takes into account not only the canal input but also the position and movement of the eyes in orbit. An example of one secondary MVST cell is shown in FIGURE 2 (see ref. 17 for other examples). In this case the input drive to the VCR would be augmented when the eyes are moving ipsilaterally and an externally applied force moves the head further to the ipsilateral side, reduced by an amount based on the ratio of the separate response sensitivities when the two movements are in opposite directions, and even eliminated when they are both directed to the contralateral side. Although the MVST cells display a variety of response characteristics, it would appear that at least some of the recorded MVST cells participate in stabilizing the intended gaze position by modulating the reflex drive to the VCR.

In man and monkey a change in the direction of gaze normally involves both eye and head movements. Combined eye-head gaze shifts and their metrics have been extensively studied in the primate and reviewed.[27-33] In acquiring an unexpected target presented in the visual field, the eyes typically move first, followed by the head in the same direction. This sequence of events is not rigid for gaze shifts made under all conditions, but a saccade frequently occurs as the head is turning. Until recently it was reasoned that the saccadic and vestibular commands summed linearly during voluntary gaze saccades. It is now accepted that the vestibular component—i.e., the VOR—is actually turned off during large amplitude gaze saccades.[34-38] One of the principal elements making up the middle leg of the VOR is the position-vestibular-pause (PVP) neuron.[12,13,39] A key identifying feature of the secondary PVP neuron is the complete cessation of the firing rate or pause during the execution of a saccade, particularly for saccades made in the direction ipsilateral to the cell's soma. For on-direction saccades the pause in the firing rate of the PVP typically precedes the saccade by 5–10 ms and outlasts the event.[12,40] The source of this powerful inhibitory input to the PVP neuron is presumably the inhibitory burst neurons,[41] which terminate extensively in the vestibular nuclei and neighboring cell groups.[39,42]

Before turning to the firing behavior of MVST cells during self-generated head movements, let's first examine what the MVST cell does not do. As discussed above, MVST cells do not carry a saccade-related signal when the head is held stationary (these experiments were conducted in animals conditioned only to this paradigm). This observation was confirmed in the experiment in which the head was unrestrained. During rapid gaze saccades with the head movement reaching velocities of 300°/s, three of the seven MVST neurons *often* exhibited either a reduction or an inhibition of the firing during a portion of the head movement; this change in the cell's firing rate was more pronounced for head movements made in the cell's off-direction (contralateral-directed head movements) than for those made in the cell's on-direction. This reduction in firing rate, however, was often difficult to evaluate because of the highly irregular or sporadic discharge behavior of the recorded MVST cells in this experiment. The neuron presented in FIGURES 3–8 is one of these neurons. When a change in firing rate occurred, the decrease in firing rate typically began after the onset of the head movement and the action potentials resumed before the head movement ended. For example, for a 200°/s head movement that lasted approximately 100 ms the cell stopped firing 12 ms after the onset of the movement and resumed 25 ms before the movement was ended or about 27 ms after peak head velocity was reached (not shown). Interestingly, the change in firing rate was not uniform for head movements made at comparable velocities and durations (compare the two off-direction head movements of about 20°/s between time 102 and 103 s in FIG. 3). This inconsistency in the firing rate as a function of head velocity for spontaneous head movements can also be seen in FIGURE 5, particularly for head movements between 50 and 200°/s (note that applied chair rotations at 50°/s in the cell's off-direction produced a silencing of the neuron). For many head movements made in this range of velocity the cell continued to fire at relatively high levels. Also evident in the figure is that for head movements > 200°/s a decrease in firing rate to < 25 imp/s occurred. Further, as shown in FIGURE 7B, a discharge modulation to an applied stimulus was still present during rapid epochs of self-generated head movements. Because the decrease in firing rate was typically brief and rarely outlasted the head movement, we prefer to use the term "inhibition" and not "pause" in firing rate to distinguish the discharge behavior of these three MVST during gaze saccades from that of the PVP neuron during ocular saccades. This apparent lack of a PVP equivalent element in the vestibular-neck pathway is intriguing at first inspection, because the spinal circuits controlling head stabilization would appear to profit from a complete removal in the reflex drive during self-generated head movements. However, as the results show in FIGURES 4 and 5, the MVST cell is not carrying a head velocity in space signal during self-generated head movements, and thus no reflex drive opposes the voluntary head movement. To what extent the brief decrease or inhibition of firing rate observed in some MVST cells actually plays in temporarily altering the stiffness of the antagonistic muscles is yet unknown, and will be the subject of future study.

Although vestibular nerve afferents have not yet been studied during both active and applied head movement, circumstantial evidence indicates that the vestibular input signal reaches the vestibular nuclei during active head movements. Out of a population of 38 neurons in this study, three secondary vestibular cells (tested but unresponsive to electrical stimulation of the spinal cord) had an equivalent response sensitivity to active head movements over the velocity range of > ± 300°/s as that to an applied head movement in the head restrained paradigm. Plotted in a manner presented in FIGURE 5, the actual and predicted responses were identical for the three cells. This finding indicates that the head velocity in space signal is carried by, if not all then at least some, vestibular nerve afferents during active head movements, and is in line with the general conclusion of Khalsa *et al.*[43] that the efferent vestibular system has little apparent influence on vestibular nerve afferents during active head movements. Clearly, a study of the firing rate of both vestibular nerve afferents and efferent vestibular neurons is required before a peripheral mechanism initiated by an intended head movement is excluded.

The MVST cell does not encode head velocity in space for self-generated head movements. The cell's firing rate was uncorrelated with head velocity in space not only for rapid, large amplitude gaze saccades but also for relatively slower, lower amplitude head movements. Khalsa *et al.*[43] recorded from 31 vestibular nuclei neurons, histologically identified by placing marking lesions in the brain stem, during both active and passive head movement. Despite the fact that it is unknown whether or not any secondary MVST cells were included in their sample, it is surprising that the two data sets are in such disagreement. No statistically significant difference in firing rate was found for head movements made voluntarily or applied, and thus all of their recorded cells responded in a predictable manner to the head velocity in space. In our sample of 38 vestibular neurons orthodromically related to the vestibular nerve, only three cells actually encoded the head velocity in space for both active and passive head movements. One possible explanation for the discrepancy of results in the two studies is that different areas of the vestibular nuclei were explored with the extracellular electrode. In the study of Khalsa *et al.*[43] it would appear that the majority of cells were recorded in areas caudal to those studied here; in fact, most of our recordings were in areas rostral to their most rostrally recorded cells (taken from their FIG. 1). If this is indeed the case, then different output and intrinsic pathways in the vestibular nuclei exist; some, such as the MVST, do not convey the head velocity in space signal, and others utilize this signal to form a central representation of the active head movement. We are currently exploring this possibility.

One of the main findings in this study is that, although the MVST cell does not encode the velocity of the head in space for voluntary movements, the MVST cell nevertheless responds to and conveys an applied perturbation of the head, even during large voluntary gaze saccades. It was not unexpected to find that the cell responded similarly during an applied head movement in the head restrained condition and an applied head movement in the head-free condition during execution of the VCR (compare FIGS. 3 and 7A). Of particular significance is the observation that the MVST cell still responds to a passive, applied stimulus during voluntary head movements. As shown in FIGURE 7B, the firing rate is lowered for this particular cell during active head movements, but a discharge modulation is nevertheless present. The functional importance of this finding is clear: To maintain head stability an applied perturbation of the head must be detected and encoded as a signal by the vestibular nerve afferents, the signal is transmitted to the MVST cell, and the MVST cell then conveys this information to the cervical spinal segments. A hyperpolarized MVST cell would be at a disadvantage to carry this signal, and thus a firing rate needs to be present on the cell. This finding also indirectly speaks against an exclusive peripheral labyrinthine mechanism that blinds the MVST cell to active head movements. The vestibular nerve afferents presumably encode the head velocity in space, which is the summation of the active and passive components of the head movement. Three secondary cells in our sample did indeed respond with an equal sensitivity to applied and self-generated head movements. However, the MVST cell sees only the passive component of the head movement, that component which is necessary for reflex stabilization of the head.

Each MVST cell was tested to a manually applied forced rotation of the head and responded with a sensitivity similar to that obtained during whole-body rotation in the head-restrained paradigm. The rationale for delivering this stimulus is twofold. First, because of mechanical limitations of the turntable, externally applied whole-body rotations could not be delivered at frequencies and velocities approaching those generated by the animal during voluntary head movements. The results show that the failure of the MVST cell to encode head velocity in space is not due to the higher frequency and higher velocity of voluntary head movements, that is, a rapidly saturating input element to the cell. And second, whole-body rotation and voluntary head movement above a stationary body both change the position of the head in space, but the latter does so by also changing the position of the neck with respect to the body. Thus, forced head rotation as an external stimulus more directly compares to the mechanical events occurring during voluntary head movement. As seen in FIGURE 8, the cell's response to forced head rotation closely approximates that obtained for whole-body rotation; and thus it appears that the neck on shoulder input contributed little, either constructively or destructively, to the cell's response to forced head rotation.

The underlying events responsible for the negation of the head velocity in space signal on MVST cells during voluntary head movements remain a matter of speculation. Although an influence by the efferent vestibular system is an attractive possibility, suitable tests have not yet been performed to identify any participation in voluntary head movements. An obvious mechanism is one that involves an efference copy of intended head movement that reaches the MVST directly through inhibitory interneuronal elements in the brain stem. Another mechanism also involves an efference copy, but acts in an on–off fashion opening or closing a gate that passes a neck reafference signal. As mentioned above, the MVST cell responded to forced head rotations as it did to whole-body rotations. This observation appears at first inspection to be at variance with the prevalent convergence of vestibular and neck afferent inputs observed in the vestibular nuclei, particularly onto vestibulospinal neurons.[44,45] However, forced head turning is an externally applied perturbation. In this scenario, the gate is closed in the absence of an intended head movement. During a voluntary head movement, the gate is opened by the voluntary motor command, and a signal proportional to the neck rotation converges onto the MVST cell to subtract the active, self-generated component of the head movement. This possibility will be explored in future experiments.

One last point needs to be addressed. As discussed earlier, many MVST cells carry an eye movement-related signal that influences the outflow of the MVST pathway during passive vestibular stimulation. None of the MVST cells examined during voluntary head movement carried eye movement-related signals, and thus our sample is incomplete. To what extent our present results generalize to the other secondary MVST cells remains to be determined.

REFERENCES

1. WILSON, V. J. & M. MAEDA. 1974. Connections between semicircular canals and neck motoneurons in the cat. J. Neurophysiol. **37:** 346–357.
2. FUKUSHIMA, K., B. W. PETERSON & V. J. WILSON. 1978. Vestibulospinal, reticulospinal and interstitiospinal pathways in the cat. Prog. Brain Res. **50:** 121–136.
3. WILSON, V. J. & B. W. PETERSON. 1988. Vestibular and reticular projections to the neck. *In* Control of Head Movement. B. W. Peterson & F. J. Richmond, Eds.: 129–140. Oxford University Press. New York.
4. ISU, N. & J. YOKOTA. 1983. Morphophysiological study on the divergent projection of axon collaterals of medial vestibular neurons in the cat. Exp. Brain Res. **53:** 151–162.
5. UCHINO, Y. & N. HIRAI. 1984. Axon collaterals of anterior semicircular canal-activated vestibular neurons and their coactivation of extraocular and neck motoneurons in the cat. Neurosci. Res. **1:** 309–325.
6. ISU, N., Y. UCHINO, H. NAKASHIMA, S. SATOH, T. ICHIKAWA & S. WATANABE. 1988. Axonal trajectories of posterior canal-activated secondary vestibular neurons and their coactivation of extraocular and neck flexor motoneurons in the cat. Exp. Brain Res. **70:** 181–191.
7. MINOR, L. B., R. A. McCREA & J. M. GOLDBERG. 1990. Dual projections of secondary vestibular axons in the medial longitudinal fasciculus to extraocular motor nuclei and the spinal cord of the squirrel monkey. Exp. Brain Res. **83:** 9–21.

8. MILES, F. A. 1974. Single unit firing patterns in the vestibular nuclei related to voluntary eye movements and passive body rotation in conscious monkeys. Brain Res. **71:** 215–224.
9. CHUBB, M. C., A. F. FUCHS & C. A. SCUDDER. 1984. Neuron activity in the monkey vestibular nuclei during vertical vestibular stimulation and eye movements. J. Neurophysiol. **52:** 724–742.
10. TOMLINSON, R. D. & D. A. ROBINSON. 1984. Signals in the vestibular nucleus mediating vertical eye movements in the monkey. J. Neurophysiol. **51:** 1121–1136.
11. MCFARLAND, J. L. & A. F. FUCHS. 1992. Discharge patterns in nucleus prepositus hypoglossi and adjacent medial vestibular nucleus during horizontal eye movement in behaving macaques. J. Neurophysiol. **68:** 319–332.
12. MCCREA, R. A., A. STRASSMAN, E. MAY & S. M. HIGHSTEIN. 1987. Anatomical and physiological characteristics of vestibular neurons mediating the horizontal vestibulo-ocular reflexes of the squirrel monkey. J. Comp. Neurol. **264:** 547–570.
13. MCCREA, R. A., A. STRASSMAN & S. M. HIGHSTEIN. 1987. Anatomical and physiological characteristics of vestibular neurons mediating the vertical vestibulo-ocular reflexes of the squirrel monkey. J. Comp. Neurol. **264:** 571–592.
14. IWAMOTO, Y., T. KITAMA & K. YOSHIDA. 1990. Vertical eye movement-related secondary vestibular neurons ascending in medial longitudinal fasciculus in cat. I. Firing properties and projection pathways. J. Neurophysiol. **63:** 902–917.
15. IWAMOTO, Y., T. KITAMA & K. YOSHIDA. 1990. Vertical eye movement-related secondary vestibular neurons ascending in medial longitudinal fasciculus in cat. II. Direct connections with extraocular motoneurons. J. Neurophysiol. **63:** 918–935.
16. SCUDDER, C. A. & A. F. FUCHS. 1992. Physiological and behavioral identification of vestibular nucleus neurons mediating the horizontal vestibuloocular reflex in trained rhesus monkeys. J. Neurophysiol. **68:** 244–264.
17. BOYLE, R. 1993. Activity of medial vestibulospinal tract cells during rotation and ocular movement in the alert squirrel monkey. J. Neurophysiol. **70:** 2176–2180.
18. WILSON, V. J., R. BOYLE, K. FUKUSHIMA, P. K. ROSE, Y. SHINODA, Y. SUGIUCHI & Y. UCHINO. 1995. The vestibulocollic reflex. J. Vest. Res. **5:** 147–170.
19. BOYLE, R. & A. K. MOSCHOVAKIS. 1993. Vestibular control of head movement in squirrel monkey: Morphology of individual vestibulospinal axons. Soc. Neurosci. Abstr. **19:** 138.
20. BOYLE, R., D. PETROVIC & J. XU. 1995. Vestibular control of head movement in squirrel monkey: Morphology of individual vestibulospinal axons. Soc. Neurosci. Abstr. **21:** 1911.
21. BRODAL, A. 1974. Anatomy of the vestibular nuclei and their connections. In Handbook of Sensory Physiology. Vol. 6. Vestibular System. H. H. Kornhuber, Ed.: 239–352. Springer. Berlin.
22. BOYLE, R., J. M. GOLDBERG & S. M. HIGHSTEIN. 1992. Inputs from regularly and irregularly discharging vestibular nerve afferents to secondary neurons in the vestibular nuclei of the squirrel monkey. III. Correlation with vestibulospinal and vestibuloocular output pathways. J. Neurophysiol. **68:** 471–484.
23. VIDAL, P. P., A. ROUCOUX & A. BERTHOZ. 1982. Horizontal eye position-related activity in neck muscles of the alert cat. Exp. Brain Res. **46:** 448–453.
24. VIDAL, P. P., J. CORVISIER & A. BERTHOZ. 1983. Eye and neck motor signals in periabducens reticular neurons of the alert cat. Exp. Brain Res. **53:** 16–28.
25. GRANTYN, A. & A. BERTHOZ. 1988. The role of tectoreticulospinal system in the control of head movement. In Control of Head Movement. B. W. Peterson & F. J. Richmond, Eds.: 224–244. Oxford University Press. New York.
26. GRANTYN, A., A. BERTHOZ, O. HARDY & A. GOURDON. 1992. Contribution of reticulospinal neurons to the dynamic control of head movements: Presumed neck bursters. In The Head-Neck Sensory-Motor System. A. Berthoz, V. Graf & P.-P. Vidal, Eds.: 318–329. Oxford University Press. New York.
27. BIZZI, E., R. E. KALIL & V. TAGLIASCO. 1971. Eye-head coordination in monkeys: Evidence for centrally patterned organization. Science **173:** 452–454.
28. BIZZI, E., R. E. KALIL, P. MORASSO & V. TAGLIASCO. 1972. Central programming and peripheral feedback during eye-head coordination in monkeys. In Cerebral Control of

Eye Movements and Motion Perception. J. Dichgans & E. Bizzi, Eds.: 220–232. Karger. Basel.

29. LANMAN, J., E. BIZZI & J. ALLUM. 1978. The coordination of eye and head movement during smooth pursuit. Brain Res. **153:** 39–53.

30. MORASSO, P., E. BIZZI & J. DICHGANS. 1973. Adjustment of saccade characteristics during head movement. Exp. Brain Res. **16:** 492–500.

31. DICHGANS, J., E. BIZZI, P. MORASSO & V. TAGLIASCO. 1974. The role of vestibular and neck afferents during eye-head coordination in the monkey. Brain Res. **71:** 225–232.

32. TOMLINSON, R. D. & P. S. BAHRA. 1986. Combined eye-head gaze shifts in the primate. I. Metrics. J. Neurophysiol. **56:** 1542–1557.

33. BIZZI, E. 1981. Eye-head coordination. *In* Handbook of Physiology. Vol. 2. The Nervous System. 1321–1335. American Physiological Society. Bethesda, MD.

34. LAURUTIS, V. P. & D. A. ROBINSON. 1986. The vestibulo-ocular reflex during human saccadic eye movement. J. Physiol. (Lond.) **373:** 209–233.

35. TOMLINSON, R. D. & P. S. BAHRA. 1986. Combined eye-head gaze shifts in the primate. II. Interactions between saccades and the vestibuloocular reflex. J. Neurophysiol. **56:** 1558–1570.

36. GUITTON, D. & M. VOLLE. 1987. Gaze control in humans: Eye-head coordination during orienting movements to targets within and beyond the oculomotor range. J. Neurophysiol. **58:** 427–459.

37. PÉLISSON, D. & C. PRABLANC. 1986. Vestibulo-ocular reflex (VOR) induced by passive head rotation and goal-directed saccadic eye movements do not simply add in man. Brain Res. **380:** 397–400.

38. TOMLINSON, R. D. 1990. Combined eye-head gaze shifts in the primate. III. Contributions to the accuracy of gaze saccades. J. Neurophysiol. **64:** 1873–1891.

39. YOSHIDA, K., R. A. MCCREA, A. BERTHOZ & P. P. VIDAL. 1982. Morphological and physiological characteristics of inhibitory burst neurons controlling horizontal rapid eye movements in the alert cat. J. Neurophysiol. **48:** 761–784.

40. FUCHS, A. F. & J. KIMM. 1975. Unit activity in vestibular nucleus of the alert monkey during horizontal angular acceleration and eye movement. J. Neurophysiol. **38:** 1140–1161.

41. HIKOSAKA, O., Y. IGUSA & H. IMAI. 1980. Inhibitory connections of nystagmus-related reticular burst neurons in the abducens, prepositus hypoglossi and vestibular nuclei in the cat. Exp. Brain Res. **39:** 301–311.

42. STRASSMAN, A., S. M. HIGHSTEIN & R. A. MCCREA. 1986. Anatomy and physiology of saccadic burst neurons in the alert squirrel monkey. II. Inhibitory burst neurons. J. Comp. Neurol. **249:** 358–380.

43. KHALSA, S. B. S., R. D. TOMLINSON, D. W. F. SCHWARZ & J. P. LANDOLT. 1987. Vestibular nuclear neuron activity during active and passive head movement in the alert rhesus monkey. J. Neurophysiol. **57:** 1484–1497.

44. BOYLE, R. & O. POMPEIANO. 1981. Convergence and interaction of neck and macular vestibular inputs on vestibulospinal neurons. J. Neurophysiol. **45:** 852–868.

45. BRINK, E. E., K. JINNAI, N. HIRAI & V. J. WILSON. 1981. Cervical input to vestibulocollic neurons. Brain Res. **217:** 13–21.

Four Convergent Patterns of Input from the Six Semicircular Canals to Motoneurons of Different Neck Muscles in the Upper Cervical Cord

Y. SHINODA,[a] Y. SUGIUCHI, T. FUTAMI,
S. KAKEI, Y. IZAWA, AND J. NA

Departments of Physiology and Otolaryngology
School of Medicine, Tokyo Medical and Dental University
1-5-45, Bunkyo-ku, Yushima
Tokyo, Japan 113

INTRODUCTION

The plane of a head movement produced by stimulation of a semicircular canal nerve parallels that of the stimulated canal.[1] This finding indicates that the signal from each semicircular canal must be distributed to a particular set of neck muscles to induce compensatory head movements. The pattern of connections between different semicircular canals and dorsal neck muscle motoneurons was first investigated by Wilson and Maeda.[2] Since then, the study of vestibulospinal connections has been dominated by reports describing connections to a specific group of motoneurons that supply large dorsal extensor muscles such as the biventer, complexus, and splenius muscles. However, it has become increasingly apparent that the large dorsal extensor muscles involved in head movement represent a highly specialized group of neck muscles.[3–5] Because more than 30 neck muscles must be controlled in proper spatial combinations to induce compensatory head movements in the same plane as the stimulated semicircular canal, it is likely that there is more than one pattern of input from the six semicircular canals to motoneurons of different neck muscles. Labyrinthine receptors responsible for vestibular inputs to neck motoneurons have been identified by examining the effect of stimulation of individual nerve branches of the vestibular nerve on motoneurons of a few neck muscles. Stimulation of individual semicircular canal nerves evokes disynaptic postsynaptic potentials (PSPs) bilaterally in neck motoneurons, regardless of whether they are excitatory or inhibitory.[2,6–8] Because of this prevalence of disynaptic excitatory and inhibitory connections between ampullary nerves and neck motoneurons, only recently has attention been given to upper cervical interneurons that may participate in the vestibulocollic reflex.

In the present study we investigate the patterns of input and the pathways from the six semicircular canals to motoneurons of various neck muscles in anesthetized cats, by recording intracellular PSPs from neck motoneurons in response to electrical stimulation of the six ampullary nerves. Some of the results have been reported previously.[9–12]

[a] Address correspondence to Dr. Yoshikazu Shinoda, Department of Physiology, School of Medicine, Tokyo Medical and Dental University, 1-5-45, Bunkyo-ku, Yushima, Tokyo, Japan 113. E-mail: yshinoda.phy1@med.tmd.ac.jp

METHODS

Experiments were performed in cats anesthetized with an intramuscular injection of ketamine (25 mg/kg) followed by intravenous injection of α-chloralose (50–60 mg/kg initial dose, supplemented with additional doses of 10–25 mg/kg with a supplementary dose of Nembutal (Abbott, Switzerland; 5–10 mg/kg) given during the course of the experiments. To stimulate ampullary nerves, bipolar stimulating electrodes were made of two fine stainless steel wires (40 μm diameter) glued together and implanted bilaterally near the anterior (ACN), lateral (LCN), and posterior (PCN) canal nerves through small holes made in the bony canals, as described by Suzuki *et al.*[13] Implantation was tested by observing eye movements elicited by stimulation of the ampullary nerves with trains of 35 pulses of 0.2 ms in duration at an interval of 2.0 ms from a constant current generator. Final electrode positions were determined by monitoring characteristic eye movements elicited by stimulation of individual ampullary nerves.[1] Thresholds of eye movements were usually 5–25 μA, and patterns of eye movements generally remained unchanged as the stimulating currents were increased three- to fivefold. Muscle nerves to different neck muscles were dissected and dorsal laminectomy was performed at C1–C4 to permit intracellular recordings from neck motoneurons. Glass microelectrodes were filled with 3 M KCl and had a resistance of 8–15 MΩ. Motoneurons were identified by their antidromic responses to stimulation of individual muscle nerves. In some experiments, lesions were made in the medial longitudinal fascicle (MLF) or the lateral vestibulospinal tract (LVST) to determine the pathways in the brain stem from the vestibular nuclei to neck motoneurons. The cerebellum overlying the floor of the fourth ventricle at the medulla was aspirated. The MLF or LVST was cut at the level of the obex with a fine blade under visual observation. After each experiment, the positions of implanted electrodes in the semicircular canals were examined under an operating microscope.

RESULTS

The pattern of connections between the six semicircular canals and motoneurons of various neck muscles was investigated by recording intracellular potentials from neck motoneurons in the upper cervical cord. Stimulation of individual canal nerves evoked either excitatory (EPSPs) or inhibitory (IPSPs) postsynaptic potentials in neck motoneurons. Virtually all neck motoneurons examined received convergent inputs from the six ampullary nerves. Motoneurons that supplied a single muscle had a homogeneous pattern of input from the six semicircular canals. Four patterns of input from the six semicircular canals to motoneurons of various neck muscles could be grouped into four patterns.

The first pattern of these four patterns was observed in motoneurons of the rectus capitis posterior (RCP) muscle. The typical response pattern of an RCP motoneuron to stimulation of the six ampullary nerves is shown in FIGURE 1A–C. Stimulation of the ACN on either side produced EPSPs, and stimulation of the PCNs on either side produced IPSPs. Stimulation of the ipsi- and contralateral LCNs produced IPSPs and EPSPs, respectively. This typical response pattern to separate stimulation of the six ampullary nerves was observed in 41 of 60 RCP motoneurons. Rare departures from the typical input pattern occurred in some RCP motoneurons. EPSPs were evoked by stimulation of the ipsilateral LCN (4.8%), and IPSPs were evoked by stimulation of the ipsilateral ACN (1.4%). These deviations from the

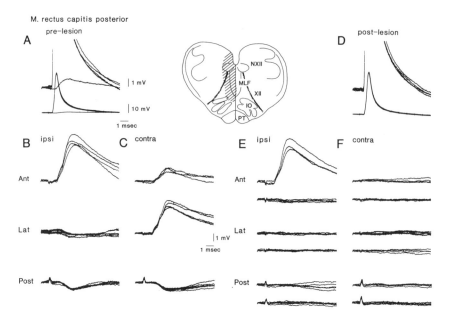

FIGURE 1. Effects of sectioning the MLF on PSPs evoked in an RCP motoneuron by stimulation of the six ampullary nerves. Antidromic spikes before (**A**) and after sectioning (**D**). Control records of PSPs evoked by stimulation of three ipsilateral (**B**) and contralateral ampullary nerves (**C**) before sectioning. Voltage and time calibrations in **C** are applied for all traces in **B, C, E,** and **F**. (**E– F**) PSPs recorded from the same motoneuron after sectioning. Stimulus strengths for all six ampullary nerves were 100 μA before and after sectioning. During intracellular recording from the same motoneuron, sectioning at the level of the obex was performed in steps mediolaterally in the MLF ipsilateral to the RCP motoneuron, and the final lesion (*hatched area, top middle*) was reconstructed on serial sections. IO, inferior olive; PT, pyramidal tract; NXII, hypoglossal nucleus; XII, hypoglossal nerve. (From Shinoda *et al.*[10] Reproduced, with permission, from the *Journal of Neurophysiology.*)

typical response pattern may be due to current spread to an adjacent ampullary nerve.

To determine the central pathways that link the six semicircular canals to neck motoneurons, a cut was made in the MLF at the level of the obex, and the effects of ampullary nerve stimulation were compared before and after the lesion. While recording intracellular potentials from the RCP motoneuron, a cut was made in the MLF ipsilateral to the recording site at the level of the obex, and the responses of the same neuron before (FIG. 1A–C) and after (FIG. 1D–F) the cut were compared. After the cut, the EPSPs evoked from the contralateral ACN and LCN disappeared, and the IPSPs from the contralateral PCN and the ipsilateral LCN and PCN also disappeared (FIG. 1E and F). However, the EPSPs evoked by ipsilateral ACN stimulation remained unchanged. A lesion was also made in the MLF contralateral to the recording site in three other experiments, but no effect of sectioning was observed for bilateral semicircular canal inputs to RCP motoneurons. Most of the EPSPs evoked by stimulation of the bilateral ACNs and contralateral LCN as well as the IPSPs evoked by stimulation of the ipsilateral PCN and LCN had latencies of less than 1.6 ms and were considered to be disynaptic.

The second pattern of input from the six semicircular canals was observed in motoneurons of the obliquus capitis inferior (OCI) muscle. The typical input pattern in an OCI motoneuron is illustrated in FIGURE 2A–C. EPSPs were evoked by stimulation of the ipsilateral ACN and PCN and the contralateral LCN, whereas IPSPs were evoked by stimulation of the contralateral ACN and PCN and the ipsilateral LCN. This typical input pattern of the PSPs was found in 36 of 44 OCI motoneurons at C1 and in 14 of 20 OCI motoneurons at C2. In the other 51 OCI motoneurons (46 at C1 and 5 at C2), the effects of stimulation of all six ampullary nerves could not be examined, the input from one or two ampullary nerves was lacking, or some deviation from this typical input pattern was found. A frequent deviation was the appearance of EPSPs evoked by stimulation of the contralateral ACN (9.5%) and IPSPs evoked by stimulation of the contralateral LCN (6.9%). The latencies of the EPSPs evoked from the ipsilateral ACN and PCN and the contralateral LCN, as well as the IPSPs from the ipsilateral LCN, indicated that most of these PSPs had latencies of 0.9–1.6 ms and could be considered disynaptic. In contrast, stimulation of the contralateral ACN induced IPSPs at latencies of 1.8 ms or longer, and these latencies were about 1.0 ms longer than the disynaptic PSPs evoked by

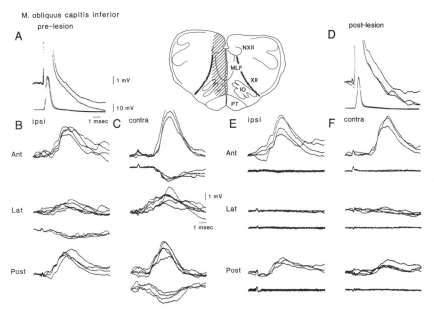

FIGURE 2. Effects of sectioning the MLF on PSPs evoked in an OCI motoneuron by stimulation of the six ampullary nerves. While recording from the same motoneuron, sectioning (*hatched area, top middle*) was performed in the medulla including the MLF ipsilateral to the motoneuron. Antidromic spike potentials recorded from the same OCI motoneuron before (**A**) and after (**D**) MLF sectioning. (**B–C**) Control records before sectioning. (**E–F**) Intracellular responses after sectioning. The depolarizing responses evoked by stimulation of the ipsilateral LCN and the contralateral ACN and PCN were reversed IPSPs (see the lower hyperpolarizing responses in **B** and **C** just after intracellular penetration) because of spontaneous diffusion of Cl⁻ from a KCl recording electrode into the cell. Lower traces in **E** and **F** are juxtacellular field potentials. (From Shinoda *et al.*[10] Reproduced, with permission, from the *Journal of Neurophysiology.*)

stimulation of other ampullary nerves. These IPSPs, therefore, were probably regarded as trisynaptic from the primary vestibular afferents.

The effects of sectioning the MLF on semicircular canal inputs were also examined in OCI motoneurons. A typical example is shown in FIGURE 2D–F. Before a cut, disynaptic EPSPs were evoked by stimulation of the ipsilateral ACN and PCN and the contralateral LCN, whereas disynaptic IPSPs were evoked by stimulation of the ipsilateral LCN and the contralateral PCN (FIG. 2B and C). Trisynaptic IPSPs were evoked by contralateral ACN stimulation (FIG. 2C). These IPSPs were reversed due to diffusion of Cl^{-1}. While recording intracellular potentials from the same OCI motoneuron (FIG. 2A and D), a cut was made in the MLF ipsilateral to the motoneuron (FIG. 2, top middle diagram). This cut eliminated the PSPs evoked by stimulation of the bilateral LCNs, but the EPSPs evoked by stimulation of the ipsilateral ACN and PCN remained almost unchanged (FIG. 2E). The trisynaptic IPSPs evoked by contralateral ACN stimulation also remained unaffected. In contrast, the disynaptic IPSPs evoked by contralateral PCN stimulation disappeared, but the trisynaptic IPSPs were not abolished (FIG. 2F). Sectioning of the medial portion of the ipsilateral MLF abolished the contralateral disynaptic effects almost completely. Sectioning the contralateral MLF before or after sectioning the ipsilateral MLF did not affect the responses in 10 experiments.

To further clarify the pathway of presumed trisynaptic inhibition, the effect of sectioning the LVST on semicircular canal inputs was examined. FIGURE 3A shows semicircular canal responses in an OCI motoneuron before (Aa) and after (Ab) sectioning the LVST. Before sectioning the LVST contralateral to the recorded motoneuron, IPSPs were evoked at 2.7 ms by stimulation of the contra-ACN and at 2.6 ms by stimulation of the contra-PCN, whereas EPSPs were evoked at 1.4 ms by stimulation of the contra-LCN (FIG. 3Aa). While recording intracellular potentials from the same OCI motoneuron, the LVST was sectioned on the side contralateral to the recorded motoneuron. The ACN- and PCN-evoked trisynaptic IPSPs disappeared after sectioning, but LCN-evoked EPSPs at 1.4 ms remained unaffected (FIG. 3Ab). The reconstructed lesion on serial sections of the medulla covered most of the LVST at the level of the hypoglossal nucleus. After sectioning the LVST, we recorded PSPs from as many motoneurons as possible. ACN stimulation did not evoke IPSPs at latencies consistent with a trisynaptic relay after sectioning the LVST in 20 of the 24 OCI motoneurons examined, and evoked only very small IPSPs in the remaining four motoneurons. LCN-evoked EPSPs were present in these motoneurons. Although the effect of sectioning the LVST on PCN-evoked trisynaptic IPSPs could not be determined in most neurons because of the presence of disynaptic IPSPs ($n = 18$), no response was evoked in the remaining six neurons as shown in FIGURE 3Ab. These results indicate that the ACN-evoked IPSPs, and probably the PCN-evoked IPSPs as well with latencies consistent with a trisynaptic relay, were conveyed via the contralateral LVST to OCI motoneurons.

To confirm that presumed trisynaptic inhibition from the contralateral vertical canal nerves is conveyed to neck motoneurons via the LVST, the effect of stimulating the contralateral LVST was examined after sectioning the bilateral MLFs (FIG. 3B). In an OCI motoneuron, stimulation of the ipsilateral primary vestibular afferents and the contra-ACN evoked EPSPs at 1.4 ms (FIG. 3Bb) and IPSPs at 2.5 ms (FIG. 3Bc), respectively. Stimulation of the contralateral LVST evoked IPSPs at a latency of 1.5 ms in the same OCI motoneuron (FIG. 3Bd). The difference in latency between the IPSPs evoked by stimulation of the contra-ACN and LVST was 1.0 ms. The stimulation electrode was confirmed histologically to be in the contralateral LVST. The difference between the latencies of the IPSPs evoked by stimulation of the contralateral vertical canal nerves and the LVST ranged from 0.4 to 1.2 ms (mean ± SD, 0.8 ± 0.2 ms, $n = 22$). The latencies of LVST-evoked IPSPs in the motoneurons ranged from 1.1 to 2.1 ms (mean ± SD, 1.5 ± 0.2 ms, $n = 37$). Because most of these IPSPs were considered to be disynaptic,[14] these findings strongly support that inhibition from the contralateral vertical canals at latencies longer than 1.8 ms is more than disynaptic. Furthermore, they suggest that the interneurons responsible for mediating these trisynaptic IPSPs are located in the spinal cord, not in the brain stem.

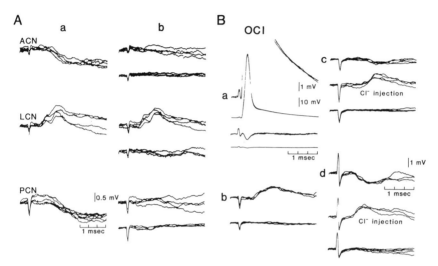

FIGURE 3. (A) Effects of sectioning the lateral vestibulospinal tract (LVST) on PSPs in an OCI motoneuron evoked by stimulation of the three contralateral canal nerves. Intracellular recording from the same motoneuron before (a) and after (b) sectioning the contralateral LVST. (B) Effects of stimulation of the contralateral LVST on an OCI motoneuron after sectioning the bilateral MLFs: (a) Antidromic spikes evoked by stimulation of the OCI muscle nerve; (b) stimulation of the ipsilateral primary vestibular afferents as a whole (200 μA); (c) stimulation of the contralateral ampullary nerves; and (d) stimulation of the contralateral LVST (150 μA). Top traces: intracellular potentials. Middle traces in Bc and Bd: reversed IPSPs after the intracellular injection of Cl⁻. Bottom traces: juxtacellular field potentials. (From Sugiuchi *et al.*[12] Reproduced, with permission, from the *Journal of Neurophysiology.*)

The results so far indicate that last-order interneurons that receive disynaptic excitation from the vertical canal nerves and monosynaptic excitation from the LVST are most likely located in the spinal cord and terminate on neck motoneurons contralateral to the vertical canal nerves. Since the LVST only projects to the ipsilateral spinal cord,[15–17] the last-order interneurons are most likely commissural neurons located in the spinal cord ipsilateral to the vertical canal nerves. To confirm that commissural neurons in lamina VIII may be last-order inhibitory interneurons, we examined the effect of microstimulation of the contralateral ventral horn on neck motoneurons (FIG. 4). Microstimulation of three different sites in the contralateral ventral horn of C1 (FIG. 4C) evoked short-latency hyperpolarization in an OCI motoneuron at C1 (FIG. 4E). This hyperpolarization was an IPSP, because injection of Cl⁻ into the cell easily reversed this hyperpolarization to depolarization (FIG. 4Ea, middle). The reversed IPSPs clearly showed the existence of a second component at

1.4 ms. By moving the stimulating electrode dorsoventrally in the ventral horn, the most effective site of stimulation was found in the ventromedial part of lamina VIII (arrowhead in FIG. 4Db). The threshold of the IPSPs evoked in this area was 25 μA, and their latency was 0.8 ms for this motoneuron. Similarly, the effective sites of stimulation for evoking such monosynaptic IPSPs in other OCI motoneurons were found mainly in the medial part of lamina VIII and sometimes in the ventromedial part of lamina VII. These effective sites were distributed rostrocaudally over the entire length of C1 and the rostral portion of C2. The latencies of these IPSPs in OCI motoneurons ranged from 0.7 to 1.8 ms (FIG. 4G) and appeared to fall into two

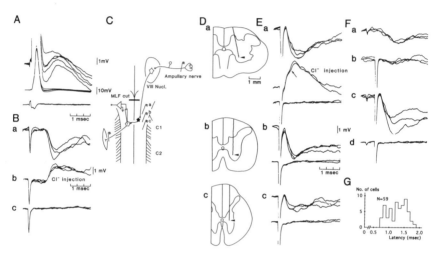

FIGURE 4. Effect of stimulation of the contralateral ventral horn on an OCI motoneuron. (**A**) Antidromic spikes evoked by stimulation of the OCI muscle nerve. (**B**) IPSPs evoked at a latency of 2.3 ms by stimulation of the contra-ACN before (**a**) and after (**b**) Cl⁻ injection. (**c**) Juxtacellular field potentials. (**C**) Schematic drawing of the experimental setup. (**D**) Stimulation sites at C1⁻ of the spinal cord. Lines and arrowheads indicate electrode tracks and the final stimulation sites, respectively. (**E**) Intracellular potentials evoked by stimulation of the contralateral spinal gray matter. Panels **a, b,** and **c** indicate the responses to stimulation at the sites indicated by the arrowheads in **a, b,** and **c** in **D.** The middle traces in **Ea** demonstrate the reversal of IPSPs after Cl⁻ injection. The arrow indicates disynaptic IPSPs. (**F**) Facilitation experiment. Weak stimulation of the ventral horn (position **b** in **D**) and the contra-ACN evoked small monosynaptic IPSPs (**b**) and small trisynaptic IPSPs (**a**), respectively. Combined stimulation with these two stimuli (stimulation of the contralateral ventral horn was applied 1.3 ms after stimulation of the contra-ACN) evoked IPSPs (**c**) larger than the algebraic sum of the two responses evoked separately. (**d**) Juxtacellular field potentials. (**G**) Latency histograms of IPSPs in OCI motoneurons evoked by stimulation of the contralateral ventral horn. (From Sugiuchi *et al.*[12] Reproduced, with permission, from the *Journal of Neurophysiology.*)

groups. The earlier group with a latency less than 1.1 ms was ascribed to monosynaptic IPSPs and the later group to disynaptic IPSPs. These findings suggest that there are commissural neurons in laminae VII and VIII that project to contralateral neck motoneurons, upon which they exert monosynaptic inhibitory effects. To verify that spinal commissural neurons are in fact the last-order inhibitory interneurons involved in trisynaptic inhibition, we investigated the effect of input from the vertical canal nerve on inhibitory commissural neurons that were in direct contact with a contralateral neck motoneuron. In preparations with bilateral MLF interruption, stimulation of the contra-ACN evoked trisynaptic IPSPs at a latency of 2.3 ms (FIG. 4B), whereas stimulation of contra-lamina VIII evoked monosynaptic IPSPs at 0.8 ms in an OCI motoneuron (FIG. 4Eb). Stimulus intensities of the contra-ACN and contra-lamina VIII were adjusted to evoke smaller IPSPs (FIG. 4Fa and b, respectively). With the same stimulus intensities, test stimuli were applied to the contra-lamina VIII at 1.3 ms after conditioning stimulation of the contra-ACN. As shown in FIGURE 4Fc, large IPSPs were evoked at 0.8 ms by the test stimulation of lamina VIII, and the amplitude of the IPSPs was much greater than the algebraic sum of the IPSPs obtained by individual stimulation of the contra-ACN and contra-lamina VIII. More specifically, the slope of the IPSPs at 0.8 ms was much steeper than that of the summed IPSPs, indicating that the monosynaptic IPSPs were facilitated by the conditioning ACN stimuli. This phenomenon should occur only if the test stimuli activated the cell bodies of last-order interneurons which mediated the response evoked by the conditioning stimuli. Furthermore, it indicates that the conditioning stimuli had a disynaptic facilitatory effect on the last-order inhibitory neurons. Therefore, the existence of this facilitation verified that at least some commissural neurons in lamina VIII receive disynaptic excitation from the ipsilateral ACN through the LVST, and have a direct inhibitory effect on the contralateral OCI motoneuron. A similar facilitatory interaction between lamina VIII-evoked and ACN-evoked IPSPs was observed in 6 of 8 OCI motoneurons examined.

The third pattern of semicircular canal input was observed in motoneurons of the sternocleido muscle. In these motoneurons, stimulation of the contralateral three canal nerves evoked disynaptic EPSPs, whereas stimulation of the ipsilateral three canal nerves evoked disynaptic IPSPs (not illustrated). These EPSPs and IPSPs were completely abolished by sectioning the MLF ipsilateral to the recorded motoneurons.

The fourth pattern of semicircular canal input was observed in motoneurons of the longus capitis (LC) muscle. These motoneurons received excitation from the bilateral PCNs and the contralateral LCN and inhibition from the bilateral ACNs and the ipsilateral LCN. This typical input pattern was found in 7 of 8 LC motoneurons at C1. The latencies of the PSPs evoked by stimulation of the canal nerves, except the contralateral ACN, were mainly less than 1.8 ms and considered to be disynaptic. The IPSPs evoked by stimulation of the contralateral ACN had latencies longer than 1.8 ms. Therefore, these IPSPs were most likely trisynaptic from the primary vestibular afferents. Sectioning of the ipsilateral MLF eliminated the PSPs evoked by individual canal nerves except the contralateral ACN, whereas sectioning of the contralateral LVST eliminated the IPSPs evoked from the contralateral ACN, but left the PSPs from the other five canal nerves unaffected.

DISCUSSION

The present study has provided evidence, by examining the effects of stimulating six ampullary nerves in each motoneuron, that virtually all motoneurons of neck muscles examined are influenced by the six semicircular canals and that motoneurons which supply a particular neck muscle have a homogeneous pattern of input from all six semicircular canals. One key assumption is that the electrical stimulation of individual canal nerves used in this study was selective and activated only the appropriate canal nerve. The position of the stimulating electrode was fixed in the site that was most effective for evoking the characteristic eye movement by stimulation of each canal nerve.[1] The patterns of input from the contralateral canal nerves to

OCI, LC, and RCP motoneurons that were examined using the method described above were consistent from one experiment to another. After each experiment, we visually confirmed that tips of stimulating electrodes were positioned correctly relative to their target ampullary nerves. These results support the reliability of our technique of selective stimulation of individual ampullary nerves. The main problems of current spread to other ampullary or macular nerves have been discussed in detail in a previous paper.[10]

The vestibulospinal connections between ampullary nerves and neck motoneurons that have been identified thus far are all disynaptic.[2,18] However, this study has shown that a trisynaptic pathway exists between ampullary nerves and neck motoneurons. Interneurons receiving vestibular input have been reported in the ventral horn of the cervical cord,[19,20] and they receive disynaptic EPSPs from the vestibular afferents.[21] Among these interneurons are commissural neurons that are activated from the contralateral labyrinth.[21,22] None of these studies provided direct evidence for the identity of the postsynaptic neurons of these interneurons. However, Sugiuchi et al.[23] have shown that commissural neurons in lamina VIII at C1–C2 receive di- or trisynaptic input from the ipsilateral vertical canal nerve and terminate on contralateral neck motoneurons. Endo et al.[24] also showed that commissural neurons receive input from vertical canals as well as from otolith organs, using natural stimulation. They found commissural neurons receiving input from the ipsilateral vertical canals as well as from the contralateral ones. The present study showed that stimulation of contralateral lamina VIII evoked predominantly monosynaptic IPSPs in neck motoneurons. These monosynaptic IPSPs were facilitated by conditioning stimulation of the contralateral ACN in OCI motoneurons. The existence of this facilitation confirmed that the last-order inhibitory interneurons responsible for mediating the trisynaptic IPSPs from the contralateral vertical canal nerves are actually commissural neurons. In the vestibulospinal system, three populations of last-order interneurons to motoneurons have been previously identified; the first consists of group Ia inhibitory interneurons, which innervate knee flexor motoneurons[25,26]; the second consists of inhibitory interneurons, which terminate on motoneurons of flexor muscles other than knee flexors[27]; and the third consists of excitatory interneurons, which innervate extensor motoneurons.[26] The commissural neurons described in this paper are the first example of identified contralateral last-order interneurons to motoneurons in the vestibulospinal system.[12,23]

This study has shown that there are four different patterns of input from the six ampullary nerves to motoneurons of various neck muscles. The first pattern, observed in RCP motoneurons, is similar to that reported for other dorsal extensor muscles by Wilson and Maeda.[2] These motoneurons receive excitation from the bilateral ACNs and the contralateral LCN, and inhibition from the bilateral PCNs and the ipsilateral LCN. The second input pattern, observed in OCI motoneurons, is entirely new. These motoneurons receive excitation from the ipsilateral ACN and PCN and the contralateral LCN, and inhibition from the contralateral ACN and PCN and the ipsilateral LCN. The third pattern is observed in sternocleidal motoneurons. These motoneurons receive excitation from the three contralateral canal nerves and inhibition from the ipsilateral canal nerves. This pattern is similar to the pattern found in neck flexor motoneurons.[6] The fourth pattern was observed in LC motoneurons. These motoneurons receive excitation from the bilateral PCNs and inhibition from the bilateral ACNs. Inputs from the LCNs are the same as in other motoneurons.

The patterns of synaptic inputs from the six semicircular canals to RCP, OCI, LC, and sternocleidal motoneurons are consistent with head movements expected in response to natural head rotation[3] and with those induced by electrical stimulation of ampullary nerves.[1] Electrical stimulation of the LCN produces head movement to the contralateral side in the horizontal plane.[1] All neck motoneurons that have been examined thus far are excited and inhibited by stimulation of the contralateral and the ipsilateral LCN, respectively. Therefore, in rotating the head to one side in the horizontal plane, all neck muscles on the contralateral side may be activated to induce compensatory head movement to the contralateral side. This result is consistent with the vestibulocollic responses of various neck muscles examined quantitatively in sinusoidal rotation.[3] Simultaneous stimulation of the bilateral ACNs and PCNs produces upward and downward head rotation on the bitemporal axis, respectively, whereas simultaneous stimulation of the unilateral ACN and PCN produces head tilt on the naso-occipital axis.[1] Bilateral RCP muscles may be maximally contracted to raise the head to the normal position during downward head rotation in the sagittal plane, and bilateral LC muscles may be maximally contracted to flex the head to the normal position during upward head rotation in the sagittal plane. However, these two muscles may not play as great a role in the development of the reflex compensatory head movement during head rotation in the frontal plane, because the inputs from the unilateral anterior and posterior semicircular canals essentially negate each other at the motoneuronal level. This qualitative nature of the input pattern from the six semicircular canals agrees with the direction of head rotation associated with maximal activation of an RCP and an LC muscle.[3] In contrast, the present pattern of ampullary inputs suggests that OCI muscles may be excited ipsilaterally and inhibited contralaterally during head tilt in the frontal plane, so that they may function in compensatory head movement on the naso-occipital axis. The OCI muscle in the cat is well developed compared with that in humans. This difference may be reflected by the much wider range of head rotation in the frontal plane in the cat. Although the OCI muscle plays a role in horizontal head rotation,[28,29] which is consistent with the present result, further analysis of EMG activities of the OCI muscle during head rotation in various directions is required to understand the functional role of this muscle in compensatory head movements.

SUMMARY

This study was performed to investigate the pattern of input and the pathways from the six semicircular canals to motoneurons of various neck muscles in anesthetized cats. Intracellular postsynaptic potentials from neck motoneurons were recorded in response to electrical stimulation of the six ampullary nerves. The results showed that motoneurons of a particular neck muscle have a homogeneous convergent pattern of input from the six semicircular canals; there are four patterns of input from the six semicircular canals to motoneurons of various neck muscles; and the trisynaptic connection between the semicircular canal nerves and neck motoneurons was identified in addition to the disynaptic connection.

REFERENCES

1. SUZUKI, J. & B. COHEN. 1964. Head, eye, body and limb movements from semicircular canal nerves. Exp. Neurol. **10**: 393–405.
2. WILSON, V. J. & M. MAEDA. 1974. Connection between semicircular canals and neck motoneurons in the cat. J. Neurophysiol. **37**: 346–357.
3. BAKER, J., J. GOLDBERG & B. PETERSON. 1985. Spatial and temporal response properties of the vestibulocollic reflex in decerebrate cats. J. Neurophysiol. **54**: 735–756.

4. RICHMOND, F. J. R. & P. P. VIDAL. 1988. The motor system: Joints and muscles of the neck. *In* Control of Head Movement. B. W. Peterson & F. J. Richmond, Eds.: 1–21. Oxford University Press. New York.

5. RICHIMOND, F. J. R., D. C. GORDON & G. E. LOEB. 1992. Heterogenous structure and function among intervertebral muscles. *In* Head-Neck Sensory-Motor System. A. Berthoz, P. P. Vidal & W. Graf, Eds.: 141–147. Oxford University Press. New York.

6. FUKUSHIMA, K., B. W. PETERSON & V. J. WILSON. 1979. Vestibulospinal, reticulospinal and interstitiospinal pathways in the cat. Prog. Brain Res. **50:** 121–136.

7. ISU, N., Y. UCHINO, H. NAKASHIMA, S. SATOH, T. ICHIKAWA & S. WATANABE. 1988. Axonal trajectories of posterior canal-activated secondary vestibular neurons and their coactivation of extraocular and neck flexor motoneurons in the cat. Exp. Brain Res. **70:** 181–191.

8. UCHINO, Y., N. ISU, T. ICHIKAWA, S. SATOH & S. WATANABE. 1988. Properties and localization of the anterior semicircular canal-activated vestibulocollic neurons in the cat. Exp. Brain Res. **71:** 345–352.

9. SHINODA, Y., Y. SUGIUCHI, T. FUTAMI, N. ANDO, T. KAWASAKI & J. YAGI. 1993. Synaptic organization of the vestibulo-collic pathways from six semicircular canals to motoneurons of different neck muscles. Prog. Brain Res. **97:** 201–209.

10. SHINODA, Y., Y. SUGIUCHI, T. FUTAMI, N. ANDO & T. KAWASAKI. 1994. Input patterns and pathways from six semicircular canals to motoneurons of neck muscles. I. The multifidus muscle group. J. Neurophysiol. **72:** 2691–2702.

11. SUGIUCHI, Y., T. FUTAMI, N. ANDO, T. KAWASAKI, Y. YAGI & Y. SHINODA. 1992. Patterns of connections between six semicircular canals and neck motoneurons. Ann. N. Y. Acad. Sci. **656:** 957–959.

12. SUGIUCHI, Y., Y. IZAWA & Y. SHINODA. 1995. Trisynaptic inhibition from the contralateral vertical semicircular canal nerves to neck motoneurons mediated by spinal commissural neurons. J. Neurophysiol. **73:** 1973–1987.

13. SUZUKI, J., K. GOTO, K. TOKUMASU & B. COHEN. 1969. Implantation of electrodes near individual vestibular nerve branches in mammals. Ann. Otol. Rhinol. Laryngol. **78:** 815–826.

14. AKAIKE, T., V. V. FANARDJIAN, M. ITO & T. OHNO. 1973. Electrophysiological analysis of the vestibulospinal reflex pathway of rabbit. II. Synaptic actions upon spinal neurones. Exp. Brain Res. **17:** 497–515.

15. NYBERG-HANSEN, R. & T. A. MASCITTI. 1964. Sites and modes of termination of fibers of the vestibulospinal tract in the cat: An experimental study with silver impregnation methods. J. Comp. Neurol. **122:** 369–388.

16. ROSE, P. K., K. WAINWRIGHT & M. NEUBER-HESS. 1992. Connections from the lateral vestibular nucleus to the upper cervical spinal cord of the cat. A study with the anterograde trace PHA-L. J. Comp. Neurol. **321:** 312–324.

17. SHINODA, Y., T. OHGAKI & T. FUTAMI. 1986. The morphology of single vestibulospinal tract axons in the lower cervical cord of the cat. J. Comp. Neurol. **249:** 226–241.

18. UCHINO, Y. & N. ISU. 1992. Properties of vestibulo-ocular and/or vestibulo-collic neurons in the cat. *In* Head-Neck Sensory-Motor System. A. Berthoz, P. P. Vidal & W. Graf, Eds.: 266–272. Oxford University Press. New York.

19. BOLTON, P. S., T. GOTO & V. J. WILSON. 1991. Commissural neurons in the cat upper cervical spinal cord. Neuroreport **2:** 743–746.

20. SCHOR, R. H., I. SUZUKI, S. J. B. TIMERICK & V. J. WILSON. 1986. Responses of interneurons in the cat cervical cord to vestibular tilt stimulation. J. Neurophysiol. **56:** 1147–1156.

21. ALSTERMARK, B., A. LUNDBERG, M. PINTER & S. SASAKI. 1987. Vestibular effects in long C3–C5 propriospinal neurons. Brain Res. **404:** 389–394.

22. BOLTON, P. S., T. GOTO & V. J. WILSON. 1993. Horizontal canal input to upper cervical commissural neurons. Exp. Brain Res. **92:** 549–552.

23. SUGIUCHI, Y., S. KAKEI & Y. SHINODA. 1992. Spinal commissural neurons mediating vestibular input to neck motoneurons in the cat cervical spinal cord. Neurosci. Lett. **145:** 221–224.

24. ENDO, K., J. KASPER, V. J. WILSON & B. J. YATES. 1994. Responses of commissural and other upper cervical ventral horn neurons to vestibular stimuli in vertical planes. J. Neurophysiol. **71:** 11–17.
25. TEN BRUGGENCATE, G., R. BURKE, A. LUNDBERG & M. UDO. 1969. Interaction between the vestibulospinal tract, contralateral flexor reflex afferents and Ia afferents. Brain Res. **14:** 529–532.
26. GRILLNER, S., T. HONGO & S. LUND. 1966. Interaction between the inhibitory pathways from the Deiters' nucleus and Ia afferents to flexor motoneurones. Acta Physiol. Scand. **68 (Suppl. 277):** 61.
27. TEN BRUGGENCATE, G. & A. LUNDBERG. 1974. Facilitatory interaction in transmission to motoneurons from vestibulospinal fibers and contralateral primary afferents. Exp. Brain Res. **19:** 248–270.
28. REIGHARD, J. & H. S. JENNINGS. 1963. Anatomy of the Cat. Henry Holt & Co. New York.
29. VIDAL, P. P., A. ROUCOUX & A. BERTHOZ. 1982. Horizontal eye position-related activity in neck muscles of the alert cat. Exp. Brain Res. **46:** 448–453.

Behavior of Primate Vestibulo-Ocular Reflex Neurons and Vestibular Neurons during Head-free Gaze Shifts[a]

J. O. PHILLIPS,[b,c] L. LING,[b] C. SIEBOLD,[d]
AND A. F. FUCHS[b]

[b]Department of Physiology and Biophysics
Regional Primate Research Center
University of Washington
Seattle, Washington 98195

[d]Abteilung Neurologie
Universität München
München, Germany

INTRODUCTION

The vestibulo-ocular reflex (VOR) and the vestibulocollic reflex (VCR) serve to stabilize the eye and head, respectively, in space, allowing stable fixation of stationary objects in the face of body movements. However, these reflexes pose a dilemma for the nervous system whenever we try to shift fixation from one point in space to another. Such gaze shifts are accomplished by a combination of eye and head movements. If the VCR were fully compensatory, the head would be unable to turn toward the new fixation point. If the VOR were fully compensatory, the eyes would never reach the intended target if that target were beyond the oculomotor range, because the head movement contribution to the gaze shift would be effectively eliminated by the VOR. Clearly, the VOR and VCR must be modified to allow accurate head-free gaze shifts to occur.

This modification could be explained by the discharge patterns of VOR and VCR interneurons and their target cells. The reflex circuitry underlying the VOR has been studied in head-fixed animals. Position-vestibular-pause cells (PVPs), which discharge with eye position and vestibular yaw stimulation and pause during saccades, receive monosynaptic input from vestibular afferents and provide monosynaptic inputs to abducens motoneurons.[1-6] Therefore, they are one of the interneurons in the shortest VOR pathway. The VOR could be affected at two different stages of this 3-neuron circuit. First, the pause in PVP activity could gate out vestibular reflexes during rapid gaze shifts involving both eye and head movements. Second, the VOR could be eliminated at the abducens motoneurons themselves, which exhibit a pause in discharge for contralateral saccades.

Behavioral evidence, however, suggests that the VOR is not simply turned on or off during the gaze shift. Large gaze (G) movements are accompanied by equally large, and very rapid, head (H) movements (FIG. 1). During the saccadic eye

[a]This work was supported by National Institutes of Health grants EY00745 and RR00166 and by a grant from the Virginia Merrill Bloedel Hearing Research Center.
[c]Address correspondence to James O. Phillips, Ph.D., Regional Primate Research Center, Box 357330, University of Washington, Seattle, WA 98195.

movement portion of the gaze shift (saccadic eye movement, FIG. 1), the eye (E) and head move in the same direction. The VOR must be suppressed at this time. However, during this period, the eye often slows as head velocity increases (FIG. 1, arrows), suggesting that VOR inhibition is not complete. After the eye stops rotating toward the target, it often counterrotates at a gain less than 1, allowing gaze to continue toward the target. This period of reduced VOR gain between the end of the

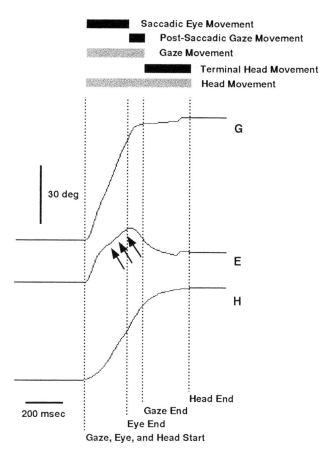

FIGURE 1. A typical primate gaze shift. Abbreviations in this and all other figures: G, gaze, the position of the eye in space; E, position of the eye in the head; H, position of the head in space. Vertical dashed lines denote beginning and end of each movement component. In this and all following figures, a downward trace represents a movement to the left.

eye and gaze movements can be as short as 12 or as long as 150 ms. After gaze has landed, the VOR is fully compensatory, and gaze is stabilized while the head movement continues. Thus, there is a progressive change of VOR gain during head-free gaze shifts.

In this report, we present preliminary evidence of how brain-stem elements known to be involved in the VOR (PVP and abducens cells) and pure vestibular neurons may contribute to the modification of vestibular reflex activity. We compare the behavior of these cells during active head-free gaze shifts with that during head-fixed gaze shifts, pursuit, and passive whole-body rotation to determine whether the head-fixed discharge properties of these cells accurately predict their behavior during head-free gaze shifts.

METHODS

Two juvenile rhesus monkeys were implanted with scleral search coils (for gaze-position recording), a head post positioned over the atlantoaxial joint (for head stabilization), and a chamber (for single-unit recording). The monkeys were then placed in the apparatus pictured in FIGURE 2, and trained to track targets for an applesauce reward. The targets could be either stepped across a two-dimensional display or moved smoothly in front of the animal with the aid of a servomotor. A food delivery tube traveled with the head of the animal, allowing it to track with the head either restrained or free to rotate in the horizontal plane. In the latter condition, head position was monitored with a potentiometer attached to a low-inertia shaft that was secured to the implanted head post. The monkey also could be rotated in the horizontal plane, either in the dark or while he fixated a target that either moved with him or remained stable in the world.

After the animals had learned to track all of the target motions with both the head fixed and free, tungsten microelectrodes were advanced into the brain stem with the use of a hydraulic microdrive. Single-unit action potentials were recorded from cells in the medial and ventrolateral vestibular nuclei, as well as the abducens nucleus. Our search stimulus was head-fixed horizontal sinusoidal whole-body rotation ($\pm 10°$, 0.5 Hz) with an earth-fixed target. Under this condition, neurons with horizontal vestibular and/or eye movement sensitivity were active; true horizontal gaze velocity cells (with equal and opposite head and eye velocity sensitivity) were not.

All isolated cells were tested with head-fixed whole-body rotation in the dark, rotation with a head-fixed target, and rotation with an earth-fixed target. The frequency and amplitude of the rotations were adjusted to simulate active head movements. Neuronal responses during head-fixed horizontal smooth pursuit (0.1–1.4 Hz, $\pm 10°$–$20°$) and during head-fixed saccades and gaze holding at various orbital eccentricities also were collected.

Eye in head, eye in space (gaze), head in space, and target position were recorded along with unit activity on VCR tape with the use of a Vetter 4000A PCM. Data were subsequently played back and digitized at 1 kHz (unit data was processed with a time resolution of 10 μs) into a Macintosh computer for off-line analysis. Analysis of the characteristics of head-fixed and head-free gaze shifts was performed using a program that displayed up to six behavioral (usually position) channels and two target channels, the derivatives of the behavioral channels (usually velocities), and unit activity. Eye, head and gaze start, end, and peak velocity were identified with velocity criteria, and the timing, position, amplitude, and velocity characteristics were compared with the unit discharge patterns. Cell responses to sinusoidal stimuli were analyzed using a separate program which determined the best least-squares sinusoidal fit to the instantaneous discharge rate of the recorded cell, eye position and velocity, and target or chair position and velocity.

Finally, cells were subjected to a trial-by-trial analysis of their discharge characteristics. We used a simple linear model of unit discharge which assumed that discharge rate was equal to the sum of eye and/or head position, velocity, and acceleration components, plus a term for the change in frequency with respect to time.

$$FR = (P_E \times A) + (V_E \times B) + (A_E \times C) + (P_H \times D)$$
$$+ (V_H \times E) + (A_H \times F) + (dFR/dt \times G) + RR \quad (1)$$

where FR is firing rate; P_E, eye position; V_E, eye velocity; A_E, eye acceleration; P_H, head position; V_H, head velocity; A_H, head acceleration; and RR, resting rate.

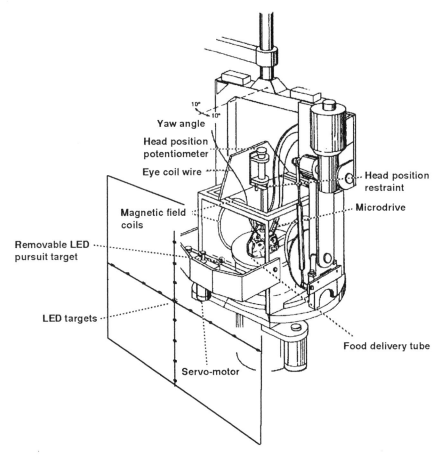

FIGURE 2. A monkey subject in the experimental apparatus. The light-emitting diode (LED) pursuit target assembly was present only when smoothly moving visual stimuli were presented.

A smoothed representation of instantaneous firing rate for each trial was obtained with the use of a Gaussian convolution of each action potential. Eye and head position, velocity and acceleration coefficients (A through F), as well as dFR/dt (G) were then adjusted using a least-squares algorithm so that the sum of the terms fit the smoothed firing rate. The resulting coefficients were then recorded, and another single-trial analysis was performed. The coefficients for each trial type were then averaged, and these were used to predict head-fixed and head-free unit responses. In many conditions, the constants could be derived directly. For example, for stable gaze holding, the eye position coefficient A could be determined from a linear regression of discharge rate versus eye position data.

RESULTS

Twenty-three cells were recorded under a sufficient number of conditions to characterize their responses to head-fixed and head-free eye and head movement. Four were pure, non-pausing vestibular neurons, 10 were horizontal PVPs, and 9 were abducens neurons.

Abducens Neurons

With the head fixed, abducens neurons discharged a burst of spikes for ipsilateral saccades, a pause for contralateral saccades, and a robust rate-position relation for different gaze fixations. During sinusoidal smooth pursuit, these cells discharged slightly in advance of ipsilateral eye position. During the passive VOR elicited by whole-body rotation, abducens cell discharge again led eye position slightly; during suppression of the VOR, firing rate remained constant. In short, their behavior was entirely consistent with their role as extraocular motoneurons or internuclear neurons projecting to medial rectus motoneurons.

Surprisingly, during active head-free gaze shifts, the discharge of abducens cells had a similar burst/pause-tonic character. Indeed, for a single trial such as that shown in FIGURE 3, abducens discharge seemed to reflect gaze velocity and position rather than eye velocity and position. During the saccadic eye movement portion of the gaze shift, the abducens neuron discharged a burst, which often continued into the postsaccadic portion of the gaze shift. At the end of the gaze shift, the discharge fell to a constant tonic rate, which was maintained throughout the head movement. This pattern is startling because the eye is counterrolling in the orbit over large excursions to compensate for the continuing head movement. Because abducens neurons control the velocity and position of the eye in the head, a burst-tonic discharge that appears best related to gaze seems to be inappropriate.

A quantitative analysis, however, shows that the head-free burst/pause-tonic pattern is a simple consequence of the head-fixed eye position and velocity sensitivity of an abducens neuron. FIGURE 4A shows the discharge pattern associated with a single gaze shift in the off direction of the abducens neuron in FIGURE 3. Each spike in the spike train indicates the occurrence of an action potential and its height is the instantaneous firing frequency during the previous interspike interval. The Gaussian-smoothed firing rate (black line) nicely reflects the firing pattern. This actual instantaneous discharge pattern is compared with a predicted firing rate based on the sum of firing rate components related to eye position and eye velocity (FIG. 4B) and eye acceleration (not shown). The coefficients for the eye position, velocity, and acceleration contributions (recall equation 1) are averaged from many trials similar to that in FIGURE 4A. Two separate least-squares fits have been determined, one from movement-associated head-free gaze shifts (shaded line), the other from head-fixed saccades (striped line). Obviously, there is very little difference between the actual smoothed data and discharge patterns based on either the head-free or fixed-head conditions. Therefore, the coefficients of the position, velocity, and acceleration components for head-fixed and head-free behavior are the same for this cell. A similar correspondence was obtained for other abducens neurons.

This modeling explains the unexpected constant discharge in FIGURE 3. In FIGURE 4B, the pause-tonic discharge pattern results because after the gaze shift the velocity of the eye decreases as the position of the eye increases. This velocity versus position trade-off produces a near constant firing rate in both FIGURES 3 and 4.

Pure Vestibular Cell

The firing of pure vestibular cells was modulated during head-free gaze shifts (FIG. 5) and during passive whole-body horizontal rotation, but not during head-

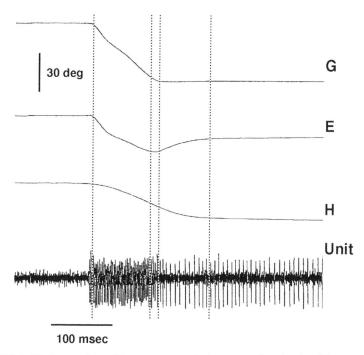

FIGURE 3. Discharge of an abducens neuron during an on-direction head-free gaze shift starting at an eccentric eye position. Vertical lines from left to right indicate gaze start, eye end, gaze end, and head end.

fixed smooth pursuit and saccades. There was no difference in the modulation of such cells when passive rotations occurred in the dark, during VOR suppression, or during tracking of a target that remained stable in the world.

The responses of a pure vestibular cell were different if the head movement was the result of an active head-free gaze shift or due to passive whole-body rotation. First, the cell in FIGURE 5 shows a weak head position sensitivity during active head movements (compare dashed line and arrow). Second, the same cell now shown in

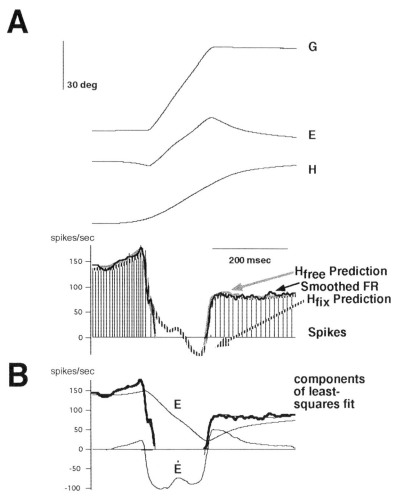

FIGURE 4. Modeling of abducens discharge in response to an off-direction head-free gaze shift. (**A**) Gaze, eye, and head position (*top panel*) are displayed with the associated spike train (*middle panel*) for a single trial. Each spike is indicated by a vertical line whose height indicates the instantaneous firing frequency of the immediately preceding interspike interval. A Gaussian convolution (Smoothed FR) of the discharge is displayed as a black line. Two curves fitted by least-squares criteria are shown. One (*shaded line*) shows the predicted discharge associated with this trial if the firing rate were the result of the sum of firing rates based on linear contributions of eye and head movement components produced with the head free (H_{free} Prediction). The contributions of the head and eye movement components (coefficients in equation 1) reflect the average of many similar trials. The second (*striped line*) predicts a discharge based on average contributions to firing rate determined in head-fixed experiments (H_{fix} Prediction). Two similar curves have been fitted for the data in FIGURES 7 and 10. (**B**) E and Ė show the time courses of the eye position and velocity contributions adjusted to fit the associated smoothed abducens discharge pattern.

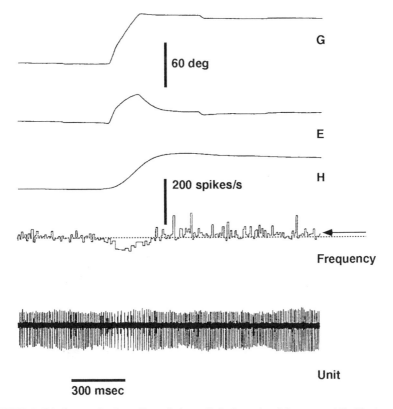

FIGURE 5. Discharge of a "pure" vestibular cell during a head-free gaze shift. Horizontal dashed line indicates the resting firing rate before the gaze shift. Horizontal arrow indicates the resting firing rate after the gaze shift.

FIGURE 6 (illustrated previously in FIG. 5) fires in phase with eye velocity during passive head rotation (FIG. 6, right). For active head rotation, however, the cell's decrease in firing leads head velocity and tends toward head acceleration (FIG. 6, left).

Our quantitative analysis (FIG. 7) confirms this impression. The predicted discharge of the cell, based on the average coefficients obtained for the head velocity and acceleration terms during head-fixed passive whole-body rotation lags the pause in smoothed firing rate. In contrast, the smoothed firing rate *is* nicely matched by a fit predicted on the basis of average velocity and acceleration coefficients obtained during head-free gaze shifts. The modeling reveals that the average head acceleration term is four times greater and the average head velocity term is one-half as great for active than for passive head movements. These data suggest that head acceleration is much more important and head velocity less important in determining the active response. Similar differences also were present in the other three "pure" vestibular neurons.

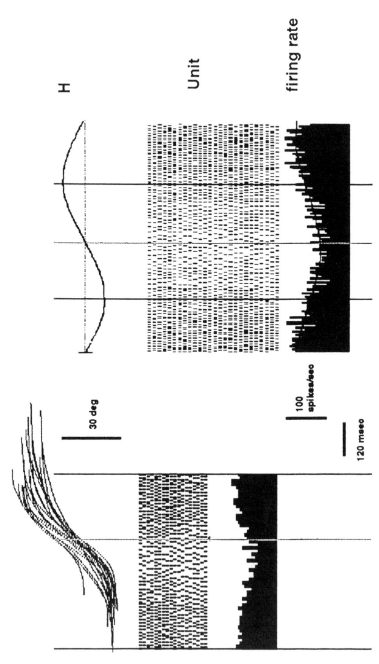

FIGURE 6. Discharge of a "pure" vestibular cell during a series of head-free gaze shifts (*right panel*) and passive whole-body rotations (*left panel*). Rasters of head position and unit discharge, and a spike frequency histogram are aligned on time of peak head velocity (*thin vertical line*).

PVP Cell

PVP cells exhibit a clear pause during many head-fixed and all head-free rapid gaze shifts (FIG. 8). For head-fixed saccades, the pause is often unreliable or directional, and the onset and duration of the pause are not well related to the onset and duration of the saccade. For head-free gaze shifts, however, the onset and

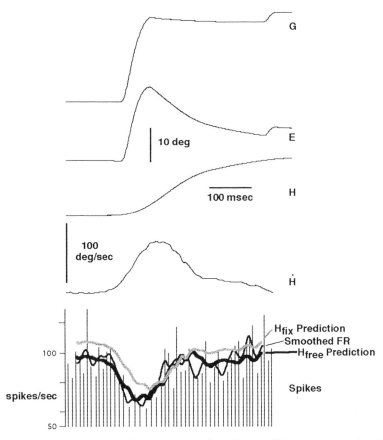

FIGURE 7. Modeling of the discharge of a "pure" vestibular cell in response to a head-free gaze shift. Gaze, eye, and head position are displayed, as is head velocity. Two predicted discharge patterns based on least-squares fits of data obtained with the head fixed (H_{fix} Prediction) and with the head free (H_{free} Prediction) have been generated using the procedures described in the legend of FIGURE 4.

duration of the pause *are* well related to the onset and duration of the gaze shift. The pause starts abruptly just before the onset of the gaze shift (FIG. 9, left panel, thin vertical line), and the peak in the smoothed firing rate is well aligned with the end of the gaze shift (FIG. 9, right panel). However, after the pause, the firing rate recovers gradually between the end of the saccade and the end of the gaze shift, as is nicely shown in FIGURE 10B. This abrupt cessation and then slow recovery in discharge parallel the changes in VOR gain discussed in the INTRODUCTION (FIG. 1).

That the slow recovery reflects a changing VOR gain is demonstrated in FIGURE 10C. Here, if the VOR gain were always 1, a predicted discharge is generated by applying the average coefficients for the head velocity and eye position components obtained during head-fixed movements to the head-free movement trajectories observed in FIGURE 10A. This curve is then compared to the smoothed firing rate of the PVP cell. The predicted firing rate based on head-fixed parameters adequately accounts for actual PVP discharge before and after the gaze shift because the two curves match rather well. However, during the interval between eye and gaze end,

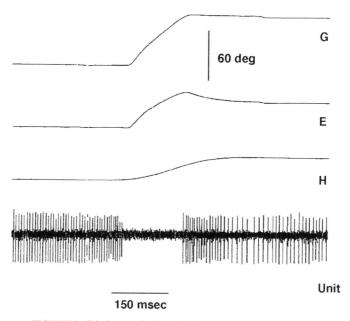

FIGURE 8. Discharge of a PVP cell during a head-free gaze shift.

the firing rate based on a perfect VOR decreases whereas the actual firing rate increases. Therefore, the increasing actual firing rate during this interval can be interpreted as reflecting a VOR gain that gradually increases to 1 at gaze end when the simulated and actual curves intersect.

Taken together, FIGURES 9 and 10 demonstrate that changes in PVP discharge do indeed parallel changes in VOR gain observed with head-free gaze shifts. PVP discharge and VOR gain are both low at the end of the saccadic eye movement and build slowly during the postsaccadic portion of the gaze shift.

DISCUSSION

We present here some preliminary results concerning the behavior of vestibular neurons and abducens neurons during active and passive head movements. As expected, the discharge patterns of abducens neurons were tightly related to

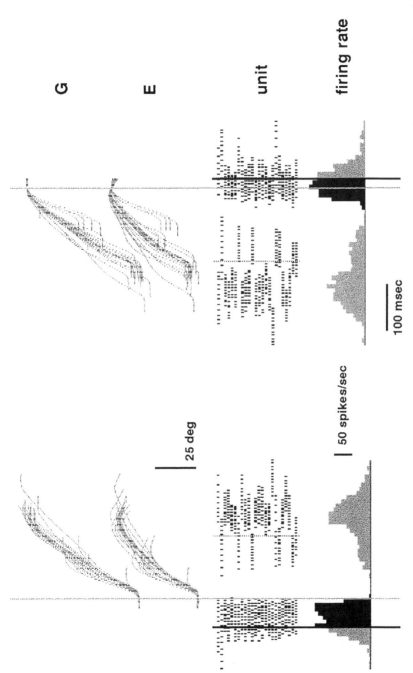

FIGURE 9. Discharge of a PVP cell during a series of head-free gaze shifts aligned on gaze start (*left panel, thin vertical line*) and gaze end (*right panel, thin vertical line*). All traces contribute to the black portions of the histograms.

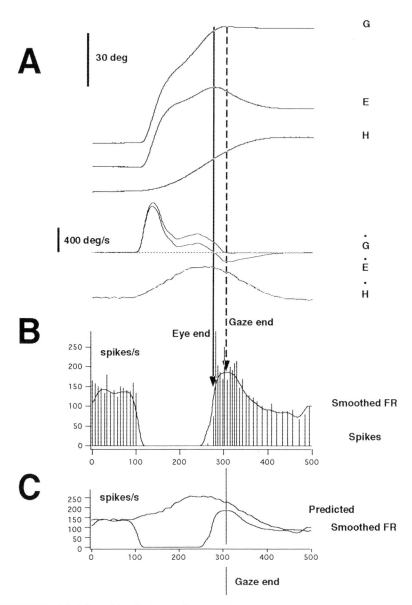

FIGURE 10. Modeling of the discharge of a PVP cell in response to a head-free gaze shift. (**A**) Dotted horizontal line indicates zero gaze or eye velocity. (**B**) Smoothed FR increases throughout the postsaccadic gaze shift, from eye end (*solid vertical arrow*) to gaze end (*dashed vertical arrow*). (**C**) A predicted discharge pattern based on least-squares fits of data obtained with the head fixed (Predicted) is compared with the smoothed firing rate (Smoothed FR). Traces were generated using the procedures described in the legend of FIGURE 4.

movement of the eyes in the head whether the head was free or fixed. However, the behavior of some neurons in the vestibular nuclei was different when the head was free or fixed.

Abducens Neurons

During head-free gaze shifts, abducens neurons unexpectedly displayed a burst-tonic discharge pattern. The firing rate appeared better correlated with rapid gaze movement than eye movement, which was undergoing the VOR (FIG. 3). Although a burst/pause-tonic discharge pattern was unexpected during head-free gaze shifts, it was entirely predicted by the head-fixed discharge properties of the cell. In particular, the steady discharge during VOR eye movements was the result of simultaneous opposite changes in eye velocity and eye position sensitivity. Therefore, and fortunately for the oculomotor system, the discharge of its motoneurons always is tightly linked to the eye movements in the orbit which they command.

The burst/pause-tonic pattern seems to be an important feature of a gaze shift whether it is made with or without head movement. Eye velocity must result reflexively from head velocity, so the eye counterrotation and head movement are matched in some way to the velocity and position sensitivities of the abducens cells. This is a feature of VOR function during head-free gaze shifts that deserves further study.

Pure Vestibular Neurons

"Pure" vestibular or vestibular-only neurons,[7] identified by their response during whole-body rotation, behave differently during active and passive head movements. Although this type of cell has not been found to project directly to the abducens nucleus in monkey,[8] it could participate in indirect VOR or VCR pathways.

The depth of modulation of the pure vestibular cell during head-free gaze shifts is different than that predicted on the basis of head-fixed gaze shifts. In FIGURE 7, the head-free prediction indicates that the difference is due to an increased (by fourfold) contribution of head acceleration and a decreased (by one-half) contribution of head velocity. The decrease in the head velocity signal carried by the pure vestibular neuron indicates that its sensitivity to vestibular stimuli, that is, head velocity, has decreased. If this cell were to participate in the indirect VOR or the VCR, its contribution would be to cause a decrease in their gains. However, there is a clear increased contribution related to head acceleration when the head is free, so in that situation, the gain of the head acceleration influence on eye movement is increased as reflected in the increased modulation seen in FIGURE 7.

The reason for the difference in the behavior of pure vestibular neurons during active and passive head rotations is unclear. Their response during passive head rotations clearly indicates that they receive a vestibular input. The discharge shown in FIGURE 5 (arrow) suggests that they may receive a weak head position input as well. During active head movements, an efference copy of the intended head movement and final head position might sum with the vestibular signal.[9] If this were the case, however, one might expect that the cells would change their resting discharge rate during head-fixed saccades, but this is not what we observe. Alternatively, pure vestibular cells might receive a neck input. Again, we might expect that if head movements were being commanded during head-fixed gaze shifts, and the monkey were generating neck muscle contractions, we might see some change in firing from the resting rates during head-free saccades; there were none. However, because we did not test these cells during head-fixed trunk rotation, we cannot be certain that a neck afferent signal was absent. Although such a test would reveal the presence of a neck input, it is likely that the neck afferent signals observed during head-fixed trunk rotation would not be the same as those present during active head rotation. In one case, the ipsilateral muscles would be generating force and shortening actively, whereas in the other case they would be shortening passively, and contralateral muscles might be undergoing lengthening contractions. Since these two situations are so dramatically different, it is unlikely that an addition of observed passively elicited neck afferent responses would help our simple model predict the actual head-free gaze related response.

PVP Neurons

Finally, we have observed that the pause and subsequent discharge of the PVP cell accurately reflects the modulation of the vestibulo-ocular reflex during head-free gaze shifts. A trial-by-trial comparison of the PVP cell discharge during head-free gaze shifts and head-fixed eye movement and passive rotations suggests that the PVP cell resumes discharging before the end of the saccadic eye movement portion of the gaze shift, continues to build its discharge during the postsaccadic gaze shift, and only displays a discharge that parallels that predicted for a passive, full gain VOR, after gaze end. This sequence matches the VOR gains predicted by behavioral observations, and is quite different from the rapid return of discharge seen following the pause of abducens cells.

It is unknown, however, what mechanism underlies these changes. Is it an intrinsic property of the PVP cell itself that its discharge recovers slowly after the pause accompanying the gaze shift? Or is PVP discharge modulated to control gaze amplitude by reducing VOR gain until gaze is directed accurately at its final position? These questions remain unanswered by our study, but they point to interesting new directions for research concerning vestibular function during natural head-free gaze movements.

REFERENCES

1. King, W. M., S. G. Lisberger, & A. F. Fuchs. 1976. Responses of fibers in medial longitudinal fasciculus (MLF) of alert monkeys during horizontal and vertical conjugate eye movements evoked by vestibular or visual stimuli. J. Neurophysiol. **39:** 1135–1149.
2. Pola, J. & D. A. Robinson. 1978. Oculomotor signals in the medial longitudinal fasciculus of the monkey. J. Neurophysiol. **41:** 245–259.
3. Ishizuka, N., H. Mannen, S. Sasaki & H. Shimazu. 1980. Axonal branches and terminations in the cat abducens nucleus of secondary vestibular neurons in the horizontal canal system. Neurosci. Lett. **16:** 143–148.
4. McCrea, R. A., A. Strassman, E. May & S. M. Highstein. 1987. Anatomical and physiological characteristics of vestibular neurons mediating the horizontal vestibulo-ocular reflex in the squirrel monkey. J. Comp. Neurol. **264:** 547–570.
5. McCrea, R. A., K. Yoshida, A. Berthoz & R. Baker. 1980. Eye movement related activity and morphology of second order vestibular neurons terminating in the cat abducens nucleus. Exp. Brain. Res. **40:** 468–473.
6. Ohgaki, T., I. S. Curthoys & C. H. Markham. Morphology of physiologically identified second-order vestibular neurons in cat, with intracellularly injected HRP. J. Comp. Neurol. **276:** 387–411.

7. FUCHS, A. F. & J. KIMM. 1975. Unit activity in the vestibular nucleus of the alert monkey during horizontal angular acceleration and eye movement. J. Neurophysiol. **38:** 1140–1161.
8. SCUDDER, C. A. & A. F. FUCHS. 1992. Physiological and behavioral identification of vestibular nucleus neurons mediating the horizontal vestibulo-ocular reflex in trained rhesus monkeys. J. Neurophysiol. **68:** 244–264.
9. PHILLIPS, J. O., L. LING, A. F. FUCHS, C. SEIBOLD & J. J. PLORDE. 1995. Rapid horizontal gaze movement in the monkey. J. Neurophysiol. **73(4):** 1632–1652.

Behavior Contingent Processing of Vestibular Sensory Signals in the Vestibular Nuclei[a]

ROBERT A. McCREA, CHIJU CHEN-HUANG,
TIMOTHY BELTON, AND GREG T. GDOWSKI

Committee on Neurobiology
Department of Pharmacological and Physiological Sciences
University of Chicago
Chicago, Illinois 60637

INTRODUCTION

The ostensible purpose of the vestibular sensory system is to inform the brain about the position and movement of the head. However, this sensory system is somewhat unusual in that sensory-motor integration occurs at the first stage of the central processing of vestibular signals. Many of the central, secondary vestibular neurons that receive direct inputs from the vestibular nerve also project directly to motoneurons and/or play an important role in a variety of motor behaviors. For example, lateral vestibulospinal tract neurons not only carry signals related to head movements, but are also phasically modulated during locomotion.[1] The secondary vestibular neurons that project to the extraocular motor nuclei carry signals related not only to ongoing head movements, but also signals related to eye position or smooth pursuit eye velocity, even in the absence of head movements.[2,3] In many instances the same central neuron serves as both a secondary sensory neuron and a constituent of an important premotor pathway. Thus, it is perhaps not surprising that many, if not most, of the neurons in the vestibular nuclei exhibit a complex combination of sensory and motor signals.[4]

In this paper we briefly describe the results of several types of experiments in which single-unit recordings were obtained from squirrel monkey central secondary vestibular neurons in different behavioral contexts. The results of these experiments show that the magnitude, and even the direction of the head movement sensory signals carried by central neurons varies under different behavioral circumstances. We conclude that the vestibular sensory signals generated by central vestibular neurons are not simply combined with other sensory and motor signals, but are *contingent* on the behavioral context in which they are generated.

METHODS

Single-unit recordings were obtained from alert squirrel monkeys trained to fixate or pursue small visual targets. During experiments, the monkey was seated on a vestibular turntable and the position of one or both eyes and the position of the head were monitored with the magnetic search coil technique. Experiments were per-

[a]This work was supported by grants EY08041 and DC02072.

formed using two different setups which allowed different types of vestibular stimulation and different types of behavioral paradigms to be used while recording from single units in the vestibular nuclei.

In one experimental setup, recordings were obtained from secondary vestibular neurons while the monkey's head was fixed to a vestibular turntable with a bolt that had been chronically implanted on the back of its head. The responses of the neurons were recorded while the monkey fixated targets that were either stationary in space or stationary with respect to the head. In other experiments using this setup, the position of the axis of turntable rotation in respect to the monkey's interaural plane was varied by positioning the monkey at different distances from the axis of rotation on a railroad mounted on top of the turntable. This configuration allowed different combinations of linear and angular head acceleration to be tested. The responses of the neurons were recorded while the monkey fixated targets that were either near (10 cm) or far (170 cm) from its head.

In the second experimental setup, the monkey's head was not fixed to the turntable, but was free to move in a yaw axis ($\pm 40°$) defined by a delrin rod positioned at roughly the C1-C2 axis. A universal joint placed in line with the delrin rod allowed a small degree of freedom in the roll and pitch planes ($\approx 10°$). Monkeys were trained to fixate or pursue a small laser spot projected onto a tangent screen 90 cm away. Generally, a combination of eye and head movements were used to pursue or fixate targets. Single-unit recordings were obtained from neurons in the vestibular nuclei.

In all experiments, secondary vestibular neurons were identified by recording the latency of synaptically evoked spikes following electrical stimulation of the ipsilateral vestibular nerve. In some experiments anodal currents were applied bilaterally to both vestibular nerves using the protocols developed by Minor and Goldberg[5] in order to functionally ablate irregular vestibular afferents. In other experiments, neurons that had axons projecting into the ascending tract of Dieters (ATD) were antidromically identified. This was done by stimulating ATD axons with a concentric bipolar stimulating electrode that was chronically implanted adjacent to the ATD at a level approximately 1 mm caudal to the ipsilateral trochlear nucleus. Many horizontal canal-related secondary VOR neurons have axons that project rostrally, but most non-ATD neurons have axons that travel in the contralateral medial longitudinal fasciculus (MLF). Secondary vestibular neurons, located ipsilateral to the stimulating electrode, which were antidromically activated and which received horizontal semicircular canal inputs, were considered to be ATD neurons whose axons terminate in the ipsilateral medial rectus subdivision of the oculomotor nucleus.[6]

RESULTS AND DISCUSSION

Changes in Signals Generated by Secondary Vestibulo-Ocular Neurons during Voluntary Cancellation of the Vestibulo-Ocular Reflex

One obvious behavioral context in which it would be advantageous to change the signal processing of central pathways related to the vestibulo-ocular reflex (VOR) is when a visual object of interest and the head are both moving together. This probably occurs most often in natural circumstances when the object being fixated is linked to the substrate on which the body is standing (e.g., a swaying tree limb or subway car). It has been known for some time that some of the cells in the vestibular nuclei, particularly those whose firing behavior is related to eye movements, show dramatic changes in their responses to vestibular stimuli when the VOR is suppressed or canceled during fixation of a head stationary target, and that many of the cells exhibiting these changes are constituents of the most direct VOR pathways.[2,3,7-9] FIGURE 1 shows the typical changes in firing behavior exhibited by two major types of VOR-related vestibular neurons when the VOR is suppressed or canceled.

The cell whose responses are illustrated in FIGURE 1A was a position-vestibular-pause (PVP) cell. PVP cells are generally considered to be important contributors to

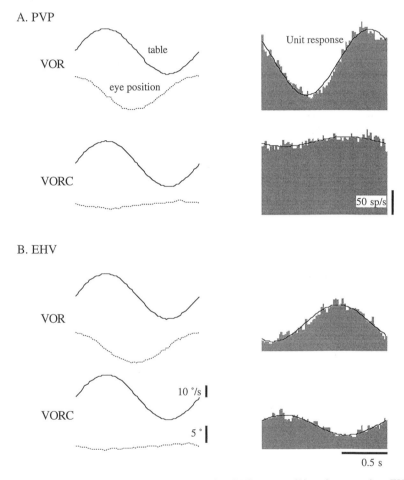

FIGURE 1. Change in the response of a secondary PVP neuron (A) and a secondary EHV neuron (B) during vestibulo-ocular reflex (VOR) cancellation. Both cells were antidromically activated following electrical stimulation of the ipsilateral ascending tract of Deiters. The top traces in both A and B show the averaged turntable velocity, eye position, and unit firing rate records obtained during VOR evoked by turntable rotation (0.7 Hz, ± 20°/s peak velocity) while a squirrel monkey fixated an earth-stationary target. Quick phases of nystagmus were not included in the averages. The bottom traces show similar records obtained while the monkey canceled the VOR by fixating a head-stationary target. The thick lines superimposed on the firing rate averages are sinusoidal fits to the modulation in firing rate.

central VOR pathways. Horizontal canal-related PVP neurons have been shown to project to the contralateral abducens nucleus and to provide excitatory inputs to abducens motoneurons.[6,10] The firing rate of most secondary horizontal PVP cells is related to ipsilateral head velocity during passive head rotation. PVPs also receive inputs related to eye movements; in particular, they pause during ocular saccades and receive inputs that are related to eye position and smooth pursuit eye velocity. The PVP cell whose firing behavior is illustrated in FIGURE 1A was activated at a short, monosynaptic latency (≤ 1.3 ms) following electrical stimulation of the vestibular nerve. This particular PVP was also antidromically activated following electrical stimulation of the ipsilateral ATD. The gain of the response generated by the PVP neuron to passive rotation was nearly four times larger when the monkey fixated an earth-stationary target than when it canceled its VOR by fixating a target that was stationary with respect to the head (FIG. 1A, top and bottom, respectively).

A second class of secondary vestibular neurons that project to the extraocular motor nuclei are even more sensitive to eye movements during smooth pursuit than PVP cells. These cells also have firing behavior that is ostensibly related to head movements during VOR cancellation and thus have been referred to as eye/head vestibular (EHV) neurons.[10,11] The vestibular signals generated by this class of secondary vestibular neurons depend on the behavioral context. The EHV cell illustrated in FIGURE 1B received monosynapic inputs from the left vestibular nerve and was antidromically activated following electrical stimulation of the ATD, which suggests that it is part of the direct premotor vestibular pathway to medial rectus motoneurons. When the monkey fixated an earth-stationary target, the cell's firing rate increased during leftward turntable rotations, as would be expected if it received inputs from the left horizontal semicircular canal. However, the preferred direction of the cell reversed when the monkey voluntarily canceled its VOR by fixating a target that was stationary with respect to the head.

The firing behavior of PVP and EHV neurons illustrated above has been frequently described. Although additional evidence would be welcome, the data available so far suggests that PVP and EHV neurons are constituents of the pathways that directly link the vestibular nerve to the extraocular motor nuclei and are probably essential components of the neural networks related to the execution and control of the VOR.[7–9,12] Some of the changes in sensitivity to vestibular stimuli observed during voluntary suppression of the VOR could be attributed to the visual or eye movement motor inputs these cells receive, although these inputs alone are probably not sufficient to explain the changes in firing behavior that occur when the VOR is canceled.[8] Regardless of the mechanisms used, it is clear that the signals generated by these sensory secondary vestibular neurons are dramatically affected by the behavioral context in which they are generated.

Single-Unit Recordings from Secondary Vestibular Neurons in Head-free Squirrel Monkeys

We recently developed techniques for obtaining stable, long-term single-unit recordings from brain stem and cerebellar neurons in squirrel monkeys that were free to move their head in the horizontal plane. One of the most striking observations in this preparation is that most of the cells in the vestibular nuclei and the cerebellar flocculus exhibit different responses to head movements that are generated actively in comparison to those generated passively.

The cell illustrated in FIGURE 2 was a "pure" vestibular neuron whose firing rate was not related to eye movements. In particular, it did not pause or burst during

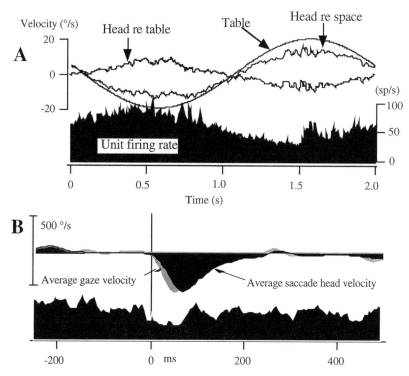

FIGURE 2. Recording from pure vestibular neuron in a head-free monkey. (**A**) Averaged head velocity responses and unit firing rate during turntable rotation. (**B**) Averaged responses during large on direction head saccades.

saccades. It is shown here because it dramatically illustrates the vast majority of the 70 vestibular neurons we have studied to date—that is, *the firing rate of most secondary vestibular neurons is not related to the velocity of active head movements.* The sensitivity of the cell to *passive* head rotation is shown in FIGURE 2A. Note that the passive rotation evokes a weak, compensatory vestibulocollic reflex (head re table trace) that slightly reduces the vestibular input to the cell (head velocity re space trace ≈ 66% of table velocity). Determined in this manner, the sensitivity of the cell to head velocity in space was 1.86 spikes/s/°/s.

The averaged records shown in FIGURE 2B were obtained during spontaneous leftward (sensory "on" direction) gaze saccades selected for a predominant contribution of head velocity to the active gaze shift. In contrast to what might be expected, the cell did not increase its firing rate, but rather was weakly inhibited during head saccades even though the average peak head velocity in space during these saccades was greater than 200°/s, and the average head acceleration was greater than 1000°/s². This was particularly obvious in this cell because it was a pure vestibular neuron—that is, it did not fire in relation to eye movements. It is important to note that although the cell was insensitive to *active* head movements, it continued to encode *passive* head movements, even during gaze saccades, although its sensitivity was reduced by nearly 75% (not shown).

Similar, although not identical, observations from other classes of secondary vestibular neurons have been made. For example, some vestibulospinal neurons respond similarly to the cell illustrated in FIGURE 2, whereas others are more inhibited during gaze saccades.[13] Most pure vestibular neurons are either weakly inhibited during on direction head saccades and head pursuit, or are unresponsive to the active component of head movements.

We are still in the process of analyzing the responses of secondary vestibular neurons that are putatively involved in the VOR. A detailed comparative analysis of the head movement-related signals generated by a PVP neuron during active and passive head movements is shown in FIGURE 3. The illustrated cell was a horizontal semicircular canal-related secondary PVP neuron in the left vestibular nucleus. It was activated at a latency of 0.8 ms following electrical stimulation of the vestibular nerve with currents of 150 μA.

FIGURE 3A shows the averaged, desaccaded response (0.99 spikes/s/°/s head velocity) of the cell during passive head rotation when the head was restrained and the monkey fixated an earth-stationary visual target (VOR). Similar to the PVP cell illustrated in FIGURE 1A, the vestibular response was reduced in amplitude to 0.22 spikes/s/°/s, during VOR cancellation (FIG. 3B). During active gaze pursuit of a target moving sinusoidally at the same frequency (0.5 Hz), the cell's sensitivity to head velocity was low (0.26 spikes/s/°/s) and in phase with *rightward* eye and head velocity, as opposed to the leftward head velocity response observed in the VOR and the VOR cancellation behavioral paradigms. The solid lines superimposed on the averaged unit responses in FIGURE 3A–C are best sinusoidal fits to the cell's firing rate corrected for its eye and neck position sensitivity (regressions plotted in FIG. 3F).

The difference in the direction and amplitude of the vestibular responses recorded during active and passive head movements was not likely due to neck afferent inputs. FIGURE 3D shows the response of the cell when the head and neck were passively twisted by forcing the head to rotate back and forth manually. FIGURE 3E shows the response of the cell when the head was held stable in space and the neck was twisted by sinusoidally rotating the body. The cell's response during forced passive head rotation and during passive neck twisting was accurately predicted by a simple model that took into account the cell's passive head velocity sensitivity, eye position, neck position, and spontaneous firing rate (solid lines superimposed on unit responses in FIG. 3D and E). Although the weak neck position sensitivity of PVP neurons has been observed in every cell of this type analyzed so far, the neck sensory signal was never strong in comparison to the vestibular sensitivity, and was always synergistic with the vestibular input. These observations, together with results such as those illustrated in FIGURE 3D and E, suggest that it is unlikely that neck afferent inputs are responsible for the difference in vestibular responses recorded during active and passive head movements observed in PVP cells. We suspect that a centrally generated head movement efference copy signal is responsible for regulating the vestibular sensitivity of PVP neurons during active head movements.

FIGURE 3G shows the firing behavior of the same PVP cell during large leftward gaze saccades containing large head movement components in the on direction of the cell. Illustrated from top to bottom are the head and gaze position records of 12 selected saccades, average head and gaze velocity, the spike rasters associated with each saccade, and the averaged response of the unit. Superimposed on the vestibular response is the same model shown in FIGURE 3D and E. Note that the firing rate of the cell invariably paused during these saccades, even though the average head velocity exceeded 100°/s.

In short, the vestibular signal generated by PVPs clearly depends on whether the

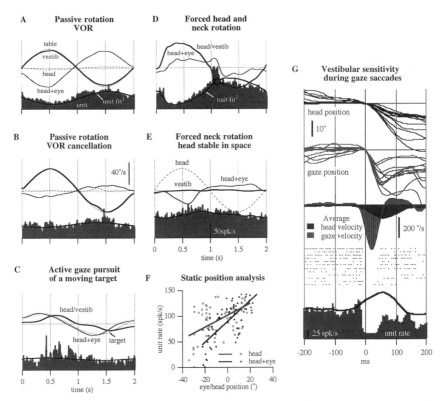

FIGURE 3. Firing behavior of a PVP unit during passive and active head movements. (A–E) Contain averaged unit rate, horizontal eye, head, table (or target), and vestibular velocity (positive values are rightward movements). Each plot is aligned on rightward head velocity. Sinusoidal fits to the unit response and the position corrected response (for eye and head sensitivity; solid, unit fit[1]) are shown in A–C. (A and B) Passive body rotation (0.5 Hz, 40°/s) during VOR and VORc, respectively. Note that the unit had a higher leftward vestibular sensitivity during VOR in comparison to VORc (0.99, 0.22, respectively). (C) Active gaze pursuit towards a sinusoidally moving target (0.5 Hz, 20°/s). Notice that the unit's response and its vestibular component (0.26) are reversed in comparison to its response during passive body rotation (A and B). (D) The response during forced passive head rotation while the body was held stationary. A model based on static eye and head position and vestibular sensitivity during VOR is shown superimposed (D, E, and G; solid, unit fit[2]) on the unit response (unit = 85 + 2.0*(head + eye) − 0.99*vestib). (E) The response during neck twisting where the body was passively rotated while the head was held stationary. (F) Plot of the unit rate during stationary epochs of spontaneous eye movements. Data for head and horizontal gaze position are shown. The best fit lines for head and horizontal gaze are shown superimposed (K_{head} = 1.2, $K_{head+eye}$ = 2.0). (G) Responses during 12 spontaneous leftward gaze saccades aligned on the initial change in gaze position. Shown are the gaze and head position for each saccade and the average gaze and head velocity. The spike raster shows the temporal response during each saccade. The average unit response is shown at the bottom with the model shown in D (superimposed).

vestibular stimulus is imposed *upon* the monkey (passive head movement) or whether the stimulus is self-generated *by* the monkey (active head movement). The vestibular sensory signal is *present* during passive head rotation, *absent* during self-generated head saccades, *reduced* during passive head movements when the VOR is voluntarily suppressed, and *reversed* in direction during active head pursuit movements. On the other hand, it is clear that the PVP premotor pathway is utilized not only for generating vestibular evoked eye movements but also for generating smooth eye movements during visual pursuit, optokinetic nystagmus, and fixation. Thus far, our data suggest that the pathway may also receive the afferent inputs underlying the cervico-ocular reflex, should the behavioral circumstance arise.

It is too early to speculate precisely how these observations fit into more general descriptive models of head and eye movement control. However, it is clear that future models of the signal processing underlying coordinated eye and head movements will require behaviorally contingent components that reflect the contingent responses of secondary VOR neurons.

Changes in the Response of Secondary Vestibulo-Ocular Neurons to Angular and Linear Head Movements as a Function of Viewing Distance

Another example of behavior-contingent processing of sensory signals by secondary vestibulo-ocular neurons is the changes in firing behavior that occur as a function of viewing distance. The eye movements required to stabilize a visual image on both foveae during angular rotation or linear translation of the head vary considerably as a function of viewing distance.[14] The gain of the VOR evoked by angular rotation of the head (AVOR) increases in squirrel monkeys as in inverse function of visual target distance. The gain of eye movements evoked by linear acceleration of the head (LVOR) is typically quite small when targets of interest are at a distance, but the gain of the LVOR increases considerably as viewing distance decreases.[15,16]

The records shown in FIGURE 4 were obtained from a secondary EHV neuron that was antidromically activated following electrical stimulation of the ATD. The figure illustrates the averaged, desaccaded eye movements and neuronal responses to sinusoidal rotation of the turntable when the monkey fixated as earth-stationary target that was 170 cm from its eyes (far target) and when it fixated a target that was only 10 cm away (near target). In FIGURE 4A, the monkey's head was centered on the axis of turntable rotation, and a small, but significant, increase occurred in both the gain of the AVOR (23%) and the gain of the unit's response (11%) when the monkey fixated the near target.

The changes in gain as a function of viewing distance were more pronounced when the axis of rotation was shifted off-center, so that a linear acceleration was added to the angular acceleration produced by turntable rotation. Both the gain and the direction of the eye movement evoked varied as a function of target distance and the axis of rotation. In FIGURE 4B, the monkey was seated 20 cm in front of the axis of rotation (Nose-out condition), producing an LVOR in the same direction as the AVOR. The gain of the evoked eye movement response increased nearly threefold during fixation of a target 10 cm away from the head. In FIGURE 4C the axis of rotation was 20 cm in front of the monkey, producing an LVOR that was opposite to the AVOR, and an eye movement that reversed in direction during near-target viewing. The traces at the bottom of FIGURE 4B and C show the calculated response of the cell to sinusoidal linear translation during fixation of near and far targets. The ATD/EHV neuron was nearly insensitive to linear translation of the head when the

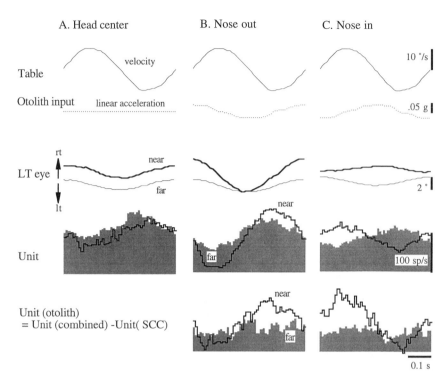

FIGURE 4. Viewing distance-dependent changes in the sensitivity of a secondary ascending tract of Dieter/eye head vestibular (ATD/EHV) neuron to semicircular canal and otolith inputs. (A–C) Averaged eye position and unit firing rate records obtained during fixation of near (10 cm) and far (170 cm) earth-stationary targets while the monkey was passively rotated by the turntable (1.9 Hz, ± 10°/s peak velocity). The filled response histograms correspond to the averaged firing rates recorded during fixation of the far target, whereas the superimposed thick lines are the averaged responses of the cell during fixation of a near target. In **A,** the monkey's head was centered on the axis of turntable rotation, and the eye movements and unit responses evoked by angular acceleration alone were recorded while the monkey fixated near and far targets. In **B** and **C,** the monkey's head was positioned 20 cm in front of (Nose out) or behind (Nose in) the axis of rotation. In **B,** the linear and angular acceleration were in the same direction, whereas in **C,** linear and angular acceleration were in opposite directions. Note that when the monkey fixated the near target, the gain of both the eye movement and the ATD/EHV unit's responses changed dramatically. The calculated responses of the unit to linear force alone (otolith input) during fixation of near and far targets are shown in the bottom traces of **B** and **C.**

target of interest was distant. But when the target was near, the change in the response of the cell was even larger than the change in the eye movement evoked by the stimulus.

It is unlikely that the changes in the gain of the AVOR and LVOR responses of secondary vestibular neurons were due to inputs related to visual following or smooth pursuit of the target. The data illustrated in FIGURE 4 were obtained during 1.9 Hz turntable rotations. Similar results were obtained when lower (0.7 Hz) and higher (4.0 Hz) rotations were used in the same cell. The fidelity of the response at

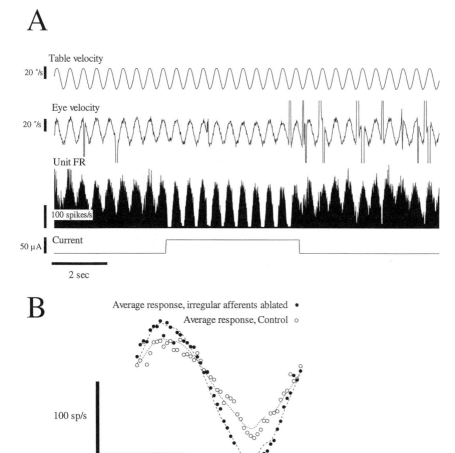

FIGURE 5. (A) Sample records from a secondary pure vestibular unit before, during, and after applying anodal currents bilaterally to the labyrinth. Anodal polarizing currents were applied during the 5-s period indicated by the current trace. In this example, the spontaneous firing rate decreased, and the response gain to turntable rotation increased when ablating currents were applied. **(B)** Averaged records of response of the unit illustrated in **A** to turntable rotation during bilateral anodal polarization of the vestibular nerves (●) and absence of polarizing currents (○).

1.9 and 4 Hz suggests that the behavior-contingent signal processing does not depend on visual following mechanisms, because visual following does not operate efficiently at these higher frequencies.[16] Apparently, the head movement signal generated by secondary vestibular neurons is parametrically adjusted to fit the kinematic requirements of the oculomotor system, presumably because they participate in the vestibulo-ocular neural network that generates compensatory eye movements whose speed and direction are dependent on behavioral context.

Functional Ablation of Vestibular Afferents Reveals Complex Processing
of Sensory Afferent Signals in the Vestibular Nuclei

The parametric adjustment of the head movement signals generated by secondary vestibular neurons would appear, at first glance, to be at odds with the anatomical fact that these cells receive direct, monosynaptic inputs from the vestibular nerve, whose vestibular signals are presumably not dependent on behavioral context. However, there are numerous ways the sensory signals generated could be modified as the behavioral context changes. The vestibular nerve is not the sole source of vestibular inputs to secondary vestibular neurons. Vestibular neurons receive inputs bilaterally from other central vestibular neurons, from the vestibulocerebellum and fastigial nucleus,[17,18] and from a variety of other areas of the brain that contain cells whose firing behavior is related to head movements (e.g., the reticular formation, the cervical spinal cord, etc.[17,19]). Consequently, it is reasonable to assume that a given secondary vestibular neuron has many synaptic inputs whose activity is related to head movements, which could be derived from several anatomical sources in addition to the vestibular nerve.

A demonstration of the apparent lack of simplicity in the anatomical organization of vestibular inputs to secondary vestibular neurons is shown in the experiment illustrated in FIGURE 5. The head movement responses of the pure vestibular cell shown in this figure were recorded in the presence and absence of 50 μA anodal currents applied bilaterally to the vestibular nerves. The effect of anodal currents applied in this manner is to silence nearly all of the irregular afferent fibers in the vestibular nerve without changing the head movement-related modulation in the firing rate of regular vestibular afferents.[5] As expected, the tonic firing rate of the cell decreased when a large fraction of the vestibular nerve was silenced (FIG. 5A). However, an unexpected finding was that ablation of irregular afferents produced an *increase* in the passive head movement sensitivity of not only this cell (FIG. 5B), but of about one-half of the cells we recorded from. A similar fraction of the cells showed a decrease in their rotational sensitivity. One obvious conclusion is that the direct contribution of vestibular nerve inputs to the head movement sensitivity of secondary vestibular neurons is small in comparison to the influence of other, polysynaptic sources of vestibular inputs. The added complexity probably exists to allow the processing of sensory signals in the vestibular nuclei to be contingent on behavioral circumstances.

CONCLUSION

In the past the comfortable assumption has often been made that the sensory signals generated within the vestibular nuclei are related primarily to signals generated by afferents in the vestibular nerves. Other sensory and motor signals that were detected were presumed to be added onto this basic sensory signal. Instead, it appears that the sensory signals generated by most central vestibular neurons are profoundly affected by the behavioral context in which they are generated.

It will apparently be necessary in the future to pay more attention to the behavioral and attentional context in which vestibular sensory signals are generated if one is to realistically assess how they are being processed centrally. For example, it is not clear what can be learned by recording eye movements or neural activity related to the vestibulo-ocular reflex under circumstances in which the reflex has no function; e.g., in the dark. It also seems unwise to rely on observations about the vestibulocollic reflex, gaze control or eye-head coordination that were made when the head was restrained from moving.

The good news is that the evidence so far indicates that signal processing in the vestibular system is not so complex that it cannot be understood if observations are made under circumstances that resemble the natural environment in which the system was designed to operate.

REFERENCES

1. ORLOVSKY, G. N. 1972. Activity of vestibulospinal neurons during locomotion. Brain Res. **46:** 85–98.
2. TOMLINSON, R. D. & D. A. ROBINSON. 1984. Signals in vestibular nucleus mediating vertical eye movements in the monkey. J. Neurophysiol. **51:** 1121–1136.
3. POLA, J. & D. A. ROBINSON. 1978. Oculomotor signals in medial longitudinal fasciculus of the monkey. J. Neurophysiol. **41:** 245–259.
4. LISBERGER, S. G. & F. A. MILES. 1980. Role of primate medial vestibular nucleus in long-term adaptive plasticity of vestibuloocular reflex. J. Neurophysiol. **43:** 1725–1745.
5. MINOR, L. B. & J. M. GOLDBERG. 1991. Vestibular-nerve inputs to the vestibulo-ocular reflex: A function-ablation study in the squirrel monkey. J. Neurosci. **11:** 1636–1648.
6. McCREA, R. A., A. STRASSMAN, E. MAY & S. M. HIGHSTEIN. 1987. Anatomical and physiological characteristics of vestibular neurons mediating the horizontal vestibulo-ocular reflex of the squirrel monkey. J. Comp. Neurol. **264:** 547–570.
7. KING, W. M., S. G. LISBERGER & A. F. FUCHS. 1976. Responses of fibers in MLF of alert monkeys to horizontal and vertical conjugate eye movements evoked by vestibular or visual stimuli. J. Neurophysiol. **39:** 1135–1149.
8. CULLEN, K. E. & R. A. McCREA. 1993. Firing behavior of brainstem neurons during voluntary cancellation of the horizontal vestibuloocular reflex. I. Secondary vestibular neurons. J. Neurophysiol. **70:** 828–843.
9. CULLEN, K. E., C. J. CHEN-HUANG & R. A. McCREA. 1993. Firing behavior of brainstem neurons during voluntary cancellation of the horizontal vestibuloocular reflex. II. Eye movement related neurons. J. Neurophysiol. **70:** 844–856.
10. SCUDDER, C. A. & A. F. FUCHS. 1992. Physiological and behavioral identification of vestibular nucleus neurons mediating the horizontal vestibuloocular reflex in trained rhesus monkeys. J. Neurophysiol. **68(1):** 244–264.
11. McFARLAND, J. L. & A. F. FUCHS. 1992. Discharge patterns in nucleus prepositus hypoglossi and adjacent medial vestibular nucleus during horizontal eye movement in behaving macaques. J. Neurophysiol. **68:** 319–332.
12. BROUSSARD, D. M. & S. G. LISBERGER. 1992. Vestibular inputs to brain stem neurons that participate in motor learning in the primate vestibuloocular reflex. J. Neurophysiol. **68(5):** 1906–1909.
13. BOYLE, R., T. BELTON & R. A. McCREA. 1996. Responses of identified vestibulospinal neurons to voluntary eye and head movements in the squirrel monkey. Ann. N. Y. Acad. Sci. This volume.
14. VIIRRE, E., D. TWEED, K. MILNER & T. VILIS. 1986. A reexamination of the gain of the vestibuloocular reflex. J. Neurophysiol. **56:** 439–450.
15. SARGENT, E. W. & G. D. PAIGE. 1991. The primate vestibulo-ocular reflex during combined linear and angular head motion. Exp. Brain Res. **87:** 75–84.
16. SNYDER, L. H. & W. M. KING. 1992. Effect of viewing distance and location of the axis of head rotation on the monkey's vestibuloocular reflex. I. Eye movement responses. J. Neurophysiol. **67:** 861–874.
17. BUTTNER-ENNEVER, J. A. 1992. Patterns of connectivity in the vestibular nuclei. Ann. N. Y. Acad. Sci. **656:** 363–378.
18. STEIN, J. & M. GLICKSTEIN. 1992. The role of the cerebellum in visual guidance of movement. Physiol. Rev. **72(4):** 967–1017.
19. FULLER, J. 1992. Neck receptors in the vestibular nuclei. *In* The Head-Neck Sensorimotor System. A. Berthoz, V. Graf & P. Vidal, Eds.: 279. Oxford University Press. New York.

Vestibular Signals in the Fastigial Nucleus of the Alert Monkey[a]

U. BÜTTNER,[b] CH. SIEBOLD, AND L. GLONTI

Department of Neurology
Ludwig Maximilians University
Munich, Germany

INTRODUCTION

The fastigial nucleus (FN), the most medial deep cerebellar nucleus, receives its Purkinje cell (PC) input from the overlying vermis. Projections are topographically organized in a way that the anterior vermis (lobules 2–5) projects to rostral FN and the posterior vermis (lobules 6–9) to caudal FN.[1] Also the nodulus (lobule 10) has been reported to project to the ventral region of FN.[2] The anterior and posterior vermis are divided by the primary fissure between lobules 5 and 6. This dividing fissure also marks some differences in connectivity. Whereas the anterior vermis is considered as part of the spinocerebellum, lobules 6 and 7 of the posterior vermis belong to the pontocerebellum. Consequently, considerable functional differences exist between the anterior vermis and lobules 6 and 7 of the posterior vermis. From anatomical[3] and electrophysiological studies[4] it is known that the anterior vermis receives a considerable vestibular input. However, only little information is available about possible vestibular sensitivities in the PCs of the anterior vermis. It is considered to be mainly involved in spinal mechanisms (gait, posture, neck), and lesions here have no effect on eye movements.[5] By contrast, all studies point to a major role of the posterior vermis (lobules 6 and 7) in eye movement control,[6] which actually led to the label "oculomotor vermis" for this structure.[7] Activity of certain neurons in the oculomotor vermis is related to saccades[8,9] and to smooth pursuit eye movements. More detailed studies including vestibular stimulation revealed that the latter neurons actually encode gaze velocity[10,11] because they are not only modulated during smooth pursuit eye movements (SPEM), but also during visual suppression of the vestibulo-ocular reflex (VOR-supp).

The functional differences of the vermis are also reflected in FN activity. Neurons in rostral FN of the monkey are modulated during vestibular stimulation but show no activity changes in relation to individual eye movements.[12,13] These "vestibular only" neurons also respond during constant velocity optokinetic stimulation.[13] However, this response probably only reflects the presence of the "velocity storage" mechanism[14] and not an involvement in eye movement generation because this response is also found in virtually all vestibular nuclei neurons including those not involved in eye movement control.[15] By contrast, neurons in caudal FN are modulated with eye movements and hence this region has been labeled fastigial oculomotor region (FOR).[16] As in the oculomotor vermis, neurons are basically saccade-[17–19] or SPEM-related.[13,20,21] According to their response pattern during combined smooth pursuit

[a]This work was supported by the Deutsche Forschungsgemeinschaft.
[b]Address correspondence to Prof. Dr. U. Büttner, Neurologische Klinik, Klinikum Grosshadern, Marchioninistr. 15, D 81377 München, Germany. E-mail: ubuettner@brain.nefo.med.uni-muenchen.de

and vestibular stimulation, the SPEM neurons can be divided into two groups. One group behaves similarly to "gaze velocity" neurons. They show no or only little modulation during the VOR, but an equal modulation during SPEM and VOR-supp. The other group of neurons has been labeled "VOR + SPEM" neurons. They are modulated during VOR-supp and SPEM, often in opposing directions, and, in contrast to the gaze velocity neurons, show their deepest modulation during the VOR.[13,20] Thus, there is ample evidence of vestibular information processing in the FN.

The findings considered thus far all refer to vestibular stimulation in the yaw plane. However, under natural conditions movements are executed in three-dimensional space, and vestibular signals have to be processed accordingly. Only very few studies have dealt with these questions. Gardner and Fuchs[12] investigated some "vestibular only" neurons during yaw and pitch stimulation. They found that a large percentage of neurons responding to yaw stimulation also responded with an increase in activity to either nose-up or nose-down pitch rotation. Neurons showed little change in activity in response to static changes in the nose-up or nose-down position, reflecting that the neurons did not receive a convergent input from otolithic organs. The aim of the present study was to further investigate the interaction of vestibular signals in the FN. It will concentrate on the effect of roll and pitch stimulation on "vestibular only" neurons in rostral FN.

METHODS

Monkeys (*Macaca mulatta*) were chronically prepared for single-unit recordings (for details see Boyle *et al.*[22]). Three-dimensional eye movements were recorded with a dual-search coil system[23] and neuronal activity with varnished tungsten microelectrodes. The FN was approached perpendicularly. During the experiment the monkey sat with its head fixed and erect in a primate chair on a vestibular turntable. Vestibular stimulation in the roll, pitch, and yaw plane consisted of sinusoidal movements (0.6 Hz, ±30–60°/s) around earth-fixed axes. In addition, intermediate positions between full roll and full pitch were investigated at 15° steps. This covered the entire range (i.e., 360°) and included the left anterior–right posterior (LARP) and right anterior–left posterior (RALP) vertical canal orientations. Torsional directions were defined according to the right-hand rule, that is, positive torsion indicating right ear down (RED). For convenience, pitch orientation was labeled 0°, orientations to the left with increasing positive values up to +90° (roll) and to the right with increasing negative values up to −90° (roll). Analysis was performed off-line. All data (neuronal activity, eye position, and stimulus signals) were stored on an FM tape recorder (Teac XR 310). Signals were digitized off-line for computer analysis with real-time occurrence of neuronal activity (spikes) and a sampling rate of 200 Hz for the remaining channels. For a given stimulus condition, neuronal activity was averaged for 7–12 cycles. Averaged neuronal responses were fitted by a least-square best sine wave, thereby determining sensitivity (imp · s^{-1}/deg · s^{-1}) and phase in relation to head velocity.

RESULTS

General Characteristics

All neurons were spontaneously active. Spontaneous activity was on average 49.8 imp/s (range, 21 to 71 imp/s) and quite irregular (interspike interval), which is in agreement with earlier studies.[12,13] It was not altered when the monkey became drowsy as judged by the eye movement recordings. The activity of the "vestibular only" neurons did not show any relation to eye movements, including smooth pursuit eye movements. In addition, it was not altered during visual suppression of the VOR (VOR-supp). Constant velocity optokinetic stimuli were not applied. No attempt was made to correlate occasional changes of activity to any body movements.

Neuronal responses were the same when vestibular stimuli were applied in the light or in complete darkness. Vestibular responses were also not altered during drowsiness. About 10–20% of neurons in rostral FN responded to vertical canal stimulation. Vestibular neurons were often grouped and in some instances up to 8–10 responsive neurons could be encountered within 2 mm.

Response Amplitude

During sinusoidal rotation at different orientations, all neurons had a preferred orientation with maximal modulation (FIG. 1A) and minimal modulation, which was usually no modulation at all (FIG. 1B). Maximal and minimal modulation occurred at orientations 90° apart (FIGS. 1 and 2). None of the neurons exhibited more than one minimum or maximum. Responses during individual cycles of stimulation were quite regular with certain fluctuations for the vast majority of neurons (FIG. 1A). Intense "waxing and waning" with the disappearance of the neuronal modulation for several cycles, as has been described for smooth pursuit related PCs in the oculomotor vermis,[10] was not encountered. With larger stimulus amplitudes and orientations close to the maximal response, most neurons (about 75%) could be silenced (cut off) during part of the cycle (FIG. 1A). With the stimulus parameters applied, the modulation was fairly sinusoidal for most neurons (FIGS. 1A and 2). Only a few neurons exhibited a clear distortion with a faster falling than rising time (skew) of neuronal activity.

For all neurons modulation (sensitivity) was a function of orientation, which could be best fitted by a sine wave (FIGS. 3 and 4). This is a consequence of the response properties of vertical canal afferents and has also been observed for vestibular nuclei neurons.[24]

Phase

The vast majority of neurons responded in phase with stimulus velocity, usually with some lead of neuronal activity, but occasionally also with some lag of 10–20° (FIG. 3). Phase relation remained constant at different orientations with a shift of 180° around the orientation with minimal or no modulation (FIGS. 3 and 4). This is also a pattern predicted from vestibular afferent behavior and found in the vestibular nuclei.[24]

Orientations

From a functional point of view there are three main orientations: pitch, roll, and 45°, the latter reflecting the vertical canal plane orientations (LARP and RALP). Since nose-down pitch or nose-up pitch rotation can lead to an activation, and the same applies for roll and canal plane orientations, eight responses are possible if related to the FN on one side: pitch down, pitch up, ipsilateral roll, contralateral roll, ipsilateral anterior canal (AC), contralateral AC, ipsilateral posterior canal (PC), and contralateral PC. Neurons were attributed to one of these eight groups. For each group neurons with an optimal orientation up to ±15° deviation were included. FIGURES 2 and 3 show an example of a vertical canal oriented neuron recorded in the right FN. It had the best modulation at −45° (right) orientation, and maximal activity

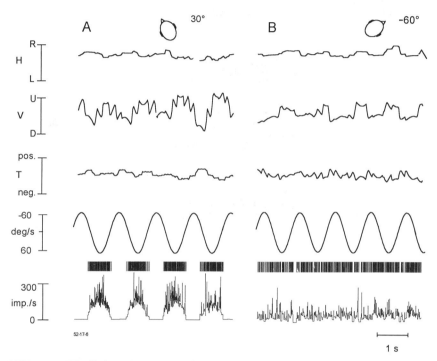

FIGURE 1. "Vestibular only" neuron in the right fastigial nucleus of the alert monkey during sinusoidal (0.6 Hz, ±60°/s) vertical stimulation of the head around an earth-fixed axis at two different orientations. In **A** the monkey's head is oriented 30° to the left from the straight ahead (pitch) orientation and in **B** 60° to the right. Traces from above: H, horizontal; V, vertical; and T, torsional eye position, head position, and instantaneous frequency. The raw data (artificial impulses) are shown above frequency. **A** shows the maximal and **B** the minimal modulation of this neuron. Orientation of **A** and **B** is 90° apart. Neuronal activity is in phase with stimulus velocity. Thus, this neuron has its best modulation during downward movements with the head oriented 30° contralaterally to the recording side and was accordingly classified as an ipsilateral anterior canal neuron. Note that vertical compensatory eye movements occur in **A**, whereas in **B**, with an orientation closer to roll, torsional compensatory eye movements are more prominent.

occurred with upward head velocity. From this it was classified as a ipsilateral posterior canal related neuron. A neuron classified as a pitch nose-down activated neuron is shown in FIGURE 4 with the maximal sensitivity at +15° (to the left) orientation. It was recorded on the right side.

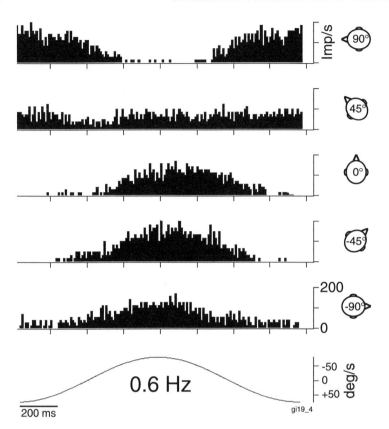

FIGURE 2. Averaged (8–12 cycles each) neuronal responses of a right fastigial nucleus neuron at different orientations during sinusoidal vertical stimulation (0.6 Hz, ±60°/s). Orientations are indicated on the right. Maximal modulation is at 45° right (−) and minimal modulation at 45° left (+). Activity is in phase with head velocity. Note the phase shift of 180° between roll left (+90°) and roll right (−90°). This neuron has its best modulation during upward movements with the head oriented 45° ipsilaterally to the recording side (ipsilateral posterior canal related neuron).

Neurons belonging to all eight groups are found in FN. More than 60% of the neurons had their optimal orientation at or close to vertical canal orientations. The remaining neurons were classified as roll or pitch neurons, the latter type being rare.

This implies that for many neurons maximal sensitivity can be related to vertical canal orientation. However, particularly the roll and pitch neurons show that vertical canal convergence is present in FN neurons. It should also be pointed out that for many vertical canal related neurons the optimal orientation was not in the 45° orientation plane but off by 15° into the pitch or roll direction.

DISCUSSION

The results clearly show that precise vestibular signals related to vertical canal stimulation are available in the fastigial nucleus. Modulation at different orientations shows a clear maximum and minimum that are 90° apart and neuronal activity is in phase with head velocity. All these features are also encountered for vertical canal related neurons in the vestibular nuclei.[24] Many neurons in FN have their optimal response along vertical canal orientations (45°). However, other neurons have their response optimum in the roll or pitch plane, which has to be the result of vertical canal convergence. There is ample evidence that such convergence is already present in the vestibular nuclei.[24] Unfortunately, little is known about the response characteristics of PCs in the anterior vermis during vertical canal stimulation because these neurons provide a major input to FN neurons. FN neurons probably also receive a direct input from the vestibular nuclei by collaterals of mossy fiber projections to the cerebellar cortex. Thus, at present it cannot be determined which inputs are the main source of activity for the vestibular-only neurons in FN. The results also show that all major orientations that can result from single vertical canal activation or vertical canal convergence are present in FN neurons. In many instances optimal responses

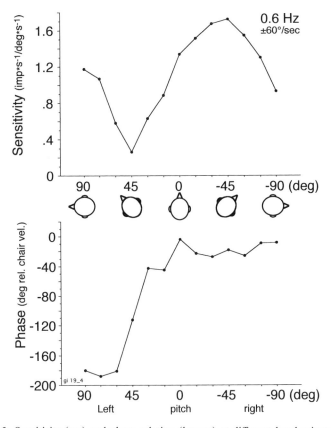

FIGURE 3. Sensitivity (*top*) and phase relation (*bottom*) at different head orientations (abscissa) during vertical rotations. Same neuron as in FIGURE 2. Sensitivity declines monotonically between maximal (−45°) and minimal (+45°) value. Data can be best fitted by a sine wave function. Phase remains constant and close to stimulus velocity except for a 180° phase shift around minimal sensitivity (+45°).

were obtained 15° off a vertical canal plane. This raises the interesting question as to whether optimal responses are grouped around the main orientations or whether FN neurons equally cover the whole spectrum of all possible orientations. Larger samples of neurons are required in order to answer this question.

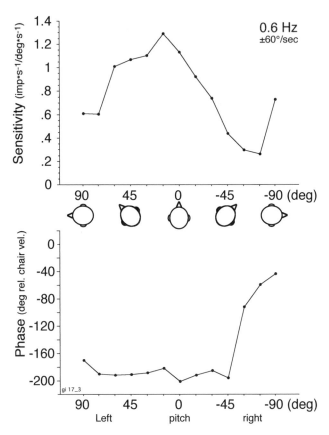

FIGURE 4. Fastigial nucleus neuron recorded on the right side with maximal modulation at +15° (*left*) and minimal modulation at −75° (*right*). All parameters as in FIGURE 3. Although slightly off the straight ahead orientation (pitch), this neuron was classified as a pitch neuron with an activity increase during nose-down movements.

Functional Considerations

Virtually all studies support the notion that FN neurons have a directional preference and that this preference is related to behavioral aspects, that is, saccade-related neurons in caudal FN have a contralateral preference in regard to burst onset.[18,19] Accordingly, lesions to caudal FN lead to contralateral saccadic hypometria and ipsilateral saccadic hypermetria.[25] Similarly, 86% of smooth pursuit related neurons in caudal FN had an activity increase during contralateral VOR-supp stimulation (type II response).[13] Lesions to caudal FN lead to an impairment of contralateral VOR-supp and the smooth pursuit related (direct) component of optokinetic nystagmus (OKN).[26] Recently, Fuchs *et al.*[21] described that 72% of smooth pursuit related neurons in caudal FN had a preferred direction contralateral and/or downward. This preference for contralateral directions is also obvious for vestibular-only neurons in rostral FN during yaw stimulation. More than 75%[12] or 87%,[13] respectively, are type II neurons. In accordance with this, lesion studies report a falling tendency of monkeys to the ipsilateral side after unilateral FN lesions.[26,27] Thus it appears that after a unilateral FN lesion, all movements to the contralateral side are too small (hypometric) and too large (hypermetric) toward the ipsilateral side. From single-unit studies it has been suggested that FN neurons provide a signal that is used to improve contralateral acceleration and ipsilateral deceleration of movements.[21] Whether this also applies for the vestibular-only neurons in rostral FN has yet to be shown.

Our results show that neurons with different orientations during vertical canal related stimulation can be encountered. Larger samples will be needed to demonstrate any preferences for specific orientations. The results clearly show that vertical canal related activity is present in the FN. They also demonstrate the presence of vertical canal interaction. However, many other and more complex possibilities of vestibular signal processing remain open and are certainly not excluded by the present data. Interactions with horizontal canal responses have to be investigated in more detail. This also applies for responses to static tilt, which have been described in the cat.[28] Ample evidence also exists for more complex spatiotemporal convergence in vestibular nuclei neurons.[29,30] It will be the aim of further studies to demonstrate or rule out such interactions for fastigial neurons.

ACKNOWLEDGMENTS

The authors wish to thank S. Langer, B. Pfreundner, M. Seiche, and I. Wendl for their assistance.

REFERENCES

1. ARMSTRONG, D. M. & R. F. SCHILD. 1978. An investigation of the cerebellar cortico-nuclear projections in the rat using an autoradiographic tracing method. I. Projections from the vermis. Brain Res. **141:** 1–19.
2. WYLIE, D. R., C. I. DE ZEEUW, P. L. DIGIORGI & J. I. SIMPSON. 1994. Projections of individual Purkinje cells of identified zones in the ventral nodulus to the vestibular and cerebellar nuclei in the rabbit. J. Comp. Neurol. **349:** 448–463.
3. KOTCHABHAKDI, N. & F. WALLBERG. 1978. Cerebellar afferent projections from the vestibular nuclei in the cat: An experimental study with the method of retrograde axonal transport of horseradish peroxidase. Exp. Brain Res. **31:** 591–604.
4. PRECHT, W., R. VOLKIND & R. H. I. BLANKS. 1977. Functional organization of the vestibular input to the anterior and posterior cerebellar vermis of cat. Exp. Brain Res. **27:** 143–160.
5. MAGNUSSON, M. & L. G. STRÖMBLAD. 1989. Voluntary and vestibular eye movements in a case of lesion restricted to the anterior vermis cerebelli. Clin. Vision Sci. **4:** 71–78.
6. BÜTTNER, U. & A. STRAUBE. 1995. The effect of cerebellar midline lesions on eye movements. Neuroophthalmology **15:** 75–82.
7. YAMADA, J. & H. NODA. 1987. Afferent and efferent connections of the oculomotor cerebellar vermis in the macaque monkey. J. Comp. Neurol. **265:** 224–241.
8. KASE, M., D. C. MILLER & H. NODA. 1980. Discharges of Purkinje cells and mossy fibres in

the cerebellar vermis of the monkey during saccadic eye movements and fixation. J. Physiol. (Lond.) **300:** 539–555.

9. HELMCHEN, CH. & U. BÜTTNER. 1995. Saccade-related Purkinje cell activity in the oculomotor vermis during spontaneous eye movements in light and darkness. Exp. Brain Res. **103:** 198–208.

10. SUZUKI, D. A. & E. L. KELLER. 1988a. The role of the posterior vermis of monkey cerebellum in smooth pursuit eye movement control. I. Eye and head movement-related activity. J. Neurophysiol. **59:** 1–18.

11. SUZUKI, D. A. & E. L. KELLER. 1988b. The role of the posterior vermis of monkey cerebellum in smooth pursuit eye movement control. II. Target velocity-related Purkinje cell activity. J. Neurophysiol. **59:** 19–40.

12. GARDNER, E. P. & A. F. FUCHS. 1975. Single-unit responses to natural vestibular stimuli and eye movements in deep cerebellar nuclei of the alert rhesus monkey. J. Neurophysiol. **38:** 627–649.

13. BÜTTNER, U., A. F. FUCHS, G. MARKERT-SCHWAB & P. BUCKMASTER. 1991. Fastigial nucleus activity in the alert monkey during slow eye and head movements. J. Neurophysiol. **65:** 1360–1371.

14. COHEN, B., V. MATSUO & T. RAPHAN. 1977. Quantitative analysis of the velocity characteristics of optokinetic nystagmus and optokinetic after-nystagmus. J. Physiol. **270:** 321–344.

15. WAESPE, W. & V. HENN. 1987. Gaze stabilization in the primate. The interaction of the vestibulo-ocular reflex, optokinetic nystagmus, and smooth pursuit. Rev. Physiol. Biochem. Pharmacol. **106:** 37–125.

16. NODA, H., S. SUGITA & Y. IKEDA. 1990. Afferent and efferent connections of the oculomotor region of the fastigial nucleus in the macaque monkey. J. Comp. Neurol. **302:** 330–348.

17. OHTSUKA, K. & H. NODA. 1991. Saccadic burst neurons in the oculomotor region of the fastigial nucleus of Macaque monkeys. J. Neurophysiol. **65:** 1422–1434.

18. FUCHS, A. F., F. R. ROBINSON & A. STRAUBE. 1993. Role of the caudal fastigial nucleus in saccade generation. I. Neuronal discharge patterns. J. Neurophysiol. **70:** 1723–1740.

19. HELMCHEN, CH., A. STRAUBE & U. BÜTTNER. 1994. Saccade-related activity in the fastigial oculomotor region of the macaque monkey during spontaneous eye movements in light and darkness. Exp. Brain Res. **98:** 474–482.

20. BÜTTNER, U. & A. F. FUCHS. 1992. Eye- and head-movement-related activity in the fastigial nucleus of the alert monkey. *In:* Vestibular and Brainstem Control of Eye, Head and Body Movements. H. Shimazu & Y. Shinoda, Eds.: 351–361. Japan Scientific Societies Press. Tokyo.

21. FUCHS, A. F., F. R. ROBINSON & A. STRAUBE. 1994. Participation of the caudal fastigial nucleus in smooth-pursuit eye movements. I. Neuronal activity. J. Neurophysiol. **72:** 2714–2728.

22. BOYLE, R., U. BÜTTNER & G. MARKERT. 1985. Vestibular nuclei activity and eye movements in the alert monkey during sinusoidal optokinetic stimulation. Exp. Brain Res. **57:** 362–369.

23. BARTL, K., CH. SIEBOLD, ST. GLASAUER, CH. HELMCHEN & U. BÜTTNER. 1996. A simplified calibration method for 3-D eye movement recordings using search-coils. Vision Res. **36:** 997–1006.

24. BAKER, J., J. GOLDBERG, G. HERMANN & B. PETERSON. 1984b. Optimal response planes and canal convergence in secondary neurons in vestibular nuclei of alert cats. Brain Res. **294:** 133–137.

25. ROBINSON, F. R., A. STRAUBE & A. F. FUCHS. 1993. Role of the caudal fastigial nucleus in saccade generation. II. Effects of muscimol inactivation. J. Neurophysiol. **70:** 1741–1758.

26. KURZAN, R., A. STRAUBE & U. BÜTTNER. 1993. The effect of Muscimol microinjections into the fastigial nucleus on the optokinetic response and the vestibulo-ocular reflex in the alert monkey. Exp. Brain Res. **94:** 252–260.

27. THACH, W. T., J. W. MINK & S. A. KANE. 1988. Fastigial, interposed, and dentate nuclei: Somatotopic organization and the movements differentially controlled by each. *In*

Neurobiology of the Cerebellar Systems: A Centenary of Ramon y Cajal's Description of the Cerebellar Circuits.: 34. Barcelona.

28. GHELARDUCCI, B. 1973. Responses of the cerebellar fastigial neurons to tilt. Pflügers Arch. **344:** 195–206.

29. BAKER, J., J. GOLDBERG, G. HERMANN & B. PETERSON. 1984a. Spatial and temporal response properties of secondary neurons that receive convergent input in vestibular nuclei of alert cats. Brain Res. **294:** 138–143.

30. ANGELAKI, D. E., G. A. BUSH & A. A. PERACHIO. 1992. A model for the characterization of the spatial properties in vestibular neurons. Biol. Cybern. **66:** 231–240.

Inverse-Dynamics Representation of Eye Movements by Cerebellar Purkinje Cell Activity during Short-Latency Ocular-Following Responses

KENJI KAWANO,[a,b] MUNETAKA SHIDARA,[a]
AYA TAKEMURA,[a] YUKA INOUE,[a] HIROAKI GOMI,[c]
AND MITSUO KAWATO[d]

[a]Neuroscience Section
Electrotechnical Laboratory
Ibaraki 305, Japan

[c]NTT Basic Research Laboratories
Kanagawa 243-01, Japan

[d]ATR Human Information Processing Research Laboratory
Kyoto 619-02, Japan

Movements of a visual scene evoke short-latency ocular-following responses.[1] In our laboratory, we have focused on understanding the neural mediation of ocular following.[2-6] Evidence from single-unit recordings and focal chemical lesions has suggested that early ocular following is mediated by a pathway that includes the medial superior temporal (MST) area of the cortex, the dorsolateral pontine nucleus (DLPN), and the ventral parafloccular (VPFL) lobes of the cerebellum. To understand how this pathway influences eye movement, a reliable method must be used to characterize the transformation from visual information to information concerning eye movements.[7] In this report, we describe the results of reconstructing the temporal firing patterns of Purkinje cells (P-cells) in the VPFL, based on the inverse-dynamics representation of eye movements.

SHORT-LATENCY OCULAR-FOLLOWING RESPONSES

To elicit ocular-following responses, we used behavioral paradigms and visual stimuli similar to those of Miles et al.[1] Briefly, monkeys faced a translucent tangent screen of white paper on which a moving random-dot pattern was back-projected. This screen subtended 85° along the vertical and horizontal meridians. The visual stimulus was a ramp movement of the pattern, and each ramp started 50 ms (in some cases, 100–300 ms) after the end of a saccadic eye movement directed to the central part of the screen (±10°). This arrangement allowed us to collect data that were generally free of saccades for at least 150 ms following the onset of the stimulus. The stimulus lasted 150 ms, then a mechanical shutter closed, and the screen was blank for 0.5–2 s while the animal remained in the dark. The shutter then reopened with

[b]Address correspondence to Dr. Kenji Kawano, Neuroscience Section, Electrotechnical Laboratory, 1-1-4, Umezono, Tsukubashi, Ibaraki 305, Japan.

the pattern in its initial position, ready for the next ramp. Ramps were presented at five speeds (10, 20, 40, 80, 160°/s) and in eight directions (right, left, up, down, and four diagonals). To keep the monkeys alert, they were given an occasional drop of fruit juice to produce fast saccades.

FIGURE 1 shows the eye movement profiles recorded from a monkey in response to downward ramp movements of 40°/s. Fifty-three milliseconds after the onset of the stimulus motion, the eye started to move. The very short response latency is a common characteristic of the ocular-following response,[1] and indicates that neural elements eliciting the response are limited in number, permitting characterization of responses at each neural element.

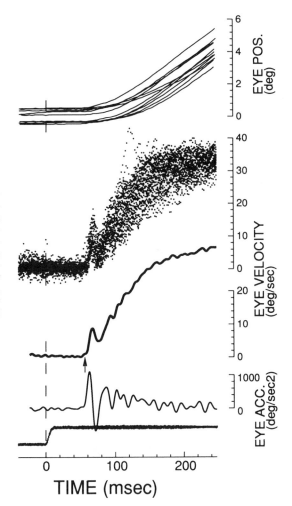

FIGURE 1. Sample ocular-following responses to multiple presentations ($n = 40$) of a 40°/s downward test ramp. Recordings, from top to bottom, indicate superimposed eye position profiles, superimposed eye velocity profiles, average eye velocity profile, eye acceleration profile, and average stimulus velocity profile. Arrow shows estimated time of response onset.

RESPONSE PROPERTIES OF P-CELLS DURING OCULAR FOLLOWING

FIGURE 2A shows a sample of responses of simple spike activity of a P-cell in the VPFL and the ocular-following responses to 160°/s downward test ramps.[3] The responses are aligned at stimulus onset. Fifty-two milliseconds after the onset of the stimulus motion, the firing rate of this neuron was increased. The eyes began moving several milliseconds after the onset of the neural responses. The directional selectivity of the P-cell was analyzed for eight directions (right, left, up, down, and four diagonals). This P-cell showed the strongest responses to the downward movements of the random-dot pattern (FIG. 2B). The neural responses to the moving visual scene at different speeds (10, 20, 40, 80, 160°/s) were studied using the downward

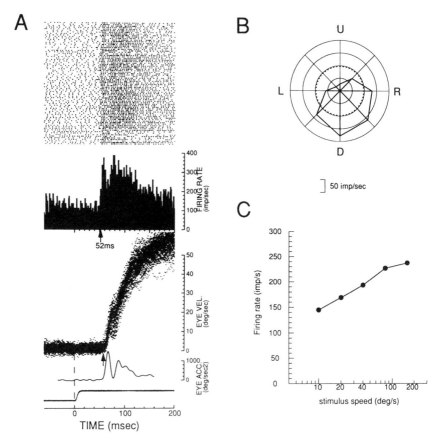

FIGURE 2. (**A**) The simple spike activity of a Purkinje cell (P-cell) in the ventral parafloccular lobe and the ocular-following responses to multiple presentations of a 160°/s downward test ramp. The responses are aligned at stimulus onset. From top to bottom, impulse rasters, peristimulus histogram, superimposed vertical eye velocity, eye acceleration, and stimulus velocity. Arrows indicate latencies. (**B**) Directional selectivity of this P-cell shown in a polar diagram. The dashed line denotes spontaneous activity level. D, down; L, left; R, right; U, up. (**C**) Speed tuning of this P-cell.

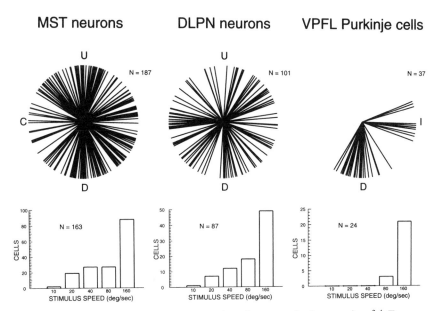

FIGURE 3. Comparison of response properties of neurons in three regions.[2-4] **Top row:** Estimated preferred directions of the neurons. **Bottom row:** Distribution of the preferred speeds of the neurons (stimulus speeds used were 10, 20, 40, 80, and 160°/s). C, contralateral; D, down; I, ipsilateral; U, up; MST, medial superior temporal; DLPN, dorsolateral pontine nucleus; VPFL, ventral parafloccular lobes.

ramps. When the stimulus speed increased, the firing frequency of the P-cell also increased (FIG. 2C).

Of 37 P-cells, characterized for directional preference during ocular following in eight directions, 11 cells responded most vigorously to the movement of the visual scene ipsilateral to the recording sides (horizontal P-cell), and 26 cells to the downward movements (vertical P-cell).[3] The directional preferences of P-cells and neurons in the MST[4] and DLPN[2] are shown in FIGURE 3 (top row). Unlike P-cells in the VPFL, no significant differences were observed regarding a preference for ipsilateral or contralateral (or for up versus down) in the MST and DLPN neurons. The optimum speeds for 24 P-cells were studied[3] (FIG. 3, bottom row), and all showed their best responses at high-stimulus speeds (especially 160°/s). Most of the MST and DLPN neurons also showed their best responses at high-stimulus speeds similar to the P-cells, but some neurons responded optimally to lower-stimulus speeds in the MST and DLPN (FIG. 3, bottom row). These results indicate a similarity between the response properties of the neurons in the MST and DLPN and, conversely, a difference between those of the neurons in the two regions and those of the P-cells in the VPFL. The latency distribution of 150 MST neurons,[4] 77 DLPN neurons,[2] and 24 VPFL P-cells[3] shown in FIGURE 4 corresponds to the stream of the information—that is, from the MST neurons to the DLPN neurons, and from the DLPN neurons to the VPFL P-cells. The difference in response latencies of neurons in the three regions, together with the differences in response properties in the neurons, suggests that MST neurons provide visual information to the VPFL via DLPN neurons, and in the VPFL the visual information is transformed into the information that determines ocular response.

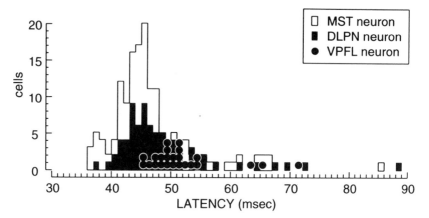

FIGURE 4. Comparison of neuronal latencies in the medial superior temporal (MST), the dorsolateral pontine nucleus (DLPN), and the Purkinje cell (P-cells) in the ventral parafloccular lobes (VPFL).[2-4] The number of neurons is plotted against the latency from the visual stimulus onset.

INVERSE-DYNAMICS REPRESENTATION
OF EYE MOVEMENTS BY P-CELLS

To characterize the response properties of the P-cells in the VPFL, we reconstructed their temporal firing patterns based on the inverse-dynamics representation of the simultaneously recorded eye movements.[7] We analyzed the temporal modulation of a P-cell response using a linear time-series multiple-regression method (FIG. 5).[7] The equation used for the analysis is as follows:

$$f(t - \Delta) = a \cdot e''(t) + b \cdot e'(t) + c \cdot e(t) + d \qquad (1)$$

where $f(t)$, $e''(t)$, $e'(t)$, $e(t)$, and Δ are the firing frequency at time t, the eye acceleration, velocity, and position at time t, and the time delay, respectively. Four coefficients (a, b, c, d) and the time delay (Δ) were estimated in such a way as to minimize the estimation error. The continuous line in the bottom tracing in FIGURE 5 shows a result of the model fitting by equation (1). A performance index "coefficient of determination" was calculated to evaluate the reliability of the model by the following equation[8]:

$$CD = 1 - \sum_t (\hat{f}(t) - f(t))^2 / \sum_t (f(t) - \bar{f})^2 \qquad (2)$$

Here, $\hat{f}(t)$ is the reconstructed P-cell firing frequency; $f(t)$ indicates the observed firing frequency pattern; and $\bar{f}$ is the averaged firing frequency during the observation period. The coefficient of determination, CD, ranges from $0 \leq CD \leq 1$, and approaches 1 when the reconstructed firing frequency is close to that observed. The CD for the fitting was 0.88, indicating that the model based on the inverse-dynamics representation of the eye movements adequately matches the temporal modulation of the P-cell response. The temporal modulation of 23 P-cells during ocular following at a stimulus velocity of 80° or 160°/s was studied by this method, and the CD was higher than 0.7 in 19 cases.[7]

The parameters for the 19 well-fitted P-cells were used in the statistical analysis.[7] The mean delay (Δ) was 7.1 ms, which was observed near the latency of the eye movements evoked by electrical stimulation,[3] suggesting that the activity of the P-cells may be used by the downstream structures as a motor command to elicit ocular following. The distribution of each coefficient is shown in FIGURE 6.[7] The mean acceleration coefficient (a) was 0.061 spikes/s per deg/s,[2] and the mean velocity coefficient (b) was 2.9 spikes/s per deg/s. The position coefficient (c) ranged from -29.6 to 0.5 spikes/s per deg, and the mean value was -12.6 spikes/s per deg.

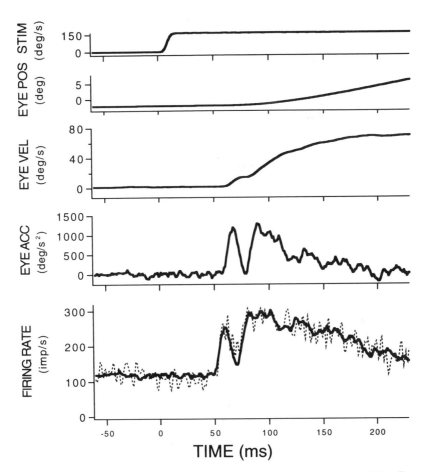

FIGURE 5. Reconstruction of the temporal pattern of firing frequency of a P-cell by a linear time-series multiple-regression method expressed by equation 1. From top to bottom, the average stimulus velocity, average eye position, average eye velocity, eye acceleration, and average firing frequency of the P-cell during ocular-following responses to multiple presentations of a 160°/s downward test ramp (*dotted line*) and the temporal pattern as reconstructed by the model (*continuous line*) are shown. Parameters used in this model were (a) 0.102 spikes/s per deg/s²; (b) 2.52 spikes/s per deg/s; (c) -15.8 spikes/s per deg; and (d) -80.7 spikes/s; Δ, 8 ms; and the coefficient of determinant was 0.88.

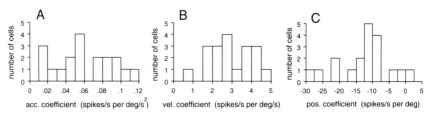

FIGURE 6. The distribution of three coefficients of the 19 P-cells in the model fitting[7]: (**A**) Acceleration coefficients, (**B**) velocity coefficients, and (**C**) position coefficients.

The mean ratio of the acceleration coefficient to the velocity coefficient (b/a) of the P-cells was 72.1, which was close to that of the motoneurons (67.4).[9] However, the mean ratio of the acceleration coefficient to the position coefficient (c/a = −294.5) of the P-cells was different from that of the motoneurons (344.8).[9] The results suggest that the firing frequency of these P-cells encodes the motor commands for the dynamic component (eye velocity and acceleration) of the ocular-following responses.

To test whether the model can be applied to a wide range of data, the responses of each P-cell at five different stimulus speeds were reconstructed by a single set of parameters. FIGURE 7 shows an example of such a fitting. A single set of parameters

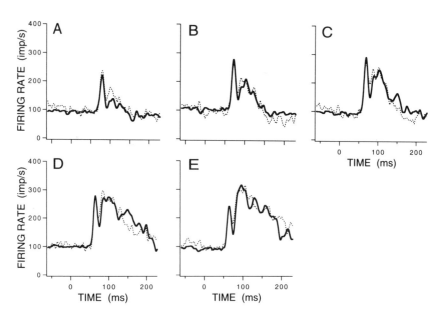

FIGURE 7. Reconstruction of temporal pattern of firing frequency of the P-cell shown in FIGURE 2 at different stimulus velocities (**A**, 10; **B**, 20; **C**, 40; **D**, 80; **E**, 160°/s). For this fitting, only one set of parameters was used: (a) 0.126 spikes/s per deg/s²; (b) 2.8 spikes/s per deg/s; (c) −17.5 spikes/s per deg; (d) −63.5 spikes/s; Δ, 8 ms; and the coefficient of determinant was 0.89. The reconstructed firing frequency profile (*continuous lines*) and raw firing frequency profile (*dotted lines*) are shown.

represents the temporal modulation of the P-cell in a wide range of stimulus speeds (CD = 0.89). Successful reconstructions of the responses at five different stimulus speeds were frequently observed in the P-cells. The CDs of 17 of the 20 P-cells were higher than 0.7 (mean ± SD, 0.80 ± 0.09). To compare the response properties of neurons in the other regions, the same analysis was applied to the responses of neurons in the MST and DLPN.[10] When a single set of parameters was used to fit the neuronal responses to five speeds, the responses of only a few neurons were successfully reconstructed. The CDs of three cells of the 9 DLPN neurons, and six of the 12 MST neurons were higher than 0.7 (mean ± SD: DLPN neurons, 0.57 ± 0.15; MST neurons, 0.61 ± 0.23). The results are consistent with the idea that the cerebellum may be responsible for the sensory-to-motor transformation to elicit ocular-following responses.

REFERENCES

1. MILES, F. A., K. KAWANO & L. M. OPTICAN. 1986. Short-latency ocular following responses of monkey. I. Dependence on temporospatial properties of visual input. J. Neurophysiol. **56:** 1321–1354.
2. KAWANO, K., M. SHIDARA & S. YAMANE. 1992. Neural activity in dorsolateral pontine nucleus of alert monkey during ocular following responses. J. Neurophysiol. **67:** 680–703.
3. SHIDARA, M. & K. KAWANO. 1993. Role of Purkinje cells in the ventral paraflocculus in short-latency ocular following responses. Exp. Brain Res. **93:** 185–195.
4. KAWANO, K., M. SHIDARA, Y. WATANABE & S. YAMANE. 1994. Neural activity in cortical area MST of alert monkey during ocular following responses. J. Neurophysiol. **71:** 2305–2324.
5. KAWANO, K., M. SHIDARA & S. YAMANE. 1990. Relation of the dorsolateral pontine nucleus of the monkey to ocular following responses. Soc. Neurosci. Abstr. **16:** 902.
6. SHIDARA, M., K. KAWANO & S. YAMANE. 1991. Ocular following response deficits with chemical lesions in the medial superior temporal area of the monkey. Neurosci. Res. **14:** S69.
7. SHIDARA, M., K. KAWANO, H. GOMI & M. KAWATO. 1993. Inverse-dynamics model eye movement control by Purkinje cells in the cerebellum. Nature **365:** 50–52.
8. HINES, W. W. & D. C. MONTGOMERY. 1972. Probability and Statistics in Engineering and Management Science, 3rd edit. Wiley & Sons. New York.
9. KELLER, E. L. 1973. Accommodative vergence in the alert monkey. Motor unit analysis. Vision Res. **13:** 1565–1575.
10. KAWANO, K., M. SHIDARA, A. TAKEMURA, Y. INOUE, H. GOMI & M. KAWATO. 1994. A linear time-series regression analysis of temporal firing patterns of cerebral, pontine and cerebellar neurons during ocular following. Jpn. J. Physiol. **44:** S219.

Influence of Sensorimotor Context on the Linear Vestibulo-Ocular Reflex[a]

GARY D. PAIGE,[b,c] GRAHAM R. BARNES,[d]
LAURA TELFORD,[b] AND SCOTT H. SEIDMAN[b]

[b]Department of Neurology
University of Rochester
Rochester, New York 14642

[d]Medical Research Council Human Movement and Balance Unit
Queen Square
London, United Kingdom

INTRODUCTION

The vestibulo-ocular reflex (VOR) functions to stabilize binocular fixation on visual targets during head movements. The VOR can conveniently be parsed into two subsystems: one that responds to angular head accelerations (the angular VOR, or AVOR) driven by the semicircular canals, and another that responds to linear head accelerations (the linear VOR, or LVOR) driven by the otolith organs. Both types of VOR are required because natural behavior includes both angular and linear head movements, and a stable image requires compensation for all. This study focuses on the human LVOR and is motivated by several important considerations. First, signals from the otolith organs that drive the LVOR are ambiguous in that they cannot distinguish linear accelerations due to linear motion from those incurred by head tilt relative to gravity. For example, a head tilt towards the left shoulder (roll-tilt) produces an equivalent signal in otolith afferents as does a prolonged horizontal linear acceleration to the right (along the interaural axis). Clearly, the eye movements required to maintain fixation for the two types of stimuli differ. Compensation for roll-tilt requires ocular torsion (or ocular counterrolling; OCR), whereas compensation for horizontal translation requires a horizontal ocular response. In fact, the ambiguity is functionally apparent in that the LVOR during interaural oscillation generates both torsional and horizontal response components simultaneously.[1] However, the torsional response is most robust during constant linear acceleration, as occurs during prolonged natural head tilt or centrifugation, and becomes progressively weaker as stimulus frequency rises.[1,2] By contrast, the horizontal response is most robust for head motion above around 0.5 Hz.[1,3–6] Thus, low-frequency linear acceleration seems to be selectively interpreted as tilt, whereas high-frequency acceleration is interpreted as translation. This study is confined to the translational LVOR, and in particular addresses the specific frequency-dependent behavior of the LVOR, as well as its interactions with visual following.

A second concern is that humans are frontal-eyed and bifoveate, which makes the geometry of eye and head movements in relation to binocular (bifoveate) fixation

[a]This research was supported by National Institutes of Health grants AG06442, RR09283, and EY07125, and a grant from Research to Prevent Blindness.
[c]Address correspondence to Dr. Gary D. Paige, Department of Neurology, University of Rochester, 601 Elmwood Avenue, Box 605, Rochester, NY 14642. E-mail: gdp@cvs.rochester.edu

critical for understanding both the goals and performance characteristics of the reflex. For any given head movement, the VOR must compensate for both the rotational and translational components to maintain binocular fixation. Proper compensation for the translational component is governed by target distance or, more accurately, fixation distance (where the two eyes are looking). Since the eyes are typically looking at a target, fixation and target distance are usually the same. Restricting attention to linear motion, the ideal compensation ocular response to a translation of magnitude, T, while fixating a target at distance, d, is proportional to arctan (T/d). If fixating a target far away, little or no eye movement is required, but as d becomes small (near fixation), ocular responses must become larger. This modulation of the LVOR by fixation distance has been repeatedly demonstrated in a variety of primate species.[3,6–11] How does the central nervous system determine fixation distance in order to properly modulate the LVOR? Evidence[8–14] suggests that the VOR (linear and angular), in some as yet unclear fashion, is linked to the vergence system, which precisely aligns the fovea of both eyes on visual targets. This influence of fixation distance on the VOR constitutes a "motor context," which modulates ongoing VOR performance, and likely reflects a high-level premotor command signal and not acutal vergence.[8,10,15] Vergence was routinely measured in these experiments and is presented in conjunction with VOR responses in RESULTS.

A third consideration is that the VOR generally operates in conjunction with visual mechanisms that also drive eye movements. These notably include the smooth pursuit system (target tracking) and the optokinetic reflex. Visual-vestibular interactions (VVI) are typically studied in two ways; when the visual image is earth-fixed (*ef*) or head-fixed (*hf*). In the former case, visually driven responses enhance the VOR, whereas in the latter case, they suppress the VOR, regardless of the nature of the head movement (i.e., rotation or translation). A fascinating feature of human VVI is an apparent modulation of VOR responses (in darkness) by the context of imagined image motion relative to the head.[16–18] That is, simply imagining that an image (or target) in darkness is *hf* or *ef* ("target context") results in a VOR attenuation or enhancement, respectively. The influence of both visual following and target context on the VOR behave with similar dynamic limitations that resemble smooth pursuit performance characteristics—both influences are limited to modest frequencies, below around 2 Hz. Although the LVOR has been studied under different conditions of VVI and target context,[3,5,7,19,20] none have directly measured fixation distance while also addressing the high-frequency behavior of the LVOR and its interactions with visual following and target context.

This study was performed to quantify the human interaural LVOR and its interactions with smooth pursuit over a range of frequencies (0.5–4.0 Hz) that is most relevant to translational reflex behavior. Contextual influences of fixation distance (i.e., vergence angle) and target motion relative to the head (real and imagined) were directly assessed.

EXPERIMENTAL METHODS

Stimulus Generation and Eye Movement Recording

Nine normal human subjects (age range, 21–49 years) participated in these experiments. Subjects were secured in a custom chair with their heads fixed by a rigid and individually molded bite bar. The chair was fixed to a servo-controlled linear sled, which generated sinusoidal translations in the IA axis at 0.5, 1.0, 2.0, and 4.0 Hz. Peak linear acceleration was held constant at 0.2 G (gravity, G = 981 cm/s^2), except at 0.5 Hz, where amplitude was limited to 0.1 G. In terms of head velocity and position, peak stimulus amplitude ranged from 31.2 to 7.8 cm/s, and from 9.94 to 0.31 cm, respectively, corresponding to the 0.5 to 4.0 Hz range of frequency.

Horizontal and vertical eye position signals were recorded binocularly using a digital video technique (Elmar Eye Tracker).[21] Calibrations were obtained by first employing a target fixation task over a range of ± 15°, and then adjusting scale factors post-hoc by assuming ideal performance during 0.5 and 1.0 Hz trials while subjects fixated visible *ef* targets. Head position was recorded using a linear potentiometer attached to the sled, and adjusted for the dynamics of the head relative to the sled.

Responses were recorded while subjects fixated *ef* visual targets at distances of 20, 45, and 135 cm, as well as *hf* targets (limited to 20 and 135 cm distances). The *ef* targets were numeric light-emitting diodes (LEDs) roughly scaled in size to account for different distances, and mounted on an array of narrow screens mounted parallel to the sled and placed at slightly different heights near eye level, such that near targets would not obstruct distant ones. The *hf* targets consisted of the projected image from an *hf* laser-LED onto these same screens. Periods of darkness were interspersed within trials at each frequency and target distance, and subjects were instructed to maintain "fixation" of the now imaginary *ef* or *hf* targets. This set of trial types yielded measures of the LVOR enhanced (*ef* targets) or suppressed (*hf* targets) by the presence of real visual targets at different distances (*ef*-LVOR and *hf*-LVOR, respectively), and by the context of imagined targets in darkness (*ief*-LVOR and *ihf*-LVOR). For convenience, in following sections of this paper we will omit "LVOR" from most labels. In short, each trial contained paired conditions, either *ef/ief* or *hf/ihf*.

Analysis of responses was derived from digitally recorded (at 100 Hz) eye and head position signals. For trials at frequencies below 2 Hz, records were differentiated, and ocular signals were smoothed and desaccaded.[22] At 2–4 Hz, response cycles without saccades were readily available and therefore were used selectively for analysis. Data from each trial were subjected to harmonic analysis on a cycle-by-cycle basis,[10] to produce response sensitivity (degrees of eye rotation per cm of head translation), phase angle, and average vergence (the mean difference between L and R horizontal eye position over the cycle). Vergence is presented in units of meter-angles (MA), which is simply the reciprocal of binocular fixation distance (in meters). Thus, 2 MA corresponds to the vergence angle required to fixate a target at 0.5-m distance. This measure is useful because it maintains geometric relevance regardless of head dimensions and thereby allows the direct comparison between results from different subjects and species.

RESULTS

Responses Related to Fixation of Earth-Fixed Targets

An example of a response to head translation at 4 Hz during an *ef/ief* trial from one subject is shown in FIGURE 1. Initially (far left in the diagram), the light is off (thick trace at top), imagined "fixation" is relatively distant, as indicated by low vergence (thick trace at bottom), and the oscillating response (eye position trace) is relatively small in amplitude. This represents a portion of the trial under *ief* conditions. When the target turns on, vergence rises steeply to match that required to fixate the now visible near target (*ef* condition), and the ocular response amplitude rises. When the light is extinguished (at around 5 s), vergence gradually declines in darkness, as the subject is unable to maintain near fixation in the absence of visual feedback. This is accompanied by a gradual decline in response amplitude. From records such as those in FIGURE 1, plots of response sensitivity against vergence for each cycle were derived. FIGURE 2 illustrates examples from trials at 4 Hz and 0.5 Hz, for both the *ef* (target on; open circles) and *ief* (dark; filled circles) conditions. The 4-Hz plot is from the same data record as in FIGURE 1. The clumping of responses, especially with the target on, corresponds to the three target distances employed. The spread of values for the near (high vergence) *ief* condition at 4 Hz reflects this subject's inability to maintain vergence after viewing the nearest target (see FIG. 1).

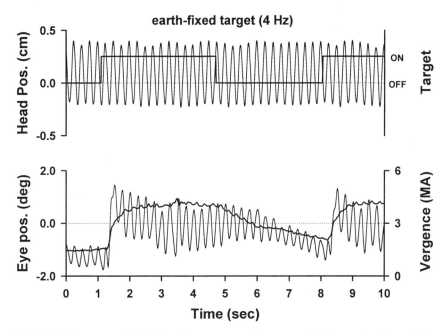

FIGURE 1. Raw record of horizontal eye movement responses (bottom pair of traces) to interaural translation at 4 Hz (thin oscillating trace in top pair; axis labeled on the left) in one subject while attempting to fixate a visible earth-fixed (*ef*) target (thick trace in top pair shows target on, as labeled on right), and when instructed to maintain fixation in darkness on the same, but now imagined, target (*ief;* target off). The response (thin oscillating trace in bottom pair; axis labeled on the left) displays evidence of modulation associated with changes in vergence (thick trace in bottom pair; axis labeled on the right), plotted in meter angles (MA).

The relationship between sensitivity and vergence was roughly linear across subjects, and for all conditions. This allows a convenient means of characterizing the response properties during head translation as a best-fit (LSF) line.[10] The solid lines in FIGURE 2 represent the geometrically ideal relationship, calculated to have a slope, S, of 0.573°/cm/MA and an intercept, I, of 0°/cm at 0 MA of vergence. The broken lines show the regression results for the *ef* and *ief* conditions. Several observations are derived from the data of FIGURE 2. First, at 4 Hz there is a positive I for both conditions. Second, the S for the *ef* condition is greater than the S for *ief*, and closer to ideal. Third, at 0.5 Hz (FIG. 2) the slope of the relationship between LVOR

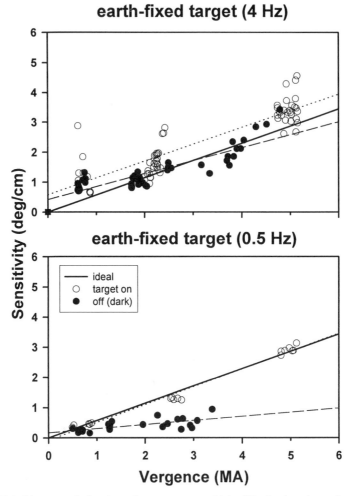

FIGURE 2. Linear vestibulocular reflex response sensitivity (°/cm), plotted as a function of vergence and on a cycle-by-cycle basis, at both 4 Hz (*upper plot*) and 0.5 Hz (*lower plot*). Open circles depict when the earth-fixed target was on (*ef* condition), whereas filled circles indicate when the target was off (imagined fixation in darkness, or *ief* condition). The thick solid lines illustrate ideal response properties while the dotted (*ef*) and dashed (*ief*) lines show best-fit lines to the data. Note the markedly reduced *ief* slope at 0.5 Hz as compared to 4 Hz, and the presence of some response sensitivity at 0 MA vergence (response intercept) in all but the *ef* condition at 0.5 Hz.

sensitivity and vergence in darkness (*ief*) is considerably reduced, and farther from ideal, as compared to that at 4 Hz.

We now focus further on LVOR and VVI frequency-response characteristics. FIGURE 3 shows mean (and SD) sensitivity slope, *S*, and phase as a function of frequency for all subjects and for all conditions (*ef*, *ief*, *hf*, *ihf*). Values for *S* were derived from regression analysis, as described above. Unlike sensitivity, phase did not display a systematic relationship with vergence, and is therefore expressed in FIGURE 3 as averages (and SDs) across vergences for each frequency and condition. For the *ef* condition, the average S at 0.5 Hz ($0.532 \pm 0.033°$/cm/MA) was close to the ideal of $0.573°$/cm/MA, but declined as frequency increased to reach $0.352 \pm 0.180°$/cm/MA at 4.0 Hz. Phase was not statistically different from zero across frequencies.

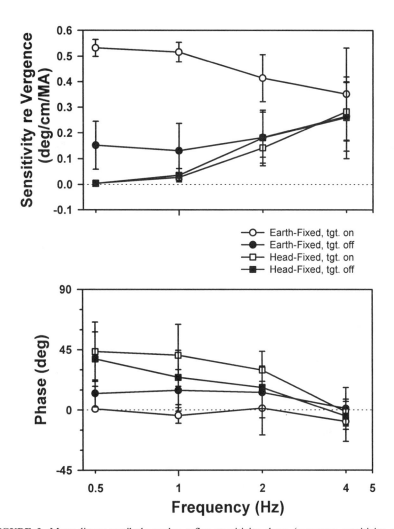

FIGURE 3. Mean linear-vestibulo-ocular reflex sensitivity slope (response sensitivity as a function of vergence) and phase, plotted as a function of stimulus frequency, for all conditions (contexts) of target motion (*see key in figure*). Error bars depict SDs. The ideal response for *ef/ief* conditions would be a slope of $0.57°$/cm/MA and phase of $0°$, and for *hf/ihf* conditions, a slope of zero.

In darkness (*ief* condition), *S* was relatively low (0.152 ± 0.093°/cm/MA) at 0.5 Hz, but climbed with rising frequency to 0.265 ± 0.135°/cm/MA at 4 Hz. Values of *S* in darkness (*ief*) were generally less than those obtained in the presence of the target (*ef*), even at 4 Hz ($p < 0.05$; paired *t* test). Phase showed a lead of +13° to +15° at all but 4 Hz, where the lead dropped to +1.2° (not significantly different from 0°). Phase values in darkness generally led those with the target present by 10–20°.

Interestingly, the mean response intercept, *I*, (sensitivity at 0 MA vergence, from regression analysis) maintained a modest value of 0.14°/cm for the *ief* condition (in darkness) at 0.5 Hz, whereas *I* for all other conditions remained near 0°/cm. *I* climbed progressively with increasing frequency to values of 0.4–0.8°/cm at 4 Hz, with large variances between subjects and conditions.

Responses Related to Fixation of Head-Fixed Targets

Response characteristics were assessed in the presence of an *hf* target and during imagined fixation (*ihf*) in darkness. Results are illustrated in FIGURE 3. In general, subjects had little difficulty suppressing eye movements at 0.5 Hz during either real or imagined fixation. Thus, both *S* (FIG. 3) and *I* were indistinguishable from zero. However, as frequency increased, *S* for both the *hf* and *ihf* conditions climbed to values that were indistinguishable from those obtained in the *ief* condition at 4 Hz (see FIG. 3). The same qualitative characteristics held for *I*. Corresponding phases displayed large leads (44° ± 22° for *hf;* 38° ± 20° for *ihf*) at 0.5 Hz, declining with increasing frequency to near zero at 4 Hz. Phases for the *ihf* condition were significantly less than those for *hf* only at 1 and 2 Hz ($p < 0.025$).

A direct comparison between *ef* and *hf* conditions is useful (see FIG. 3). For both response sensitivity and phase, differences between *ef* and *hf* (target on) were greatest at 0.5 Hz ($p < 0.001$; paired *t* test, for both slope and phase) and declined with increasing frequency. The differences became statistically insignificant by 4 Hz ($p > 0.1$), indicating a loss of visual influence on eye movements at high frequency. The same qualitative characteristics applied to differences between *ief* and *ihf* conditions (in darkness). Differences were statistically significant for *S* only at 0.5 Hz ($p < 0.005$) and 1 Hz ($p < 0.05$), and for phase only at 0.5 Hz ($p < 0.005$). This suggests that the influence of imagined target motion, like that of real visual targets, is limited to modest frequencies.

DISCUSSION

These experiments have quantified the frequency-dependent response properties of the LVOR and its interactions with visually-driven eye movements and sensorimotor context. The latter comprises at least two forms that operate in darkness—an influence of viewing distance as reflected by binocular vergence angle, and an influence of imagined target motion in space. Both of these contextual influences were quantified. The frequency bandwidth addressed, 0.5–4.0 Hz, may appear to many as surprisingly limited and high. However, this range is based on previous experiments in monkeys[1] and humans,[8] which suggest that influences of viewing distance on the LVOR are robust during oscillations of 3–5 Hz or during transient accelerations,[9,11] but weak at more modest frequencies.[5,19] This is in concert with the notion that the LVOR operates as a set of parallel and frequency-dependent reflexes, a low-frequency tilt-LVOR, which may also act to enhance a failing AVOR below 0.1 Hz,[23,24] and a high-frequency translational-LVOR,[1,6,9,25] which is robust at and above roughly 0.5 Hz. The current results specifically address the range relevant to the translational LVOR. The horizontal ocular responses recorded are consistent with a compensatory reflex that generates binocular eye movements that help maintain binocular fixation in space during interaural linear motion. A relevant psychophysical observation is that all subjects reported subjective sensations of interaural translational motion throughout the series of trials, and never experienced tilt. This is in contrast to low-frequency linear acceleration in the same laboratory using the same device (see Seidman and Paige, this volume), which induces sensations of tilt, not translation.

Our findings specifically address the dynamics of the translational LVOR across frequency, and as a function of context (fixation and target motion), and demonstrate its surprisingly high-pass characteristics. Regardless of the context of imagined target motion, LVOR responses in darkness maintain the greatest sensitivities, with phase angles near 0°, at the highest frequency, and display decreasing sensitivity and rising phase leads as frequency declines to 0.5 Hz. The influence of vergence angle (as a measure of viewing distance) is likewise greatest at 4 Hz, and is reduced to near zero as frequency drops to 0.5 Hz. Similar findings have been recently obtained from monkey subjects.[25]

These data bridge the literature by replicating attributes of findings from several laboratories, each studying the LVOR under different conditions of linear motion, frequency, and fixation distance. This is not to argue that vergence angle is the only signal relevant to viewing distance that can influence LVOR responses. Accommodation of the intraocular lens is known to modify the LVOR in monkeys,[9] but has not been demonstrably important in humans.[6,8] Monocular target distance cues may be of interest, but could not explain results obtained in darkness, except perhaps indirectly by constituting another potential contextual variable. One confounding concern is that measured vergence angle potentially represents the sum of different driving signals. For example, vergence is driven by binocular disparity, but also indirectly through interactions from intraocular accommodation (accommodative convergence). However, optical manipulation of accommodation does not influence the vergence effect on the LVOR, as studied during vertical linear oscillation.[6,8] Nevertheless, there remains the possibility for other, as yet unidentified, variables related to viewing distance and vergence that remain to be quantified.

In contrast to the influence of vergence on the LVOR, which is strongest at the highest frequencies, the influence of imagined target motion is limited to lower frequencies, and becomes inconsequential as frequency increases to 4 Hz. This is true even in the presence of real targets, because the LVOR slopes under *ef* and *hf* conditions, as well as *ief* and *ihf* conditions, converge at 4 Hz. These features resemble actual and imagined visual influences on the AVOR.[16–18,26–28] These AVOR studies, together with the current data on the LVOR, imply that the influence of imagined target motion on the VORs generally follows pursuit-like dynamics.

One common observation in LVOR studies[8–11] using transient or high-frequency stimuli is the presence of a response even at zero vergence (the intercept). In other words, the LVOR maintains a small response to linear motion even though none is required to maintain binocular fixation in space, since zero vergence connotes fixation of an infinitely far target. Indeed, any response under these conditions actually generates retinal image slip. An earlier interpretation of this "positive intercept" phenomenon is that it serves to match the overall performance of the LVOR to its ideal requirements better than if the intercept were zero.[10] This can be appreciated in FIGURE 2, which includes the best-fit line segment (slope and intercept are both represented) to the data along with the ideal (slope of 0.573°/

cm/MA and intercept of 0°/cm). In this subject, the *ef* response at 4 Hz is consistently above the ideal across the range of vergence, but in the *ief* case the line intersects the ideal at around 3 MA of vergence, indicating a binocular fixation distance of 33 cm. This intersection corresponds to perfect reflex performance; that is, where the LVOR response matches requirements. On average, that point occurs at fixation distances between 33 and 73 cm across all conditions (target motion contexts). Thus, the LVOR seems optimized to maintain fixation stability at roughly arms length. Further, as vergence extends from this distance in either direction, the error accumulated is quite small. In contrast, if the intercept were zero, ideal performance would exist only for fixation of far targets, and would become progressively erroneous as vergence increased. This would be especially troublesome at 4 Hz, where the mean LVOR response slope is less than ideal even in the presence of an *ef* target. Indeed, the slopes average 61% of ideal under *ef* conditions, and 46% in darkness (both *ief* and *ihf* conditions). Interestingly, these values in darkness are considerably greater than those reported in the human LVOR previously.[6,8,11] The difference may reside in the remarkable frequency-dependence of the vergence influence; even a shift from 4 to 3 Hz provides a noticeable decline in the effect.

Another provocative observation regarding the positive intercept in the LVOR is that it exists even at lower frequencies. At 0.5 Hz, the slope and intercept under *ief* conditions are significantly different from zero, and account for a modest LVOR response in darkness at this frequency. By contrast, under *ihf* conditions, *S* (the vergence influence) disappears while *I* maintains a small value. This implies that some LVOR sensitivity exists which cannot be removed under a context that tends to suppress it, and further, that this response component is not vergence-dependent. We do not sufficiently know the frequency response of the LVOR below 0.5 Hz, but can speculate that it is likely to be different for the response slope (vergence effect) and intercept (perhaps a more primordial phenomenon). In addition, we speculate that the same residual response that underlies the intercept at 0.5 Hz and above extends to lower frequencies of linear acceleration, and it is this component of the LVOR that has been typically recorded in most studies of the LVOR.

REFERENCES

1. PAIGE, G. D. & D. L. TOMKO. 1991. Eye movement responses to linear head motion in the squirrel monkey. I. Basic characteristics. J. Neurophysiol. **65:** 1170–1182.
2. LICHTENBERG, B. K., L. R. YOUNG & A. P. ARROTT. 1982. Human ocular counterrolling induced by varying linear accelerations. Exp. Brain Res. **48:** 127–136.
3. SKIPPER, J. J. & G. R. BARNES. 1989. Eye movements induced by linear acceleration are modified by visualisation of imaginarty targets. Acta Otolaryngol. (Suppl.) **468:** 289–293.
4. TOKITA, T., H. MIYATA, M. MASAKI & S. IKEDA. 1981. Dynamic characteristics of the otolithic oculomotor system. Ann. N. Y. Acad. Sci. **374:** 56–68.
5. OAS, J. G., R. W. BALOH, J. L. DEMER & V. L. HONRUBIA. 1992. The effect of target distance and stimulus frequency on horizontal eye movements induced by linear acceleration on a parallel swing. Ann. N. Y. Acad. Sci. **656:** 874–876.
6. PAIGE, G. D. 1989. The influence of target distance on eye movement responses during vertical linear motion. Exp. Brain Res. **77:** 585–593.
7. BALOH, R. W., K. BEYKIRCH, V. HONRUBIA & R. D. YEE. 1988. Eye movements induced by linear acceleration on a parallel swing. J. Neurophysiol. **60:** 2000–2013.
8. PAIGE, G. D. 1991. Linear vestibulo-ocular reflex (LVOR) and modulation by vergence. Acta Otolaryngol. (Suppl.) **481:** 282–286.
9. SCHWARZ, U. & F. A. MILES. 1991. Ocular responses to translation and their dependence on viewing distance. I. Motion of the observer. J. Neurophysiol. **66:** 851–863.

10. PAIGE, G. D. & D. L. TOMKO. 1991. Eye movement responses to linear head motion in the squirrel monkey. II. Visual-vestibular interactions and kinematic considerations. J. Neurophysiol. **65:** 1183–1196.

11. BUSETTINI, C., F. A. MILES, U. SCHWARZ & J. R. CARL. 1994. Human ocular responses to translation of the observer and of the scene: Dependence on viewing distance. Exp. Brain Res. **100:** 484–494.

12. HINE, T. & F. THORN. 1987. Compensatory eye movements during active head rotation for near targets: Effects of imagination, rapid head oscillation and vergence. Vision Res. **27:** 1639–1657.

13. VIIRRE, E., D. TWEED, K. MILNER & T. VILIS. 1986. A reexamination of the gain of the vestibuloocular reflex. J. Neurophysiol. **56:** 439–450.

14. SNYDER, L. H. & W. M. KING. 1992. The effect of viewing distance and location of the axis of head rotation on the monkey's vestibulo-ocular reflex: I. Eye movement responses. J. Neurophysiol. **67:** 861–874.

15. SNYDER, L. H. & W. M. KING. 1992. Changes in vestibulo-ocular reflex (VOR) response anticipate changes in vergence angle. Vision Res. **32:** 569–575.

16. BARR, C. C., L. W. SCHULTHEIS & D. A. ROBINSON. 1976. Voluntary, non-visual control of the human vestibulo-ocular reflex. Acta Otolaryngol. (Stockh.) **81:** 365–375.

17. FURST, E. J., J. M. GOLDBERG & H. A. JENKINS. 1987. Voluntary modification of the rotatory induced vestibuloocular reflex by fixating imaginary targets. Acta Otolaryngol. (Stockh.) **103:** 232–240.

18. BARNES, G. R. 1988. Head-eye co-ordination: Visual and nonvisual mechanisms of vestibulo-ocular reflex slow-phase modification. Prog. Brain Res. **76:** 319–328.

19. SHELHAMER, M., D. M. MERFELD & J. C. MENDOZA. 1995. Effect of vergence on the gain of the linear vestibulo-ocular reflex. Acta Otolaryngol. (Suppl.) In press.

20. ISRAËL, I. & A. BERTHOZ. 1989. Contribution of the otoliths to the calculation of linear displacement. J. Neurophysiol. **62:** 247–263.

21. DISCENNA, A. O., V. DAS, A. Z. ZIVOTOFSKY, S. H. SEIDMAN & R. J. LEIGH. 1995. Evaluation of a video tracking device for measurement of horizontal and vertical eye rotations during locomotion. J. Neurosci. Methods **58:** 89–94.

22. PAIGE, G. D. & E. W. SARGENT. 1991. Visually-induced adaptive plasticity in the human vestibulo-ocular reflex. Exp. Brain Res. **84:** 25–34.

23. RUDE, S. A. & J. F. BAKER. 1988. Dynamic otolith stimulation improves the low frequency horizontal vestibulo-ocular reflex. Exp. Brain Res. **73:** 357–363.

24. TOMKO, D. L., C. WALL III, F. R. ROBINSON & J. P. STAAB. 1988. Influence of gravity on cat vertical vestibulo-ocular reflex. Exp. Brain Res. **69:** 307–314.

25. TELFORD, L., S. H. SEIDMAN & G. D. PAIGE. 1994. Linear vestibulo-ocular reflex (LVOR) as a function of frequency and amplitude. Neurosci. Abstr. **20:** 567.

26. MCKINLEY, P. A. & B. W. PETERSON. 1985. Voluntary modulation of the vestibuloocular reflex in humans and its relation to smooth pursuit. Exp. Brain Res. **60:** 454–464.

27. KASTEEL-VAN LINGE, A. & A. J. J. MAAS. 1990. Quantification of visuo-vestibular interaction up to 5.0 Hz in normal subjects. Acta Otolaryngol. (Stockh.) **110:** 18–24.

28. PAIGE, G. D. 1994. Senescence of human visual-vestibular interactions: Smooth pursuit, optokinetic, and vestibular control of eye movements with aging. Exp. Brain Res. **98:** 355–372.

Organizational Principles of Otolith- and Semicircular Canal–Ocular Reflexes in Rhesus Monkeys[a]

DORA E. ANGELAKI[b,c] AND BERNHARD J. M. HESS[d]

[b]Department of Surgery (Otolaryngology)
University of Mississippi Medical Center
2500 North State Street
Jackson, Mississippi 39216-4505

[d]Department of Neurology
University Hospital
Zurich, CH-8091 Switzerland

INTRODUCTION

In contrast to a single functional role of semicircular canal–ocular reflexes in terms of gaze stabilization during rotatory head movements, otolith-ocular reflexes are quite diverse and comprise a number of different phenomena, most of which have not been put into a clear functional context. Otolith-ocular reflexes include counter-rolling of the eyes during roll tilts,[1–4] a steady-state compensatory nystagmus during constant velocity off-vertical axis rotations,[5] a low-frequency enhancement of vestibulo-ocular reflex (VOR) dynamics during earth-horizontal axis oscillations,[6–7] changes in the orientation and dynamics of canal-ocular reflexes as a function of head orientation relative to gravity,[8–9] as well as context-specific ocular reflexes during translational motion.[10–12] Among these different reflex actions, the best understood in terms of function is the otolith contribution to horizontal and vertical gaze stabilization during linear translations.[10–13]

In a series of recent studies, we have sought to characterize further the primate otolith-ocular reflexes in an attempt to find the common principles underlying these diverse observations. For this, we recorded three-dimensional eye movements during earth-vertical and off-vertical axis rotations in the yaw, pitch, and roll planes. We found that the various otolith-ocular phenomena can be considered in terms of three distinct otolith-ocular systems: (1) a translational VOR, which is functionally equivalent to the semicircular canal angular VOR; (2) a system that dynamically modulates primary eye position as a function of head orientation relative to gravity; and (3) an inertial vestibular system that detects absolute head motion in space. The latter two systems, which code head orientation relative to gravity and angular velocity in space, are probably primarily involved in spatial orientation and motor coordination rather than gaze stabilization per se.

[a]This work was supported by grants from the National Institutes of Health (EY10851), the National Aeronautics and Space Administration (NAGW-4377), the Air Force Office of Scientific Research (F49620), and the Swiss National Science Foundation (31-32484.91).
[c]Corresponding author; e-mail: dea@fiona.umsmed.edu

METHODS

Experiments were performed in rhesus monkeys that were chronically prepared with skull bolts to restrain the head during experiments. The animals were implanted with dual-search coils for three-dimensional eye movement recordings using the magnetic search coil technique (details of these procedures are provided elsewhere[8–9]). The coil signals and the turntable position signals were digitized at a rate of 833 Hz and stored on the hard disk of a PC for off-line analyses. Calibration of eye coil signals was based on an *in vitro* procedure to determine the coil sensitivities and an *in vivo* procedure in which the animal was asked to fixate target lights for fluid reward. Three-dimensional eye position (vector E with components E_{tor}, E_{ver}, and E_{hor}) and eye angular velocity (vector Ω with components Ω_{tor}, Ω_{ver}, and Ω_{hor}) were expressed in head-centered Cartesian coordinates as rotation vectors. The coordinate system was defined by the orientation of the magnetic fields relative to the animal's head, which was restrained in a standard 15° nose-down position. Horizontal eye movements were described as rotations about the head vertical axis (leftward positive). Similarly, vertical eye movements were described as rotations about the interaural axis (downward positive), and torsional eye movements as rotations about the naso-occipital axis (positive for rotation of the upper pole of the eye towards the right ear). To estimate slow-phase velocity, eye position was digitally differentiated and fast phases of nystagmus were removed based on time and amplitude windows set for the second derivative of the magnitude of the eye velocity vector.

During rotation in the yaw, pitch and roll planes, the VOR was studied using two different experimental protocols: (1) Constant velocity rotations at different velocities ranging from ±37°/s to ±184°/s, and (2) sinusoidal oscillations at different frequencies (0.01–1.14 Hz) and peak displacements: ±5° (1.14 Hz), ±18° (0.53 Hz), ±45° (0.21 Hz), ±90° (0.10 or 0.05 Hz), ±180° (0.10 or 0.05 Hz), ±450° (0.02 Hz), and ±900° (0.01 Hz). The axis of rotation in these experiments was either earth-vertical or earth-horizontal (to examine the contribution of the otolith system to the VOR).

Eye position (during constant velocity rotation) and slow phase eye velocity (during both constant velocity rotation and sinusoidal oscillations) were quantified by fitting sinusoidal functions describing either head position or angular head velocity responses.[14–15] Gain and phase were subsequently calculated from the fitted equations and the stimulus parameters.

RESULTS

Dependence of Torsional and Vertical Eye Position on Head Orientation in Space

As the head rotates at constant velocity about an earth-horizontal yaw axis (barbecue rotation), linear acceleration varies sinusoidally along each of the interaural and naso-occipital axes. The frequency of these sinusoidal stimulus components is proportional to the velocity of rotation. For example, a rotation at 58°/s would correspond to a frequency of $(58°/s)/(360°) = 0.16$ Hz. During earth-horizontal axis rotation at constant velocity about the head yaw axis, a characteristic pattern of torsional and vertical eye position modulations was present in addition to a steady-state horizontal nystagmus that was compensatory to the velocity of head rotation (FIG. 1). These torsional and vertical eye position modulations were roughly sinusoidal and phase-locked to head position relative to gravity. Peak-to-peak modulation of eye position was large for all velocities, amounting to about 25°–30°. Torsional eye

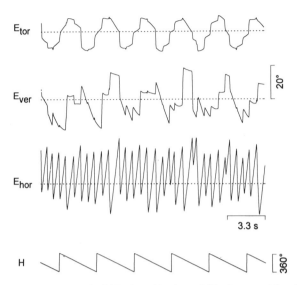

FIGURE 1. Torsional (E_{tor}), vertical (E_{ver}), and horizontal (E_{hor}) eye position during constant velocity yaw rotation at $110°/s$ about an earth-horizontal axis. Dotted lines mark zero eye position and velocity. H, head position (turntable potentiometer resets every $360°$).

position was zero in prone and supine positions (at zero-crossing and reset of turntable potentiometer) and maximal in ear-down positions. When the head was left ear-down, the eyes rotated in the positive direction (i.e., the left eye intorted and the right eye extorted). Vertical eye position modulation was phase shifted by approximately $90°$ relative to torsional modulation. Thus, it was minimal (negative, i.e., upward) in prone and maximal (positive, i.e., downward) in supine positions.

The large modulations of torsional eye position correspond to the traditional counterrolling of the eyes as the head changes orientation relative to gravity in the roll plane (i.e., when there is a non-zero gravity component along the interaural axis). Similar modulations of vertical eye position (counterpitching) are observed when the head changes orientation in the pitch plane, that is, when there is a gravity-component along the naso-occipital axis.[16] Because barbecue (yaw) rotation imposes a sinusoidally varying gravity stimulus along both the interaural and naso-occipital axes, both counterrolling and counterpitching are observed. These eye movements were only in part achieved through slow phase modulation, in contrast to what one might expect for eye movements that stabilize torsional and vertical gaze as, for example, in rabbits.[17] In particular, during high rotational speeds, most of the modulation in torsional and vertical eye position was achieved through saccadic eye movements (e.g., $110°/s$, FIG. 1). Thus, the evoked combination of slow and fast eye movements rarely resulted in a nystagmus, but rather in a pattern of alternating of fast and slow eye movements in the same direction, as shown in FIGURE 1, particularly for torsional eye movements.

Because a major portion of the eye position changes was achieved through saccadic eye movements, the modulation of torsional and vertical slow-phase eye velocity was small, even for lower velocities when a rather regular nystagmus was observed (e.g., $58°/s$, FIG. 2). There was also a small modulation of horizontal slow-phase velocity that was phase locked to head position relative to gravity. This modulation corresponds to a horizontal translational vestibulo-ocular reflex whose sensitivity was low in the conditions of the present experiments.

The sensitivity and phase of each of the torsional and vertical eye position and slow-phase eye velocity modulations were evaluated by fitting a sinusoid to each component separately. Mean sensitivity and phase values ($\pm$SD) of the eye position and slow-phase velocity modulation are illustrated in FIGURE 3 and FIGURE 4 for torsional and vertical eye movements, respectively. We found that: (1) Peak eye position modulation remained constant as a function of frequency and tightly phase-locked to head position (with gravity along the interaural head axis for peak E_{tor} and along the naso-occipital axis for peak E_{ver}). Thus, these modulations in torsional and vertical eye position represent a dynamic rather than a static response as it was believed thus far. (2) The derivatives of E_{tor} and E_{ver} should exhibit increasing gains with frequency and phase leads of 90° relative to head position. Instead, the sensitivity of slow-phase eye velocity was small and independent of frequency. This discrepancy in the temporal properties of $E_{tor}(E_{ver})$ and $\Omega_{tor}(\Omega_{ver})$ reflects the fact that the modulation of $E_{tor}(E_{ver})$ was largely due to fast eye movements which do not contribute to slow-phase eye velocity.

The head position–dependent modulations in torsional and vertical eye position were by no means limited to constant velocity rotations. They were present whenever there was a static or dynamic reorientation of the head relative to gravity. For example, yaw oscillations at 0.53 Hz ($\pm$18°) about an earth-horizontal axis resulted in a systematic modulation of torsional eye position that was mostly achieved through fast eye movements (FIG. 5). This modulation seems to depend little on semicircular canal input because it was also present after inactivation of all semicircular canals. Because the amplitude of head displacement was small and centered in supine position, a systematic sinusoidal modulation was only present in torsional eye position (in response to a component of gravity along the interaural axis proportional

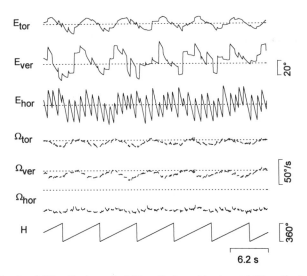

FIGURE 2. Torsional (E_{tor}, Ω_{tor}), vertical (E_{ver}, Ω_{ver}), and horizontal (E_{hor}, Ω_{hor}) eye position and slow-phase eye velocity (fast phases removed) during constant velocity yaw rotation about an earth-horizontal axis at 58°/s. Dotted lines mark zero eye position and velocity. H, head position (turntable potentiometer resets every 360°).

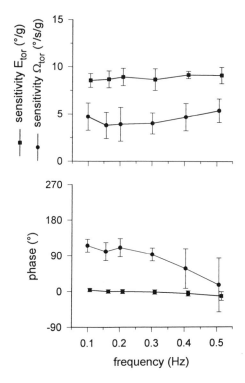

FIGURE 3. Sensitivity and phase of mean torsional eye position (E_{tor} in °/g, *squares*) and slow-phase eye velocity (Ω_{tor} in °/s/g, *circles*) during constant velocity yaw rotation as a function of frequency ($f = \omega/2\pi$, where ω is the velocity of rotation). Response phase has been expressed relative to head position. Mean values ±SD ($n = 5$).

to the sine of the rotation angle). During this motion, the component of gravity along the naso-occipital axis varied in proportion to the cosine of the rotation angle (which can be approximated as a constant); thus only a static positive (downward) deviation of the eyes was present throughout the motion.

These results suggest the following: (1) The counterrolling of the eyes during roll tilts does not represent solely a static otolith-ocular reflex, but rather a phenomenon that occurs during both static and dynamic otolith stimulation. (2) A similar vertical reflex (referred to as counterpitching) exists during pitch tilts. Furthermore, tilts about intermediate axes result in modulation of both torsional and vertical eye position as a function of head orientation in space. (3) Mean torsional and vertical eye position is adjusted via both fast and slow eye movements such that slow-phase eye velocity changes minimally. (4) Most likely, this systematic gravity-dependent modulation of three-dimensional eye position is unrelated to the classical concept of gaze stabilization. Rather, this otolith-ocular reflex seems to emerge from a need to adjust the coordinates of primary eye position in relation to some, yet unknown, motor coordination and orientation principles (see below).

Vestibular Detection of Angular Velocity

The horizontal steady-state nystagmus during constant velocity off-vertical axis yaw rotation (e.g., FIGS. 1 and 2) is not phase-locked to head position but rather proportional to head velocity. The same is true for constant velocity pitch and roll rotations, which elicit a steady-state compensatory vertical and torsional nystagmus, respectively.[15] These responses represent the ability of the otolith system to independently detect the velocity of rotation as the head moves dynamically relative to gravity.[5,18]

Independent otolith-ocular responses to head position and angular velocity are not only limited to constant velocity rotation. Sinusoidal oscillations with peak-to-peak amplitudes of more than 360° constitute a stimulus where the wave forms of head position (H) and head velocity (Ḣ) differ (see FIG. 6, bottom traces). During such large amplitude oscillations, the period of one revolution of the head in space varies within a single head velocity cycle, such that vestibulo-ocular responses to both head position and velocity can be independently assessed. Under these conditions, two independent reflex responses are elicited during low-frequency sinusoidal oscillations about an earth-horizontal axis (FIG. 6): Responses (in this case, horizontal) to head angular velocity, which follow the head velocity waveform of the stimulus (Ḣ), and responses to head position, which follow closely the waveform of head position (H), and are represented by the "wiggles" in each response component. In intact animals, both otolith and semicircular canal activity contribute to the generation of these head velocity responses (FIG. 6A). However, the large horizontal head velocity response in an animal with all semicircular canals inactivated demonstrates that a large proportion of the vestibulo-ocular signals that generate these responses in intact animals originate from the otolith organs (FIG. 6B).

Thus, otolith-ocular responses compensatory for head angular velocity are elicited during both sinusoidal oscillations and constant velocity rotations about off-vertical axes. The frequency selectivity of these otolith-ocular responses in an animal with plugged semicircular canals are illustrated for yaw and roll rotations in

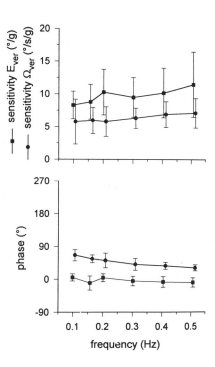

FIGURE 4. Sensitivity and phase of mean vertical eye position (E_{ver} in °/g, *squares*) and slow-phase eye velocity (Ω_{ver} in °/s/g, *circles*) during constant velocity yaw rotation as a function of frequency ($f = \omega/2\pi$, where ω is the velocity of rotation). Response phase has been expressed relative to head position. Mean values ±SD ($n = 5$).

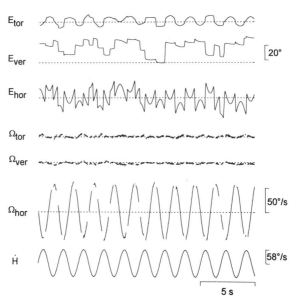

FIGURE 5. Torsional (E_{tor}, Ω_{tor}), vertical (E_{ver}, Ω_{ver}), and horizontal (E_{hor}, Ω_{hor}) eye position and slow-phase eye velocity (fast phases removed) during sinusoidal oscillations about an earth-horizontal axis, 0.53 Hz ± 18° (±58°/s). Dotted lines mark zero eye position and velocity. H, head velocity (turntable tachometer output).

FIGURES 7A and 8A, respectively. Responses were large (gains of 0.4) and compensatory to head velocity (i.e., response phase was close to zero) during oscillations at very low frequencies. As frequency increased, gains progressively declined and phase lags were introduced. This dynamic behavior is consistent with a low-pass filter, in accordance with the sluggish build-up and decay of the steady-state slow-phase eye velocity during constant velocity off-vertical rotation. The low-pass filtered otolith-ocular and the high-pass filtered semicircular canal-ocular dynamics are perfectly matched such that during yaw, pitch or roll rotation about earth-horizontal axes VOR is perfectly compensatory throughout the frequency range in animals with intact semicircular canals (FIGS. 7B and 8B; filled circles: earth-horizontal axis rotation; open circles: earth-vertical axis rotation).

In conclusion, there seems to exist a separate set of otolith-ocular responses that are proportional to angular head velocity as the animal dynamically reorients relative to gravity. These velocity signals are relayed to the VOR after being low-pass filtered and result in (1) a steady-state compensatory nystagmus during constant velocity rotation and (2) an improvement in the low-frequency VOR dynamics during sinusoidal oscillations about off-vertical axes. Contrary to results in rabbits[17] and previous postulations for primates,[11,19] these otolith-ocular responses are completely independent of the modulations of torsional and vertical eye position and slow-phase eye velocity that are phase locked to head position relative to gravity. Whatever the functional role of these velocity responses is, their presence in the VOR is directly related to the function of "velocity storage" and its various vestibulo-ocular manifestations.

DISCUSSION

Schematically, the vestibulo-ocular system can be subdivided into three function-ally distinct subsystems as illustrated in FIGURE 9. Short-latency semicircular canal and otolith afferent signals generate compensatory eye movements to stabilize gaze. The canal-ocular reflexes elicit eye movements compensatory to head angular velocity whereby semicircular canal afferents convey signals proportional to a head-fixed angular velocity vector **v**. Similarly, translational otolith-ocular reflexes elicit eye movements compensatory to head translation. These reflexes originate from primary otolith afferent signals which detect linear accelerations of the head (vector **a**). The gain of these reflexes is dependent on parameters related to binocular fixation, such as target distance and eccentricity.[10,12] They also account for differences between the axis of head and eye rotation in order to keep the eyes on target during eccentric rotations.[20,21] Both of these reflexes comprise the traditional VORs whose function is short-latency, high-frequency gaze stabilization during a combination of angular and linear (translational) head motion.

Inertial Vestibular Processing

Vestibulo-ocular signals originating from both the semicircular canals and the otolith organs are also used to compute head motion in space (inertial processing,

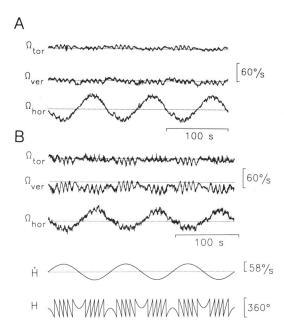

FIGURE 6. Torsional (Ω_{tor}), vertical (Ω_{ver}), and horizontal (Ω_{hor}) slow-phase eye velocity elicited by sinusoidal yaw oscillations at 0.01 Hz $\pm$ 900° ($\pm$58°/s) about an earth-horizontal axis. (**A**) Responses in an intact rhesus monkey. (**B**) Responses in a rhesus monkey after inactivation of all six semicircular canals. Ḣ, head velocity (turntable tachometer output); H, head position (potentiometer output reset every 360°). Dotted lines mark zero eye velocity.

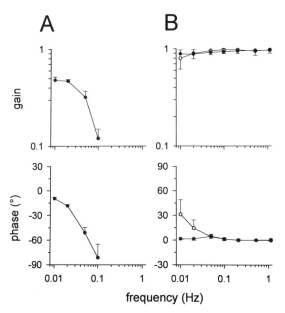

FIGURE 7. Frequency response of the horizontal vestibulo-ocular reflex. (**A**) Gain and phase during low-frequency earth-horizontal axis oscillations of an animal after inactivation of all six semicircular canals. (**B**) Gain and phase of intact animals during earth-vertical (*open circles*) and earth-horizontal (*filled circles*) axis rotation in complete darkness. Mean values ±SD ($n = 7$).

FIG. 9). Head-fixed semicircular canal afferent inputs (v) are centrally transformed into angular head velocity in space (Ω_c) based on a spatial transformation T_G that differs for horizontal and vertical canal activity: For lateral semicircular canals, Ω_c signals are generated by rotating head-fixed semicircular canal activity towards the gravity vector; for vertical semicircular canals, Ω_c signals are generated through a projection of vertical canal activity onto the direction of gravity.[8,9,22] As illustrated in FIGURES 1, 2, and 6, the otolith system is able to detect the velocity of head rotation during off-vertical axis rotations, most likely through a correlation of gravity and jerk signals.[18,23–25] Because this estimation of angular velocity is based on gravity information, the otolith system detects inertial angular velocity Ω_o,—that is, absolute head velocity in space. Inertial vestibular signals (Ω_c and Ω_o) contribute to slow-phase eye velocity after being low-pass filtered by a leaky integrator. We previously proposed that inertial vestibular signals are primarily involved in head control and perhaps motor coordination of gaze, head, and body posture.[8–9] Even though the function of these inertial vestibular signals is probably not strictly oculomotor, they are nevertheless relayed to the VOR, possibly through a gaze control mechanism in association with the immobilized head and neck during a typical laboratory VOR testing.

The existence of inertial vestibular signals can account for a series of observations, which often have been collectively referred to as "velocity storage": (1) The steady-state compensatory nystagmus during constant velocity rotation and the low-frequency improvement in VOR dynamics during sinusoidal oscillations about off-vertical axes represent the static and low-frequency contribution of Ω_o to VOR slow-phase velocity.[15] (2) The changes in the time constant and spatial orientation of the VOR either during centrifugation or after fast short-lasting head tilts reflect the spatially transformed vestibular signals Ω_c.[8,9] (3) The peculiar velocity storage-related steady-state nystagmus that is generated during constant velocity rotation about an earth-vertical axis while simultaneously oscillating about a nested earth-horizontal axis (e.g., "pitch-while-rotating") results from inertial processing of vestibular signals Ω_c.[9,26]

Thus, a number of seemingly independent experimental observations associated with velocity storage in the VOR are in fact the result of the same functional processing, that is, of a vestibular computation of absolute motion of the head in space. The cerebellar nodulus and/or ventral uvula seem to be directly involved in the computation of inertial vestibular signals: Surgical lesions of these cerebellar areas eliminate (1) the steady-state nystagmus during constant velocity rotation and the low-frequency enhancement of VOR dynamics during sinusoidal oscillations about off-vertical axes;[27] (2) the ability of the VOR to adjust its spatial orientation as a function of head orientation in space;[9] and (3) the generation of the steady-state nystagmus during the combined rotation/oscillation paradigms (e.g., "pitch-while-rotating").[9]

Gravity-dependent Modulation of Primary Eye Position

A third distinct class of otolith-ocular reflexes detects the orientation of the head in space and accordingly adjusts the torsional and vertical coordinates of three-

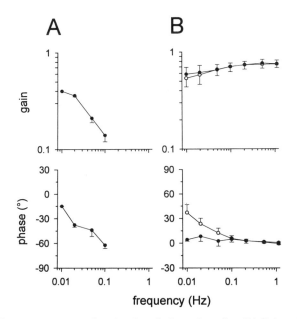

FIGURE 8. Frequency response of torsional vestibulo-ocular reflex. (**A**) Gain and phase during low-frequency earth-horizontal axis oscillations of an animal after inactivation of all six semicircular canals. (**B**) Gain and phase of intact animals during earth-vertical (*open circles*) and earth-horizontal (*filled circles*) axis rotation in complete darkness. Mean values ±SD ($n = 7$).

dimensional eye position. The torsional changes in mean three-dimensional eye position correspond to the traditional counterrolling of the eyes during static roll tilts which has been repeatedly described over several decades.[2-4,28] These torsional and vertical changes in mean eye position are identical to responses that Paige and Tomko[11] described as "tilt linear vestibulo-ocular responses" during mid- and high-frequency linear translation. Our results add several important aspects in the quantitative properties and functional relevance of these reflexes: (1) In primates, the relevant parameter in "tilt" otolith-ocular responses (i.e., torsional eye movements in response to linear acceleration along the interaural axis and vertical eye movements in response to linear acceleration along the naso-occipital axis) is eye position and not slow-phase eye velocity, as previously assumed. (2) The peak-to-peak modulation of mean torsional and vertical eye position is large (25–30°) and remains constant for frequencies at least up to 0.5 Hz, contrary to similar observations in rabbits where amplitudes of torsional and vertical eye position modulations drop sharply with frequency, accompanied by large phase lags at frequencies above

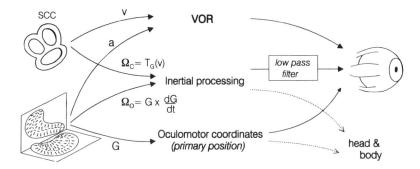

FIGURE 9. Synopsis of otolith-ocular reflexes: (1) Head-fixed semicircular canal angular velocity signals (v) and translational acceleration signals from otolith organs (a) generate functionally compensatory VORs. (2) Mutually perpendicular jerk and gravitational signals from the otolith organs (coding angular velocity $\Omega_o \sim G \times dG/dt$) and spatially transformed angular semicircular canal signals $\Omega_c = T_G(v)$ contribute to the detection of angular head motion in space. (3) Gravity signals from otolith afferents (G) control the vertical and torsional coordinates of primary eye position as a function of head orientation in space.

approximately 0.1 Hz.[17,29] (3) The modulation of torsional and vertical eye position in primates is achieved through a coordinated interaction of both slow and fast (saccadic) eye movements, in contrast to the assumption that ocular counterrolling represents a slow-phase response. (4) These torsional and vertical otolith-ocular responses in primates are totally independent of the low-frequency VOR enhancement during off-vertical axis rotations (FIG. 6). Again, this result is different from previous postulations that it was the "tilt" otolith-ocular reflexes that were responsible for the improvement in low-frequency VOR dynamics.[11,19] It is of interest that this observation represents another difference between rabbits and monkeys: In contrast to monkeys, it is in fact the modulation of torsional and vertical eye position that is responsible for the gain enhancement and reduction in phase lag of the respective VORs during earth-horizontal axis rotations in rabbits.[17,30]

Based on these results, it appears that the function of primate torsional and vertical eye position modulations as the head changes orientation in space has little to do with gaze stabilization. It rather appears that these otolith-ocular reflexes might be related to an orienting response. Spontaneous and visually guided eye movements in primates and humans have been shown to be confined to two rotational degrees of freedom. Based on this constraint in eye movement kinematics, a unique eye position (primary position) exists which allows one to define mutually orthogonal coordinates to parametrize all permissible spontaneous or visually guided eye movements. Primary position represents an important oculomotor parameter in the intrinsic representation of three-dimensional eye movements.[31,32] Detailed analysis of such responses has suggested that primary eye position and consequently the oculomotor coordinates of three-dimensional eye movements dynamically depend on head orientation in space.[33] The simple dynamics of these torsional and vertical eye position modulations for frequencies up to 0.5 Hz suggest that the otolith system might exert a direct (i.e., not dynamically processed) effect onto the neural circuitry that controls primary eye position and generates three-dimensional eye movements.

Translational Vestibulo-Ocular Reflexes

Since translational VORs are treated in more detail in a different chapter in this volume (see Paige *et al.*), we will not address their properties here. However, as part of a general outline of otolith-ocular reflexes, it is important to briefly discuss some basic organizational principles. For example, the signal processing underlying generation of translational otolith-ocular responses is still largely unknown. One line of speculation considers the signal processing in translational VOR as a mere replica of angular VOR processing, thereby proposing that linear acceleration signals from primary otolith afferents are centrally integrated to compute linear velocity (FIG. 10A). Similar to angular velocity signals from the semicircular canals, linear velocity would be subsequently processed by the oculomotor neural integrator such that eye movements compensatory to linear displacement could be generated. However, such a double integration scheme has consequences that cannot be reconciled with experimental data: In contrast to experimental findings, for example, a double integration would predict a translational VOR with low-pass filtered properties exhibiting gains that decrease with frequency and phase lags that increase with frequency. This is true even if one considers that only the most irregularly firing (phasic) otolith afferents are involved in generating translational responses.

The double integration idea originated from the assumption that otolith signals should be centrally processed in much the same way as semicircular canal signals. Along the lines of the Skavenski and Robinson[34] approach, one simply expects two integrations (each contributing a phase shift of $-90°$) in order to convert linear acceleration to linear displacement signals, which would drive eye position in a similar way as head angular velocity signals are thought to control eye position during angular VORs. The same temporal shift could, however, also be achieved by replacing the first integration by a differentiation and reversing the sign. In this case, central signals would exhibit gains that increase with frequency (consistent with coding of jerk), whereas temporal phase would be the same as after the first processing step in the double integration scheme (i.e., phase-shifted through $-90°$ from linear acceleration). Accordingly, the same neural integrator could convert central otolith signals into eye position commands (FIG. 10B). Of course, it should be added that these cascade, seemingly opposite, operations (i.e., differentiation followed by integration) do not cancel since they are both non-ideal (i.e., leaky) with different time constants.

What is the evidence, however, that translational otolith-ocular signals follow a conceptually similar central processing as that which has been demonstrated for semicircular canal–ocular reflexes? At present none. In contrast, there are at least three main differences in the functional and computational aspects of otolith-borne translational responses compared to semicircular canal-borne rotational VORs: First, in the angular VOR the first integration is due to peripheral mechanical dynamics such that primary semicircular canal afferents already code for head angular velocity. No such mechanical integration is present for the otolith system: regularly and less regularly firing primary otolith afferents code for linear acceleration in the frequency range of at least up to 2 Hz.[35] Second, semicircular canal

A Double integration hypothesis

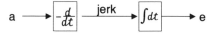

B Jerk-integration hypothesis

C Distributed spatio-temporal processing

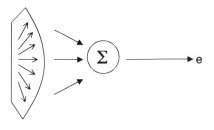

FIGURE 10. Signal processing in translational otolith-ocular reflexes. (**A**) Double-integration hypothesis: linear acceleration (a) is integrated to linear velocity (v_l), which is subsequently converted to eye position (e). (**B**) Jerk-integration hypothesis: linear acceleration (a) is high-pass filtered and sign-reversed before converted to eye position (e) through the neural integrator. (**C**) Distributed spatiotemporal processing: otolith afferent signals are summed in a spatiotemporal fashion to generate the dynamics of translational VORs.

afferents code angular velocity along three approximately orthogonal directions corresponding to the activation directions of the semicircular canals. In contrast, each primary otolith afferent codes for a different direction of linear acceleration in space. Third, the required eye rotation for proper gaze stabilization due to angular head motion is kinematically equivalent to the head rotation (after correction for differences in the axes of rotation). In contrast, a required eye rotation during linear translation must compensate for a head translation: This requires a nontrivial transformation, which is a function of viewing distance and gaze eccentricity. The need for binocular coordination is bound to generate unique spatiotemporal properties of the underlying otolith-ocular connectivity. For example, the same linear acceleration stimulus (along the naso-occipital axis, for example) could elicit no eye movement, a purely vertical eye movement, a purely horizontal eye movement or a combination of both.[10]

Due to the lack of any experimental data regarding neuronal responses to linear translation, our understanding of the translational otolith-ocular computations is still rudimental. Even though it might be appealing at first sight, it may prove unrealistic to attempt to conceptualize the organization of the translational otolith-ocular reflexes in analogy to the semicircular canal-ocular reflexes given the distinctly different properties of the otolith system. In fact, the translational VOR dynamics could also be generated simply by considering that otolith afferents with different dynamics and different spatial specificity linearly converge onto second- or higher-order vestibular cells. Along this line, the phasic dynamics of the reflex could arise from spatiotemporal summation of primary otolith afferent responses (FIG. 10C).

In conclusion, our present understanding of the dynamic organization of translational otolith-ocular reflexes is certainly rudimental. Any attempt to model the dynamics or any other aspect of the complex organization of these responses would necessarily suffer from the complete lack of knowledge of the basic computational and neurophysiological principles that underlie these reflexes. Single-unit data from the brain stem and cerebellar areas are urgently needed before any serious modeling effort be undertaken to untangle these computations. Any of the three schemes outlined in FIGURE 10 (and possibly additional ones) will have to be modified and detailed before the basic characteristics of translational otolith-ocular reflexes can be simulated. Once the basic otolith-ocular processing is determined, binocular three-dimensional eye position commands have to be incorporated into the basic circuitry in order to account for the strong dependence of these reflexes on binocular coordination. In addition to the involved spatiotemporal properties of translational VORs, the large complexity and diversity of the otolith-ocular system in general presents a challenge to our understanding of the underlying computational principles that need not necessarily follow similar principles as in semicircular canal–ocular reflexes.

REFERENCES

1. COLLEWIJN, H., J. VAN DER STEEN, L. FERMAN & T. C. JANSEN. 1985. Human ocular counterroll: Assessment of static and dynamic properties from electromagnetic scleral coil recordings. Exp. Brain Res. **59:** 185–196.
2. DIAMOND, S. G., C. H. MARKHAM, N. E. SIMPSON & I. S. CURTHOYS. 1979. Binocular counterrolling in humans during dynamic rotation. Acta Otolaryngol. **87:** 490–498.
3. KELLOGG, R. S. 1965. Dynamic counterrolling of the eye in normal subjects and in persons with bilateral labyrinthine defects. NASA SP-77: 195–202.
4. HANNEN, R. A., M. KABRISKY, C. R. REPLOGLE, V. L. HARTZLER & P. A. ROCCAFORTE. 1966. Experimental determination of a portion of the human vestibular system response through measurement of eyeball counterroll. IEEE Trans. Biomed. Eng. **13:** 65–70.
5. CORREIA, M. J. & K. E. MONEY. 1970. The effect of blockage of all six semicircular canal ducts on nystagmus produced by dynamic linear acceleration in the cat. Acta Otolaryngol. **69:** 7–17.
6. TOMKO, D. L., C. WALL III, F. R. ROBINSON & J. P. STAAB. 1988. Influence of gravity on cat vertical vestibulo-ocular reflex. Exp. Brain Res. **69:** 307–314.
7. RUDE, S. A. & J. F. BAKER. 1988. Dynamic otolith stimulation improves the low frequency horizontal vestibulo-ocular reflex. Exp. Brain Res. **73:** 357–363.

8.   ANGELAKI, D. E. & B. J. M. HESS. 1994. Inertial representation of angular motion in the vestibular system of rhesus monkeys. I. Vestibulo-ocular reflex. J. Neurophysiol. **71:** 1222–1249.jm
9.   ANGELAKI, D. E. & B. J. M. HESS. 1995. Inertial representation of angular motion in the vestibular system of rhesus monkeys. II. Otolith-controlled transformation that depends on an intact cerebellar nodulus. J. Neurophysiol. **73:** 1729–1751.
10. PAIGE, G. D. & D. L. TOMKO. 1991a. Eye movement responses to linear head motion in the squirrel monkey II. Visual-vestibular interactions and kinematic considerations. J. Neurophysiol. **65:** 1183–1196.
11. PAIGE, G. D. & D. L. TOMKO. 1991b. Eye movements responses to linear head motion in the squirrel monkey. I. Basic characteristics. J. Neurophysiol. **65:** 1170–1182.
12. SCHWARZ, U. & F. A. MILES. 1991. Ocular responses to translation and their dependence on viewing distance. I. Motion of the observer. J. Neurophysiol. **66:** 851–864.
13. PAIGE, G. D., G. R. BARNES, L. TELFORD & S. H. SEIDMAN. 1996. Influence of sensorimotor context on the linear vestibulo-ocular reflex. Ann. N. Y. Acad Sci. This volume.
14. ANGELAKI, D. E. & B. J. M. HESS. Three-dimensional organization of otolith-ocular reflexes in rhesus monkeys. I. Linear acceleration responses during off-vertical axis rotations. J. Neurophysiol. In press.
15. ANGELAKI, D. E. & B. J. M. HESS. Three-dimensional organization of otolith-ocular reflexes in rhesus monkeys. II. Inertial detection of angular velocity. J. Neurophysiol. In press.
16. HASLWANTER, T., D. STRAUMANN, B. J. M. HESS & V. HENN. 1992. Static roll and pitch in the monkey: Shift and rotation of Listing's plane. Vision Res. **32:** 1341–1348.
17. BARMACK, N. H. 1981. A comparison of the horizontal and vertical vestibulo-ocular reflexes of the rabbit. J. Physiol. **314:** 547–564.
18. ANGELAKI, D. E. 1992a. Two-dimensional coding of linear acceleration and the angular velocity sensitivity of the otolith system. Biol. Cybern. **67:** 511–522.
19. SARGENT, E. W. & G. D. PAIGE. 1991. The primate vestibulo-ocular reflex during combined linear and angular head motion. Exp. Brain Res. **87:** 75–84.
20. VIIRRE, E., D. TWEED, K. MILNER & T. VILIS. 1986. A reexamination of the gain of the vestibuloocular reflex. J. Neurophysiol. **56:** 439–450.
21. SNYDER, L. H. & W. M. KING. 1992. Effect of viewing distance and location of the axis of head rotation on the monkey's vestibuloocular reflex. I. Eye movement responses. J. Neurophysiol. **67:** 861–874.
22. ANGELAKI, D. E., B. J. M. HESS & J. I. SUZUKI. 1995. Differential processing of semicircular canal signals in the vestibuloocular reflex. J. Neurosci. **15:** 7201–7216.
23. ANGELAKI, D. E. 1992b. Detection of rotating gravity signals. Biol. Cybern. **67:** 523–533.
24. HAIN, T. C. 1986. A model of the nystagmus induced by off vertical axis rotation. Biol. Cybern. **54:** 337–350.
25. HESS, B. J. M. 1992. Three-dimensional head angular velocity detection from otolith afferent signals. Biol. Cybern. **67:** 323–333.
26. HESS, B. J. M. & D. E. ANGELAKI. 1993. Angular velocity detection by head movements orthogonal to the plane of rotation. Exp. Brain Res. **95:** 77–83.
27. ANGELAKI, D. E. & B. J. M. HESS. 1995b. Lesion of the nodulus and ventral uvula abolish steady-state off-vertical axis otolith response. J. Neurophysiol. **73:** 1716–1720.
28. WOELLNER, R. C. & A. GRAYBIEL. 1959. Counterrolling of the eyes and its dependence on the magnitude of gravitational or inertial force acting laterally on the body. J. Appl. Physiol. **14:** 632–634.
29. BAARSMA, E. A. & H. COLLEWIJN. 1975. Eye movements due to linear accelerations in the rabbit. J. Physiol. **245:** 227–247.
30. BARMACK, N. H. & V. E. PETTOROSSI. 1988. The otolith origin of the vertical vestibuloocular reflex following bilateral blockage of the vertical semicircular canals in the rabbit. J. Neurosci. **8:** 2827–2835.
31. CRAWFORD, J. D. & T. VILIS. 1991. Axes of eye rotation and Listing's law during rotations of the head. J. Neurophysiol. **65:** 407–423.

32. CRAWFORD, J. D. & T. VILIS. 1992. Symmetry of oculomotor burst neuron coordinates about Listing's plane. J. Neurophysiol. **68:** 432–448.
33. HESS, B. J. M. & D. E. ANGELAKI. 1995. Dynamic control of primary position and Listing's coordinates as a function of head position in space in rhesus monkeys. Soc. Neurosci. Abstr. **21:** 1199.
34. SKAVENSKI, A. A. & D. A. ROBINSON. 1973. Role of abducens neurons in vestibuloocular reflex. J. Neurophysiol. **36:** 724–738.
35. FERNANDEZ, C. & J. M. GOLDBERG. 1976. Physiology of peripheral neurons innervating otolith organs of the squirrel monkey. III. Response dynamics. J. Neurophysiol. **39:** 996–1008.

Modeling the Organization of the Linear and Angular Vestibulo-Ocular Reflexes[a]

THEODORE RAPHAN,[b,c] SUSAN WEARNE,[b,c]
AND BERNARD COHEN[c,d]

[b]Institute of Neural & Intelligent Systems
Department of Computer and Information Sciences
Brooklyn College of the City University of New York
Brooklyn, New York 11210

[c]Department of Neurology
[d]Department of Biophysics and Physiology
Mount Sinai School of Medicine
New York, New York 10029

INTRODUCTION

Locomotion in a gravitational environment activates the otoliths and semicircular canals and excites the linear and angular vestibulo-ocular reflexes (lVOR and aVOR). This generates gaze movements which tend to compensate for head movement and to align eye orientation in space with the direction of the gravito-inertial acceleration (GIA) vector. Eccentric rotation on a centrifuge elicits composite responses of the aVOR and lVOR through angular rotation and by dynamically changing the orientation and magnitude of the GIA with respect to the subject vertical.[1–7] A technique frequently used to extract the compensatory component of the lVOR during centrifugation has been to subtract the horizontal eye velocity trace when subjects have their backs to the direction of motion from that when they face the motion.[3,6,7] This subtractive technique, which presumably eliminates the contribution of the aVOR, is based on the assumption that ocular responses to linear and angular acceleration linearly combine and obey superposition.

The idea that the lVOR and aVOR superpose has some support from responses of squirrel monkeys to sinusoidal oscillation on a centrifuge.[8] However, studies in rhesus monkeys during optokinetic after-nystagmus (OKAN) have shown that combinations of angular and linear acceleration stimuli do not necessarily superpose. Time constants of horizontal OKAN and postrotatory nystagmus in side down positions vary depending on whether eye velocity is directed toward or away from gravity.[9,10] Specifically, the time constant of horizontal OKAN is longer during head tilts that reorient the eye velocity axis by inducing downward vertical cross-coupled components, than during head tilts that induce upward vertical components.[9] These results during static head tilts can be modeled as a modification of the parameters of the system matrix characterizing velocity storage in three dimensions.[9,11] Consistent with this finding, when long-duration centripetal accelerations induce significant tilts of the GIA vector, the lVOR and aVOR responses in rhesus and cynomolgus monkeys also do not superpose.[12] Whether parameter modifications during OKAN

[a]This work was supported by grants EY 04148, NS 00294, and PSC-CUNY Award 666329.

when the head is tilted can explain the interaction of the aVOR and the IVOR during centrifugation has not been systematically studied. It is also not known whether a model of the IVOR–aVOR interaction which implements dynamic parameter variation can explain the data in humans.

The aim of this paper is to present a model that relates the characteristics of the IVOR to the response dynamics of otolith primary afferents and the characteristics of central vestibular and oculomotor neurons and explains how the IVOR and aVOR of monkeys and humans combine during linear and angular accelerations on a centrifuge.

METHODS

Animals were prepared at sterile surgery under anesthesia with dual search coils to record three-dimensional eye orientation.[13,14] Voltages proportional to the horizontal and vertical components of eye orientation were transduced by the frontal coil. Voltages proportional to the torsional component of eye orientation were transduced by a coil placed on top of the eye.

Eye movements were induced by optokinetic stimulation, by angular acceleration about an earth vertical axis with the animal either centered or at a 26-cm radius from the axis of rotation (eccentric rotation), or by rotating the animal at 60°/s in yaw about an axis tilted 60° with respect to the spatial vertical. The implanted eye was centered in the magnetic fields. Alertness was maintained by administration of amphetamine sulfate (0.3 mg/kg) intramuscularly, 30 min prior to testing.

Monkeys were rotated about a vertical axis at 40°/s² to a constant angular velocity of 400°/s, either with the head centered with respect to each rotation axis or at the end of the centrifuge arm. During centrifugation, they either faced the direction of motion or had their backs to motion. To calibrate yaw, pitch, and roll axis eye movements, animals were rotated about a spatial vertical axis at 30°/s in the presence of a lighted, textured visual surround in upright, side down, and prone positions. It was assumed that horizontal and vertical gains were close to unity in this condition.[14-16] Roll gains were assumed to be 0.6 when rotation was around a nasooccipital axis aligned with the spatial vertical[15,17] (see ref. 18 for calibration and computation of eye position and velocity in head coordinates).

Eye position data were sampled at a rate of 600 Hz per channel using the DAOS data acquisition system (Mycon Technology) running on a 386-based PC AT. Before sampling, eye position data were prefiltered by an 8-pole Butterworth filter with a corner frequency of 30 Hz. Slow-phase eye velocity was obtained by transforming the eye velocity vector to head coordinates and removing saccades with an order statistic filter.[19]

Horizontal time constants were estimated by fitting a sum of two exponential functions, representing the cupula and velocity storage modes. The cupula time constant was constrained to 4 s,[20,21] while the time constant of velocity storage was estimated from the parameters of the second exponential. The velocity storage integrator was approximated as a piecewise linear system.[9,11,16,22]

Eye position and velocity vectors were referenced to a right-handed, head-fixed coordinate frame (FIG. 1). The X, Y, and Z axes are the pitch, roll, and yaw axes, respectively. Eye velocities were computed in head coordinates by finding the Euler angles from the coil voltages and using standard methods for finding eye velocity from the Euler angles and their derivatives.[18] Eye velocities to the left (ω_Z), down

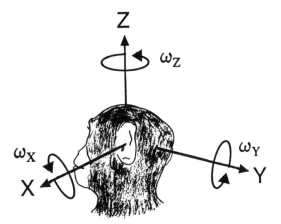

FIGURE 1. Definition of coordinate system for eye movements and stimuli. The head coordinate frame is right-handed with the positive X axis (pitch) pointing out the left ear, the positive Y axis (roll) pointing out the back of the head, and the positive Z axis (yaw) pointing out the top of the head. The positive directions of angular velocity vectors aligned with these axes correspond to angular rotations indicated by the circular arrows.

(ω_X), and counterclockwise (from the animal's point of view) (ω_Y) are represented in the figures by positive (upward) deflections in the eye velocity traces.

RESULTS: MODELING THE lVOR–aVOR INTERACTION

Conceptual Basis of the Model and Its Organization

The model of how otolith and canal processing are combined to generate the lVOR, aVOR, and their interaction due to interaural acceleration comprises two major subsystems (FIG. 2): one driven by linear head acceleration, A_X, and the other driven by angular head velocity, ω_Z. The semicircular canals respond to ω_z and generate the aVOR. The aVOR subsystem of the model has been adapted from Raphan *et al.*[16] (FIG. 2). The otoliths respond to the composite linear acceleration vector, GIA (the vector sum of A_x and gravity, A_z), and generate the regular and irregular activity of the afferents, Y_1 through Y_N (OTOLITH PROCESSING, FIG. 2, top left). The firing pattern of the afferents will be referred to as the otolith afferent activity vector. It is postulated that the central vestibular system extracts information about the linear motion of the head and the orientation of the yaw axis relative to the GIA vector from this afferent activity vector. Mechanisms that extract information related to head motion and change gaze position in accordance with changes in head position are defined as compensatory. Those that extract the orientation of the head yaw axis relative to the GIA and reorient yaw axis related response vectors with the GIA are defined as orientation mechanisms.

The orientation mechanism is modeled by a neural network, β_{OY} (FIG. 2), which operates on the otolith afferent activity vector to determine orientation of the body vertical, relative to the GIA. It generates orientation commands which would tend to

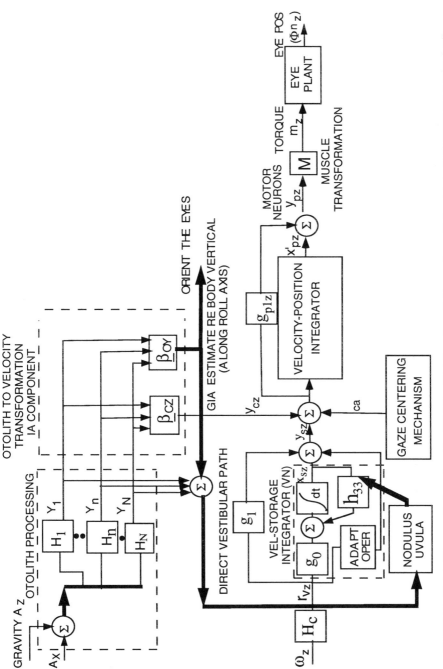

FIGURE 2. Model of linear vestibulo-ocular reflex (lVOR) and its interaction with the angular vestibulo-ocular reflex (aVOR). See text for details.

align GIA related vectors with the GIA. When the head and body are fixed, it would tend to align the yaw axis of the eye with the GIA. This mechanism produces responses such as ocular counterrolling and reorientation of the yaw axis eigenvector of velocity storage through the nodulus.[23] It also is responsible for modifying the time constant of velocity storage (FIG. 2, heavy line through h_{33}) which is related to orientation misalignments of the GIA and the head yaw axis. The specifics of this network and how it is related to the otolith afferent activity vector are beyond the scope of this paper.

The characteristics of the compensatory network can be derived by considering the functional requirements of the compensatory lVOR. Because the end organ senses head acceleration, the compensatory lVOR requires two integrations to drive the motoneurons that code the position of the eyes to compensate for the head motion. No specialized motoneurons drive the linear and angular VORs,[24] and a common velocity-position integrator provides the appropriate matching for the oculomotor plant dynamics.[25,26] The compensatory lVOR must therefore share the velocity-position integrator with the aVOR, necessitating an earlier integration of the linear acceleration signal sensed by the otoliths, which then drives the final common integrator. This integration must be implemented by processing the otolith afferent activity vector.

Otolith Afferent Processing

Fernandez and Goldberg[27–29] identified a range of otolith afferents which they classified on the basis of regularity of firing frequency. Regularly firing afferents had an approximately constant gain with respect to acceleration from D.C. to 2.0 Hz and a phase close to zero that declined monotonically after about 0.1 Hz (FIG. 3A). To a trapezoid of linear acceleration, the corresponding temporal response followed the stimulus closely with a small decline over a 90-s interval during the constant velocity phase (FIG. 3B). Irregularly firing afferents had a rising gain and a rising and falling phase characteristic, with a small phase lead of about 30° over the same frequency range (FIG. 3C). During the acceleration trapezoid, the firing rate of irregularly discharging afferents peaked at a higher level and had a greater initial decline (FIG. 3D), but with approximately the same dominant time constant as the regular afferents.

The overall transfer function for each otolith afferent class can be modeled by cascading three systems given by $H(s) = H_I H_V H_M$ (cf. refs. 27–29). The term H_I represents a long time constant integrative process, H_M represents the mechanical transduction process, and H_V represents a velocity-sensitive process. We have assumed that there are three poles in the combined transfer function $H(s)$, representing modes common to all afferents. That is, all afferents possess a long time constant integrative mode, $1/(s + h_I)$, a mechanical mode, $1/(s + h_M)$, and a velocity-sensitive integrative mode, $1/(s + h_V)$. The numerators in the transfer functions of different afferents effect the degree of compensation, giving rise to the different afferent classes.

The transfer function for a regular afferent is given by:

$$H(s) = \frac{(s + 0.022)(s + 0.099)(s + 15)}{(s + 0.025)(s + 0.1)(s + 10)} \tag{1}$$

The amplitude and phase characteristics for equation 1 (FIG. 3E) closely approximate the regular afferent data of Fernandez and Goldberg[27–29] (FIG. 3A). A small phase lead is found at low frequencies and a phase lag that increases at higher

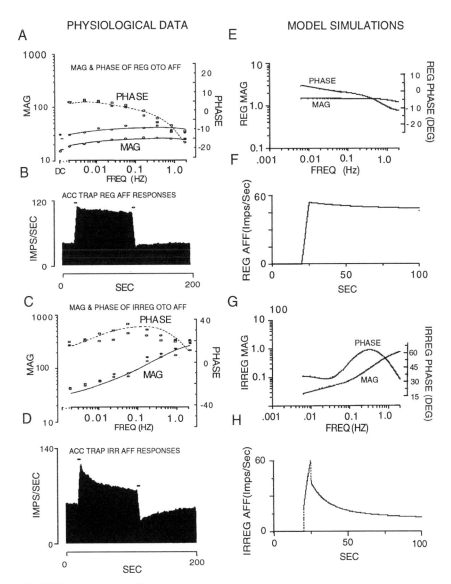

FIGURE 3. Comparison of frequency domain and time domain responses of regular (**A** and **B**) and irregular (**C** and **D**) otolith afferents with corresponding model predictions (**E** and **F**). Physiological data from Fernandez and Goldberg.[27-29]

frequencies. The amplitude response increases slightly at low frequencies but remains fairly constant over the range of frequencies considered (compare FIG. 3A and 3E). The response to a trapezoid of acceleration also followed the stimulus closely with a small decline over a 90-s interval in the constant velocity phase (FIG. 3F) and simulated the data of FIGURE 3B.

The irregular afferent transfer function is given by:

$$H(s) = \frac{(s + 0.01)(s + 0.05)(s + 0.5)}{(s + 0.025)(s + 0.1)(s + 10)} \tag{2}$$

The gain curve has less than unity slope due to the alternating pole-zero structure of the transfer function. This characterizes the transfer function of these afferents and approximates the experimental data (compare FIG. 3G and C). The phase of the transfer function given by equation 2 reaches 60°, whereas that of the experimental data reaches only 40°. The ramp response of an irregular afferent (FIG. 3D) is also fit by this model (FIG. 3H).

Equations 1 and 2 represent third-order systems with common poles and different zeros. The differences between the data and model could be reduced if a higher-order alternating pole-zero system were used. This would introduce a range of integrators for each afferent class. All otolith afferents would therefore have the appropriate dynamical modes to allow extraction of an integrative process for implementing the compensatory lVOR.

The integration is implemented by the subsystem OTOLITH TO VELOCITY TRANS-FORMATION IA COMPONENT (FIG. 2) operating on the otolith afferent activity vector produced by interaural acceleration. It linearly superposes the components of the activity vector through the neural network β_{CZ}, generating the neural velocity command, y_{cz}. The signal, y_{cz}, is summed with the neural velocity command, y_{sz}, from the combined activation of the DIRECT VESTIBULAR PATH and VELOCITY STORAGE INTEGRATOR associated with the aVOR. The combined signal, $y_{cz} + y_{sz}$, drives the velocity-position integrator (VEL-POS INTEGRATOR) and direct pathway, g_{plZ}, which activates the motoneurons to orient the eyes (EYE PLANT). Thus, the first integration in the compensatory aVOR is performed by the semicircular canals and velocity storage with its direct pathway. The first integration in the lVOR is performed by the otolith afferents and the neural network β_{CZ}. The second integration is performed by the velocity-position integrator which is common to the aVOR and lVOR.

Simulation of the Linear VOR

The frequency response of the compensatory lVOR of squirrel monkeys subjected to interaural sinusoidal linear acceleration has a rising gain and declining phase for frequencies above 0.5 Hz[30] (Paige, personal communication, 1994). Below 0.5 Hz, the gain is small and the phase is erratic[30] (Paige, personal communication, 1994). An appropriate choice of the β_{CZ} parameters predicted the dominant gain and phase characteristics for frequencies above 0.5 Hz (FIG. 4A). The model also simulated the human lVOR response to a bell of linear acceleration. For this stimulus, eye velocity in the human rose following a small delay, reaching a peak value at the peak stimulus velocity. Eye velocity then decayed to a steady-state value. The peak value of compensatory eye velocity varied inversely with viewing distance[31] (FIG. 4B).

The effects of different viewing distances were simulated by adjusting the gain of the otolith-to-velocity transformation (multiplying the β_{CZ} vector by a constant) according to viewing distances of 1, 2, 3, and 4 m^{-1} (FIG. 4D). The shapes and characteristics of the simulated responses approximated the human data (compare FIG. 4B and C). In order to fit the human responses, the lVOR gains obtained from simulating the frequency domain data from the squirrel monkey (FIG. 4A and B) had to be multiplied by an order of magnitude factor. The reason for the discrepancy in

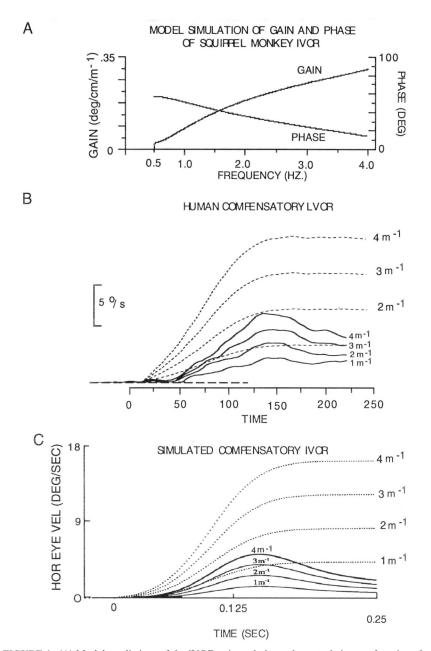

FIGURE 4. (**A**) Model predictions of the IVOR gain and phase characteristics as a function of frequency. The model parameters were chosen to approximate average gain and phase behavior of the IVOR in squirrel monkeys normalized with respect to viewing distance[30] (also, Paige, personal communication, 1994). The gain was doubled to obtain the correct response magnitude for the experiment described in FIGURE 5. (**B**) Human compensatory IVOR to bell of interaural linear acceleration, with four different viewing distances.[3] (**C**) Response of the model to a bell of linear acceleration at four viewing distances (1, 0.5, 0.33, and 0.25 m). Data on human compensatory IVOR from Bussetini *et al.*[31]

gains is not known, but may be due to differences in experimental conditions and the attempt to extrapolate squirrel monkey data to human responses. Regardless, the fact that we could predict the gain and phase characteristics of otolith units, extract the gain and phase characteristics of the lVOR response in squirrel monkeys, and from this predict the dominant characteristics of the lVOR response in humans in this simple manner, suggests that the lVOR is structured according to the principles utilized in this realization.

Simulation of Combined Linear and Angular Accelerations during Centrifugation

For rotation about a vertical axis, horizontal eye velocity rose during the period of angular acceleration to a peak value of close to $200°/s$. During the constant velocity period, eye velocity decayed with a time constant of approximately 14 s. Vertical and roll components of eye velocity were approximately zero throughout the stimulus. In contrast, eccentric rotation on the centrifuge changed the direction of the GIA vector with respect to the head and increased its magnitude. This changed the orientation and dynamic characteristics of eye velocity. Horizontal eye velocity rose during the angular acceleration and then decayed approximately exponentially during constant velocity rotation (FIG. 5A). A vertical component of eye velocity, ω_x, was induced such that the eye velocity vector reoriented toward the tilted GIA (FIG. 5A). The main differences in eye velocity responses were between facing and back-to-motion conditions. The eye velocity had a more curved buildup and faster decay when facing than when back to motion (FIG. 5B and C). These differences indicate a shorter horizontal time constant when facing motion than when back to motion.

The model (FIG. 2) was used to test whether the time constant variation of velocity storage was responsible for the facing/back asymmetries in velocity profiles. Because the GIA angle increases as the centrifuge accelerates, we expected a dynamic reduction in the horizontal time constant during centrifugation. The equation for the reduction in time constant as a function of tilt angle was obtained from OKAN data obtained during static head tilts (FIG. 5D and E). Linear fits to the OKAN time constants for leftward, rightward, left ear down, and right ear down conditions were obtained by regression analysis (FIG. 5D and E). By incorporating these functions to modulate the time constant of velocity storage dynamically, the simulations (solid black curves, FIG. 5B and C) overlaid the data (FIG. 5B and C, shaded regions) with negligible error.

The ability to predict centrifuge data from time constant data during OKAN (FIG. 5B and C, solid lines) demonstrates that the spatial properties of velocity storage are the same during dynamic as during static GIA variations. The close predictions of the centrifuge data by the aVOR model with time constant variation suggests that the direct contribution of the compensatory lVOR is minimal in these monkeys. This is in accordance with the low gain of the lVOR at low frequencies found in squirrel monkeys.[30]

Using dynamic time constant variations and the compensatory lVOR, we attempted to fit human responses to centrifugation. Although good fits were obtained to a typical human response during on-axis rotation by including an adaptation operator,[32] time constant variation and the compensatory lVOR alone could not adequately fit previously recorded human response to centrifugation[5,6] (FIG. 6A). In humans, back to motion eye velocity (FIG. 6B) is significantly smaller than when centered (FIG. 6A) or during facing motion.[5,6] The back to motion traces are characterized by a sharp truncation in peak eye velocity and a reduced time constant.

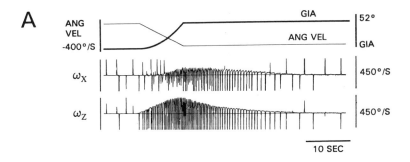

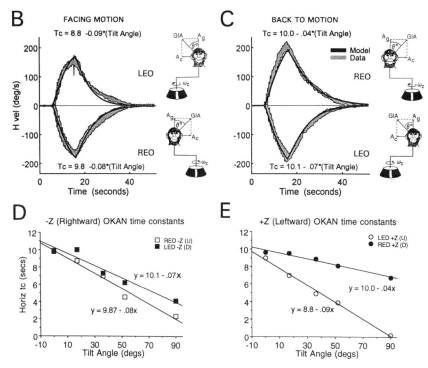

FIGURE 5. (**A**) Eye velocity response to angular acceleration of $40°/s^2$ on a centrifuge. The response is characterized by a buildup and decay of horizontal eye velocity (ω_Z) as well as vertical eye velocity (ω_X). (**B**) The horizontal eye velocity of overlaid traces during facing motion (**B**, shaded traces) for left ear out (LEO) and right ear out (REO) were fit by the model of the aVOR when the time constant of velocity storage was made to decline dynamically as a function of GIA tilt relative to the head (**B**, solid line overlaying data). Similar fits were obtained during back to motion (**C**). The time constant as a function of angle between head yaw and GIA direction used to fit the data for leftward and rightward eye velocities are shown above and below the data. The time constant variation as a function of GIA direction relative to the head was consistent with the corresponding time constants obtained during horizontal OKAN with the head tilted (**D** and **E**). The open symbols indicate horizontal time constants during upward cross-coupling (U); the filled symbols represent time constants measured during downward cross-coupling (D). Each symbol represents measurement of one time constant.

To fit these data, we included a gaze-centering mechanism which generates an eye velocity component, (FIG. 2, ca), dependent on the direction and magnitude of the beating field. This signal increases nonlinearly with the buildup of the IVOR eye velocity command signal, and causes the sharp truncation of eye velocity that was observed when back to motion.[6] This important nonlinearity is present in the IVOR

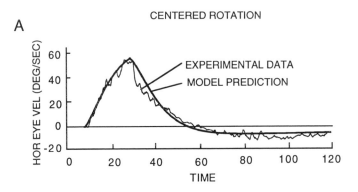

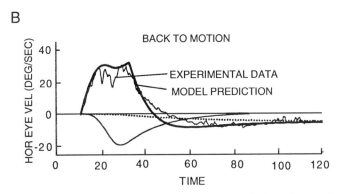

FIGURE 6. Model simulations (*heavy line*) overlaying human horizontal eye velocity data during centered rotation and centrifugation. During centered rotation (**A**), eye velocity builds up and decays with a time constant equal to that of velocity storage driven by the eighth nerve output. The undershoot is due to adaptation. For back to motion centrifugation (**B**), the eye velocity could not be predicted from the superposition of the IVOR and aVOR component responses. It was necessary to include a velocity component due to effects of beating field, called the "center of attention" component. Inclusion of this component produced an appropriate "clamping" in the simulated peak eye velocity, which corresponds closely to the profile of the data. (From Wearne.[6])

of humans but not in monkeys. Thus, the monkey response to centrifugation is characterized by a low-gain compensatory IVOR and a dominant time constant variation. The human response is characterized by three components: dynamic time constant variation in the aVOR, an eye velocity component from the center of attention mechanism, ca, and one from the direct compensatory IVOR, y_{cz} (FIG. 6B).

DISCUSSION

This study has shown that the dominant behavior of the IVOR can be modeled from the response characteristics of otolith afferents to linear acceleration. Responses to linear acceleration on a sled and to centrifugation were simulated. Model simulations suggest that linear acceleration affects the aVOR in two ways: by direct activation of the compensatory IVOR which superposes with the aVOR, and by dynamic modification of the time constants of velocity storage as the GIA vector tilts with respect to the head. In cynomolgus and rhesus monkeys, orientation effects of linear acceleration on velocity storage adequately explained the responses to centrifugation, showing that the compensatory IVOR plays a negligible role. This is different from that in humans, where changes in beating field are more pronounced[6] and, according to the model, significantly affect compensatory eye velocity.

Based largely on the high-frequency gain characteristics of the IVOR, it has been argued that the time derivative of linear acceleration, or linear jerk, is the driving signal.[33–36] Dynamic analysis of the spatiotemporal responses of central vestibular neurons to linear acceleration in different head planes of decerebrate and anesthetized rats[35,36] has recently been used in support of this view. By characterizing central neural response properties in two rather than one dimension, a linear jerk signal can be represented as the minor axis (S_{min}) of a "response ellipse" that characterizes the spatiotemporal properties of broadly tuned semicircular canal related neurons.[35–37] Because the jerk-related S_{min} signal is 180° out of phase with head velocity, it has been postulated that this signal could generate horizontal eye velocity "that is compensatory (i.e., opposite in polarity) to linear head velocity."[35] However, this formulation only applies to sinusoids, and it would not be true for a ramp of acceleration. It is conceptually and mathematically incorrect to utilize a derivative as a substitute for an integral, and it does not explain the response characteristics of the IVOR under all circumstances. Moreover, the utilization of a derivative of acceleration to drive the IVOR would be counter to its compensatory function. According to the model (FIG. 2), weighted combinations of regular and irregular unit classes are linearly combined to generate the frequency characteristics of the IVOR. The response ellipse associated with central units could be explained as being due to the linear combination of otolith afferents having different polarization angles needed for implementing the integration process. This makes it unlikely that jerk is the driving signal for the IVOR. An attractive feature of the model is its ability to simulate the IVOR under a wide range of circumstances without using a derivative of acceleration, i.e., jerk.

An underlying postulate of the model (FIG. 2) was that there are two aspects of the VOR that maintain spatial constancy of gaze. Mechanisms such as the aVOR and the compensatory IVOR, which generate neural gaze signals to counter the movement of the head, are compensatory mechanisms. Those that resolve differences between an internal sense of the body vertical (yaw axis) with the externally generated GIA vector are orientation mechanisms. This is done by reorienting spatially-based vectors in the central nervous system to the GIA. One example is the alignment of the yaw eigenvector of velocity storage of the aVOR with the GIA.[9,11] In this process, the dominant eigenvalues, that is, the inverse of the time constants of velocity storage, are altered[9,11] through parametric control via the nodulus.[23] The orientation-dependent variation in the horizontal time constant as a function of the GIA proved to be a key factor in understanding the effects of linear acceleration on the aVOR in rhesus and cynomolgus monkeys. Differences in horizontal eye velocity during facing and back to motion centrifugation in squirrel monkeys[7] may also be explained by direction-dependent horizontal or vertical time constant asymmetries.

The concept of an orientation mechanism also sheds light on the behavior of ocular counterrolling. One major theoretical question regarding ocular counter-rolling has been how the central nervous system resolves ambiguous tilt and translation signals during combined GIAs.[38–43] In the absence of additional sensory information, the equivalence between gravity and linear acceleration precludes any distinction being made between them purely on the basis of primary otolith signals. Although we have not modeled the effects of linear acceleration on ocular counter-rolling, a network (B_{OY}) has been proposed that defines the relationship between linear acceleration and ocular counterrolling. When the head is statically tilted, the orientation mechanism acts to align the axis out the top of the eye, i.e., the yaw axis of the eye, with the GIA. Generally, any rotation of the GIA relative to the body vertical would tend to align the yaw axis of the eye with the GIA, if the head is fixed. This would lead to ocular counterrolling during linear interaural acceleration and forward or back to motion on a centrifuge.

From the point of view of the model, the so-called tilt-translation ambiguity is only an ambiguity in terms of the laws of physics and Einstein's equivalence principle; no ambiguity exists regarding how the vestibular system processes the signals generated in the otolith afferents by the linear acceleration vector. Orientation commands arise from the direction of the composite GIA vector and compensatory movements from the estimated motion extrapolated from the GIA. The simulations suggest that all afferents are necessary to produce the compensatory lVOR response. By analogy, we postulate that all afferents contribute to the orienting response.

Human responses to centrifugation were different from those in the monkey, and could not be explained by either an orientation-dependent time constant change or the addition of a compensatory lVOR response. There was, however, a significant shift in the beating field of the induced nystagmus in humans that moved the eyes toward the quick phase side of the lVOR.[6] This was not observed in our studies on monkeys. The beating field effect, which was incorporated into the model as a "gaze centering mechanism," suggests that a dominant effect of the lVOR in humans can also be thought of as an orienting mechanism which tends to orient the eyes toward the quick phase side. This modulates eye velocity in accordance with the change in the beating field.

Thus, the model provides a basis for understanding both the monkey and the human lVOR and its interaction with the aVOR in terms of the compensatory and orientation effects of linear acceleration. Although we have not quantitatively modeled the orientation mechanism in terms of the otolith afferent activity vector, we have established a conceptual basis for doing this by analogy with the compensatory lVOR.

SUMMARY

A one-dimensional mathematical model of the compensatory linear vestibulo-ocular reflex (lVOR) was developed. The model was based on the concept that to effect oculomotor compensation, linear head acceleration sensed by the otoliths must be integrated twice to form the angular position-related signal required by the motoneurons. This contradicts the postulate that linear acceleration is differentiated to generate "jerk," which is then used to drive the compensatory lVOR. The transfer characteristics of different otolith afferent classes[27] were modeled by a transfer function with a common modal structure and different degrees of compensation. Both the time and frequency domain behavior of regular and irregular otolith afferents were simulated. The outputs of the various afferent classes were super-posed by a linear filter to generate the velocity command which drives the oculomo-tor velocity-position integrator. The model was used to simulate the dominant gain and phase characteristics of the compensatory lVOR in monkey[30,44] and the dynamic characteristics of the compensatory human lVOR response for brief periods of linear acceleration on a sled.[31] The model was then combined with the velocity storage-based model of the angular vestibulo-ocular reflex (aVOR) to simulate the eye velocity response to centrifugation in monkey and man. The model suggests that the orientation response that modifies the time constants of the velocity storage integra-tor is the dominant aspect of the response to linear acceleration in monkey. Human responses, on the other hand, are dominated by an effect of the beating field, which modifies the eye velocity command to the oculomotor system.

ACKNOWLEDGMENT

We would like to thank Victor Rodriguez for technical assistance in making the figures.

REFERENCES

1. LANSBERG, M. P., F. E. GUEDRY & A. GRAYBIEL. 1965. Effect of changing resultant linear acceleration relative to the subject on nystagmus generated by angular acceleration. Aerosp. Med. **36:** 456–460.
2. CRAMPTON, H. C. 1966. Does linear acceleration modify cupular deflection? *In* Second Symposium on the Role of the Vestibular Organs in Space Exploration. NASA. Washington, D.C. SP-115.: 169–184.
3. YOUNG, L. R. 1967. Effects of linear acceleration on vestibular nystagmus. *In* Third Symposium on the Role of the Vestibular Organs in Space Exploration. NASA SP-152.
4. ANGELAKI, D. E. & J. H. ANDERSON. 1991. The vestibulo-ocular reflex in the cat during linear acceleration in the sagittal plane. Brain Res. **543:** 347–350.
5. CURTHOYS, I. S., S. L. WEARNE, M. J. DAI, G. M. HALMAGYI & J. R. HOLDEN. 1992. Linear acceleration modulates the nystagmus induced by angular acceleration stimulation of the horizontal canal. Ann. N.Y. Acad. Sci. **656:** 716–724.
6. WEARNE, S. 1993. Spatial orientation of the human linear and angular vestibulo-ocular reflexes during centrifugation. Ph.D. thesis. University of Sydney. Australia.
7. MERFELD, D. M. & L. R. YOUNG. 1995. The vestibulo-ocular reflex of the squirrel monkey during eccentric rotation and roll tilt. Exp. Brain Res. **106:** 111–122.
8. SARGENT, E. W. & G. D. PAIGE. 1991. The primate vestibulo-ocular reflex during combined linear and angular head motion. Exp. Brain Res. **87:** 75–84.
9. DAI, M., T. RAPHAN & B. COHEN. 1991. Spatial orientation of the vestibular system: Dependence of optokinetic after nystagmus on gravity. J. Neurophysiol. **66:** 1422–1438.
10. RAPHAN, T., M. DAI & B. COHEN. 1992. Spatial orientation of the vestibular system. Ann. N.Y. Acad. Sci. **656:** 140–157.
11. RAPHAN, T. & D. STURM. 1991. Modelling the spatiotemporal organization of velocity storage in the vestibuloocular reflex by optokinetic studies. J. Neurophysiol. **66:** 1410–1420.
12. WEARNE, S., T. RAPHAN & B. COHEN. 1994. Differential effects of compensatory gaze of interaural (IA) linear acceleration in monkey and man. Soc. Neurosci. Abstr. **20:** 1194.
13. JUDGE, S. J., B. J. RICHMOND & F. C. CHU. 1980. Implantation of magnetic search coils for measurement of eye position: An improved method. Vision Res. **20:** 535–538.
14. ROBINSON, D. A. 1963. A method of measuring eye movement using a scleral search coil in a magnetic field. IEEE Trans. Biomed. Eng. **10:** 137–145.

15. CRAWFORD, J. D. & T. VILIS. 1991. Axes of eye rotation and Listing's law during rotations of the head. J. Neurophysiol. **65:** 407–423.
16. RAPHAN, T., V. MATSUO & B. COHEN. 1979. Velocity storage in the vestibulo-ocular reflex arc (VOR). Exp. Brain Res. **35:** 229–248.
17. HENN, V., D. STRAUMANN, B. J. M. HESS, T. HASLWANTER & N. KAWACHI. 1992. Three-dimensional transformation from vestibular and visual input to oculomotor output. Ann. N. Y. Acad. Sci. **656:** 166–180.
18. YAKUSHIN, S. B., M. J. DAI, J.-I. SUZUKI, T. RAPHAN & B. COHEN. 1995. Semicircular canal contribution to the three-dimensional vestibulo-ocular reflex: A model-based approach. J. Neurophysiol. In press.
19. ENGELKIND, E. J. & K. W. STEVENS. 1990. A new approach to the analysis of nystagmus: An application for order statistic filters. Aviat. Space Environ. Med. **61:** 859–864.
20. WAESPE, W., B. COHEN & T. RAPHAN. 1983. Role of the flocculus and paraflocculus in optokinetic nystagmus and visual-vestibular interaction: Effects of lesions. Exp. Brain Res. **50:** 9–33.
21. FERNÁNDEZ, C. & J. M. GOLDBERG. 1971. Physiology of peripheral neurons innervating semicircular canals of the squirrel monkey. Response to sinusoidal stimulation and dynamics of peripheral vestibular system. J. Neurophysiol. **34:** 661–675.
22. RAPHAN, T. & B. COHEN. 1985. Velocity storage and the ocular response to multidimensional vestibular stimuli. *In* Adaptive Mechanisms in Gaze Control; Facts and Theories. A. Berthoz & G. Melvill Jones, Eds. vol. 1: 123–143. Elsevier. Amsterdam.
23. WEARNE, S., T. RAPHAN & B. COHEN. 1996. Nodulo-uvular control of central vestibular dynamics determines spatial orientation of the angular vestibulo-ocular reflex. N. Y. Acad. Sci. This volume.
24. WILSON, V. J. & G. MELVILL-JONES. 1979. Mammalian Vestibular Physiology. Plenum Press. New York.
25. ROBINSON, D. A. 1975. A quantitative analysis of extraocular muscle cooperation and squint. Invest. Ophthalmol. **14:** 801–825.
26. SKAVENSKI, A. A. & D. A. ROBINSON. 1973. Role of abducens neurons in vestibuloocular reflex. J. Neurophysiol. **36:** 724–738.
27. FERNÁNDEZ, C. & J. M. GOLDBERG. 1976. Physiology of peripheral neurons innervating otolith organs of the squirrel monkey. II. Directional selectivity and force response relations. J. Neurophysiol. **39:** 985–995.
28. FERNÁNDEZ, C. & J. M. GOLDBERG. 1976. Physiology of peripheral neurons innervating otolith organs of the squirrel monkey. I. Response to static tilts and to long duration centrifugal force. J. Neurophysiol. **39:** 970–984.
29. FERNÁNDEZ, C. & J. M. GOLDBERG. 1976. Physiology of peripheral neurons innervating otolith organs of the squirrel monkey. III. Response dynamics. J. Neurophysiol. **39:** 996–1008.
30. PAIGE, G. D. 1996. Influence of sensorimotor context on the linear vestibulo-ocular reflex. Ann. N. Y. Acad. Sci. This volume.
31. BUSETTINI, C., F. A. MILES, U. SCHWARZ & J. CARL. 1994. Human ocular responses to translation of the observer and of the scene: Dependence on viewing distance. Exp. Brain Res. **100:** 484–494.
32. YOUNG, L. R. & C. M. OMAN. 1969. Model for vestibular adaptation to horizontal rotation. Aerosp. Med. **40:** 1076–1080.
33. NIVEN, J. I., W. C. HIXSON & M. J. CORREIA. 1966. Elicitation of horizontal nystagmus by periodic linear acceleration. Acta Otolaryngol. **62:** 429–441.
34. HAIN, T. C. 1986. A model of the nystagmus induced by off vertical axis rotation. Biol. Cybern. **54:** 337–350.
35. ANGELAKI, D. E., G. A. BUSH & A. A. PERACHIO. 1993. Two-dimensional spatiotemporal coding of linear acceleration in vestibular nuclei neurons. J. Neurosci. **38:** 1053–1060.
36. BUSH, G. A., A. A. PERACHIO & D. E. ANGELAKI. 1993. Encoding of head acceleration in vestibular neurons. I. Spatiotemporal response properties to linear acceleration. J. Neurophysiol. **69:** 2039–2055.
37. SCHOR, R. H. & D. E. ANGELAKI. 1992. The algebra of neural response vectors. Ann. N. Y. Acad. Sci. **656:** 190–204.

38. MAYNE, R. 1974. A systems concept of the vestibular organs. *In* Handbook of Vestibular Physiology. Vestibular System. H. H. Kornhuber, Ed. vol. 6, part 2: 493–580. Springer-Verlag. New York.
39. LICHTENBERG, B. K., L. R. YOUNG & A. P. ARROTT. 1982. Human ocular counterrolling induced by varying linear accelerations. Exp. Brain Res. **48:** 127–136.
40. MARKHAM, C. H. 1989. Anatomy and physiology of otolith-controlled ocular counterrolling. Acta Otolaryngol. Suppl. **468:** 263–266.
41. PAIGE, G. D. & D. L. TOMKO. 1991. Eye movement responses to linear head motion in the squirrel monkey. I. Basic characteristics. J. Neurophysiol. **65:** 1170–1182.
42. PAIGE, G. D. & D. L. TOMKO. 1991. Eye movement responses to linear head motion in the squirrel monkey. II. Visual-vestibular interactions and kinematic considerations. J. Neurophysiol. **65:** 1183–1196.
43. HESS, B. J. M. & N. DIERINGER. 1991. Spatial organization of linear vestibulo-ocular reflexes of the rat: Responses during horizontal and vertical linear acceleration. J. Neurophysiol. **66:** 1805–1818.
44. TELFORD, L., S. H. SEIDMAN & G. D. PAIGE. Linear vestibulo-ocular reflex as a function of frequency and amplitude. Soc. Neurosci. Abstr.: 567.

Nodulo-Uvular Control of Central Vestibular Dynamics Determines Spatial Orientation of the Angular Vestibulo-Ocular Reflex[a]

SUSAN WEARNE,[b,c] THEODORE RAPHAN,[b,c]
AND BERNARD COHEN[b,d]

[b]Department of Neurology
[d]Department of Biophysics and Physiology
Mount Sinai School of Medicine
New York, New York 10029

[c]Institute of Neural and Intelligent Systems
Department of Computer and Information Sciences
Brooklyn College of the City University of New York
Brooklyn, New York 11210

INTRODUCTION

Behavioral data following lesions of the brainstem demonstrate that orientation of the axis of the angular vestibulo-ocular reflex (aVOR) to the spatial vertical is mediated by velocity storage and does not involve the direct vestibular pathway. Lesion and electrical stimulation studies indicate that this spatial orientation is under the control of the nodulus and ventral uvula. Longitudinal Purkinje cell zones in the nodulus and uvula of the rabbit comprise individual modules whose olivocerebellar afferents and corticonuclear efferents are tuned to axes that lie close to those of the semicircular canals. Zones determined by olivocerebellar afferents in the nodulus and uvula of the rhesus monkey have a similar organization (see Voogd[1] for review). From these morphologic data and from anatomic and behavioral results following selective lesions of the nodulus and uvula, we propose that the three-dimensional dynamics of the velocity storage system are determined by functionally independent modules of the nodulus and ventral uvula, each controlling the time constants of velocity storage about a single semicircular canal-related axis.

Spatial Orientation of the aVOR

The dynamics of vestibular nystagmus, optokinetic nystagmus (OKN), and optokinetic after-nystagmus (OKAN) are sensitive to the direction of gravito-inertial acceleration (GIA).[2–14] Tilting the GIA vector with respect to the subject during vestibular or optokinetic nystagmus reorients the axis of the compensatory eye velocity.[3,15,16] In particular, the yaw axis component of the eye velocity vector tends to align with the GIA, and the time constants of all components are modified according

[a]This work was supported by grants NS00294, EY04148, and EY01867 and PSC-CUNY Award 666329.

364

to the tilt of the GIA with respect to the head yaw axis. The combination of these processes, which we term spatial orientation of the aVOR, has been demonstrated in many primate species, including rhesus, cynomolgus, and squirrel monkeys[3,7,8,13–15,17–20] and humans.[4–6,11,21,22]

Spatial orientation of the aVOR has been modeled as a reduction in the time constant of the dominant horizontal component, an increase in the torsional and/or vertical time constants, and the appearance of orthogonal vertical or torsional "cross-coupled" components.[16] Together, these processes shift the axis of eye rotation away from the head vertical toward the GIA and change its dynamic characteristics. Several studies have postulated that the central velocity storage mechanism is responsible for spatial orientation of the aVOR, whereas the direct visual and vestibular pathways are insensitive to changes in the GIA,[13,16,22] but there has been no empirical test of this hypothesis. Midline lesions of the dorsal rostral medulla caudal to the abducens nucleus abolish velocity storage, leaving the direct vestibular and optokinetic paths intact (see Katz *et al.*[23] for review). Such discrete lesions afford the possibility for a direct test of this postulate.

In the first part of this study, we analyzed three-dimensional eye movements in midline-sectioned rhesus monkeys to assess the relative contributions of the central velocity storage mechanism and the direct visual and vestibular pathways to spatial orientation of the aVOR.

Neural Substrate of aVOR Orientation

The nodulus and ventral uvula have been implicated in control of the three-dimensional dynamic characteristics of velocity storage. Electrical stimulation of the nodulus and lobule 9d of the ventral uvula reduces the horizontal time constant of OKAN or vestibular nystagmus.[24] A similar reduction occurs when the head is tilted rapidly during post-rotary nystagmus ("tilt dumping")[8,13,20,25–28] or when subjects view a relative stationary visual surround during vestibular nystagmus or OKAN ("light dumping").[29–31] Ablation of the nodulus and ventral uvula abolishes both light dumping and tilt dumping in rhesus monkeys, and increases the horizontal time constant.[26] Cross-coupled vertical and torsional components induced during axis reorientation also depend upon the nodulus and uvula.[32,33]

Little is known of the mechanism by which the nodulus and uvula control spatial orientation of the aVOR. Central interaction of visual, vestibular, and oculomotor systems requires that their sensorimotor transformations be effected in a common reference frame.[34] Electrophysiologic studies in the rabbit flocculus and inferior olive have established that this intrinsic reference frame is closely aligned with the normals to the planes of the three semicircular canals.[35–39] The nodulus and uvula likely utilize the same coordinate system in controlling the orientation of the aVOR. Analogous to the modular structure of other parts of the cerebellum,[40–45] the nodulus and uvula are organized in sagittally oriented zones, determined by discrete olivocerebellar inputs and discrete corticonuclear projections to the vestibular and deep cerebellar nuclei.[1,46–56] In rabbit, olivocerebellar afferents convey visual and vestibular signals in coordinates close to those of the semicircular canals to different zones of the nodulus and ventral uvula,[35,39,53–55,57,64] (see Voogd[1] for review). Efferents of these canal-related zones target non-VOR relay regions of superior vestibular nucleus (SVN) and medial vestibular nucleus (MVN)[46]—i.e., those regions which do not project to the extraocular motornuclei. We refer to these regions as peripheral SVN (SVN_p) and peripheral MVN (MVN_p). These regions correspond approximately to the locations of commissural connections mediating velocity storage,[23,65] (see Büttner-Ennever[66] for review) and to the locations of canal-related "vestibular-only" (VO) neurons,[67] which are believed responsible for producing velocity storage.[68,69] These data suggest that the nodulus and uvula control the three-dimensional dynamics of velocity storage in coordinates closely aligned with those of the semicircular canals. In the second part of this study, we correlated complete and discrete lesions of the nodulus and uvula in rhesus monkeys with deficits of VOR orientation in specific spatial planes to test this hypothesis.

METHODS

Nine juvenile rhesus (*Macaca mulatta*) monkeys were used in these studies. Anatomic and behavioral data from three animals will be described in detail. An abridged description of the experimental, anatomic, and surgical methods is given below.

Experimental Paradigms

Eye movements were induced by optokinetic stimulation, by angular acceleration about an earth vertical axis with animals either centered or 26 cm eccentric from the axis of rotation (centrifugation), or by rapidly reorienting the animal during post-rotatory vestibular nystagmus. Optokinetic stimulation at 40°/s or 60°/s about the animal's yaw axis was given with the head upright or tilted 45° or 90° ear down. Animals were also tested when prone or supine. During centrifugation, animals were accelerated at 10°/s² to a final angular velocity of 400°/s, inducing a 52° tilt of the GIA vector relative to gravity. The steady-state angular velocity was maintained for up to 120 s or until eye velocity decayed to zero. By positioning the animals either tangentially or radially with respect to the direction of motion, centripetal acceleration could be directed along either the interaural or the naso-occipital axis during yaw axis centrifugation. Reorientation during post-rotatory nystagmus (tilt dumping) was performed by rotating the animals in yaw at 60°/s about a spatial vertical axis, until the per-rotatory nystagmus had decayed to zero. Rotation was then stopped, inducing post-rotatory nystagmus. Two seconds later, the animal was reoriented by rotating through 90° to the ear down or prone/supine position. Light dumping was performed by exposing the animal to a relative stationary surround during vestibular nystagmus or OKAN.

Measurement of Three-Dimensional Eye Orientation

Three-dimensional eye orientation was recorded using dual search coils implanted on either the left or the right eye. Voltages proportional to horizontal and vertical eye position were transduced by a frontal coil placed concentrically around the iris; voltages proportional to the torsional component of eye orientation were transduced by a coil sutured under the superior rectus on the top of the eye.[70,71] The monkey's head and the field coils were fixed to the primate chair.

Coordinates and Notation

With the monkey erect, the yaw axis was aligned with gravity, and the horizontal stereotaxic plane was aligned with the gravitational horizontal. The three-dimensional components of the vestibular stimuli and the oculomotor responses were referenced to the right-handed Cartesian coordinate system shown in FIGURE 1A. The X, Y, and Z axes denote the interaural (positive left), naso-occipital (positive backward), and dorsoventral (positive up) axes of the head, respectively. Three-dimensional eye orientation was represented as Euler angles. The components of the eye velocity vector in head coordinates, symbolized $\omega = [\omega_x, \chi_y, \omega_z]$ and denoting vertical, torsional, and horizontal rotations, were obtained directly from the Euler angles and their derivatives.[72,73]

The relationship between the coordinate frames used to describe neural responses in the rabbit and oculomotor responses in the monkey is indicated in FIGURE 1B. The dashed lines show the visual sensitivity axes[e] of neurons in the left nodulus and in subnuclei of the right inferior olive of the rabbit. Complex spike activity of

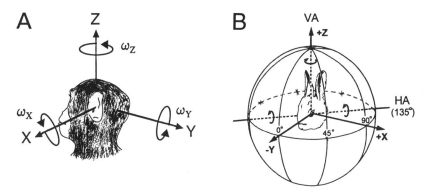

FIGURE 1. (A) Right-handed coordinate frame to which components of the eye velocity vector are referred. Positive direction of rotation about each axis is defined according to the right-hand rule, as leftward yaw ($+\omega_Z$), downward pitch ($+\omega_X$), and counterclockwise roll ($+\omega_Y$), from the animal's point of view. (B) Intrinsic coordinate frame used to describe maximal sensitivity axes for visual modulation of neurons in the left nodulus and right inferior olive of the rabbit (after Simpson and Graf[36]), and the head reference frame used to measure eye movements in this paper [+X, −Y, +Z]. The excitatory direction for complex spike responses of Purkinje cells in the left nodulus is indicated by the curved arrows about axes VA and HA (135°). The positive pole of the HA (135°) axis is thus rotated 45° clockwise about the +Z axis.

Purkinje cells in the rabbit nodulus is tuned to optokinetic stimulation about a vertical axis, VA, or about a horizontal axis, HA (135°). The VA axis is aligned with the +Z head axis while the positive pole of the HA (135°) axis is rotated counterclockwise about the +Z axis by 135° from the forward pointing pole of the naso-occipital (−Y) axis. Thus, the VA axis is aligned approximately with the axis of the lateral canals, and the HA (135°) axis is aligned with the axis of the ipsilateral (left) anterior canal and contralateral (right) posterior canal.[36,39,46] The VA and the HA (135°) are the predominant axes represented on visual climbing fibers in the left nodulus.[36,46,74] Complex spike responses tuned to optokinetic stimulation about the axis of the ipsilateral posterior canal are represented in the contralateral nodulus. By contrast, complex spike responses to angular acceleration aligned with the axes of the

[e]The sensitivity axis of a neuron is that axis around which head or surround rotation causes maximal modulation of its firing rate.

ipsilateral posterior canal (PC) and ipsilateral anterior canal (AC) are both represented in the ipsilateral nodulus.[54,55,57]

EFFECTS OF MIDLINE MEDULLARY SECTION ON VELOCITY STORAGE

In accordance with previous results,[23,65,66,75,76] interruption of crossing axons in the rostral medulla in M613 abolished velocity storage. The lesion was in the midline just caudal to the abducens nuclei. It extended approximately 2 mm below the surface of the 4th ventricle. The rostral portion of the lesion was angled slightly to the

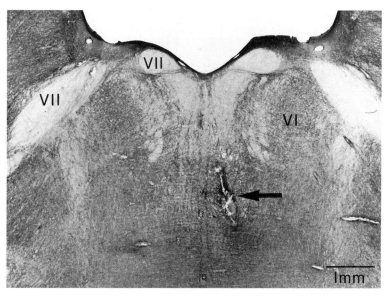

FIGURE 2. Coronal section from immunostained material used in the reconstruction of FIGURE 3A, showing the most rostral extension of the midline medullary section in M613. The lesion (*arrow*) is just to the left of the midline, angled slightly left, and starts below the genu of the facial nerve and the abducens nuclei. It is ventral and medial to the abducens rootlets that lie in the medial portions of the abducens nuclei at this level.

left. It lay under decussating fibers between the abducens nuclei and was medial and ventral to the abducens rootlets (FIG. 2, arrow). Oligosynaptic pathways responsible for the short-latency aVOR that course through the region of the abducens nuclei would have been spared by this lesion. The extent of the lesion, reconstructed on a 0.75 mm lateral parasagittal schematic, is shown in FIGURE 3A. Commissural connections likely to be involved in mediating velocity storage[23,66,68] that would have been severed by this lesion are shown in FIGURE 3B.

The gain of the short-latency (direct) aVOR was not diminished by the midline section. Instead, small but nonsignificant increases were observed postoperatively in both aVOR and OKN gains. In response to a 60°/s step of angular velocity, the average aVOR gain increased from 0.88 ± 0.06 preoperatively to 0.94 ± 0.11 postoperatively for leftward slow phases, and from 0.71 ± 0.04 preoperatively to

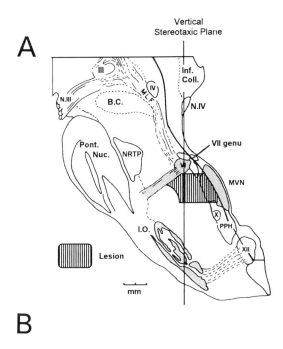

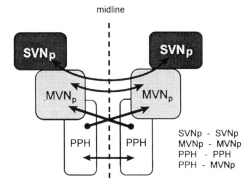

FIGURE 3. (A) Sagittal reconstruction demonstrating the extent of lesion in M613. The lesion was reconstructed from coronal sections similar to that shown in FIGURE 2. Although the lesion was in the midline, it is plotted on a sagittal section drawn 0.75 mm from the midline to aid in identification of surrounding brain-stem structures. The vertical striped region corresponds to the lesioned area. It lies between the medial vestibular nuclei (MVN) and prepositus hypoglossi (PPH). Rostrally, the lesion extended just caudal to the abducens nucleus (VI) and rootlets. (B) Commissural connections between PPH and non-VOR relay zones of SVN (SVN$_p$) and MVN (MVN$_p$) hypothesized to mediate velocity storage (after Büttner-Ennever,[66] Katz *et al.*[23] and Yokota *et al.*[68]). III, oculomotor nucleus; N III, third cranial nerve; BC, brachium conjunctivum; Inf. Coll., inferior colliculus; IV, trochlear nucleus; N IV, fourth cranial nerve; MLF, median longitudinal fasciculus; NRTP, nucleus reticularis tegmenti pontis; Pont. nuc., pontine nuclei; VII genu, genu of seventh cranial nerve; X, dorsal vagus nucleus; XII, glossopharyngeal nucleus; I.O., inferior olive. SVN$_p$, SVN peripheral, non-VOR relay areas of SVN; MVN$_p$, MVN peripheral, non-VOR relay areas of MVN.

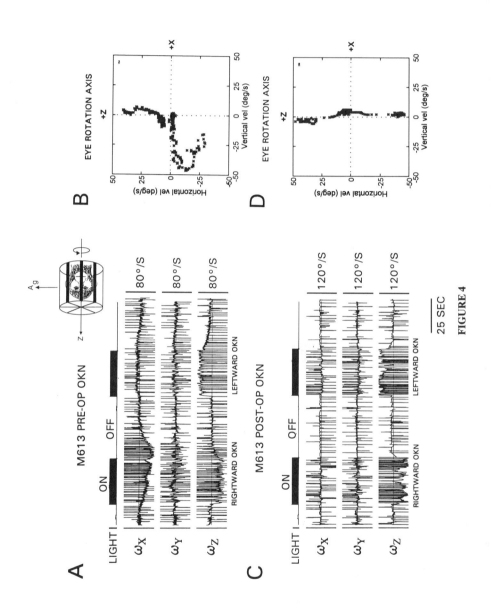

FIGURE 4

0.79 ± 0.01 postoperatively for rightward slow phases. The postoperative gain of horizontal OKN in response to 60°/s steps of surround velocity (FIG. 4C) was unchanged from its preoperative level (FIG. 4A). Mean OKN gains increased from 0.59 ± 0.4 preoperatively to 0.71 postoperatively for leftward slow phases, and from 0.56 ± 0.12 preoperatively to 0.63 postoperatively for rightward slow phases. Neither increase was significant. These data indicate that the lesion did not involve the direct VOR and OKN pathways.

The horizontal VOR time constant during angular velocity steps of 60°/s was initially asymmetric with a leftward preponderance. Postoperatively, it fell from 19.1 ± 2.7 s to 5.8 ± 2.1 s for leftward slow phases, and from 7.6 ± 2.1 s to 5.4 ± 0.2 s for rightward slow phase eye velocities. Both effects were significant (paired t tests: mean leftward decrease = 13.29 s, p = .001; mean rightward decrease = 2.15 s, p < .001). These postoperative values are close to the average time constant of activity recorded from primary semicircular canal afferents in squirrel monkeys.[77-80]

All other oculomotor functions related to velocity storage were correspondingly affected. Horizontal OKAN, which was prominent before lesion (FIG. 4A, trace ω_Z), was lost after surgery (FIG. 4C). The horizontal OKAN time constant decreased from 12.8 ± 2.9 s to 1.7 ± 0.6 s during leftward OKAN (mean decrease = 11.01 s, p = .011) and from 8.1 ± 1.9 s to 1.8 ± 0.2 s during rightward OKAN (mean decrease = 6.3 s, p = .018). The animal was able to hold lateral gaze in darkness and in light, demonstrating that the velocity-position integrator had not been affected by the midline lesion, and that the short time constants were not attributable to deficiencies in the velocity-position integrator. These results collectively indicate that the midline section had abolished velocity storage in M613, sparing direct pathways from the semicircular canals and the visual system responsible for rapid compensatory eye movements.

EFFECTS OF MIDLINE SECTION ON ORIENTATION OF EYE ROTATION AXES

In addition to a compensatory horizontal nystagmus, optokinetic stimulation in yaw with the head tilted typically produces orthogonal vertical and torsional components of eye velocity. Because both direct and velocity storage paths are excited during OKN in normal animals, their relative contributions to axis reorientation cannot be assessed unequivocally on behavioral grounds, raising the possibility that

←
―――

FIGURE 4. OKN and OKAN before (A and B) and after (C and D) midline section in M613. From top to bottom, the data traces are stimulus (light ON/OFF), vertical eye velocity (ω_x), roll eye velocity (ω_Y), and horizontal eye velocity (ω_Z). The phase plane graphs (B and D) were generated by plotting the horizontal component of the eye velocity vector, ω_Z, against the vertical component ω_X. The decaying portions of eye velocity, starting 2 s after the end of OKN and continuing until eye velocity reached zero, were used in these graphs. Responses for $+Z$ rotation are shown above the abscissa, and responses for $-Z$ rotation below the abscissa. Stimulus velocities were 40°/s in A and 60°/s in C. (A) Preoperatively, M613 had normal OKN and OKAN with a longer horizontal time constant during downward ($+\omega_X$) than upward ($-\omega_X$) cross-coupling. Strong upward cross-coupling was present during both OKN (light ON period) and OKAN (light OFF period), producing a strong shift in the eye velocity axis of the phase plane graph B. (C) Postoperatively, OKAN was abolished (ω_Z trace) and no cross-coupling to vertical was present during either the OKN or OKAN periods. Despite the higher stimulus velocity in the postoperative traces (60°/s), the OKN gain was not affected by the lesion. The eye rotation axis remained aligned with the Z axis (D).

the direct OKN path might contribute to axis reorientation. In the preoperative example shown in FIGURE 4A and B, with the animal in the ear-down position, the axis of eye rotation shifted primarily in the roll plane toward alignment with the tilted GIA (FIG. 4A, trace ω_X; 4B). Typical of many monkeys,[18,81] M613 had a significant up > down vertical asymmetry, producing larger roll-plane axis shifts for upward ($-\omega_x$) than for downward ($+\omega_x$) coupled components. As in humans,[22] strong cross-coupling was also present during OKN (light ON period), preoperatively.

Following abolition of velocity storage with loss of OKAN, no cross-coupling of OKN was present, either during roll-plane (FIG. 4C and D) or pitch-plane head tilts, and the eye velocity vector decayed purely along the Z axis in each of the paradigms tested. Centrifugation induced similar results: the eye velocity vector, now produced solely by the direct vestibular pathway, remained in head coordinates and did not shift toward the GIA. These data demonstrate that spatial orientation of the aVOR is mediated through velocity storage, and that the direct vestibular and optokinetic paths are insensitive to the direction of the GIA.

LESIONS OF NODULUS AND UVULA

The nodulus and uvula can be subdivided into parasagittal zones comprising strips of Purkinje cells, innervated by a particular subnucleus of the inferior olive and projecting to particular cerebellar or vestibular target nuclei.[41,48,82] Based on the sensitivity axes of their olivocerebellar afferents, the zones of the nodulus and uvula in rabbit are organized in semicircular canal coordinates (FIG. 5). Climbing fiber afferents have been identified functionally as visual (optokinetic) or vestibular, aligned approximately with the axis of one of the three semicircular canals (FIG. 1B). Optokinetic signals about a vertical axis (VA OKN) originate from the caudal dorsal cap (cdc), whereas optokinetic signals tuned approximately to the axis of the ipsilateral anterior canal [horizontal axis, HA (135°) OKN] originate from the rostral dorsal cap (rdc) and ventrolateral outgrowth (vlo).[35,37,39,55,58–60,74] Vestibular signals aligned with the anterior and posterior canal axes (AC and PC VOR signals) project from the beta nucleus of the inferior olive.[57,59–62,83] Utricular signals project from the dorsomedial cell column (DMCC).[53] No VA vestibular signals from the lateral semicircular canals have been recorded on climbing fiber afferents to the nodulus or uvula.[54,55]

The sagittal zones created by the olivocerebellar system coincide with the longitudinally organized corticonuclear efferent system.[48] In rabbit, Wylie and colleagues[46] have correlated the climbing fiber zones of the ventral surface of the nodulus with Purkinje cell projections to the vestibular and deep cerebellar nuclei (FIG. 5). In a variety of species, nodular Purkinje cells target the non-relay zones of the vestibular nuclei, specifically peripheral and dorsal SVN,[46,56,84] and non-VOR relay regions of MVN, including caudal MVN[46,51,56,85,86] and portions of rostral MVN[56] (McCrea, personal communication, 1995) (FIG. 5). These projection regions correspond to the locations of posterior and anterior canal-related VO neurons in SVN_p and horizontal canal-related VO neurons in rostral areas of MVN_p that are believed responsible for the production of velocity storage.[68,69] They also coincide with the location of terminations of commissural fibers which are believed to mediate velocity storage[23,66,68] (cf. FIG. 5 and FIG. 3B).

Anatomic data of Gerrits and Voogd[1] indicate that the rhesus monkey nodulus has a similar organization to that of the rabbit. Four sagittal zones, based on four white matter compartments innervated by discrete subnuclei of the contralateral inferior olive have been distinguished.[1] We have designated these as zones 1–4 (FIG.

6A; FIG. 9)./ In rhesus monkey, the most medial zone (zone 1), which comprises two subzones, extends from the midline to 0.8 mm lateral in the formalin-fixed nodulus and uvula (FIG. 6A) and receives climbing fiber input from the beta nucleus medially and the cdc laterally. Zone 1 therefore corresponds to the first and second zones in the rabbit (FIG. 5). The second zone (zone 2), which extends from 0.8 to 2.4 mm

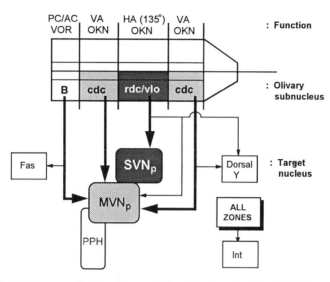

FIGURE 5. Modular organization of the ventral nodulus, based on the distribution of olivocerebellar afferents and corticonuclear efferents. Four white-matter compartments of the ventral nodulus of the rabbit with function of climbing fiber input (*above*) and projections to the vestibular and deep cerebellar nuclei (*below*), from the data of Wylie and colleagues.[46] SVN_p and MVN_p refer to non-VOR relay regions of the superior and medial vestibular nuclei. Dark shading indicates zones of the nodulus and vestibular nuclei tuned to vertical canal-related axes. Light shading indicates zones tuned to VA or lateral canal-related axes. All of the arrows below represent corticonuclear projections. The heavy arrows to SVN_p and MVN_p represent projections postulated to be important for control of spatial orientation of velocity storage: The two cdc zones (VA OKN) project to MVN_p and the rdc/vlo zone [HA (135°) OKN] to SVN_p and the dorsal Y group. *Abbreviations*: B, beta nucleus; cdc, caudal dorsal cap; rdc, rostral dorsal cap; vlo, ventrolateral outgrowth; Fas, fastigial nucleus; Int, interposed nucleus; PPH, prepositus hypoglossi; Dorsal Y, dorsal Y group; PC/AC VOR, vestibular signals aligned with the axes of the posterior and anterior canals; HA and VA OKN, optokinetic signals aligned with horizontal and vertical axes. (Adapted from Wylie *et al.*[46])

through both dorsal and ventral lamellae of the nodulus and into the uvula (FIG. 6A), was labeled from injections which included the vlo and rostral beta nucleus. Similar to the rabbit, the nodular projection is probably restricted to climbing fibers from the vlo, while fibers from the rostral beta nucleus may extend into the uvula.[1] Zone 3, innervated by the cdc, extends from 2.4 to 3.2 mm and is restricted to the nodulus. An

---

/The olivocerebellar projection zones indicated in FIGURES 6A and 9 were inferred from injections which included several olivary subnuclei, and cannot be identified unambiguously on this basis.[1] For this reason, olivary subnuclei indicated as projecting to zones in FIGURE 9 represent the most likely projections, by analogy with the organization in rabbit.

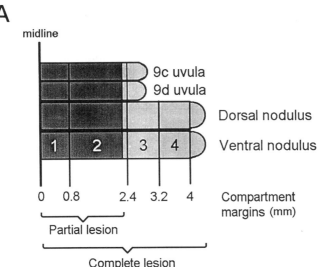

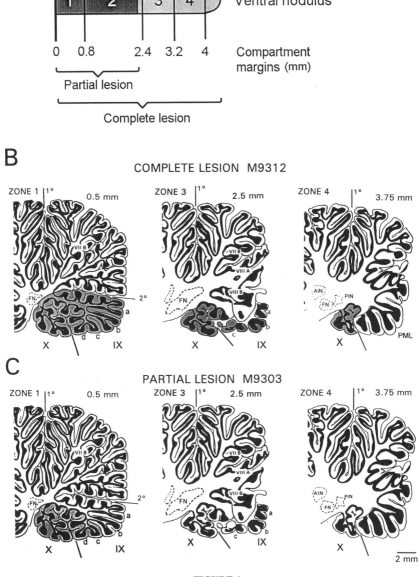

FIGURE 6

auxiliary projection to this zone from the beta nucleus cannot be excluded, but is unlikely in the nodulus.[1] Zone 4 extends from 3.2 to 4 mm lateral in the nodulus. Its olivocerebellar afferents are currently unidentified in rhesus monkey, but by analogy with the lateral zone in rabbit, probably include the DMCC medially and rostral medial accessory olive (rMAO) laterally in the dorsal lamella, and the cdc as a lateral extension of zone 3, in the ventral lamella of the nodulus.[52,59,60]

Description of Nodulo-Uvular Lesions

Two types of lesion were performed. Complete nodulo-uvulectomy ablated zones 1–4 of the nodulus (FIG. 6A and B). The uvular lesion was complete in lobules 9c and 9d, but lobules 9a and 9b were left intact laterally (FIG. 6B). Partial nodulo-uvulectomy was also performed, in which zones 1 and 2 of the nodulus and ventral uvula (lobules 9c and 9d) were removed, but zones 3 and 4 of the nodulus were spared (FIG. 6A and C). This left intact the lateralmost 1.6–1.8 mm of the nodulus (zones 3 and 4) and a narrow lateral strip of zone 2. Lobules 9a and 9b of the uvula were intact medially, as were the lateral tips of lobules 9c and 9d (FIG. 6C).

OCULOMOTOR EFFECTS OF COMPLETE AND PARTIAL LESIONS OF NODULUS AND UVULA

The results of complete and partial lesions (TABLE 1) were characterized in terms of three primary effects:

TABLE 1. Differential Effects of Complete and Partial Lesions

Complete Lesion	Partial Lesion
• Loss of cross-coupling	• Loss of cross-coupling
• Loss of dynamic control of vertical and roll tc's	• Loss of dynamic control of vertical and roll tc's
• Loss of dynamic control of horizontal tc.	• NO loss of dynamic control of horizontal tc.

Loss of cross-coupling. The ability to reorient the axis of eye velocity to the GIA was reduced or lost in both completely and partially lesioned animals. Phase plane graphs from M9312 (complete lesion) during facing and back to motion centrifugation demonstrate this postoperative loss (FIG. 7A). The top row shows a roll plane

←———————————————————————————————

FIGURE 6. (A) Schematic representation of a coronal section indicating complete and partial lesions of nodulus and uvula with respect to sagittal zones defined by anatomic data of Voogd[1] in rhesus monkey. (B and C) Normal rhesus monkey sagittal sections[89] at 0.5 mm (zone 1), 2.5 mm (zone 3), and 3.75 mm (zone 4) from the midline, with superimposed shaded regions indicating the extent of complete lesion in M9312 (B) and the partial lesion in M9303 (C). Because the lesions were symmetric, only one side is shown in the reconstruction. The central regions of lobules 9d and 10 of the caudal vermis were removed en bloc, extending almost to the lateral margins of the uvula. Zones 3 and 4 of the nodulus were removed in the completely lesioned animals and were intact in the partially lesioned animals. Lobules 9a and 9b were spared in medial zones in the partially lesioned animals, together with the lateral tips of lobules 9c and 9d, and a thin lateral strip of nodular zone 2.

view of the eye rotation axis during centrifugation which tilts the GIA by 52° in the roll plane. Preoperatively (filled circles), the axis of eye rotation aligned approximately with the GIA. After surgery (open circles), no reorientation was present during centrifugation with either the right or the left ear out.

Similar results were obtained during OKAN with the head tilted by 90°, before (open circles) and after (filled circles) surgery (phase plane graphs, FIG. 7B; M9303, partial lesion). Axis shifts before surgery were asymmetric, reflecting a prominent up/down asymmetry in this animal, as in M613 (FIG. 4A). Before surgery, the eye velocity axis tilted through 90° when the vertical cross-coupled component was upward (FIG. 7B, lower left panel, filled circles; FIG. 7B, upper right panel, filled circles). After surgery, axis reorientation was greatly reduced (open circles), but a residual vertical response was present, producing a small shift of the eye velocity axis in the direction of the GIA. A similar loss or reduction in axis reorientation was also reported by Angelaki and Hess[12,33] following nodulo-uvulectomy in rhesus monkeys. It is possible that the residual cross-coupling may have originated in lateral parts of the uvula, and the thin section of zone 2 of the nodulus that were spared in partially lesioned animals.

Loss of control of vertical and roll time constants. Six animals were tested with vertical vestibular and optokinetic steps about a spatial vertical axis; only three animals (1 completely lesioned; 2 partially lesioned) were tested with roll steps about a spatial vertical axis. With the animals upright, side down, prone or supine, vertical and roll time constants were short and no longer depended on head orientation,[3,18,81] demonstrating a loss of sensitivity to the GIA. The vertical VOR time constant fell from a preoperative level of 16.2 s to 5.2 s postoperatively (FIG. 8A, left), and the roll time constant fell from 10.7 s to 3.5 s for rotation about a vertical axis (FIG. 8A, right). Both values are close to the time constant of the peripheral afferents.[78] Thus, dynamic control of the vertical and roll time constants was lost after surgery in both completely and partially lesioned monkeys, and the yaw axis orientation vector of velocity storage no longer shifted towards the pitch/roll axes with the animals in side down or prone/supine positions.

Angelaki and Hess[12] also reported an impairment in the dynamics of the low-frequency torsional VOR following complete or partial nodulo-uvulectomy in rhesus monkeys, but found no corresponding effect on the dynamics of the vertical VOR. Inasmuch as vertical time constants were reduced in each of our lesioned monkeys, the reason for these discrepant findings is not clear. Based on our results and the morphologic organization of the caudal vermis with respect to the inferior olive, it is unlikely that the nodulus and uvula selectively control the dynamics of torsional eye movements.

Loss of dynamic control of horizontal time constant. Horizontal VOR time constants increased significantly in completely lesioned animals from a mean of 25.1 s before operation to 49.4 s after surgery ($p = .048^*$; FIG. 8B). Similar increases were obtained for OKAN time constants. The long horizontal time constants were accompanied by periodic alternating nystagmus that could be elicited in darkness by giving low-amplitude vestibular or optokinetic stimuli. The mean period of the periodic alternating nystagmus was ≈ 150 s. Concurrently, completely lesioned animals lost their ability to reduce or dump horizontal slow-phase velocity during per- or postrotatory nystagmus or OKAN in response to exposure to a self-stationary visual surround.[26]

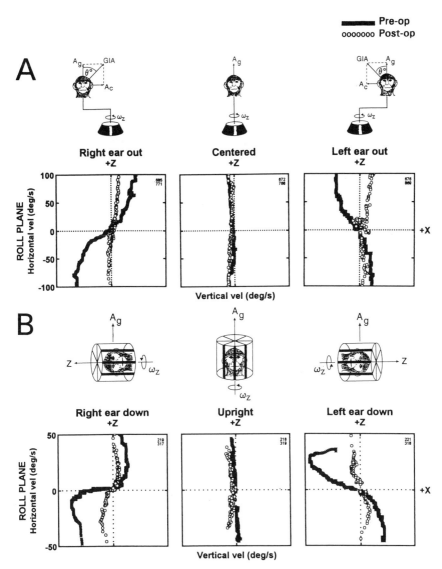

FIGURE 7. Comparison of three-dimensional eye movements in completely and partially lesioned monkeys. These phase plane graphs were generated by plotting the horizontal component of eye velocity against the vertical component. Only the decaying portion of eye velocity is plotted, from the onset of constant centrifuge velocity until the eye velocity had decayed to zero. (**A**) Completely lesioned monkey M9312—eye rotation axis during facing and back to motion centrifugation which tilts the GIA through 52° in the monkey's roll plane. Preoperatively (*filled circles*), the eye velocity axis gradually aligned with the GIA. Postoperatively (*open circles*) axis reorientation was abolished. (**B**) Partially lesioned monkey M9303 during OKAN with head tilted 90° in the roll plane. Postoperatively, cross-coupling was greatly reduced, but not completely abolished in this monkey.

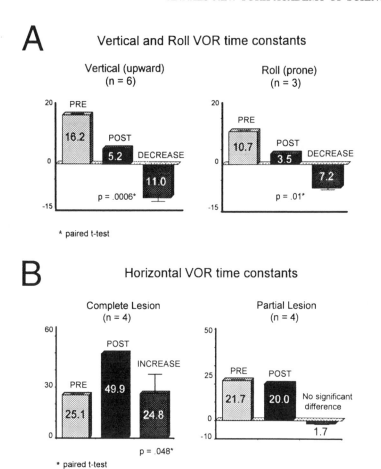

FIGURE 8. Effects of nodulo-uvulectomy on VOR time constants during rotation at 60°/s around a spatial vertical axis. The bars show means of all animals in each group; t-bar above indicates standard deviations. *p*-values indicate statistical significance levels for paired *t* tests. **(A)** Vertical (upward only) and roll (prone only) VOR time constants during rotation in pitch and roll, respectively. No differences were apparent between complete and partially lesioned animals, and data from both groups were combined. Postoperatively, time constants were reduced. **(B)** Complete lesions (*left graph*) caused an increase in mean horizontal time constants postoperatively. Partial lesion (*right graph*) had no effect on the mean horizontal time constant.

Before nodulo-uvulectomy, horizontal OKAN or vestibular time constants on initial testing averaged 21.7 s in the partially lesioned group. During testing some animals habituated, reducing the horizontal time constant.[87] Following partial nodulo-uvulectomy, this habituation was lost, and the time constant returned to the initial pre-lesion level (mean 20 s) (FIG. 8B), but did not exceed this level, as in the completely lesioned group. These animals could also reduce or "dump" the horizontal time constant during head tilts, centrifugation, and exposure to a self-stationary visual surround. Thus, although ablation of the central 2 mm of the nodulus and uvula abolished cross-coupling from yaw to pitch or roll and the ability to change the vertical and roll time constants dynamically, it did not affect the animal's ability to change the dynamics of horizontal eye velocity in response to tilts of the GIA. We conclude that the processes involved in controlling orientation through the vertical and torsional time constant and in control of the horizontal time constant are anatomically and functionally separable. These results provide a behavioral correlate for functional specificity in individual zones of the nodulus and uvula, and support for the modular model of cerebellar function.[40,48]

HYPOTHESIZED CONTROL OF SPATIAL ORIENTATION BY SEMICIRCULAR CANAL-RELATED MODULES OF THE NODULUS AND UVULA

We conclude that vertical and roll time constants and components of the cross-coupled response are modulated by central portions of the nodulus and uvula whereas the horizontal time constant is controlled by sagittal zones in lateral

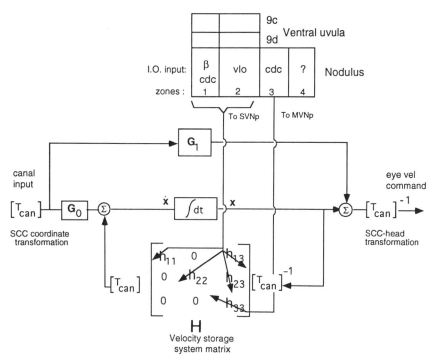

FIGURE 9. Model of three-dimensional control of orientation and dynamics of velocity storage system by canal related zones of nodulus and ventral uvula. G_0: Gain matrix in integrator pathway; G_1: Direct vestibular pathway gain matrix; T_{can}: matrix of head to canal coordinate transformation; H: velocity storage system matrix shown in head coordinates, and transformed by the similarity transformation $[T_{can}][H][T_{can}]^{-1}$ into the canal coordinates of the system. See text for further details.

portions of the nodulus. Insofar as zones identified on the basis of olivary input in the monkey have corresponding functions and efferent projections to those demonstrated in the rabbit, we postulate that the nodulus and uvula control spatial orientation of velocity storage by projecting from canal-related Purkinje cell zones to regions of SVN_p and MVN_p containing canal-related VO neurons. FIGURE 9 formalizes this hypothesis. The direct vestibular pathway with gain matrix, (G_1), which is independent of gravity, is not controlled by the nodulus and uvula. All central processing is performed in semicircular canal coordinates. The matrix T_{can} represents the transformation from head coordinates to semicircular canal coordinates, and T_{can}^{-1} the inverse transformation from canal to head coordinates.[72,88] The velocity storage system matrix, [H], is shown in head coordinates in order to simplify the representation and demonstrate the upper triangular structure of the matrix. The similarity transformation $[T_{can}][H][T_{can}]^{-1}$ transforms this matrix into the canal coordinates used by the central vestibular system. The aVOR integrator pathway is under parametric control by the nodulus and uvula. Zones 1 and 2 modulate anterior and posterior canal-related VO neurons in SVN_p, to control the vertical and roll time constants ($1/h_{11}$ and $1/h_{22}$), and the horizontal to vertical (h_{13}) and horizontal to roll (h_{23}) cross-coupling parameters. The parameter h_{13}, for example, determines the extent to which input signals aligned with the Z axis of the head will excite the vertical mode of velocity storage. Zone 3 modulates horizontal canal-related VO neurons in MVN_p, to control the horizontal time constant, $1/h_{33}$. Control of the horizontal time constant is independent of cross-coupling between axes. In this scheme, the eigenvalues (inverse time constants) and cross-coupling parameters of the velocity storage system matrix are controlled by the central vertical canal-related zones of the nodulus and uvula (zones 1 and 2), whereas the horizontal eigenvalue is controlled by the lateral, horizontal canal-related zone (zone 3) of the nodulus. According to this organizational structure and consistent with our data, anatomically discrete zones in the nodulus and uvula can function independently to control the orientation of eye movements.

ACKNOWLEDGMENTS

We thank Dr. Gay Holstein and Dr. Jan Voogd for providing us with data, assistance, and critical advice on the preparation and interpretation of our anatomic results, and Dr. John Simpson for invaluable discussion. Special thanks to Victor Rodriguez for technical assistance and assistance in assembling the figures.

REFERENCES

1. VOOGD, J. 1996. Organization of the vestibulocerebellum. Ann. N.Y. Acad. Sci. This volume.
2. RAPHAN, T. & B. COHEN. 1986. Multidimensional organization of the vestibulo-ocular reflex (VOR). *In* Adaptive Processes in Visual and Oculomotor System. E. L. Keller & D. S. Zee, Eds.: 285–292. Pergamon Press. New York.
3. RAPHAN, T. & B. COHEN. 1988. Organizational principles of velocity storage in three dimensions: The effect of gravity on cross-coupling of optokinetic after-nystagmus. Ann. N. Y. Acad. Sci. **545:** 74–92.
4. CRAMPTON, H. C. 1966. Does linear acceleration modify cupular deflection? *In* Second Symposium on the Role of the Vestibular Organs in Space Exploration, Ed. NASA. SP-115.: 169–184. Washington, D.C.
5. LANSBERG, M. P., F. E. GUEDRY & A. GRAYBIEL. 1965. Effect of changing resultant linear

acceleration relative to the subject on nystagmus generated by angular acceleration. Aerosp. Med. **36:** 456–460.

6. CURTHOYS, I. S., S. L. WEARNE, M. J. DAI, G. M. HALMAGYI & J. R. HOLDEN. 1992. Linear acceleration modulates the nystagmus induced by angular acceleration stimulation of the horizontal canal. Ann. N. Y. Acad. Sci. **656:** 716–724.

7. MERFELD, D. M. & L. R. YOUNG. 1995. The vestibulo-ocular reflex of the squirrel monkey during eccentric rotation and roll tilt. Exp. Brain Res. **106:** 111–122.

8. MERFELD, D. M., L. R. YOUNG, G. D. PAIGE & D. L. TOMKO. 1993. Three dimensional eye movements of squirrel monkeys following postrotatory tilt. J. Vestib. Res. **3:** 123–141.

9. CLEMENT, G. & C. E. LATHAN. 1991. Effect of static tilt about the roll axis on horizontal and vertical optokinetic nystagmus and optokinetic after-nystagmus in humans. Exp. Brain Res. **84:** 335–341.

10. GIZZI, M., S. RUDOLPH, B. COHEN & T. RAPHAN. 1992. The representation of the spatial vertical in human optokinetic nystagmus. Ann. N. Y. Acad. Sci. **656:** 843–846.

11. HARRIS, L. R. & G. R. BARNES. 1987. Orientation of vestibular nystagmus is modified by head tilt. *In* The Vestibular System: Neurophysiologic and Clinical Research. M. D. Graham & J. L. Kemink, Eds.: 539–548. Raven Press. New York.

12. ANGELAKI, D. E. & B. J. M. HESS. 1995. Inertial representation of angular motion in the vestibular system of rhesus monkeys. II. Otolith-controlled transformation that depends on an intact cerebellar nodulus. J. Neurophysiol. **73:** 1729–1751.

13. ANGELAKI, D. E. & B. J. M. HESS. 1994. Inertial representation of angular motion in the vestibular system of rhesus monkeys. I. Vestibuloocular reflex. J. Neurophysiol. **71:** 1222–1249.

14. MERFELD, D. M., L. R. YOUNG, D. L. TOMKO & G. D. PAIGE. 1991. Spatial orientation of VOR to combined vestibular stimuli in squirrel monkeys. Acta Otolaryngol. Suppl. **481:** 287–292.

15. DAI, M. J., T. RAPHAN, B. COHEN & C. SCHNABOLK. 1991. Spatial orientation of velocity storage during post-rotatory nystagmus. Soc. Neurosci. Abstr. **17:** 314.

16. RAPHAN, T. & D. STURM. 1991. Modelling the spatiotemporal organization of velocity storage in the vestibuloocular reflex by optokinetic studies. J. Neurophysiol. **66:** 1410–1420.

17. MERFELD, D. M. 1990. Spatial orientation on the squirrel monkey: An experimental and theoretical investigation. Ph.D. thesis, MIT. Cambridge, MA.

18. DAI, M., T. RAPHAN & B. COHEN. 1991. Spatial orientation of the vestibular system: Dependence of optokinetic after nystagmus on gravity. J. Neurophysiol. **66:** 1422–1438.

19. DAI, M. J., T. RAPHAN & B. COHEN. 1992. Characterization of yaw to roll cross-coupling in the three-dimensional structure of the velocity storage integrator. Ann. N. Y. Acad. Sci. **656:** 829–831.

20. RAPHAN, T., S. WEARNE & B. COHEN. 1994. Static and dynamic effects of gravito-inertial acceleration (GIA) on spatial orientation of velocity storage. Soc. Neurosci. Abstr. **20:** 1195.

21. WEARNE, S. 1993. Spatial orientation of the human linear and angular vestibulo-ocular reflexes during centrifugation. Ph.D. thesis, University of Sydney. Australia.

22. GIZZI, M., T. RAPHAN, S. RUDOLPH & B. COHEN. 1994. Orientation of human optokinetic nystagmus to gravity: A model based approach. Exp. Brain Res. **99:** 347–360.

23. KATZ, E., J. M. B. V. DE JONG, J. A. BÜTTNER-ENNEVER & B. COHEN. 1991. Effects of midline medullary lesions on velocity storage and the vestibulo-ocular reflex. Exp. Brain Res. **87:** 505–520.

24. SOLOMON, D. & B. COHEN. 1994. Stimulation of the nodulus and uvula discharges velocity storage in the vestibulo-ocular reflex. Exp. Brain Res. **102:** 57–68.

25. RAPHAN, T., B. COHEN & V. HENN. 1981. Effects of gravity on rotatory nystagmus in monkeys. Ann. N. Y. Acad. Sci. **374:** 44–55.

26. WAESPE, W., B. COHEN & T. RAPHAN. 1985. Dynamic modification of the vestibulo-ocular reflex by the nodulus and uvula. Science **228:** 199–201.

27. BENSON, A. J. 1974. Modification of the response to angular accelerations by linear accelerations. *In* Handbook of Sensory Physiology. H. Kornhuber, Ed. Vol. 6: 281–320. Springer. Berlin.

28. COHEN, B., I. KOZLOVSKAYA, T. RAPHAN, D. SOLOMON, D. HELWIG, N. COHEN, M. SIROTA & S. YAKUSHIN. 1992. Vestibuloocular reflex of rhesus monkeys after spaceflight. J. Appl. Physiol. 73(2): 121S–131S.
29. COHEN, B., V. MATSUO & T. RAPHAN. 1977. Quantitative analysis of the velocity characteristics of optokinetic nystagmus and optokinetic after-nystagmus. J. Physiol. (Lond.) 270: 321–344.
30. COHEN, B., V. HENN, T. RAPHAN & D. DENNETT. 1981. Velocity storage, nystagmus, and visual vestibular interactions in humans. Ann. N. Y. Acad. Sci. 374: 421–433.
31. WAESPE, W., B. COHEN & T. RAPHAN. 1983. Role of the flocculus and paraflocculus in optokinetic nystagmus and visual-vestibular interaction: Effects of lesions. Exp. Brain Res. 50: 9–33.
32. COHEN, B., S. WEARNE, T. RAPHAN & H. REISINE. 1994. Functional independence of nodular and uvular microzones controlling spatial orientation of velocity storage. Soc. Neurosci. Abstr. 20: 1191.
33. ANGELAKI, D. E. & B. J. M. HESS. 1994. The cerebellar nodulus and ventral uvula control the torsional vestibulo-ocular reflex. J. Neurophysiol. 72: 1443–1447.
34. COHEN, B. 1988. Representation of three-dimensional space in the vestibular, oculomotor, and visual systems. Ann. N. Y. Acad. Sci. 545: 239–247.
35. LEONARD, C. S., J. I. SIMPSON & W. GRAF. 1988. The spatial organization of visual messages in the flocculus of the rabbit's cerebellum. I. Typology of inferior olive neurons of the dorsal cap of Kooy. J. Neurophysiol. 60: 2073–2090.
36. SIMPSON, J. I. & W. GRAF. 1985. The selection of reference frames by nature and its investigators. In Adaptive Mechanisms in Gaze Control; Reviews of Oculomotor Research. A. Berthoz & G. M. Jones, Eds. 1: 3–16. Elsevier. Amsterdam.
37. GRAF, W., J. I. SIMPSON & C. S. LEONARD. 1988. The spatial organization of visual messages in the flocculus of the rabbit's cerebellum. II. Complex and simple spike responses of Purkinje cells. J. Neurophysiol. 60: 2091–2121.
38. SIMPSON, J. I., J. VAN DER STEEN & J. TAN. 1992. Eye movements and the zonal structure of the rabbit flocculus. In The Cerebellum Revisited. R. Llinas & C. Sotelo, Eds. Springer-Verlag. New York.
39. SIMPSON, J. I., W. GRAF & C. LEONARD. 1981. The coordinate system of visual climbing fibers to the flocculus. In Progress in Oculomotor Research. A. F. Fuchs & W. Becker, Eds.: 475–484. Elsevier. New York.
40. ITO, M. 1984. The Cerebellum and Neural Control. Raven Press. New York.
41. VOOGD, J. 1964. The Cerebellum of the Cat. Structure and Fiber Connections. Ph.D. thesis, University of Leiden. The Netherlands.
42. OSCARSSON, O. 1979. Functional units of the cerebellum—Sagittal zones and microzones. Trends Neurosci. 2: 143–145.
43. OSCARSSON, O. 1969. The sagittal organization of the cerebellar anterior lobe as revealed by the projection patterns of the climbing fiber system. In Neurobiology of Cerebellar Evolution and Development. R. Llinas, Ed.: 525–537. American Medical Association. Chicago, IL.
44. VOOGD, J., N. M. GERRITS & D. T. HESS. 1986. Parasagittal zonation of the cerebellum in macaques: An analysis based on acetylcholinesterase histochemistry. In Cerebellum and Neuronal Plasticity. M. Glickstein, C. Yeo & J. Stein, Eds.: 15–39. Plenum. New York.
45. GROENWEGEN, H. J. & J. VOOGD. 1977. The parasagittal zonation within the olivocerebellar projection. I. Climbing fiber distribution in the vermis of the cat cerebellum. J. Comp. Neurol. 174: 417–488.
46. WYLIE, D. R., C. I. DE ZEEUW, P. L. DIGIORGI & J. I. SIMPSON. 1994. Projections of individual Purkinje cells of identified zones in the ventral nodulus to the vestibular and cerebellar nuclei in the rabbit. J. Comp. Neurol. 349: 448–463.
47. WALBERG, F., T. NORDBY & E. DIETRICHS. 1987. The olivonodular projection: A re-examination based on folial cerebellar implants. Neurosci. Lett. 81: 82–88.
48. VOOGD, J. & F. BIGARÉ. 1980. Topographical distribution of olivary and corticonuclear fibers in the cerebellum. A review. In The Inferior Olivary Nucleus: Anatomy and Physiology. J. Courville, C. C. D. Montigny & Y. Lamarre, Eds.: 207–234. Raven Press. New York.

49. VOOGD, J. 1989. Parasagittal zones and compartments of the anterior vermis of the cat cerebellum. *In* The Olivocerebellar System in Motor Control. Exp. Brain Res. Suppl. 17. P. Strata, Ed.: 3–19. Springer-Verlag. New York.

50. VOOGD, J. 1982. The olivocerebellar projection in the cat. *In* The Cerebellum: New Vistas. S. L. Palay & V. Chan-Palay, Eds.: 135–161. Springer-Verlag. New York.

51. SHOJAKU, H., Y. SATO, K. IKARASHI & T. KAWASAKI. 1987. Topographical distribution of Purkinje cells in the uvula and the nodulus projecting to the vestibular nuclei in cats. Brain Res. **416:** 100–112.

52. TAN, J., N. M. GERRITS, R. NANHOE, J. I. SIMPSON & J. VOOGD. 1995. Zonal organization of the climbing fiber projection to the flocculus and nodulus of the rabbit. A combined axonal tracing and acetylcholinesterase histochemical study. J. Comp. Neurol. **356:** 23–50.

53. BARMACK, N. H. & M. H. FAGERSON. 1994. Vestibularly-evoked activity of single neurons in the dorsomedial cell column of the inferior olive in rabbit. Soc. Neurosci. Abstr. **20:** 1190.

54. BARMACK, N. H., M. FAGERSON, B. J. FREDETTE, E. MUGNAINI & H. SHOJAKU. 1993. Activity of neurons in the beta nucleus of the inferior olive of the rabbit evoked by natural vestibular stimulation. Exp. Brain Res. **94:** 203–215.

55. BARMACK, N. H. & H. SHOJAKU. 1992. Representation of a postural coordinate system in the nodulus of the rabbit cerebellum by vestibular climbing fiber signals. *In* Vestibular and Brain Stem Control of Eye, Head, and Body Movement. H. Shimazu & Y. Shinoda, Ed.: 331–338. Japan Scientific Societies Press. Tokyo.

56. HAINES, D. E. 1977. Cerebellar corticonuclear and corticovestibular fibers of the flocculonodular lobe in a prosimian primate (*Galago senegalensis*). J. Comp. Neurol. **174:** 607–630.

57. BARMACK, N. H. & H. SHOJAKU. 1989. Topography and analysis of vestibular-visual climbing fibre signals in the rabbit cerebellar nodulus. Soc. Neurosci. Abstr. **15:** 180.

58. TAKEDA, T. & K. MAEKAWA. 1984. Collateralized projection of visual climbing fibers to the flocculus and nodulus of the rabbit. Neurosci. Res. **2:** 125–132.

59. KATAYAMA, S. & N. NISIMARU. 1988. Parasagittal zonal pattern of olivo-nodular projection in rabbit cerebellum. Neurosci. Res. **5:** 424–438.

60. BALABAN, C. D. & R. T. HENRY. 1988. Zonal organization of olivo-nodulus projections in albino rabbits. Neurosci. Res. **5:** 409–423.

61. ALLEY, K., R. BAKER & J. I. SIMPSON. 1975. Afferents to the vestibulo-cerebellum and the origin of the visual climbing fibers in the rabbit. Brain Res. **98:** 582–589.

62. BARMACK, N. H., R. W. BAUGHMAN, P. ERRICO & H. SHOJAKU. 1993. Vestibular primary afferent projections to the cerebellum of the rabbit. J. Comp. Neurol. **327:** 521–534.

63. SATO, Y. & N. M. BARMACK. 1985. Zonal organization of olivocerebellar projections to the uvula in rabbits. Brain Res. **359:** 281–292.

64. KANO, M. S., M. KANO & K. MAEKAWA. 1990. Receptive field organization of climbing fiber afferents responding to optokinetic stimulation in the cerebellar nodulus and flocculus of the pigmented rabbit. Exp. Brain Res. **82:** 499–512.

65. DEJONG, J. M. B. V., B. COHEN, V. MATSUO & T. UEMURA. 1980. Midsagittal brainstem sections: Effects on ocular adduction and nystagmus. Exp. Neurol. **68:** 420–442.

66. BÜTTNER-ENNEVER, J. A. 1992. Patterns of connectivity in the vestibular nuclei. Ann. N. Y. Acad. Sci. **656:** 363–378.

67. FUCHS, A. F. & J. KIMM. 1975. Unit activity in the vestibular nucleus of the alert monkey during horizontal angular acceleration and eye movement. J. Neurophysiol. **38:** 1140–1161.

68. YOKOTA, J. I., H. REISINE & B. COHEN. 1992. Nystagmus induced by electrical microstimulation of the vestibular and prepositus hypoglossi nuclei in the monkey. Exp. Brain Res. **92:** 123–138.

69. REISINE, H. & T. RAPHAN. 1992. Neural basis for eye velocity generation in the vestibular nuclei during off-vertical axis rotation. Exp. Brain Res. **92:** 209–226.

70. JUDGE, S. J., B. J. RICHMOND & F. C. CHU. 1980. Implantation of magnetic search coils for measurement of eye position: An improved method. Vision Res. **20:** 535–538.

71. ROBINSON, D. A. 1963. A method of measuring eye movement using a scleral search coil in a magnetic field. IEEE Trans. Biomed. Electron. **10:** 137–145.

72. YAKUSHIN, S. B., M. J. DAI, J.-I. SUZUKI, T. RAPHAN & B. COHEN. 1995. Semicircular canal

contribution to the three-dimensional vestibulo-ocular reflex: A model-based approach. J. Neurophysiol. In press.

73. GOLDSTEIN, H. 1980. Classical Mechanics. 2nd edit. Addison-Wesley. Reading, MA.

74. KANO, M., M. S. KANO, M. KUSUNOKI & K. MAEKAWA. 1990. Nature of optokinetic response and zonal organization of climbing fiber afferents in the vestibulocerebellum of the pigmented rabbit. II. The nodulus. Exp. Brain Res. **80:** 238–251.

75. CHERON, G., P. GILLIS & E. GODAUX. 1986. Lesions in the cat prepositus complex: Effects on the optokinetic system. J. Physiol. **372:** 95–111.

76. BLAIR, S. M. & M. GAVIN. 1981. Brainstem commissure and control of time constant of vestibular nystagmus. Acta Otolaryngol. **91:** 1–8.

77. FERNÁNDEZ, C. & J. M. GOLDBERG. 1971. Physiology of peripheral neurons innervating semicircular canals of the squirrel monkey. II. Response to sinusoidal stimulation and dynamics of peripheral vestibular system. J. Neurophysiol. **34:** 661–675.

78. GOLDBERG, J. M. & C. FERNANDEZ. 1971. Physiology of peripheral neurons innervating semicircular canals of the squirrel monkey. I. Resting discharge and response to angular accelerations. J. Neurophysiol. **34:** 635–660.

79. GOLDBERG, J. M. & C. FERNANDEZ. 1971. Physiology of peripheral neurons innervating semicircular canals of the squirrel monkey. III. Variations among units in their discharge properties. J. Neurophysiol. **34:** 676–684.

80. BÜTTNER, U. & W. WAESPE. 1981. Vestibular nerve activity in the alert monkey during vestibular and optokinetic nystagmus. Exp. Brain Res. **41:** 310–315.

81. MATSUO, V. & B. COHEN. 1984. Vertical optokinetic nystagmus and vestibular nystagmus in the monkey: Up-down asymmetry and effects of gravity. Exp. Brain Res. **53:** 197–216.

82. VOOGD, J. 1969. The importance of fiber connections in the comparative anatomy of the mammalian cerebellum. *In* Neurobiology of Cerebellar Evolution and Development. R. Llinas, Ed.: 493–514. American Medical Association. Chicago, IL.

83. SHOJAKU, H., N. H. BARMACK & K. MIZUKOSHI. 1991. Influence of vestibular and visual climbing fiber signals on Purkinje cell discharge in the cerebellar nodulus of the rabbit. Acta Otolaryngol. Suppl. **481:** 242–246.

84. ANGAUT, P. & A. BRODAL. 1967. The projections of the "vestibulocerebellum" onto the vestibular nuclei in the cat. Arch. Ital. Biol. **105:** 441–479.

85. BRODAL, A. & P. BRODAL. 1985. Observations on the secondary vestibulocerebellar projections in the macaque monkey. Exp. Brain Res. **58:** 62–74.

86. WALBERG, F. & E. DIETRICHS. 1988. The interconnection between the vestibular nuclei and the nodulus: A study of reciprocity. Brain Res. **449:** 47–53.

87. COHEN, H., B. COHEN, T. RAPHAN & W. WAESPE. 1992. Habituation and adaptation of the vestibulo-ocular reflex: A model of differential control by the vestibulo-cerebellum. Exp. Brain Res. **90:** 526–538.

88. ROBINSON, D. A. 1982. The use of matrices in analyzing the three dimensional behavior of the vestibulo-ocular reflex. Biol. Cybern. **46:** 53–66.

89. MADIGAN, J. & M. CARPENTER. 1971. Cerebellum of the Rhesus Monkey. Atlas of Lobules, Laminae and Folia in Sections. University Park Press. London.

Whole-Body Rotations Enhance Hippocampal Theta Rhythmic Slow Activity in Awake Rats Passively Transported on a Mobile Robot[a]

VLADIMIR V. GAVRILOV,[b,c] SIDNEY I. WIENER,[b,d]
AND ALAIN BERTHOZ[b]

[b]CNRS-Collège de France
Laboratoire de Physiologie de la Perception et de l'Action UMR-C 9950
15, rue de l'Ecole de Médecine
75270 Paris, Cedex 06 France

[c]Institute of Psychology
Russian Academy of Sciences
13, Yaroslavskaya Street
129366 Moscow, Russia

INTRODUCTION

Many species of animals have the ability to navigate to a goal that cannot be seen at the moment that the displacement movements are initiated. The neural basis of this behavior has been the subject of intensive research in the last decade. The hippocampal system has been a focus of these efforts because of the navigational deficits found after hippocampal lesions in humans[1] and in animal models.[2] Another reason for interest in the hippocampus is the remarkable finding that in rats neural activity in this structure is correlated with the position of the animal in the environment and also with active displacements. Rat hippocampal place cells (pyramidal cells of the CA1 and CA3 regions) discharge as the rat occupies a small portion (about 5–10% of the total area) of its environment.[3] Within the same animal, different place cells have been shown to be selective for different locations, and the fields of as few as a dozen such neurons can span a small testing chamber.[4] Shifting the position of cues in the environment can induce firing fields to change positions in register with these cues. However, this is not a simple sensory response because such spatial selectivity persists in the absence of such cues.[5,6] More recently, we have shown that inertial cues (which can be detected with the somatosensory and vestibular systems) can also influence the spatially selective discharges of place cells.[7] We propose that this information is acquired during active displacements and can incrementally update hippocampal representations of body position; this would be a neural basis for "path integration."[8]

[a]This work was supported by CNES, Human Frontiers, EEC/ESPRIT/BRA 6615 MUCOM, CNRS Programme Cognisciences. V.V.G. received a grant from the Fondation pour la Recherche Médicale. S.I.W. was supported by a Fogarty Institute/INSERM Senior Fellowship, CNRS Poste Rouge, NATO Senior Fellowship, Fondation Fyssen, Fondation pour la Recherche Médicale.
[c]V.V.G. was on leave from the Institute of Psychology, Moscow.
[d]Corresponding author. E-mail: sw@ccr.jussieu.fr

The present study is focused on the analysis of those components of hippocampal electroencephalographic (EEG) activity that are strongly correlated with locomotion. Several principal types of slow electrical activity are recorded in the hippocampus including the theta rhythm, small amplitude desynchronized, and also large amplitude irregular activity (LIA). Of particular interest here is the theta rhythm (4–12 Hz in rats) which is generated at two principal sites, the CA1 pyramidal layer and in the dentate gyrus,[9] and can be triggered by stimulation of certain brain-stem areas as well as the medial septum. Only the atropine-resistant theta (7–12 Hz) is associated with so-called type I movements, especially walking, running, and jumping.[10] Because it is these movements that bring the rat from one location to another, and thus lead to the successive activation of different place cells, type I theta is of particular interest for better understanding the neural basis of the representation of space. However, little is known about the role and relative importance of different types of sensory information in generating hippocampal theta EEG because of the difficulties in presenting controlled sensory stimuli to the unrestrained animals used in these studies.

In order to determine the role of inertial cues on hippocampal spatial representations, we have recorded single-unit and EEG activity from high-impedance electrodes (1–5 MOhm glass micropipettes) placed in the hippocampus.[11] To eliminate possible influences of locomotor activity on hippocampal theta activity, rats were trained to remain awake while immobilized in a sling and headholder and then displaced passively on a mobile robot. In several of these recording sessions we noted tendencies for augmented hippocampal theta EEG during passive displacements of the rats. To confirm this, the experiments were repeated in six recording sessions with an electrode configuration designed for higher resolution recordings of hippocampal theta activity.[12] In summary, this study attempted to answer two fundamental questions: (1) Is high-frequency theta activity, usually associated with active locomotion and other type I behaviors, also observed in passively displaced animals? and (2) if so, how does inertial information modulate this activity?

METHODS

Recordings of EEG were obtained from two adult male Long-Evans hooded rats. During a one-month period, the rats were trained to be restrained and suspended in a cloth sling which permitted all four limbs to protrude freely. The rats were water deprived during this adaptation period. Drops of water were delivered in a small reservoir mounted below the muzzle of the rat. Water was available during the training sessions and also for a short period at the end of the day in order to maintain body weight at 80% of the normal value. Lapping the water was considered as a behavioral criterion that a rat was ready for the following stage of training. Training consisted of three stages: initial adaptation to restriction in the sling, then adaptation to passive displacements on a robot, and, finally, after surgical implantation of the electrodes, to displacements with the head fixed. The latter stage took about one week.

Motion Parameters

The rats were passively translated and rotated on a mobile computer-driven robot (Robosoft, Bayonne, France) within a square arena (3 × 3 m) surrounded by black curtains at the sides and above (FIG. 1). The robot was programmed to accelerate and decelerate in one second; other movements were at constant velocities (FIG. 2). The rats were rotated clockwise (CW) or counterclockwise (CCW) by angles ranging from 360° to 1080° at several speeds (50, 100, or 300 deg/s) in the center of the arena and near each wall (FIG. 1). The robot's linear displacements within the arena for this series are shown in FIGURE 1 as dashed lines. The robot made 5-s pauses between successive movements. A video system monitored the displacements of the robot from the positions of red and blue light bulbs mounted on a scaffold above the rat. These signals were used for synchronization of the EEG data. All movement sequences were repeated in light and in darkness. For experi-

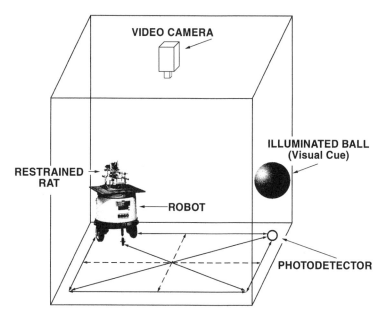

FIGURE 1. Schematic representation of experimental apparatus and protocol. Attached to the top of the mobile computer-driven robot is the restraining system, which maintained the head of the rat fixed; the body was suspended in a sling. The experiments were performed in a 3 × 3 m arena surrounded by darkroom curtains on the four walls and top. The videocamera was positioned at the center at the top of the tent. Dashed lines show trajectories of the robot. The lit ball was removed from the arena in experiments in darkness.

ments performed in darkness, all lights were turned off, all curtains were closed, and the field of view of the rat was occluded with a small piece of darkroom curtain. In light conditions, a curtain at one side of the arena was opened permitting a large number of objects in the illuminated room outside the arena to be visible.

Optokinetic Stimulation

In order to test for possible correlations of hippocampal theta EEG with eye movements as well as with visual stimulation, the restrained rat was moved to the

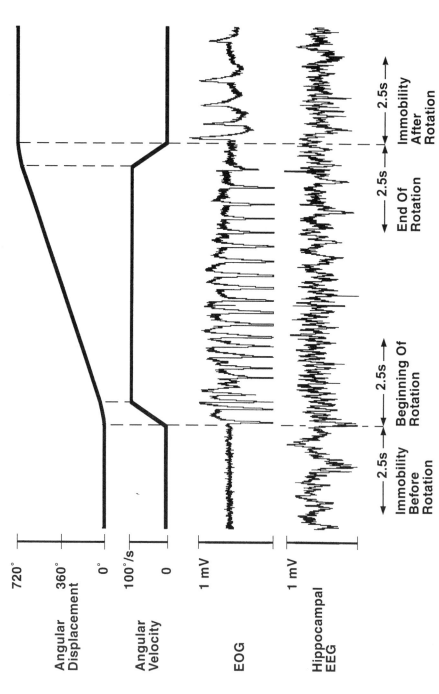

FIGURE 2. Hippocampal EEG and eye movement (EOG) recordings prior to, during, and after two full rotations at speed 100 deg/s. Above are

center of the darkened arena. A planetarium-like projector was mounted above the rat on a frame attached to the robot. The visual field was rotated around the vertical axis at speeds of 12, 25, 50, and 80 deg/s both CW and CCW for 2-min periods each. Successive rotations were interrupted by 10- to 30-s delays. Nystagmus was recorded with silver/silver chloride ball electrodes placed on the inner canthus of each eye.

Surgical Procedure

Prior to surgery, rats were tranquillized with 0.1 mL xylazine (Rompun, 2%) followed with 60 mg/kg pentobarbital intraperitoneally for anesthesia. The skull was exposed and five tiny screws were anchored in it to secure two large screws adapted to maintain a light-weight Plexiglas platform[13] that would be installed later, just prior to each recording session. This platform was a support for a light-weight electrode driver,[13] as well as for electrical connectors; it also had receptacles for bars which stably fixed the head of the rat. A screw in the occipital bone served as an electrical ground and as a reference for recordings.

EEG Recordings

Monopolar recordings of hippocampal EEG were made with Teflon-coated silver wires (200 μm in diameter) with insulation removed about 0.3 mm from the tip. The electrode was one of a twisted pair with 0.5 mm intertip distance. These were stereotaxically lowered into the dentate gyrus at coordinates 3.8 mm posterior and 1.5 mm to the left to bregma and at a depth of 3.5 to 4.5 mm from the outer surface of the skull. During implantation, the depth was selected under guidance from on-line monitoring of theta EEG activity. Brain electrical activity was passed through FET current amplifiers, then a differential AC amplifier (A-M Systems Model 1700; filter settings 0.1 Hz–1 kHz), and was sampled on a 386DX-33 personal computer through a CED 1401 interface (Cambridge, UK). The sampling rate was 500 Hz.

Data Analysis

The CED Spike2 macro environment was used for data analysis programs. EEG spectral characteristics during passive rotation and linear displacements were analyzed over four 2.5-s intervals: just before and after the beginning, and just before and after the end of the displacement (FIG. 2). The fast Fourier transforms of the slow electrical activity corresponding to these intervals were averaged for all repetitions of each respective type of displacement. We compared the relative power of the theta band between different conditions (e.g., beginning versus end of each type of movement, each type of movement in light versus in darkness, etc.). Paired *t* tests compared the relative power measured in these conditions for each of the respective frequencies in the theta band. Shifts in peak frequency in the theta band are not reported here.

Histological Procedure

To mark recording sites, at the end of the experiments the rats were heavily sedated with pentobarbital, and 20 μamp DC current was passed through the

IMMOBILE | ROTATION | IMMOBILE

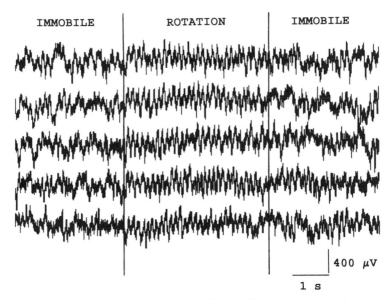

400 μV

1 s

FIGURE 3. Five traces of hippocampal EEG activity recorded over the course of an experimental session lasting about 20 min. In the 10-s intervals shown, the vertical dashed lines mark the beginning (*left*) and end (*right*) of the whole-body rotation of the rat on the robot. (From Gavrilov *et al.*[11] Reproduced, with permission, from *Neuroscience Letters.*)

recording electrode for 5 s. Rats were then given a lethal dose of pentobarbital and perfused with 0.9% NaCl, followed by 4% formalin. The brain was conserved in 30% sucrose solution, then frozen, cut into 50-μm sections, and stained with cresyl violet for observations of electrode position.

RESULTS

There was a marked increase in high-frequency theta hippocampal EEG in the restrained rats during passive rotations and translations. The onset of theta EEG was clearly synchronized with the beginning of the movements (FIGS. 2 and 3) and, in some cases, continued only to stop abruptly at the end of the movements (FIG. 3). The power in the 7–8.5 Hz frequency band increased significantly (paired t test, $p < .05$) in the initial 2.5 s of rotations in comparison with measurements made during immobility, both preceding and following the movements (FIG. 4; see also FIG. 2). Note that this, and all of the changes in EEG power described below, occur in the high-frequency theta band. This same increase in power of the theta EEG was found for translations (FIG. 5) although this was limited to a single histogram bin at 7.5 Hz. Other analyses showed that the power in the theta band was significantly greater during rotations than during translations; this is apparent in comparisons of FIGURES 4 and 5. In light the relative power at 7.5 Hz was increasingly higher for faster rotation speeds (FIG. 6). In darkness this velocity-dependent augmentation in power was replicated in both the 7.5- and 8-Hz frequency bands. No significant differences were found in theta power when the rat was subjected to successively faster translations (not shown). For all of these effects, the recordings in darkness replicated those of the light sessions. Thus it is unlikely that visual sensory inputs influenced the amplitude of the hippocampal theta EEG.

In our protocol, the passive whole-body movements of the restrained rats induced head movements that, in turn, are known to elicit ocular nystagmus. We

ROTATION IN LIGHT

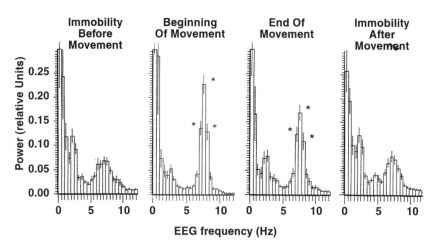

ROTATION IN DARKNESS

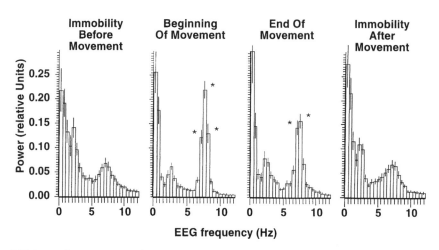

FIGURE 4. Power spectra of hippocampal EEG during passive rotations in light and in darkness. Data were averaged over 55 trials for the intervals shown in FIGURE 2. In light conditions, one of the arena curtains was opened to allow the rat to see objects in the room. X-axis, EEG frequency scale (Hz); bin width, 0.47 Hz; y-axis, values of spectral power in relative units. Error bars are standard errors of mean; asterisks are to the right of the bins in the theta type I band that were significantly different in comparisons between recordings during rotation and immobility (*t* test, $p < .05$).

TRANSLATION IN LIGHT

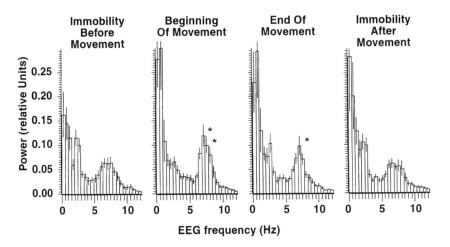

TRANSLATION IN DARKNESS

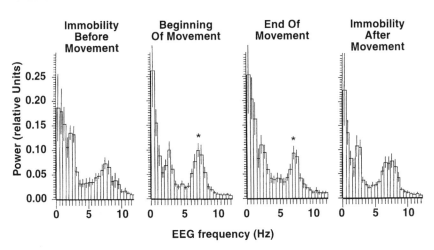

FIGURE 5. Hippocampal EEG power spectra averages over 32 passive translations in light and in darkness. Results are from the same experimental session as in FIGURE 4. Intervals and analyses were similar to those of FIGURE 4.

attempted to dissociate these respective influences by studying the relation between eye movements and theta spectral power. During optokinetic stimulation, there were significant increases in the power in the high-frequency theta band, as compared with measures in darkness (not shown). No significant increases in theta power were found when the visual field was rotated at progressively higher velocities. Taken together, these data suggest that oculomotor activity, especially nystagmus evoked by optokinetic as well as vestibular stimuli, is correlated with high-frequency theta in

ROTATION IN LIGHT

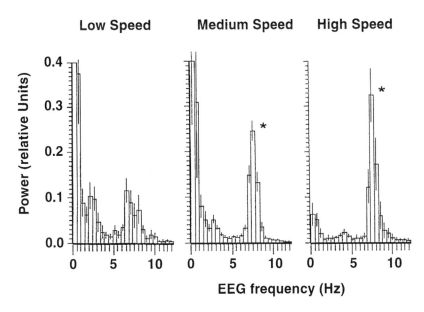

ROTATION IN DARKNESS

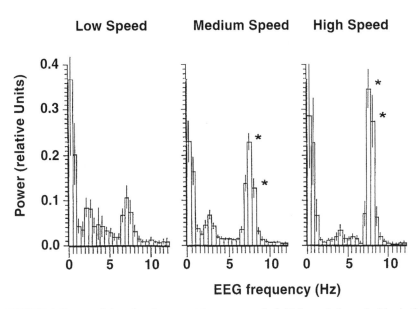

FIGURE 6. Increased theta band power at three progressively higher rotation velocities in the same recording session. Data are from the first 2.5 s of passive rotations. Low speed was 50 deg/s ($n = 8$), medium was 100 deg/s ($n = 40$), and high speed was 300 deg/s ($n = 7$).

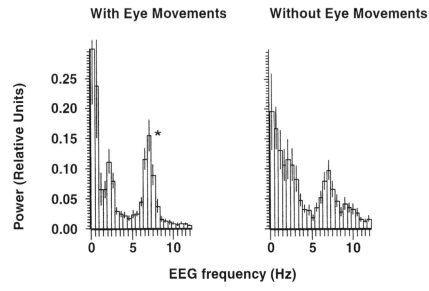

FIGURE 7. Spectral characteristics of hippocampal EEG in a restrained rat subjected to optokinetic stimulation with a planetarium-like projector. Averaged power spectrum ($n = 21$) of 2.5 s hippocampal EEG measurements accompanied with eye movements (*left*) and without eye movements (*right*). Data were combined from trials with optokinetic stimulation at speed 12 deg/s and 80 deg/s; no significant differences were found in measures made at the two speeds.

rats. Furthermore, in data obtained during optokinetic stimulation, theta power was significantly greater in trials when nystagmus was present than in those where it was absent (FIG. 7).

We compared hippocampal EEG recorded at the beginning of rotations to that measured while the robot was immobile after the same rotations. As shown in FIGURE 2, nystagmus was found in both of these intervals. However, the spectral power at 7.5 Hz was significantly lower after the end of the rotations than it was after rotation onset (FIG. 8). This suggests that the augmentation in theta power is not a simple vestibular response and is not correlated in a simple manner with nystagmus inasmuch as the rat had experienced the same (nystagmus-eliciting) acceleration forces (albeit in opposite directions) at the beginning and end of the rotations (FIG. 2). An uncoupling of nystagmus and hippocampal theta EEG is also evidenced in the second half of the rotation of FIGURE 2, where nystagmus continues, but theta is diminished. The significantly greater theta power at the beginning of movements in FIG. 8 suggests that, in addition to eye movements, other cues related to self-movements also influence the augmentation in power of theta hippocampal EEG.

DISCUSSION

The theta EEG in the 6–9 Hz range that was studied here has been associated in previous work with what were called "voluntary" movements of the animal such as running and jumping,[10] whereas only the 4–7 Hz theta frequency band has been observed during immobility of the animal.[14] These results have been replicated so frequently that the behavioral categories type I and type II have been used interchangeably to describe the corresponding high and low theta frequency bands. In contrast with this, our results show that robust high-frequency type I theta occurs not only in freely moving rats, but also in awake immobilized animals. We found that the power of the hippocampal EEG in the 6–9 Hz theta band was enhanced particularly during certain types of passive whole-body movements. This seems to be correlated with nystagmus as well as with activation of the vestibular and somatosensory systems that sense inertial stimuli and signal self-movements. We will first interpret our results in light of previous findings and then briefly discuss how whole-body movements and hippocampal theta EEG may figure in spatial navigation processing.

Rotations

In our study, whole-body rotations induced increases in theta power in the 7–8.5 Hz frequency range. Although Winson[15] also reported that whole-body rotation led to increases in theta power, this was shown only in curarized rats for theta EEG at a lower frequency (type II) band than that measured here. However, because type II theta is absent in the freely moving animal, it is less likely to be associated with processing of self-displacement information for navigation. The increased amplitude of this low-frequency, atropine-sensitive type II hippocampal theta EEG could be explained by the observations of Horii *et al.*[16] that electrical stimulation of the round window as well as caloric stimulation in urethane-anesthetized rats leads to increased levels of hippocampal acetylcholine. Despite the fact that cholinergic inputs to hippocampus from the medial septum drive the theta rhythm, this mechanism is

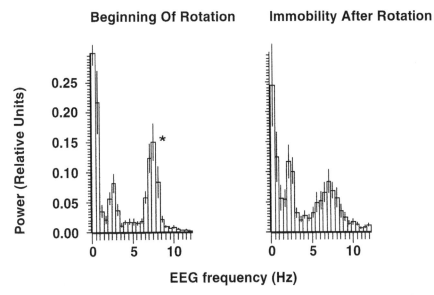

FIGURE 8. Nystagmus episodes in darkness. Comparison of theta band EEG after acceleration at the beginning of rotation versus deceleration at the end of rotation. Trials were selected for prominent nystagmus (*n* = 18).

unlikely to be related to the effects described here because the high-frequency theta that we recorded corresponds to the atropine-resistant EEG associated with type I behaviors.

The increases in theta power recorded here were progressively more dramatic at higher velocity rotations. This result recalls Vanderwolf's finding[10] in freely moving rats that theta amplitude was greater for "more vigorous, large-scale movements." However, the present data do not support his interpretation of theta-correlated movements as "voluntary" because all of the movements in our study were passive.

Translations

Arnolds et al.[17,18] studied hippocampal theta EEG in dogs and cats in several conditions including walking on a treadmill and passive translations on a cart. One of their principal findings was that upon the onset of displacements the theta EEG increased in peak frequency by increments ranging from 0.5 to over 2 Hz. These increases in the magnitude of higher frequency theta were also observed in passively translated dogs and cats. In agreement with the results found here, no significant increases in theta amplitude occurred at higher velocity translations. This is in contrast with the velocity dependency that we found during passive rotations.

In the study of Arnolds et al.[18] in the cat, eye movements (EOG) and ponto-geniculo-occipital (PGO) waves were recorded as indicators of saccadic eye movements. However, the data analyses and interpretations of this work rely principally upon the PGO waves. In their FIGURE 3,[18] it is evident that the onset of hippocampal theta EEG is synchronous with the onset of eye movements, as indicated by the EOG trace. Both of these occurred at the beginning of the passive translation of the cat.

Eye Movements

Several different reports point to influences on hippocampal theta EEG by eye movements. Sakai et al.[19] briefly described hippocampal theta changes in one encéphale isolé cat following caloric stimulation. It is not clear, however, whether this result is a type II theta response to vestibular sensory inputs like the results of Winson[15] or whether it is related to vestibular-evoked eye movements, or both. The data of Arnolds et al.[18] (FIG. 2) in the alert immobile cat show that the onset of a train of theta EEG waves is synchronous with the onset of eye movements as evidenced by EOG traces. Rapid eye movement sleep is another situation where strong correlations between theta activity and eye movements are found.[10,20]

Vestibular Stimulation

During rotations like the ones shown in FIGURE 3, the theta rhythmic activity was restricted to the period when the rat was rotated. This would suggest that sensory (vestibular) inputs are correlated with theta activity. However, despite the fact that accelerations and decelerations associated with the onset and the end of the rotations were approximately equal in magnitude (FIG. 2), theta synchrony occurred only after the beginning of and during the movement (FIG. 8). This suggests that the presence of high-frequency theta EEG is related to the actual state of movement of the animal, whether or not the movements are actually generated by the rat. Thus it seems that theta power increases are affected both by eye movements and inertial (vestibular and somatosensory) stimuli associated with rotations.

The contributions of vestibular cues for navigation have been described by several authors. Animals and humans that have been passively displaced in the absence of visual and auditory inputs can return independently to the point of origin, and this is disrupted by lesions of the vestibular system.[21,22] Other neurophysiological experiments have shown that the hippocampus has access to self-movement information.[7,23,24]

However, the actual role of the hippocampal theta rhythm in updating hippocampal spatial representations remains elusive. Spatially and behaviorally selective discharges of principal neurons of hippocampal CA1 are in synchrony with the theta rhythm.[25] O'Keefe and Recce[26] report that the timing of the first spike of each successive burst from a given hippocampal place cell undergoes precession in its phase relation with the ongoing theta activity. A similar relation has been shown for sniffing and theta in rats.[27] Models of hippocampal function (e.g., McNaughton *et al.*[28]; Burgess *et al.*[29]) have employed the theta rhythm as a kind of clock for synchronizing sequences of repeated computations by the neuronal circuitry.

One possible function for the triggering of the onset of theta rhythm with whole-body movements could be to reset the theta rhythm,[30] presumably to assure continued updating of hippocampal representations of self-position. The results concerning the association of theta with nystagmus suggest another possibility: each fast-phase eye movement represents, in effect, the shift of the local view field across the retina. Perhaps this requires hippocampal synchronization, again as a type of resetting function. This, too, would be expected to call into action the circuitry involved in spatial representations and to bring the new field of view in concordance with the hippocampal representation of the current position of the animal.

ACKNOWLEDGMENTS

Thanks to V. Korshunov for helpful comments and loan of the electrode driver, A. Reber for help with eye movement recordings, S. Lemarchand for animal care, M.-A. Thomas for histology, A. Treffel for construction of restraint apparatus and robot accessories, O. Trullier for assistance with recordings, and F. Lacloche for assistance with illustrations.

REFERENCES

1. MILNER, B. 1972. Disorders of learning and memory after temporal lobe lesions in man. Clin. Neurosurg. **19:** 421–446.
2. MORRIS, R. G. M., P. GARRUD, J. N. P. RAWLINS & J. O'KEEFE. 1982. Place navigation in rats with hippocampal lesions. Nature **297:** 681–683.
3. O'KEEFE, J. A. 1976. Place units in the hippocampus of the freely moving rat. Exp. Neurol. **51:** 78–109.
4. WIENER, S. I., C. A. PAUL & H. EICHENBAUM. 1989. Spatial and behavioral correlates of hippocampal neuronal activity. J. Neurosci. **9:** 2737–2763.
5. O'KEEFE, J. & A. SPEAKMAN. 1987. Single unit activity in the rat hippocampus during a spatial memory task. Exp. Brain Res. **68:** 1–27.
6. QUIRK, G. O., R. U. MULLER & J. L. KUBIE. 1990. The firing of hippocampal place cells in the dark depends on the rat's recent experience. J. Neurosci. **10:** 2008–2017.
7. WIENER, S. I., V. KORSHUNOV, R. GARCIA & A. BERTHOZ. Inertial, substratal and landmark cue control of hippocampal CA1 place cells. Eur. J. Neurosci. **7:** 2206–2219.
8. WIENER, S. & A. BERTHOZ. 1993. Forebrain structures mediating the vestibular contribution during navigation. *In* Multisensory Control of Movement. A. Berthoz, Ed.: 427–456. Oxford University Press. Oxford, UK.

9. WINSON, J. 1974. Patterns of hippocampal theta rhythm in the freely moving rat. Electroencephalogr. Clin. Neurophysiol. **36:** 291–301.
10. VANDERWOLF, C. H. 1969. Hippocampal electrical activity and voluntary movement in the rat. Electroencephalogr. Clin. Neurophysiol. **26:** 407–418.
11. GAVRILOV, V. V., S. I. WIENER & A. BERTHOZ. 1995. Enhanced hippocampal theta EEG during whole body rotations in awake restrained rats. Neurosci. Lett. **197:** 239–241.
12. ROBINSON, T. E. 1980. Hippocampal rhythmic slow activity (RSA; theta): A critical analysis of selected studies and discussion of possible species-differences. Brain Res. Rev. **2:** 69–101.
13. KORSHUNOV, V. 1995. Miniature microdrive for extracellular recording of neuronal activity in freely moving animals. J. Neurosci. Methods **57:** 77–80.
14. FOSTER, T. C., C. A. CASTRO & B. L. MCNAUGHTON. 1989. Spatial selectivity of rat hippocampal neurons: Dependence on preparedness for movement. Science **244:** 1580–1582.
15. WINSON, J. 1976. Hippocampal theta rhythm. I. Depth profiles in the curarized rat. Brain Res. **103:** 57–70.
16. HORII, A., N. TAKEDA, T. MOCHIZUKI, K. OKAURA-MOCHIZUKI, Y. YAMAMOTO & A. YAMATODANI. 1994. Effects of vestibular stimulation on acetylcholine release from rat hippocampus: An in vivo microdialysis study. J. Neurophysiol. **72(2):** 605–611.
17. ARNOLDS, D. E. A. T., F. H. LOPES DA SILVA, W. AITINK & A. KAMP. 1979. Hippocampal EEG and behaviour in dog. II: Hippocampal EEG correlates with elementary motor acts. Electroencephalogr. Clin. Neurophysiol. **46:** 571–580.
18. ARNOLDS, D. E. A. T., F. H. LOPES DA SILVA, P. BOEIJINGA, A. KAMP & W. AITINK. 1984. Hippocampal EEG and motor activity in the cat: The role of eye movements and body acceleration. Behav. Brain Res. **12:** 121–135.
19. SAKAI, K., K. SANO & S. IWAHARA. 1973. Eye movements and hippocampal theta activity in cats. Electroencephalogr. Clin. Neurophysiol. **34:** 547–549.
20. LEUNG, L-W. S., F. H. LOPES DA SILVA & W. J. WALDMAN. 1982. Spectral characteristics of the hippocampal EEG in the freely moving rat. Electroencephalogr. Clin. Neurophysiol. **54:** 203–219.
21. BERITOFF, J. S. 1965. Neuronal mechanisms of higher vertebrate behavior. Little, Brown and Co. New York.
22. MILLER, S., M. POTEGAL & L. ABRAHAM. 1983. Vestibular involvement in a passive transport and return task. Physiol. Psychol. **11:** 1–10.
23. O'MARA, S. M., E. T. ROLLS, A. BERTHOZ & R. P. KESNER. 1994. Neurons responding to whole-body motion in the primate hippocampus. J. Neurosci. **14:** 6511–6523.
24. SHARP, P. E., H. T. BLAIR, D. ETKIN & D. B. TZANETOS. 1995. Influences of vestibular and visual motion information on the spatial firing patterns of hippocampal place cells. J. Neurosci. **15:** 173–189.
25. OTTO, T., H. EICHENBAUM, S. WIENER & C. G. WIBLE. 1991. Learning-related patterns of CA1 spike trains parallel stimulation parameters optimal for inducing hippocampal long-term potentiation. Hippocampus **1(2):** 181–192.
26. O'KEEFE, J. & M. L. RECCE. 1993. Phase relationship between hippocampal place units and the EEG theta rhythm. Hippocampus **3(3):** 317–330.
27. MACRIDES, F., H. EICHENBAUM & W. B. FORBES. 1982. Temporal relation between sniffing and the limbic theta rhythm during odor discrimination reversal learning. J. Neurosci. **2:** 1705–1717.
28. MCNAUGHTON, B. L., L. L. CHEN & E. J. MARKUS. 1991. "Dead reckoning," landmark learning, and the sense of direction: A neurophysiological and computational hypothesis. J. Cognit. Neurosci. **3(2):** 190–202.
29. BURGESS, N., J. O'KEEFE & M. RECCE. 1993. Using hippocampal 'place cells' for navigation, exploiting phase coding. *In* Advances in Neural Information Processing Systems. S. J. Hanson, C. L. Giles & J. D. Cowan, Eds. vol. 5. Morgan Kaufmann. San Mateo, CA.
30. VINOGRADOVA, O. S., E. S. BRAZHNIK, V. F. KITCHIGINA & V. S. STAFEKHINA. 1993. Acetylcholine, theta-rhythm and activity of hippocampal neurons in the rabbit. IV. Sensory stimulation. Neuroscience **53:** 993–1007.

Vestibular and Visual Cues in Navigation: A Tale of Two Cities

JAMES J. KNIERIM,[a] WILLIAM E. SKAGGS,
HEMANT S. KUDRIMOTI, AND BRUCE L. McNAUGHTON

Arizona Research Laboratories
Division of Neural Systems, Memory, and Aging
University of Arizona
384 Life Sciences North Building
Tucson, Arizona 85724

A traveler visits Kyoto, Japan, for the first time, and he decides to take a walk to explore the city. After meandering up and down the city streets, he decides that it is time to head back to the hotel. Not recognizing any landmarks in this new environment, his internal "sense of direction," which was continually updated as he wandered around, nonetheless provides a rough idea of which way to go in order to get to the hotel. As he proceeds in that direction, wondering if he has gotten lost once again, he finally comes upon a street corner that he recognizes from his outward journey, and is reassured that he is headed in the right direction.

At another time, the same traveler finds himself in New York City, where he grew up and which he knows very well. Leaving a restaurant on 64th Street, he confidently heads west toward Third Avenue to walk back to his hotel, engrossed in conversation. As he comes to the next street corner, he is taken aback when he recognizes that the street is Second Avenue, rather than Third. Suddenly, his whole perception of the orientation of the world, and where he is in it, rotates 180°, as he realizes that he has actually been walking east and must turn around to reach his destination.

This tale of two cities illustrates some of the basics of navigation and spatial learning that are the subject of this paper. Increasing behavioral and neurophysiological evidence indicates that mammalian navigation is based on a complex interplay of two broad classes of spatial cues: external sensory cues, such as visual landmarks, and internally generated signals (idiothetic cues), such as vestibular signals, about the animal's self-motion in the environment.[1] However, the exact nature of this interplay is still largely unknown. Do mammals preferentially use one type of cue over the other? Are any such preferences dependent on the exact cues available, on the exact navigational task, or on the prior experience of the animal? These questions have been addressed in several behavioral and neurophysiological studies, often with conflicting results. This paper reviews some of these studies and then reviews a neurophysiological and computational model developed over the past few years by McNaughton and colleagues,[2–5] which may account for many of the discrepancies in the literature. The model proposes that the hippocampus and related structures constitute a path integration system—that is, a navigation system that uses self-motion cues to maintain and update a vector representation of the animal's current distance and bearing relative to a starting location. In this model, the primary driving force on the head direction cell system, which serves as an "internal compass" for the rat, is the vestibular system. The role of external sensory information, such as visual landmarks, is to recalibrate the path integrator when it drifts out of calibration. Importantly, the model proposes that this role of visual input is a learned phenomenon, and it is thus potentially dependent on many aspects of the animal's prior

[a] Corresponding author.

experience. We report on some physiological studies that demonstrate such experience-dependence in the hippocampal place cell system and the thalamic head direction cell system, and suggest that this plasticity is the underlying cause of the varying results in the literature.

BEHAVIORAL STUDIES

Many studies have shown that rodents use both visual[6–10] and vestibular[11–17] cues to navigate efficiently. For example, if one arm of a plus (+)-shaped maze is consistently baited with food, rats will learn to go quickly to that arm when they are started at any of the other three arms. If the array of prominent landmarks surrounding the maze is rotated 90°, however, the rats will now choose the corresponding arm rotated 90° from the original goal arm, demonstrating that they were using the visual cues to locate the goal.[6] Other studies, however, show that rodents do not need these cues to navigate efficiently. A gerbil, for example, can search randomly for a displaced pup in the complete absence of external sensory cues, and then head directly back to its nest once it has found the pup.[11] This path integration ability was shown to be controlled largely by vestibular cues: if the platform containing the nest and gerbil was rotated abruptly while the gerbil searched for the pup, then the gerbil would compensate for this rotation and head back to the original nest location; however, if the rotation was very slow, below vestibular threshold, the gerbil would not compensate and would head toward the new nest location. Other studies have demonstrated that damage to the vestibular organs or vestibular nuclei can cause severe disruptions in various navigation tasks.[13,14,16,17]

It is not clear, however, whether animals primarily use path integration or visual landmarks for navigation, and whether under certain conditions the animals may switch from one strategy to another. Studies by Alyan and Jander[18] and by Etienne and colleagues[1,19–22] have addressed this question by incorporating probe trials in their tasks, in which visual information is made to conflict with idiothetic information. The studies by Alyan and Jander[18] suggest that mice rely initially on path integration mechanisms and ignore visual cues when these cues conflict; however, as the number of trials increases, the visual information eventually comes to predominate over the idiothetic information. Etienne's work, however, suggests the opposite, in that their hamsters relied predominantly on visual cues in early probe trials, and only after repeated "errors" did they begin to disregard the visual cues and rely on their path integration mechanisms.[21] Thus, these two studies, using similar (although not identical) procedures, arrived at very different results, illustrating the complex nature of the interaction between visual and vestibular cues. Furthermore, Etienne's work demonstrates that even the influence of visual cues alone can be quite complex, because it appears that not all visual cues are equally effective in controlling the animal's spatial behavior.[22] This difference in visual cue effectiveness may explain some of the variability seen between different studies in assessing the relative influences of visual landmarks and path integration.

NEUROPHYSIOLOGICAL STUDIES

The one brain structure most often identified with spatial learning and navigation in mammals is the hippocampus. Lesions to the hippocampal formation consistently impair performance in spatial learning tasks, while sparing other forms of learning.[23]

In addition, the most striking correlate of hippocampal cell firing is the spatial location of the animal.[24] These two sets of findings led O'Keefe and Nadel[23] to propose that the hippocampus formed a cognitive map of the environment, whereby organisms learn to navigate in familiar and unfamiliar environments. Nonetheless, after 25 years of research, the exact nature of the driving inputs to place cells is still not well understood. Most studies of their properties have focused on the role of external sensory cues (mostly visual cues) in controlling the spatial selectivity of these cells, and they have shown that place cells can be controlled by salient visual landmarks. For example, if a rat is trained to locate food on a +-shaped maze[7,25] or to forage for randomly scattered food pellets in a high-walled apparatus,[26] place cells are usually bound to the visual cues in the environment, in that rotation of these cues causes an equal rotation of the firing locations of place cells. However, visual input is not necessary in order for place cells to demonstrate normal spatial selectivity. If the salient visual cues are removed[7] or if the lights are extinguished entirely,[27–29] place cells retain their appropriate firing locations, provided that the rat had its bearings before the visual input was removed.

Another type of cell that has been linked to spatial navigation is the head direction cell, which was first discovered in the postsubiculum[30,31] and which has been identified subsequently in numerous brain areas.[32–36] These cells fire at high rates when an animal's head is pointed in a particular direction, regardless of the spatial location of the animal, and thus they presumably underlie an animal's internal sense of direction. Like place cells, head direction cells can be controlled by salient visual cues,[31] but they also maintain their directional tuning when the cues are removed or when the lights are extinguished, at least for a few minutes.[31,32,35] Under these conditions, both place cells and head direction cells presumably use idiothetic cues to maintain their firing selectivities.

The early studies that demonstrated visual cue control over place cells performed the cue rotations while the animal was removed from the environment. A number of more recent studies performed these manipulations in the presence of the rat, and the results have been more variable. Most of these experiments intentionally introduced a conflict between the directional information provided by idiothetic cues and the directional information provided by visual cues. For example, Chen and colleagues[35] rotated the visual cues in darkness while the rat was still in the experimental room. When the lights were turned back on, the rat perceived that the visual environment was rotated, but it had experienced no similar rotation from idiothetic cues. Under these conditions, most posterior cortical head direction cells did not rotate their tuning curves with the visual cues, but instead remained bound to the rat's inertial reference framework. Similarly, Sharp and colleagues[37] performed a variety of manipulations designed to give the rat different directional information from vestibular and visual cues while rats foraged for food in a high-walled cylinder with visual cues on the walls. In some experiments, they rotated the walls and the floor (with the rat), under conditions of light or darkness, and in other experiments they rotated only the floor or only the walls. Their recordings from hippocampal place cells showed a strong interaction between the visual and vestibular cues: when the two cues provided the same information to the rat, the behavior of place cells was consistent; however, when the two cues provided conflicting information, sometimes the firing of the place cells was tied to the visual cues, sometimes it was tied to the vestibular cues, and sometimes the firing properties changed altogether. Overall, some studies suggested that visual cues usually predominate over vestibular cues[31,36,38]; others suggested that idiothetic cues predominate,[33,35,39] while others showed an influence of both types of cues that is seemingly unpredictable from trial to trial, but may be related to the degree of the discrepancy between the two sources of directional information.[37,40,41]

A MODEL OF THE HIPPOCAMPAL SYSTEM
AS A PATH INTEGRATION SYSTEM

Over the past few years, McNaughton and colleagues have developed a computational and neurophysiological model of the hippocampus and related structures that may help to account for the variability seen in both behavioral and physiological studies of the relative influences of visual and vestibular cues.[2-5] The model proposes that the hippocampus is primarily a path integration system and that the primary drive upon place cells and head direction cells is from vestibular and other idiothetic sources. Because this is an inertially based system, it is prone to cumulative error. The model proposes that the role of visual landmarks is to recalibrate the system when it drifts. This recalibration ability is a learned phenomenon, built up through exploration of a new environment. Thus, in a completely novel environment, visual cues should have little or no effect on the firing properties of place cells and head direction cells, but their influences will become stronger as the rat explores and becomes familiar with the environment, until eventually the visual cues are able to correct errors in the system due to drift in the vestibular system.

Let us first discuss how the rat's internal direction sense is updated. The model comprises four classes of cells (FIG. 1). *Head direction cells* are represented by the outer ring of cells, where each cell's preferred firing direction is represented by that cell's position in the ring. *Vestibular cells* detect right and left rotations of the head in the azimuthal plane. *Rotation cells,* represented by the inner two rings, fire only when they receive input simultaneously from vestibular cells and from their corresponding head direction cells; thus these cells represent the combination of a particular head direction and a particular change (right turn or left turn) in that head direction. Finally, *visual cells,* which represent particular local views of the landmarks visible at each head direction in the environment, have modifiable synapses onto the head direction cells.

When an animal is facing north, the "north" head direction cells are active, but the vestibular and rotation cells are silent. Excitatory connections between cells representing similar head directions and inhibitory connections (not shown) between cells representing different directions ensure that there is a single peak of population activity representing one head direction. When the animal turns its head 90° to the right, the "right" vestibular neurons detect this motion and begin to fire, which in turn causes the "right × north" rotation cell to begin firing. Because the connections of the rotation cells back onto the head direction cells are asymmetric, displaced in the direction of head rotation, the peak of the population activity of the head direction cells shifts in that direction. When the animal's head turn stops, the vestibular cells and rotation cells cease firing, and the head direction cell peak activity remains at its new location (east). In this way, the animal's sense of direction is updated purely on the basis of idiothetic information.

During exploration, however, the simultaneous firing of head direction cells and the visual cells that represent the landmarks currently visible to the rat strengthen the modifiable connections between these cells. If there is a consistent mapping between particular head directions and particular visible landmarks, then these connections will continue to strengthen, until they become strong enough to override the vestibular input. Thus, when the vestibular system begins to accumulate error over time, causing the head direction cells to drift out of calibration, the visual input is able to override the vestibular input and recalibrate the system.

These principles are illustrated at the beginning of this paper. The traveler in Kyoto is in a totally unfamiliar environment, and as he wanders, he is maintaining his sense of direction relative to his hotel purely by means of path integration. The many visual landmarks are of little use, because he has not had the time to learn the directions associated with the landmarks. Instead, he must rely on his internal direction sense to head back, until he finally comes upon a landmark that is

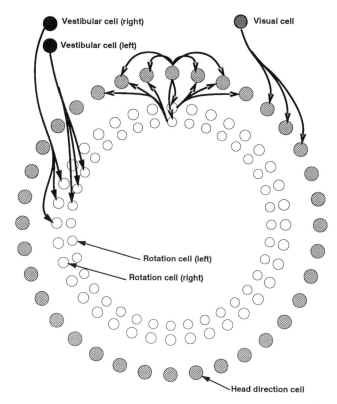

FIGURE 1. A model of the rat's internal sense of direction. (From Skaggs *et al.*[4] Reproduced, with permission, from the MIT Press.)

associated with a particular direction, and he is reassured he is going the right way. In contrast, in the very familiar environment of New York, the traveler is still using his internal direction sense to guide his initial heading direction as he leaves the restaurant and believes he is heading west. When he recognizes the street corner as Second Avenue, however, this visual input causes a sudden reorientation of his sense of direction, and his perception of the orientation of the world shifts 180°; presumably, the visual cues caused his "west" cells to shut off and his "east" cells to start firing.

One prediction from this model is that, if no stable relationship exists between the visual landmarks and the animal's internal direction sense, then no strong associations would form between the visual cells and the head direction cells, and thus the visual landmarks would not exert strong control over the head direction cells. This prediction was confirmed in an experiment in which we intentionally disoriented one group of rats before each entry into a high-walled cylinder with a single white cue card.[42] Each time the rat entered the environment, its direction sense was presumably set at some arbitrary direction relative to the visual cue. A second group of rats was not disoriented, but instead was allowed to maintain a consistent sense of direction relative to the visual cue. After extensive training, we then disoriented both groups of rats and recorded simultaneously the firing of hippocampal place cells and anterior thalamic head direction cells. The results showed clearly that the visual cue had much weaker control over these cells in the rats that had always been disoriented during training than in the control group of rats. In the former group, place fields and head direction tuning curves often rotated relative to the visual cue both between and within sessions; these rotations were much less frequent in the control rats. Importantly, the head direction cells and the place cells were always tightly coupled to each other; whenever the place cells rotated relative to the visual cue, simultaneously recorded head direction cells rotated by the same amount.

Recently, McNaughton and colleagues[5] used the same principles embodied in this model of the rat's sense of direction to expand the model and incorporate two-dimensional translations of the head in addition to rotations. Briefly, the model proposes that the rat's two-dimensional position in space can be updated by self-motion cues in a manner similar to the updating of head direction. Five classes of cells comprise this model. The rat's location in space is encoded by the firing of hippocampal *place cells,* whereas *head direction cells* encode the rat's current heading in the environment. These two classes of cells connect to a third class, which encodes the combination of a particular place and a particular head direction. *Self-motion cells,* a variety of which are found in different cortical areas,[43] modulate the activity of these *place-direction cells,* such that they fire only when the rat is at a particular location and heading and is in motion. These properties have been reported in cells of the subiculum and postsubiculum.[44,45] If the place-direction cells have asymmetric contacts back onto the place cell system, biased in the direction that the rat is heading (analogous to the asymmetric contacts of the rotation cells onto head direction cells), then this system could serve as a path integrator, whereby self-motion cues continually update the animal's representation of direction (in the head direction cell system) and location (in the place cell system). The place system will also be subject to cumulative error, however, and it is proposed that modifiable synapses from *visual cells* onto the place cells can, with experience, override the idiothetic input when it drifts out of calibration.

Although current data are insufficient to prove or disprove these models, we believe that the principles underlying them—that the hippocampus is primarily a path integration system, controlled by vestibular and other idiothetic cues, with a learned role of visual landmarks to correct for cumulative error—account to a large degree for many otherwise puzzling and conflicting experimental results, some of which were outlined above. The large degree of variability seen in studies that tried to tease apart the relative influences of visual versus vestibular cues may well be due to the experience-dependent nature of the visual cue control, proposed in the above models and verified experimentally.[42] It is evident that mammalian navigational abilities result from a complex interaction between idiothetic and external sensory cues, and the models reviewed in this paper may provide a useful conceptual framework for understanding this interaction at the behavioral, neurophysiological, and computational levels.

REFERENCES

1. ETIENNE, A. S. 1992. Navigation of a small mammal by dead reckoning and local cues. Curr. Dir. Psychol. Sci. **1:** 48–52.
2. MCNAUGHTON, B. L., L. L. CHEN & E. J. MARKUS. 1991. "Dead reckoning," landmark learning, and the sense of direction: A neurophysiological and computational hypothesis. J. Cognit. Neurosci. **3:** 190–202.
3. MCNAUGHTON, B. L., J. J. KNIERIM & M. A. WILSON. 1995. Vector encoding and the vestibular foundations of spatial cognition: Neurophysiological and computational mechanisms. *In* The Cognitive Neurosciences. M. Gazzaniga, Ed.: 585–595. MIT Press. Cambridge, MA.
4. SKAGGS, W. E., J. J. KNIERIM, H. S. KUDRIMOTI & B. L. MCNAUGHTON. 1995. A model of the neural basis of the rat's sense of direction. *In* Advances in Neural Information Processing Systems, Vol. 7. D. S. Touretzky, G. Tesauro & T. K. Leen, Eds.: 173–180. MIT Press. Cambridge, MA.
5. MCNAUGHTON, B. L., C. A. BARNES, J. L. GERRARD, K. GOTHARD, M. W. JUNG, J. J. KNIERIM, H. KUDRIMOTI, Y. QIN, W. E. SKAGGS, M. SUSTER & K. L. WEAVER. 1996. Deciphering the hippocampal polyglot: The hippocampus as a path integration system. J. Exp. Biol. **199:** 173–185.
6. O'KEEFE, J. & D. H. CONWAY. 1980. On the trail of the hippocampal engram. Physiol. Psychol. **8:** 229–238.
7. O'KEEFE, J. & A. SPEAKMAN. 1987. Single unit activity in the rat hippocampus during a spatial memory task. Exp. Brain Res. **68:** 1–27.
8. SUZUKI, S., G. AUGERINOS & A. H. BLACK. 1980. Stimulus control of spatial behavior on the eight-arm maze in rats. Learn. Motiv. **11:** 1–18.
9. COLLETT, T. S., B. A. CARTWRIGHT & B. A. SMITH. 1986. Landmark learning and visuo-spatial memories in gerbils. J. Comp. Physiol. A **158:** 835–851.
10. ZOLADEK, L. & W. A. ROBERTS. 1978. The sensory basis of spatial memory in the rat. Anim. Learn. Behav. **6:** 77–81.
11. MITTELSTAEDT, M. L. & H. MITTELSTAEDT. 1980. Homing by path integration in a mammal. Naturwissenschaften **67:** 566–567.
12. DOUGLAS, R. J. 1966. Cues for spontaneous alternation. J. Comp. Physiol. Psychol. **62:** 171–183.
13. POTEGAL, M., M. J. DAY & L. ABRAHAM. 1977. Maze orientation, visual and vestibular cues in two-maze spontaneous alternation of rats. Physiol. Psychol. **5:** 414–420.
14. MILLER, S., M. POTEGAL & L. ABRAHAM. 1983. Vestibular involvement in a passive transport and return task. Physiol. Psychol. **11:** 1–10.
15. MATTHEWS, B. L., K. A. CAMPBELL & S. A. DEADWYLER. 1988. Rotational stimulation disrupts spatial learning in fornix-lesioned rats. Behav. Neurosci. **102:** 35–42.
16. MATTHEWS, B. L., J. H. RYU & C. BOCKANECK. 1989. Vestibular contribution to spatial orientation. Acta Otolaryngol. (Stockh.) Suppl. **468:** 149–154.
17. OSSENKOPP, K.-P. & E. L. HARGREAVES. 1993. Spatial learning in an enclosed eight-arm radial maze in rats with sodium arsanilate-induced labyrinthectomies. Behav. Neural Biol. **59:** 253–257.
18. ALYAN, S. & R. JANDER. 1994. Short-range homing in the house mouse, *Mus musculus*: Stages in the learning of directions. Anim. Behav. **48:** 285–298.
19. ETIENNE, A. S., R. MAURER & F. SAUCY. 1988. Limitations in the assessment of path dependent information. Behaviour **106:** 81–111.
20. ETIENNE, A. S., S. JORIS, R. MAURER & E. TERONI. 1990. Enhancing the impact of visual extra-maze cues in a spatial orientation task. Behav. Brain Res. **38:** 199–210.
21. ETIENNE, A., S. J. LAMBERT, B. REVERDIN & E. TERONI. 1993. Learning to recalibrate the role of dead reckoning and visual cues in spatial navigation. Anim. Learn. Behav. **21:** 266–280.
22. ETIENNE, A. S., S. JORIS-LAMBERT, C. DAHN-HURNI & B. REVERDIN. 1995. Optimizing

visual landmarks: Two- and three-dimensional minimal landscapes. Anim. Behav. **49:** 165–179.
23. O'KEEFE, J. & L. NADEL. 1978. The hippocampus as a cognitive map. Clarendon Press. London.
24. O'KEEFE, J. & J. DOSTROVSKY. 1971. The hippocampus as a spatial map: Preliminary evidence from unit activity in the freely-moving rat. Brain Res. **34:** 171–175.
25. O'KEEFE, J. & D. H. CONWAY. 1978. Hippocampal place units in the freely moving rat: Why they fire where they fire. Exp. Brain Res. **31:** 573–590.
26. MULLER, R. U. & J. L. KUBIE. 1987. The effects of changes in the environment on the spatial firing of hippocampal complex-spike cells. J. Neurosci. **77:** 1951–1968.
27. MCNAUGHTON, B. L., B. LEONARD & L. CHEN. 1989. Cortical-hippocampal interactions and cognitive mapping: A hypothesis based on the reintegration of the parietal and inferotemporal pathways for visual processing. Psychobiology **17:** 230–235.
28. QUIRK, G. J., R. U. MULLER & J. L. KUBIE. 1990. The firing of hippocampal place cells in the dark depends on the rat's recent experience. J. Neurosci. **10:** 2008–2017.
29. MARKUS, E. J., C. A. BARNES, B. L. MCNAUGHTON, V. L. GLADDEN & W. E. SKAGGS. 1994. Spatial information content and reliability of hippocampal CA1 neurons: Effects of visual input. Hippocampus **4:** 410–421.
30. TAUBE, J. S., R. U. MULLER & J. B. RANCK, JR. 1990. Head direction cells recorded from the postsubiculum in freely moving rats. I. Description and quantitative analysis. J. Neurosci. **10:** 420–435.
31. TAUBE, J. S., R. U. MULLER & J. B. RANCK, JR. 1990. Head direction cells recorded from the postsubiculum in freely moving rats. II. Effects of environmental manipulations. J. Neurosci. **10:** 436–447.
32. MIZUMORI, S. J. Y. & J. D. WILLIAMS. 1993. Directionally selective mnemonic properties of neurons in the lateral dorsal nucleus of the thalamus of rats. J. Neurosci. **13:** 4015–4028.
33. WIENER, S. I. 1993. Spatial and behavioral correlates of striatal neurons in rats performing a self-initiated navigation task. J. Neurosci. **13:** 3802–3817.
34. CHEN, L. L., L.-H. LIN, E. J. GREEN, C. A. BARNES & B. L. MCNAUGHTON. 1994. Head direction cells in the rat posterior cortex. I. Anatomical distribution and behavioral modulation. Exp. Brain Res. **101:** 8–23.
35. CHEN, L. L., L.-H. LIN, C. A. BARNES & B. L. MCNAUGHTON. 1994. Head direction cells in the rat posterior cortex. II. Contributions of visual and ideothetic information to the directional firing. Exp. Brain Res. **101:** 24–34.
36. TAUBE, J. S. 1995. Head direction cells recorded in the anterior thalamic nuclei of freely moving rats. J. Neurosci. **15:** 70–86.
37. SHARP, P. E., H. T. BLAIR, D. ETKIN & D. B. TZANETOS. 1995. Influences of vestibular and visual motion information on the spatial firing patterns of hippocampal place cells. J. Neurosci. **15:** 173–189.
38. GOODRIDGE, J. P. & J. S. TAUBE. 1995. Preferential use of the landmark navigation system by head direction cells in rats. Behav. Neurosci. **109:** 1–13.
39. WIENER, S. I., V. A. KORSHUNOV, R. GARCIA & A. BERTHOZ. 1995. Inertial, substratal and landmark cue control of hippocampal CA1 place cell activity. Eur. J. Neurosci. **7:** 2206–2219.
40. ROTENBERG, A., J. KUBIE & R. MULLER. 1993. Variable coupling between a stimulus object and place cell firing fields. Soc. Neurosci. Abstr. **19:** 357.
41. KNIERIM, J. J., H. S. KUDRIMOTI & B. L. MCNAUGHTON. 1994. Dynamics of visual cue control over head direction cells and place cells. Soc. Neurosci. Abstr. **20:** 1207.
42. KNIERIM, J. J., H. S. KUDRIMOTI & B. L. MCNAUGHTON. 1995. Place cells, head direction cells, and the learning of landmark stability. J. Neurosci. **15:** 1648–1659.
43. MCNAUGHTON, B. L., S. J. Y. MIZUMORI, C. A. BARNES, B. J. LEONARD, M. MARQUIS & E. J. GREEN. 1994. Cortical representation of motion during unrestrained spatial navigation in the rat. Cereb. Cortex **4:** 27–39.
44. SHARP, P. E. & C. GREEN. 1994. Spatial correlates of firing patterns of single cells in the subiculum of the freely moving rat. J. Neurosci. **14:** 2339–2356.
45. SHARP, P. E. 1996. Multiple spatial/behavioral correlates for cells in the rat postsubiculum: Multiple regression analysis and comparison to other hippocampal areas. Cereb. Cortex **6:** 238–259.

Subjective Sensation during Interaction between Horizontal Vestibular and Vertical Pursuit Stimulation

VICENTE HONRUBIA,[a] ALAN GREENFIELD,[a]
CLIFFORD LAU,[b] AND ANGUS RUPERT[c,d]

[a] UCLA Division of Head and Neck Surgery
CHS 62-132
10833 Le Conte Avenue
Los Angeles, California 90095

[b] Office of Naval Research
Arlington, Virginia 22217

[c] NASA—Johnson Space Center
Houston, Texas 77058

Vestibular function is a sensorimotor integration process that facilitates the maintenance of gaze, posture, equilibrium, and the perception of head position and motion. This report documents the results of studies in human subjects concerning the relationship between the perception of moving objects, the vestibular subjective sensation of motion (VSSM), and associated eye movements during interactive visual and vestibular stimulation.

Studies concerning mechanisms of eye movement control have shown that both visual and vestibular input, working simultaneously, are necessary for proper gaze stabilization throughout the range of normal head movement.[1-3] The visual tracking of small moving targets depends on the smooth pursuit (SP) system, whose function is to maintain objects of visual interest centered on the fovea of the retina. The operation of SP is optimal when object motion is of low velocity and low frequency. The SP functions as a closed loop velocity servo system with the effective stimulus being the retinal slip velocity, which is equal to the difference between the object velocity and the eye tracking velocity.[4] Motion of the head is detected in the inner ear by the hair cells functioning as transducers.[5,6] The inner ear responses are coded in terms of head velocity during natural head movements because of underlying mechanical and physiological processes and subsequent biological signal transformation in the nervous system.[1,7] The operation of the vestibular system is critical for producing compensatory vestibulo-ocular reflexes (VOR) to maintain stable gaze during head motion of high velocities and/or high frequencies. In everyday activities, with diverse motion of objects and of the head, the maintenance of gaze is the result of the complementary interaction of the visual and vestibular systems working together in ways that are becoming well understood in regard to the production of reflexes.[1,8,9]

The joint function of the vestibular and visual systems provides the information necessary for the perception of self-motion, of the relative motion between objects, and of the motion of objects in relation to the self, data that is necessary for orientation during human navigation. In contrast to the reflexes, the psychophysical

[d] Mailing address: Angus Rupert, M.D., Code 22 NAMRL, Pensacola, FL 32508-1046.

mechanisms of visual and vestibular interaction are poorly understood. One difficulty associated with the psychophysical phenomena is that accepted methods to quantify the VSSM are not available. In contrast to the evaluation of hearing and vision, for example, the VSSM is not part of the clinical evaluation of vestibular patients.[2]

Many situations lead to illusions of motion (e.g., circularvection, oculogyration, etc.).[10–12] One type of illusion, which has been described by us, occurs when the perception of the velocity of a small visual target (VT) moving sinusoidally in the horizontal plane is predictably affected by rotational vestibular and optokinetic stimulation.[13,14] In these experiments, the VT appears to travel for a shorter duration when it moves in the direction of the body's angular acceleration or against the direction of the optokinetic drum. Both vestibular and optokinetic stimuli resulted in a sensation of body motion (by the phenomenon of circularvection during optokinetic stimulation).

It was then postulated that the brain judges the motion of objects in relation to the self in a relativistic manner. The brain operates as if there is an egocentric sense against which the motion of the world is evaluated. The steady-state condition of this internal reference center (IRC) can be changed by physiological stimulation of the vestibular or visual motion detectors. The following relation describes the operation of this center:

$$V_{ss} = V_p - IRC, \qquad (1)$$

where V_{ss} is the perceived object velocity, V_p is the head-referenced target velocity, and IRC is the velocity of the world as perceived by the brain during vestibular or optokinetic stimulation. The difference between V_{ss} and V_p is a measure of the effect of vestibular and optokinetic inputs in the IRC or, in other words, a measure of how these stimuli affect the perception of the world by the brain.

In order to expand the information about the operation of the IRC, the sinusoidal VT trajectory was placed in a vertical orientation. This experimental paradigm allowed the generalization of equation 1 to a vector form. In addition, vestibular stimulation was provided by sinusoidal head rotation at a frequency that more closely approximated normal head movements. Let us define $\vec{V}_{VOR}$ as the slow component VOR velocity associated with sinusoidal head rotation. If both stimuli are executed concurrently, we then can write

$$\vec{V}_{ss} = \vec{V}_p - \vec{V}_{VOR} \qquad (2)$$

as a generalization of equation 1. In the present experiment, it was expected that an error will occur in the perception of motion of a vertically moving VT during horizontal vestibular stimulation. Under the influence of the visual (vertical) and vestibular (horizontal) stimuli, it is anticipated that the perceived VT trajectory will be tilted and that this error can be compensated by tilting the trajectory of this target away from true vertical. We hypothesized that the magnitude of horizontal eye velocities resulting from the tracking of this target after tilt is predicted by the magnitude of the slow component of the VOR during identical vestibular stimulation without any visual cues. During the evaluation of this hypothesis, it was found that the data provided information about the mechanism and a new approach to the quantitative measurement of the VSSM.

METHODS

Eye Movement Recording

Ten healthy young male subjects participated in this study. Subjects were not informed of the psychophysical nature of the experiment prior to testing. Subjects were fitted with standard electro-oculographic (EOG) electrodes. These were placed monocularly in the vertical plane and bitemporally in the horizontal plane. EOG amplifiers with a cutoff frequency of 100 Hz were used. Although care was taken in the placement of the electrodes so as to record only movement in the horizontal or vertical plane by the appropriate electrode pair, slight misalignment could occur in spite of efforts to relocate the electrodes when necessary.

Eye movements were calibrated by moving the VT ± 15° in the horizontal plane and ± 8° in the vertical plane.[15,16] The scale of the chart recorder was adjusted to give a deflection of approximately 1 mm/° at the time of calibration. Eye movements during calibration were recorded by the chart recorder. A precise calibration factor was digitally recorded in each data file. This process was repeated at least five times during every test session before every set of test conditions to compensate for EOG changes.

The tracking capability of each subject in the horizontal and vertical planes was measured at the beginning of each test session. For vertical tracking, the VT was made to move sinusoidally in the vertical plane at a peak velocity of 12°/s and a frequency of 0.2 Hz. For horizontal tracking, the VT was made to move sinusoidally in the horizontal plane at a peak velocity of 24°/s and a frequency of 0.2 Hz.

Stimulus Presentation and Eye Movement Measurement

Subjects were seated in a rotatory chair mounted on a voltage controlled servo motor. Rotation occurred in the horizontal plane. Chair velocity was measured by means of a tachometer. Subjects were restrained with seatbelts and leg and head restraints. A flat black planar surface was mounted on the chair and placed in the center of the subjects' field of vision, 30 inches from the center of the head, for the purpose of projecting a VT. The chair was placed in a light-tight darkened experimental chamber. Communication between subjects and operators was accomplished by means of an intercom. Handles equipped with electronic switches (subjective sensation switches) were located on the end of each armrest of the rotatory chair. The switches were used by the subjects to indicate their perceived direction of self-rotation.

The VT was created by a laser beam projected into a system of mirrors mounted on galvanometers. The motion of one mirror generated the vertical motion of the VT while the motion of another, oriented at right angles to the first, generated the horizontal motion. The amplitude of the command signal sent to the horizontal galvanometer could be continuously adjusted by the operator to give motion between 0 and 24°/s. Computer programs were written to simultaneously activate the chair and the VT motion at any desired frequency with independent amplitudes and phase values.

A Macintosh computer was used to control the experimental apparatus and to acquire and store data. Custom software (MacEyeball©[17]) was used to operate the computer. The computer recorded the command signals controlling the vertical movement of the VT, the chair tachometer signal, vertical and horizontal eye position signals, and a response indicating the subject's perceived direction of self-motion. Data was digitized at 204.8 Hz.

In addition to the computer, a digital chart recorder (Gould TA4000 8 channel) provided a hard-copy record of the experiment. The TA4000 recorded the command signals to the laser galvanometers, the chair tachometer signal, vertical and horizontal eye position signals, a response indicating the subject's perceived direction of self-motion, and the laser power command signal.

Measurement Conditions

Each subject was rotated sinusoidally and without any visual stimuli at a frequency of 0.2 Hz for 150 s. This test was divided into three segments, each 50 s in length. Each segment used a different rotational stimulus peak velocity, 14, 21, and 28°/s. The order in which these segments were presented was randomized. A subset of six subjects was instructed to press the subjective sensation switches to indicate perceived direction of self-motion.

Three interactive tests were designed to evaluate the hypothesis of equation 2. In the FULL cycle tests, the laser power was always on. The rotational chair was driven sinusoidally at a frequency of 0.2 Hz and at one of the following three randomly presented peak velocities: 14, 21, or 28°/s. The vertical motion of the VT was sinusoidal with a frequency of 0.2 Hz and a peak velocity of 12°/s. The horizontal motion of the VT was sinusoidal with a frequency of 0.2 Hz and a peak velocity that could range between 0 and 24°/s. The combination of vertical and horizontal VT motions produced a linear trajectory with an angle from the vertical between 0 and 63°. Command signals were synchronized so that as the chair moved to the left, the VT moved up and to the right, and as the chair moved to the right, the VT moved down and to the left. The trajectory of the VT may be written in vector form as a function of time (t),

$$V_{VT}(\hat{i} \tan \theta \sin \omega t + \hat{j} \sin \omega t), \tag{3}$$

where $V_{VT} = 12°/s$, $\omega = 2\pi \cdot 0.2$ Hz, θ is the angle of inclination with the vertical and $\hat{i}$ and $\hat{j}$ are unit vectors in the horizontal and vertical planes, respectively. The velocity of the rotatory chair may be similarly expressed as

$$-V_c \hat{i} \sin \omega t, \tag{4}$$

where $V_c = 14$, 21, or 28°/s, presented as described earlier.

In the UP and DOWN cycle tests, all of the stimulus parameters were identical to those in the FULL cycle tests with the exception of the laser power control. In the UP cycle test, the laser was turned on during chair movement to the left as the VT moved up, and off as the chair moved to the right. In the DOWN cycle test, the laser was turned on during chair movement to the right as the VT moved down, and off as the chair moved to the left. These half-cycle tests were intended to isolate the measurement of eye movement responses to the right or to the left.

In each test, an error in the perceived motion of a vertically moving VT was created by horizontal vestibular stimulation. The underlying principles guiding the design and execution of these experiments are schematically described in FIGURE 1.

Equation 2 predicts that subjects will perceive a VT trajectory that is other than vertical. With the subsequent addition of a horizontal component to $\vec{V}_P$, it is expected that $\vec{V}_{VOR}$ can be negated and $\vec{V}_{ss}$ be made purely vertical. In FIGURE 1, A describes the characteristics of the stimuli and eye responses expected during an isolated vertical pursuit test. Diagram B describes stimuli and responses during horizontal head rotation in the dark. The arrows show the trajectories during the quarter cycle when the VT moves with increasing velocity upwards and when the rate table moves with increasing velocity toward the left. Diagrams C and D depict the relations of the stimuli and of the responses during conditions of interactive visual and vestibular stimulation. In addition, the lower diagrams show solid arrows indicating the expected direction of the imaginary $\vec{V}_{ss}$. In C, the $\vec{V}_{ss}$ is shown inclined to the left as predicted by equation 2 due to the interaction of the visual and vestibular stimuli. Eye movement trajectories in C are vertical because of the visual suppression of the

VOR. That is, there is no horizontal component in the eye movement response. However, if the VT trajectory is tilted to the right, as in D, the $\vec{V}_{ss}$ perception will became vertical when the horizontal component of the eye-movement trajectory $\vec{V}_p$ is equal to the eye movement during VOR stimulation (e.g., diagram B). The magnitude of $\vec{V}_p$ in the horizontal plane can be measured and is what we call the interaction velocity. According to equation 2, the magnitude of the interaction velocity is indistinguishable from eye velocities measured during rotation in the dark using identical rotatory stimuli.

For each interaction test, the VT trajectory was initially placed in the vertical plane. Subjects were told to track the VT during the test and given 20 or 25 s to view it

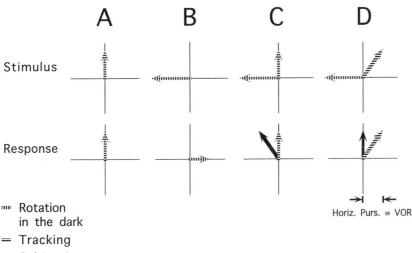

FIGURE 1. Schematic representation of stimulus-response expectations underlying our experiments. **A** involves only laser tracking in the vertical direction; **B** represents horizontal vestibular stimulation only, with no targets for fixation; **C** is a superposition of the first two cases; and **D** represents the situation after inclination of the visual target (VT) trajectory so that it appears vertical to the subject. "Horiz. Purs." indicates the magnitude of the horizontal component; it is expected that this will be equal to the response in **B**. Tracking stimuli and responses are indicated by arrows shaded with a horizontal pattern. Vestibular stimuli and responses are indicated by arrows shaded with a vertical pattern. Subjective responses are shown by solid arrows.

in the vertical plane. At the end of this period, subjects were asked to indicate by voice whether the trajectory appeared tilted left, tilted right, or was vertical. The tilt of the VT trajectory was then adjusted by the operator and the subject was again queried. This process was repeated several times using a random order of converging angles. Several reports of vertical might be found in a given test.

The initial adjustment to the horizontal VT controller was about half the rotatory head velocity taking into consideration the approximated 0.5 VOR gain of normal subjects as experienced in the laboratory. The VT velocity was adjusted to either a more leftward or rightward direction in random order to verify the accuracy of the report. The magnitude of the horizontal vector and hence the angle of tilt was recorded in the computer file, along with all the other experimental signals. The time at which the subjective verticality was reported was noted in the hard-copy record. The procedure was repeated several times during the 30-cycle duration of the test, usually providing three opportunities for appreciation of subjective verticality measurements.

Interaction tests were grouped in the following order: FULL cycle, UP cycle, and DOWN cycle. There were three of these groups for each subject. Each group corresponded to one of the randomly presented rotatory chair peak velocities.

For six subjects, another FULL cycle test was performed with a peak rotatory chair velocity of 28°/s at the end of the protocol. During this test, subjects were instructed to use the subjective sensation switches to indicate their direction of self-rotation.

Data Analysis Software

Several software programs were created in the LabVIEW programming language for use in this experiment. A program to view and print raw MacEyeball data, the *data viewer,* was written. A second program (*data splitter*) was made to divide long MacEyeball data files into individual smaller segments. A program for manual removal of fast components from the horizontal EOG channel was created (*the cumulator*). This program reconstructs a position record of slow components by removing fast components and replacing them with a fit that connects the end points of the two adjacent slow components. The result is a cumulative record of eye position. Finally, a program was written to analyze the response from the subjective sensation switches. This program would search the subjective sensation record and identify the time of the beginning and end of perceived left and right motions for each cycle of chair motion.

Data Analysis Procedure

Data analysis was accomplished from records stored in standardized computer files and by using paper records made by the chart recorder. The tracking ability of subjects in the horizontal plane was evaluated by comparing saccade free sinusoidal responses with peak-to-peak VT trajectory amplitudes so as to compute gain. Eye movements during vertical SP were deemed to be unreliable because of the inherent inaccuracy of such EOG measurements. They are affected by the artifactual effect of eyelid movement during eye blinking.[18] They were nonetheless recorded and measured in all tests. As expected, these measurements reflected more variation than the horizontal recordings.

The data *splitter* was used to divide the VOR response (no interaction) into three segments distinguished by rotatory chair peak velocity. The horizontal EOG channel of each segment was analyzed with the data *cumulator.* The resulting records were analyzed in terms of trends and inspected for peak-to-peak sinusoidal amplitudes which were converted to response velocities.

To analyze the interactive tests (FULL, UP, and DOWN cycle), segments of data where subjects reported a vertical VT trajectory were identified by cycle number and placed in separate files to be analyzed. FULL cycle tests yielded one peak velocity for each segment. UP and DOWN cycle tests (HALF cycle tests) each yielded two peak velocities for each segment. One value was obtained for eye movements while the VT was visible, and another for eye movements while the VT was not visible and analyzed accordingly (see above).

Data from the subjective sensation switches was evaluated as described above. The perceived times when motion to the right or left began (RB or LB) and when it ended (RE or LE) were recorded for rotation in the dark and for FULL cycle interaction. These FULL cycle tests were conducted with a rotatory chair peak velocity of 28°/s. Each of these sets of measurements (RB, LB, RE, LE) were converted to phases with respect to the rotatory chair motion and means and standard deviations were computed within a given test. The FULL cycle tests were divided to obtain results BEFORE and AFTER inclination of the VT trajectory away from true vertical.

RESULTS

Eye Movements

Vestibulo-Oculomotor Responses

An example of eye-movement responses during VOR testing is shown in FIGURE 2. FIGURE 2A, labeled horizontal EOG, is a trace of the eye position during horizontal rotations in the dark. This response shows nystagmic eye movements consisting of slow and fast components. For every cycle of head rotation, the direction of the slow component is opposite to the velocity of the head as shown in FIGURE 2F. In the vertical plane, no appreciable movements were related to the periodic movement of the head (FIG. 2C). The vertical eye position records have been edited to eliminate the corneoretinal potential variations associated with eye blinks that are common in the EOG recordings in the vertical plane.[18] Also shown in this figure are responses indicating direction of subjective self-motion as recorded by hand switches under the subject's control (FIG. 2E). Clockwise motion is shown by an upward trace deflection; counterclockwise motion is shown by a downward trace deflection.

Visual-Oculomotor Response

Smooth pursuit tracking was tested in every subject with both horizontally and vertically moving stimuli. Tracking responses in the horizontal plane yielded a mean gain of 0.97 with a standard deviation of 0.06. This result indicates that subjects were capable of tracking a VT as required for a test of interaction between VOR and horizontal SP tracking. The mean gain of vertical tracking was found to be 0.91 with a standard deviation of 0.22. Vertical eye measurements were not used in the evaluation of our hypothesis for reasons described above.

Visual-Vestibular Interaction

The goal of these experiments is to compare eye velocities measured during rotation in the dark with corresponding eye velocities measured during visual-vestibular interaction at a time when the subject reported a vertical VT trajectory. This goal was accomplished in three different tests under the headings of FULL, UP, and DOWN cycles of interaction.

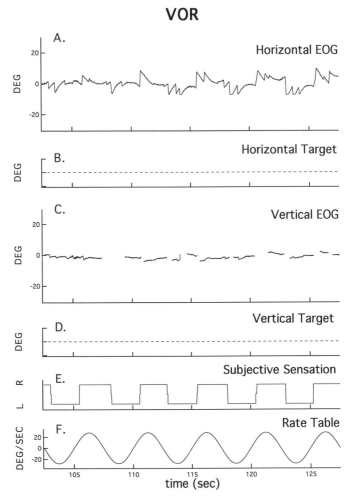

FIGURE 2. Vestibulo-ocular reflexes. Raw data from rotation in the dark. (**A**) A standard horizontal electro-oculographic (EOG) response to rotation in the dark showing a typical nystagmus with a combination of fast and slow components. (**B**) Dashed line indicates that the visual target (VT) is off so that no tracking or fixation stimulus of any kind is found in the horizontal plane. (**C**) Shows relatively little vertical EOG response due to the horizontal stimulus. (**D**) Dashed line indicates that the VT is off so that no tracking or fixation stimulus of any kind is found in the vertical plane. (**E**) Shows the subject's perception of self-motion as recorded by the electronic switches located on the armrests of the rotatory chair. (**F**) Displays a rate table motion of 0.2 Hz and 28°/s peak velocity.

Full-cycle visual-vestibular interaction. During these tests, the subjects were exposed to rotatory chair motion and VT motion simultaneously. No visual stimuli were present other than the VT. An example of the data recorded during chair rotations at 28°/s peak velocity is shown in FIGURE 3. The rate table and the vertical VT motion started simultaneously. As indicated in FIGURE 1, the phase relationship was such that counterclockwise head velocity was in phase with upward VT velocity (see FIG. 3D and F). Records of eye movements are shown in FIGURE 3A (horizontal EOG) and 3C (vertical EOG). During these tests, the subject's perception of the VT motion is a straight VT trajectory, which, due to the relative phases of the interactive stimuli, appears tilted to the left. The horizontal EOG traces shown during the first two

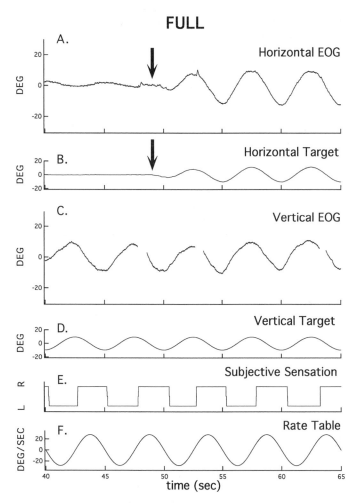

FIGURE 3. Raw data from a FULL cycle test. (**A**) Shows horizontal pursuit at the time when the visual target (VT) trajectory is inclined away from true vertical to subjective vertical. (**B**) The record in **A** is a response to **B** which indicates how the horizontal component of VT motion is modified by the operator to create an oblique VT trajectory. (**C**) Shows constant amplitude vertical pursuit. (**D**) The record in **C** is a response to **D** which indicates the fixed amplitude vertical component of VT motion. (**E**) Shows the subject's perception of self-motion as recorded by the electronic switches located on the armrests of the rotatory chair. (**F**) Displays a rate table motion of 0.2 Hz and 28°/s peak velocity.

cycles of response are almost straight traces with small sinusoidal position modulation due to a slight misalignment of the horizontal electrodes. At the time indicated by the arrows, the trajectory of the VT was inclined toward the right by the introduction of the command signal in the horizontal controlling galvanometer (see FIGS. 3A and B). The horizontal EOG records reflect the presence of a vector in that plane with large sinusoidal horizontal eye movements. Notice that the magnitude of the vertical vector remains unchanged and in phase with the horizontal vector. Both the VT and the eye trajectory have a rightward trajectory during upward motion and a leftward trajectory during downward motion. The inclination of the VT was changed until the subject indicated that the light appeared to move vertically.

FIGURE 3E (subjective sensation) shows a simultaneously recorded trace regarding subjective sensation of self-motion. Subjects reported motion responses that corresponded with the phase of the head velocity motion.

Half-cycle visual-vestibular interaction. During these tests, the subjects were exposed to rotatory chair motion and only a half cycle of VT visibility. In one experiment, the VT was visible only during its upward motion (UP cycle) and, in the other experiment, the VT was visible only during its downward motion (DOWN cycle).

An example of the records obtained in these experiments is shown in FIGURE 4. The data was obtained during UP cycle interaction. FIGURE 4A shows horizontal eye response during the transition period when the VT trajectory is changed from true vertical to subjective vertical. Tracking is evident during periods when the VT is visible. Nystagmus from the VOR response is present when the VT is not visible. During the first two cycles, when the VT was visible and strictly vertical, the horizontal eye trace is flat while the vertical trace shows upward SP motion; compare the target trajectories in the horizontal and vertical planes. During the horizontal nystagmic response, no vertical eye movement occurred, and the vertical eye trace (FIG. 4C) is flat except for the times when there were eye blinks that have been edited. During the last three cycles, as the horizontal command signal to the VT appears (FIG. 4B), a horizontal SP response alternates with the horizontal nystagmic response. There is no indication of discontinuity except at those moments when a fast component is associated with the VOR nystagmic response. The vertical eye movements remain unchanged. There is tracking during the appearance of the vertical VT and a flat response during the time of darkness *and* horizontal nystagmic responses.

Analysis of Horizontal Eye Movements

Vestibulo-Oculomotor Responses (Rotation in the Dark)

A summary of eye-velocity measurements from the 10 subjects is shown in FIGURE 5A. The response peak angular velocity is indicated for each test magnitude. The slope of the linear regression line is 0.47 ($r = 0.58$, $n = 30$). The mean gain values were also computed for each of the three head-velocity stimuli (0.47, 0.42, 0.47) independently. These gains were not statistically different from one another when subjected to a one-factor repeated ANOVA ($p > 0.05$), and thus the slope of the regression line is representative of the gain for all tests.

Visual-Vestibular Interaction

FULL cycle visual-vestibular interaction. The values of the horizontal eye movement velocity at the time of subjective verticality for all the subjects at each of the

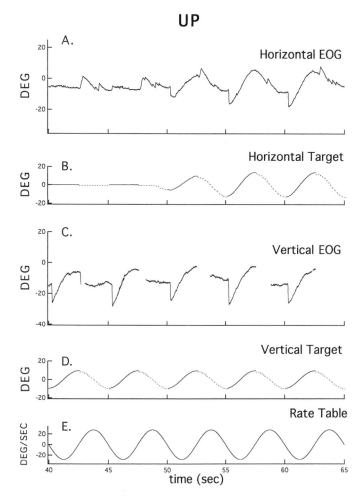

FIGURE 4. Raw data from an UP cycle test. (**A**) Shows horizontal pursuit at the time when the visual target (VT) trajectory is inclined away from true vertical to subjective vertical. Nystagmus is evident during periods when the VT is not visible. (**B**) The record in **A** is a response to **B** which indicates how the horizontal component of VT motion is modified by the operator to create an oblique VT trajectory. Dashed lines indicate periods when the VT is not visible. (**C**) Shows pursuit in the vertical plane when the VT is visible and a flat response when it is not. (**D**) The record in **C** is a response to **D** which indicates the fixed amplitude vertical component of VT motion. Again, dashed lines indicate periods when the VT is not visible. (**E**) Displays a rate table motion of 0.2 Hz and 21°/s peak velocity.

three rotatory velocities are shown in FIGURE 5D. The least square regression line through the data has a slope of 0.61 (r = 0.58, n = 28). A comparison of the values of the VOR responses in the dark and of the interaction velocity is shown in FIGURE 5G. The slope of the regression line is 0.91 (r = 0.73, n = 28). The confidence interval (±0.35) indicates that the slope is not different from 1.0. Thus, although

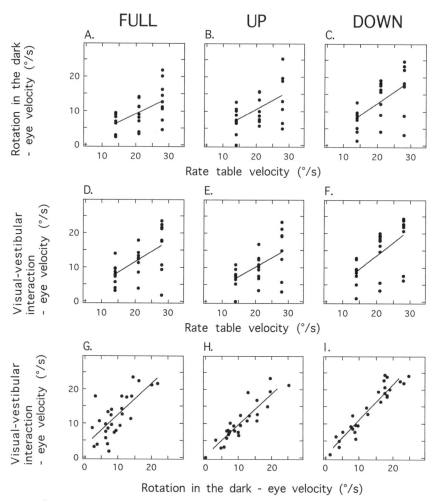

FIGURE 5. Data for one test paradigm shown in each column: FULL (*left*), UP (*middle*), and DOWN (*right*). First row shows eye velocity measured during rotation in the dark plotted against the rotatory chair velocity. Second row shows visual-vestibular interaction eye velocity plotted against the rotatory chair velocity. Third row shows visual-vestibular interaction eye velocity plotted against eye velocity measured during rotation in the dark. Each plot has undergone linear regression analysis. The resultant slopes (m), correlation coefficients (r), and number of points (n) are: (**A**) m = 0.47 (r = 0.58, n = 30); (**B**) m = 0.53 (r = 0.53, n = 27); (**C**) m = 0.68 (r = 0.61, n = 28); (**D**) m = 0.61 (r = 0.58, n = 28); (**E**) m = 0.55 (r = 0.56, n = 27); (**F**) m = 0.78 (r = 0.64, n = 28); (**G**) m = 0.91 (r = 0.73, n = 28); (**H**) m = 0.90 (r = 0.90, n = 27); and (**I**) m = 1.04 (r = 0.95, n = 28).

values of the VOR and interaction test responses varied among subjects, the clear correlation between the responses suggests that their individual variations reflect internal operating differences rather than errors associated with the experimental procedures.

Half-cycle visual-vestibular interaction. Horizontal eye velocities were calculated separately during the UP and DOWN cycle tests at the time of the subjective vertical perception of the VT for each subject. Thus, each of the UP or DOWN cycle visual-vestibular interaction tests yielded two sets of eye-velocity data. The first set contains measurements from the nystagmic response while rotating in the dark. The second set corresponds to the visual-vestibular interaction measurement. FIGURE 5B and C show the individual nystagmic response results plotted against each rotational velocity and the calculated linear regression lines. Slopes are 0.53 ($r = 0.53, n = 27$) and 0.68 ($r = 0.61, n = 28$), for the UP and for the DOWN cycle tests, respectively. The z-transformations of the correlation coefficients indicate that the two slopes are not significantly different.[19] The result of visual-vestibular interaction measurements are shown in FIGURE 5E and F. The slope of the least square lines are 0.55 ($r = 0.56$, $n = 27$) and 0.78 ($r = 0.64, n = 28$) for the UP and DOWN cycle data, respectively. Finally, comparisons between the measurements obtained with the VT visible and with the VT extinguished for each of the UP and DOWN cycle tests are shown in FIGURE 5H and I. The slopes of the regression lines are 0.90 ($r = 0.90, n = 27$) and 1.04 ($r = 0.95, n = 28$) for the UP and DOWN data respectively. The slopes are not statistically significantly different from 1 as indicated by the confidence intervals of the slopes (± 0.18 and ± 0.14, respectively). The correlation coefficients indicate a significant positive relationship between the visual interaction data and the nystagmic measurements. In spite of the variability in the individual interactive and VOR nystagmic responses, the correlation coefficients strongly suggest the consistency of the performance of individuals to match their illusionary images to the values of their individual VORs.

Subjective Sensation of Self-Motion

Subjects were instructed during rotatory testing to activate the right-hand switch for the duration of the time that they felt they were moving to the right and the left-hand switch for the duration of the time they felt motion to the left. These times were converted to phases relative to the rotatory chair stimulus and averaged for each subject. This procedure was carried out in six subjects during rotation in the dark and during FULL cycle visual-vestibular interaction tests, both with a 28°/s rotatory chair peak velocity. During FULL cycle interactive tests, two sets of data were obtained. The first set was obtained when the subject was fixating on the vertically moving VT at the initial part of the test, and the second set after the VT was adjusted for subjective verticality.

There are three sets of phase measurements: One for rotation in the dark, one for interaction before tilt, and one for interaction after tilt (FIG. 6). Each set contains measurements corresponding to RB, RE, LB, and LE. One-factor repeated ANOVAs were performed to compare the measurements of each set with the corresponding measurements of the other two sets. In each of these four comparisons, p was found to exceed 0.05, indicating that no statistically recognizable difference was found between corresponding sets of measurements.

A further calculation was performed to estimate the threshold of the subjects for vestibular sensation. First, all of the RB phases were averaged. The result was 31.2°. Assuming a 400-ms reaction time,[20] a phase correction of 29.5° is obtained at a frequency of 0.2 Hz. The corrected RB phase is then 1.7°, which corresponds to a stimulus threshold of 0.8°/s. Similar computations for RE, LB, and LE data give threshold values of 2.4°/s, 1.8°/s, and 1.8°/s, respectively. All of these values fall within the expected range for normal subjects.[21]

DISCUSSION

The relationship between horizontal eye velocities during rotation in the dark (no VT present) and during simultaneously vertical visual and horizontal vestibular stimulation in three distinct paradigms—FULL, UP, and DOWN cycle visual-vestibular

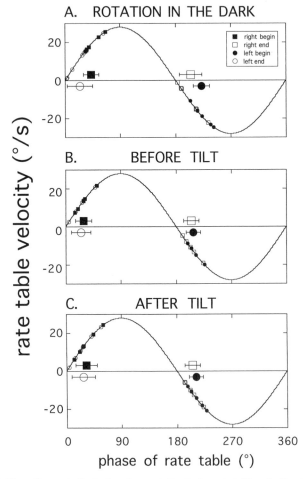

FIGURE 6. These figures indicate the phase relative to the rate table velocity at which subjects indicated a change in their direction of rotation. Both individual subject responses and mean and standard deviations are indicated. **(A)** Data acquired during rotation in the dark at a rate table peak velocity of 28°/s. **(B)** Data acquired during the FULL cycle interaction test *before* the visual target (VT) trajectory was inclined to compensate for the illusion of tilt. **(C)** Data acquired during the FULL cycle interaction test *after* the VT trajectory was inclined to compensate for the illusion of tilt. The legend indicates phases obtained from the following data: RB, time when the subject perceived rotation to the right to begin; RE, time when the subject perceived rotation to the right to end; LB, time when the subject perceived rotation to the left to begin; and LE, time when the subject perceived rotation to the left to end.

interaction—provides qualitatively consistent results among subjects. In each of these paradigms, there is an error in the perception of motion of the vertically moving VT during horizontal vestibular stimulation. This error can be compensated by tilting the trajectory of this target away from true vertical. In each case, we have shown that the magnitude of horizontal eye velocities resulting from the tracking of this inclined target at subjective vertical is predicted by the magnitude of the slow component of the VOR during identical vestibular stimulation without visual cues. The results are consistent with the hypothesis stated in equation 1 that the perception of a VT motion (V_{real}) is made in relationship to an IRC.

The vectorial representation of these relationships, as in equation 2, is clearly justified by the results illustrated in FIGURE 5, which demonstrate that the steady-state conditions of the IRC are dependent on the vestibular system during horizontal rotations. A pragmatic interpretation of the data is to think that the visual motion sensation can be quantitatively thought of as the result of the "physical" interaction between the real VT velocity and the brain's appreciation of the subject's motion. That is, the VT is evaluated relative to the subject's head, but with an important circumstance that the "subject" velocity is computed to be equal to VOR and not to the head velocity. Then it could be inversely argued that the $\overrightarrow{VOR}$ provides an estimation of the $\overrightarrow{VSSM}$. The following identity seems to be true:

$$\overrightarrow{VSSM} = -\overrightarrow{VOR} \tag{5}$$

Therefore, if the VOR is an objective measurement of the VSSM, other systems, such as vision and proprioception, need to cooperate to provide the correct head-velocity sensation that is underestimated by the VSSM at the frequencies and velocities tested. The present results point to the need to document further the contribution of other systems to the brain centers which make possible error-free navigation. These results also give evidence of the interaction that must exist between the various systems to provide information adequate for orientation.

Measurements of self-motion perception using VOR during rotation in the dark and during interaction before and after inclination of the VT trajectory are statistically indistinguishable. The psychophysical experience of motion is independent of the oculomotor response and is chiefly determined by head motion, i.e., vestibular stimulation. In other words, the sensation of self-motion is unaffected by the visual interaction, suggesting that the pathways to the centers for vestibular sensation are different from those that regulate VOR responses. It is likely they are also independent of other reflexes such as neck or proprioceptive inputs.[22] Most, if not all, of the vestibular second-order neurons that receive primary vestibular inputs, also receive visual inputs.[23] A subset of second-order neurons that project to higher centers for VSSM must exist. These neurons no doubt receive the same input from the vestibular periphery as those mediating the VOR, since the VSSM and VOR have comparable dynamics.[22,24] That is, they are likely innervated by an aggregate of primary afferents with distributed physiological properties. The VSSM continues to be in phase with the sinusoidal head movement while the eye trajectory is completely suppressed, but where do the VSSM signals depart from the VOR signals? It is evident that the VSSM is coded in terms of head velocity just as the motion of objects is coded in terms of their velocity through the retinal slip signal acting as the SP system input.[3,4,25] During interactive tests, subjects' perception of VT movement was in phase with the velocity of the VT and the subjects' VSSM was in phase with the head angular velocity, not the angular acceleration. It was also found that the timing of the subjects' perception of a change in rotational direction is consistent with the known value of the sensation threshold to a purely vestibular stimulus and that this perception is uninfluenced by the condition of the VT or the associated eye movements.

Although vestibular psychophysical research has been difficult in the past, the use of interactive stimuli offers new avenues to objectively evaluate vestibular subjective sensation. The progress of this approach suggests that related areas (i.e., optokinetic stimuli, neck reflexes, etc.) should also be investigated.

REFERENCES

1. ROBINSON, D. A. 1981. Control of eye movements. *In* Handbook of Physiology, The Nervous Component, part 2. V. B. Brooks, Ed.: 1275–1320. Williams and Wilkins. Baltimore, MD.
2. BALOH, R. W. & V. HONRUBIA. 1990. Clinical Neurophysiology of the Vestibular System. 2nd edit. F. A. Davis Co. Philadelphia, PA.
3. LISBERGER, S. G., E. J. MORRIS & L. TYCHSEN. 1987. Visual motion processing and sensory-motor integration for smooth pursuit eye movements. Annu. Rev. Neurosci. **10**: 97–129.
4. HORRIDGE, G. A. 1966. Study of a system, as illustrated by the optokinetic response. Symp. Soc. Exp. Biol. **20**: 179–198.
5. HUDSPETH, A. J. 1985. The cellular basis of hearing: The biophysics of hair cells. Science **230(4727)**: 745–752.
6. STEINHAUSEN, W. 1927. Über Sichtbarmachung and Funktinosprüfung der Cupula terminalis in den Bogengangsampullen der Labyrinthes. Arch. Gesamte Physiol. **217**: 747–755.
7. GOLDBERG, J. M. & C. FERNANDEZ. 1975. Vestibular mechanisms. Annu. Rev. Physiol. **37**: 129–162.
8. LAU, C. G. Y. 1978. Modeling of visual-vestibular interaction and the fast components of nystagmus. PhD thesis. University of California, Santa Barbara. Santa Barbara, CA.
9. ROBINSON, D. A. 1977. Vestibular and optokinetic symbiosis: An example of explaining by modeling. *In* Control of Gaze by Brain Stem Neurons. R. Baker & A. Berthoz, Eds.: **1**: 49–58. Elsevier/North-Holland Biomedical Press. Amsterdam.
10. WHITESIDE, T. C. D., A. GRAYBIEL & J. I. NIVEN. 1965. Visual illusions of movement. Brain **88**: 193–210.
11. POST, R. B. 1986. Induced motion considered as a visually induced oculogyral illusion. Perception **15(2)**: 131–138.
12. BRANDT, T., J. DICHGANS & E. KOENIG. 1973. Differential effects of central verses peripheral vision on egocentric and exocentric motion perception. Exp. Brain Res. **16(5)**: 476–491.
13. HONRUBIA, V., R. KHALILI & R. W. BALOH. 1992. Optokinetic and vestibular interactions with smooth pursuit. Psychophysical responses. Ann. N.Y. Acad. Sci. **656**: 739–746.
14. HONRUBIA, V., R. KHALILI, C. G. LAU & R. W. BALOH. 1992. Optokinetic and vestibular interactions with smooth pursuit: Psychophysical responses. Acta Otolaryngol. **112(2)**: 163–169.
15. FENN, W. O. & J. B. HURSH. 1937. Movements of the eyes when the lids are closed. Am. J. Physiol. **118**: 8–14.
16. POWSNER, E. R. & K. S. LION. 1950. Testing eye muscles. Electronics **23**: 96–99.
17. DEMER, J. L. 1992. Mechanisms of human vertical visual-vestibular interaction. J. Neurophysiol. **68(6)**: 2128–2146.
18. BARRY, W. & G. MELVILL-JONES. 1965. Influence of eye lid movement upon electrooculographic recording of vertical eye movements. Aerosp. Med. **36**: 855–858.
19. COHEN, J. & P. COHEN. 1983. Applied Multiple Regression/Correlation Analysis for the Behavioral Sciences. 2nd edit. L. Erlbaum Associates. Hillsdale, NJ.
20. ZACHARIAS, G. L. & L. R. YOUNG. 1981. Influence of combined visual and vestibular cues on human perception and control of horizontal rotation. Exp. Brain Res. **41(2)**: 159–171.
21. VON BÉKÉSY, G. 1955. Subjective cupulometry. AMA Arch. Otol. **61**: 16–28.

22. MERGNER, T., G. ROTTLER, H. KIMMIG & W. BECKER. 1992. Role of vestibular and neck inputs for the perception of object motion in space. Exp. Brain Res. **89(3):** 655–668.
23. WAESPE, W. & V. HENN. 1987. Gaze stabilization in the primate. The interaction of the vestibulo-ocular reflex, optokinetic nystagmus, and smooth pursuit. Rev. Physiol. Biochem. Pharmacol. **106:** 37–125.
24. HONRUBIA, V., H. A. JENKINS, R. W. BALOH, H. R. KONRAD, R. D. YEE & P. H. WARD. 1982. Comparison of vestibular subjective sensation and nystagmus responses during computerized harmonic acceleration tests. Ann. Otol. Rhinol. Laryngol. **91(5 Pt. 1):** 493–500.
25. YOUNG, L. R. 1971. Pursuit eye tracking movements. *In* The Control of Eye Movements. P. Bach-Y-Rita & C. C. Collins, Eds.: 429–443. Academic Press. New York.

In Vivo–in Vitro Correlations in the Central Vestibular System: A Bridge Too Far?[a]

P. P. VIDAL,[b] A. BABALIAN,[b] N. VIBERT,[b]
M. SERAFIN,[c] AND M. MÜHLETHALER[c]

[b]Laboratoire de Physiologie de l'Action et de la Perception
CNRS-Collège de France, UMR C 9950
15 rue de l'Ecole de Médecine
75270 Paris cedex 06, France

[c]Département de Physiologie
Centre Médical Universitaire
1 rue Michel Servet
1211 Genève 4, Switzerland

INTRODUCTION

The neuronal operations underlying gaze and postural control have been the object of intense studies for the past 30 years. Several approaches were employed successfully to investigate the neuronal networks involved. Extracellular recordings in the behaving animal have been used to assess the function of each subgroup of neurons. Morphological and electroanatomical methods have led to a precise description of their connectivity. Post-spike trigger averaging and intracellular injection of dyes in the alert animal have been useful to link the morphological results with functional data. Finally, this experimental knowledge was used to elaborate theoretical models that satisfactorily described the neuronal computations necessary to control gaze and posture. Nevertheless, it should be stressed that an important, and often implicit, hypothesis is present in all these studies: the various computations necessary to control gaze, such as the integration of the velocity signal, or the velocity storage mechanisms, are emerging properties of the neuronal networks under scrutiny. However, this assumption may not be entirely correct.

For the past 15 years, *in vitro* studies on slices have demonstrated that individual neurons of vertebrates are endowed with nonlinear membrane properties, which confer to them complex integrative properties.[1] Furthermore, multiple pre- and postsynaptic receptors responding to various neurochemical compounds have been shown to deeply influence the time course and the mode of response of a given neuron to its various inputs. It is therefore not surprising that previous studies in invertebrates have demonstrated that the intrinsic membrane properties and the neuropharmacological characteristics of each of the various neuronal groups had to be taken into account in order to understand the sensorimotor transformations in these species. By contrast, in vertebrates, the respective contributions of the emerging properties of a network as opposed to the specific properties of its individual components, that is, the neurons (and the glial cells), are still largely open to question.

[a]This work was supported by grants from the CNRS (PIC), the Ministère des Affaires Etrangères, the Fondation de la Recherche Médicale, and the CNES.

This is due mainly to various limitations of slice preparations that will now be briefly summarized.

The functional identification of the neurons under study is usually quite complicated on slices: the lack of functionally meaningful discharge, the difficulty of using proper antidromic and orthodromic activations, and problems such as current spread and axon reflexes are not easy to overcome. Furthermore, due to the limited thickness of the slice (usually up to 600 μm), most of the recorded neurons are probably axotomized and must have lost part of their dendritic trees.

Some of these problems can be solved by using complex *in vitro* preparations. To our knowledge three of them have been quite successfully used in our field of interest: the *in vitro* whole brain (IWB) of the frog,[2] of the lamprey,[3–7] and, more recently, of the guinea pig.[8] These preparations allow one to correctly identify the neurons and to control the extracellular medium. Nevertheless, deafferentation from sensory inputs in the case of the frog and guinea-pig IWB precludes the use of natural visual and vestibular stimulation. The possibility of overcoming this problem by inducing nystagmus or saccades using electrical stimulations of the primary vestibular and visual afferents remains to be proven in these preparations. On the other hand, natural vestibular stimulation had been successfully used in the lamprey IWB.[5–7] However, this preparation has some other limitations compared with the frog and guinea-pig IWB.

Finally, it should be mentioned that whether *in vivo* or *in vitro,* electrophysiological techniques obviously have their limits. For example, the number of described receptors of each neuromediator at play in the vestibular system[9] has dramatically increased during the past years. Indeed, using methods of molecular biology, it became possible to identify the individual subunits that compose these receptors, and to describe the various combinations within a class of receptors.[9] This receptor heterogeneity cannot be neglected because their various subclasses—for example, N-methyl-D-aspartate (NMDA) receptors—can have widely different distributions in the brain and can induce different effects on the neurons, once activated. Unhappily, very few specific agonists and antagonists have yet been described for most of these receptor subclasses, which precludes the study of their functional implications with electrophysiological methods. Nevertheless, recent morphological methods such as *in situ* hybridization[10] can help to tackle this problem by monitoring the expression of the messenger RNA leading to the synthesis of receptors in various behavioral context.

Given these methodological limitations, it is clear that to solve the issue of the respective contributions of the emerging properties of a network, as opposed to the individual properties of its constituent elements, will require the combination of various complementary neurobiological methods in different types of *in vivo* and *in vitro* preparations. This paper illustrates some of the successes and failures we have encountered by using such strategies to explore the guinea-pig central vestibular system.

PROPERTIES OF MEDIAL VESTIBULAR NUCLEUS NEURONS ON SLICES

In slices, using the intrinsic membrane properties as criteria, the medial vestibular nucleus neurons (MVNn) were categorized into two main classes[11,12]: type A MVNn (about 30% of the recorded cells) and type B MVNn (about 50% of the recorded cells). A small and nonhomogeneous cell group, type C MVNn (about 20% of the recorded cells), could also be distinguished, but those were not investigated in detail.

Type A MVNn had wider action potentials than type B MVNn, followed by a deeper and single after-hyperpolarization (AHP). This large AHP was followed by a delayed return to the baseline following hyperpolarizing current pulses. Type A MVNn exhibited small high-threshold calcium spikes that could be potentiated by barium, and a 4-AP resistant A-like conductance.

Type B MVNn had a double-component AHP, an early fast one and a delayed slower and larger one, presumed to be due to a combination of different voltage- and calcium-dependent potassium conductances. Type B MVNn had large high-threshold calcium spikes, prolonged calcium-dependent plateau potentials as well as subthreshold persistent sodium conductances (plateau potentials). Finally, a subpopulation of type B MVNn displayed low-threshold calcium spikes[13] (LTS). Both cell types had very regular resting discharges.[11,12]

We have also reported the occurrence of spontaneous rhythmic bursts in type B MVNn which could be induced by various mechanisms. They can occur spontaneously. They could also be triggered by long-lasting perfusion with NMDA,[14] apamin[15] (a selective blocker of one type of Ca^{2+}-dependent K^+ conductance), or by a high Mg^{2+}/low Ca^{2+} artificial cerebrospinal fluid.[15] In the latter cases the bursting activity is insensitive to APV, but is abolished by TTX or blocked by bath application of 20–50 μM of ouabain, a blocker of the sodium pump. The frequency of the bursts was voltage-dependent in all cases.

As clear-cut as they look, the results obtained on slices are not easy to interpret in a functional context:

1. Type C MVNn, which represent a sizable part of the MVNn, may represent either a whole subpopulation of MVNn with intermediate characteristics, or a pool of deteriorated cells.

2. The origin of the MVNn resting discharge in slices is unknown. It could depend on the presence of intrinsic membrane properties driving the membrane toward the threshold.

3. It is difficult to correlate our *in vitro*-based classification of the MVNn with the different subtypes of vestibular neurons that have been described *in vivo*. Type A and type B MVNn cannot be distinguished in slice on the basis of their resting discharge, which is regular for both cell types. This precludes attempts to link type A and type B MVNn studied on slice with the regular and irregular MVNn recorded *in vivo*. Moreover, we failed to identify MVNn as second-order vestibular neurons on slices following electrical stimulation of the vestibular nerve. Indeed, we never succeeded in preserving vestibular afferents from the stump of the eighth nerve to the vestibular nuclei in a 500-μm slice, whatever its orientation.

4. Some of the nonlinear neuronal properties observed on slices might be very useful to explain certain aspects of information processing in the vestibular network. For example, plateau potentials[11,12] could be the cornerstone of the various neuronal integrators. On the other hand, it is clear that on slices, deafferented, axotomized neurons could display very unusual behaviors.

5. Although infusion of apamin into the vestibular nuclei in alert guinea pig induced oscillatory head and eye movements,[15] which corroborate its effect on slices, it is not clear whether such oscillations are spontaneously occurring in the behaving animal.

This list can look somewhat discouraging. Nevertheless, as we will see, the guinea-pig IWB preparation can help to tackle some of these problems. Before trying to correlate the *in vivo* and *in vitro* properties of the vestibular neurons, we will briefly describe the activity of the second-order MVNn in the alert guinea pig.

PROPERTIES OF MEDIAL VESTIBULAR NUCLEUS NEURONS *IN VIVO*

We recently quantified the discharge of identified type I second-order MVNn using horizontal sinusoidal vestibular stimulations (0.1 to 3 Hz, 40°/s peak velocity) in the alert head-fixed guinea pig,[16] during rapid eye movement (REM) sleep and during vestibular adaptation. In the alert state, second-order MVNn can be segregated according to the regularity of their resting discharges. During natural vestibular stimulations, they code head velocity, and some of them exhibit a sensitivity to the horizontal component of eye position. In addition, some MVNn pause during quick phases of the vestibular nystagmus oriented ipsilaterally to the recording side, and burst during quick phases oriented contralaterally. These results indicate that MVNn, in the guinea pig, behave quite similarly to those in the cat and monkey.

The gain of the horizontal vestibulo-ocular reflex (VOR) was adaptively modified by inducing a visuovestibular conflict[16]: sinusoidal rotations (0.05 and 0.1 Hz, 20°/s peak velocity) were applied to head-restrained guinea pigs in the light, while the visual scene was stabilized relative to its head. Second-order MVNn responses were tested in darkness before and after 30-, 60-, and 90-min training periods. In all the MVNn tested ($n = 7$) the gain of the neuronal response was decreased by 30 to 50% after vestibular adaptation. In addition, the adaptive changes were frequency selective (2 out of 2 neurons tested). To our knowledge, this is the first demonstration that second-order vestibular neurons do change their gain during VOR adaptation.

In other types of experiments, we quantified guinea-pig's eye movements during wakefulness and sleep. In particular, we described a possibly new type of eye movement, i.e., 10 Hz oscillations of high amplitude (max. 30°) and high velocity (max. 1000°/s) during REM sleep episodes.[17] We also demonstrated that the neck muscle twitches occurring in that state were synchronized with ocular oscillations. On the other hand, it is well established that some MVNn neurons contact monosynaptically the extraocular and neck motoneurons. Therefore, in order to elucidate whether the membrane oscillations described *in vitro* in MVNn could be relevant for the discharge patterns of these cells during REM sleep, we have recorded several identified type I second-order MVNn during this state of vigilance. Our recordings demonstrated that these cells did not oscillate in parallel with eye oscillations and muscle twitches, while their discharges were still shaped by vestibular stimulations and pauses occurring during REMs oriented to the recording side. In other words, the putative functional relevance of the ability of the MVNn to oscillate *in vitro* remains to be proven. A key to the understanding of these *in vitro* oscillations may be the rhythmic discharge of the central vestibular neurons recorded during fictive locomotion in guinea pig,[18] cat,[19] and lamprey.[4]

We can now examine how the guinea-pig IWB can help to correlate some of the *in vivo* characteristics of the MVNn with the properties of these cells demonstrated in the slice preparation.

GAZE CONTROL–RELATED NEURONAL NETWORK IN THE IWB: FIELD POTENTIAL RECORDINGS

Viability of the Vestibular Network in the IWB

To explore the viability of the vestibular networks in the IWB, we have recorded the field potentials evoked in various brain-stem structures following the electrical stimulation of several cranial nerves (vestibular, optic, and extraoculomotor nerves). Field potential recordings have the advantage to test the responsiveness of big populations of neurons. Furthermore, the characteristics of the field potentials can be easily compared to the data previously recorded *in vivo,* in alert and acute preparations. FIGURES 1 and 2 illustrate some of our results. As can be seen in FIGURE 1A, the orthodromic field potential evoked in the vestibular nuclei by single-shock stimulation of the ipsilateral eighth nerve exhibits exactly the same characteristics in terms of shape, amplitude, and depth profile as in alert preparations. The latency of the response is also comparable to that recorded in the alert guinea pig, taking into account the lower (29 °C) than normal (38 °C) temperature of the IWB. This important point was checked by progressive warming of the IWB to 38 °C under Nembutal, Droperidol perfusion: at 38 °C the latency of the response in the IWB became similar to that *in vivo.*

The similarities between the field potential characteristics recorded in the IWB and *in vivo* were checked for the other types of field potentials listed below:

- Positive oligo-synaptic field potential evoked in the contralateral vestibular nucleus by stimulation of the eighth nerve (commissural inhibition)

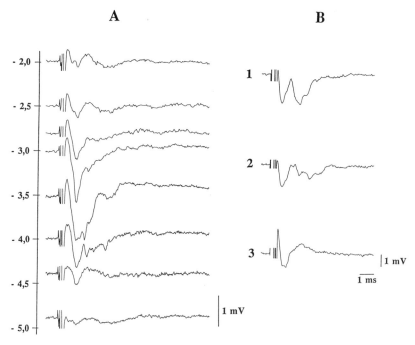

FIGURE 1. (A) Depth profile of the extracellular field potential evoked by stimulation of the ipsilateral vestibular nerve in the medial vestibular nucleus. Numbers on vertical bar indicate the localization of the recording electrode in millimeters with respect to the ventral surface of the brain stem (the *in vitro* whole brain is positioned upside down). (B) Extracellular field potentials evoked by stimulation of the ipsilateral vestibular nerve in the medial vestibular nucleus: Effect of perfusion with a high magnesium–0 calcium-containing Ringer solution. 1, Control orthodromic field potential; 2, 15 min following the perfusion; and 3, 30 min following the perfusion. Note progressive decrease of the synaptic component and persistence of the presynaptic afferent volley.

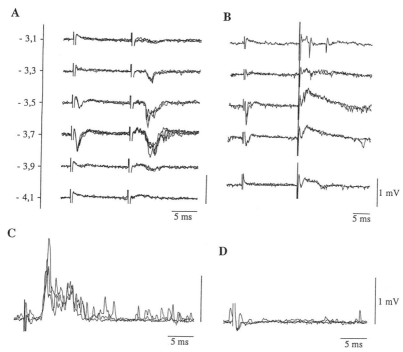

FIGURE 2. (A) Depth profile of the extracellular field potential recorded in the abducens nucleus following stimulation of the ipsilateral abducens nerve (first shock), and stimulation of the contralateral vestibular nerve (second shock). Numbers on vertical bar indicate the localization of the recording electrode in millimeters with respect to the ventral surface of the brain stem. (B) Depth profile of the extracellular field potentials recorded in the abducens nucleus evoked by stimulation of the ipsilateral abducens nerve (first shock), and stimulation of the ipsilateral vestibular nerve (second shock). (C) Extracellular activity of the abducens nerve, recorded with a suction electrode positioned on the stump of the abducens nerve, following stimulation of the contralateral vestibular nerve. (D) Absence of extracellular activity in the abducens nerve, checked with a suction electrode positioned on the stump of the abducens nerve, following stimulation of the ipsilateral vestibular nerve.

- Disynaptic negative field potentials evoked in the contralateral abducens (FIG. 2A, second shock), ipsilateral and contralateral oculomotor nuclei following stimulations of the eighth nerve (direct disynaptic excitatory pathways of the VOR)
- Disynaptic positive field potentials evoked in the ipsilateral abducens (FIG. 2B, second shock) following stimulation of the eighth nerve (direct disynaptic inhibitory pathway of the VOR)
- Antidromic field potentials evoked in the abducens (FIG. 2A and B, first shock) and oculomotor nuclei following stimulations of the abducens and oculomotor nerves, respectively.

Finally, we investigated with suction electrodes the gross activity of the abducens (FIG. 2C and D) and oculomotor nerves following stimulation of the eighth nerve. The characteristics and the latencies of multiunit recordings of the extraoculomotor motoneurons confirm and extend the results obtained with the field potentials.

Altogether, these results demonstrate three important points: (1) At least some neuronal groups underlying gaze control (extraocular motoneurons, first- and second-order vestibular neurons, type II inhibitory interneurons, etc.) survive in the IWB. (2) Their functional connectivity is well preserved, which allows identification of various cell groups (see above). (3) The field potential recordings in the IWB permit one to precisely localize some structures like the abducens nucleus (less than 1 mm^3). This provides us with convenient landmarks to localize various neuronal groups underlying the gaze control. For example, it was possible to determine from which part of the vestibular complex the recordings were obtained (mainly the MVN in the present experiments).

Nature of the Synaptic Transmission between the First- and Second-order Vestibular Neurons

Once the survival of the vestibulo-ocular network was assessed, the pharmacology of synaptic transmission between first- and second-order vestibular neurons was investigated. We monitored changes of field potentials evoked by stimulation of the vestibular nerve in the vestibular nuclei, following perfusions with CNQX (6-cyano-7-nitro-quinoxaline-2-3-dione), a selective antagonist of the AMPA/kainate receptors, APV (D-L-2-amino-5-phosphonovaleric acid), a selective antagonist of the NMDA receptors, or a high magnesium–0 calcium-containing Ringer solution which blocks synaptic transmission. CNQX abolishes the major part of the field potential, confirming the dominating role of AMPA (α-amino-3-hydroxy-5-methyl-4-isoxazolepropionic acid) receptor-mediated glutamatergic transmission between first- and second-order vestibular neurons. APV abolished a sizable, but variable part of the remaining field potential in most of our recordings. This strongly suggests NMDA receptor-mediated transmission. However, its contribution is apparently quite variable and can be even absent in certain groups of second-order vestibular neurons. A minor synaptic field potential often persisted under CNQX and APV perfusion, but was blocked by the high magnesium–0 calcium-containing solution. This demonstrates that another, unidentified neuromediator could also play a significant role in the synaptic transmission between primary afferents and second-order vestibular neurons. Finally, the perfusion with the high magnesium–0 calcium-containing Ringer solution revealed the existence of a negativity induced by the arrival of the presynaptic volley in the vestibular nucleus (FIG. 1B, second and third trace). In normal Ringer solution (FIG. 1A, 1B$_1$ first trace), or *in vivo,* presence of this volley, which is often buried in the negative wave of the field potential, may prevent an exact determination of the onset of the postsynaptic component.

GAZE CONTROL–RELATED NEURONAL NETWORKS IN THE IWB PREPARATION: INTRACELLULAR RECORDINGS

We will not detail here the intracellular recordings obtained from abducens and oculomotor motoneurons. They confirm the results obtained with the field potentials concerning the integrity of the vestibulo-ocular pathways in the IWB. We will focus on the intracellular recordings that were conducted in the medial vestibular nucleus. These results are clear-cut and can be summarized as follows:

1. It is possible to retrieve type A, type B (Fɪɢ. 3, upper and lower left traces) and type C MVNn (not shown) in the IWB. This means that our previous classification determined on slices was not artifactual, despite possible damage of cells due to the slicing procedure.
2. In contrast to our recordings on slices, where all the MVNn have a regular spontaneous discharge, the MVNn exhibit resting activities of various regularity in the IWB. Interestingly, type A MVNn recorded so far in the IWB had a regular discharge (Fɪɢ. 3, upper left trace) rate whereas that of type B MVNn was irregular (Fɪɢ. 3, lower left trace). As seen in the next paragraph, these results could be important to bridge the gap between the data obtained on slices and in the alert animal. Furthermore, most of the regular type A MVNn and irregular type B MVNn were identified as second-order vestibular neurons (Fɪɢ. 3, upper and lower right traces).

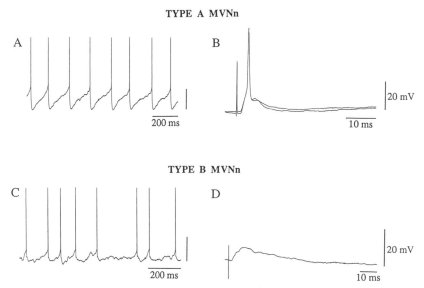

FIGURE 3. Regular (**A**) and irregular (**C**) resting-discharge of type A and type B medial vestibular nucleus neurons (MVNn), respectively, identified as second-order vestibular neurons by the monosynaptic excitatory postsynaptic potentials in response to stimulation of the vestibular nerve (**B** and **D**).

3. The predominant role of the glutamatergic synaptic transmission between first- and second-order vestibular neurons was confirmed by intracellular recordings. We have monitored transformations of EPSPs evoked by vestibular nerve stimulation following perfusion with CNQX (a selective antagonist of the AMPA/kainate receptors), APV (a selective antagonist of the NMDA receptors), and a Ringer solution of high magnesium–0 calcium concentrations (blockade of the synaptic transmission). CNQX abolished a large part of the EPSPs at monosynaptic latency (about 1.6 ms), confirming the important

role of the AMPA receptors in the synaptic transmission between first- and second-order vestibular neurons. APV could block a variable part of the EPSPs which remained after CNQX perfusion, but, as for the field potentials, this was not always the case. This indicates a variable contribution of NMDA receptors. Interestingly, the latency of the NMDA receptor-mediated component of the vestibular synaptic field potential and the underlying NMDA component of the EPSP amounted to about 1.8 ms, which is also compatible with monosynaptic delay. On the other hand, recent current-clamp experiments on slices in the rat[20] have demonstrated that the latency of NMDA receptor-mediated component in presumed second-order vestibular neurons following stimulation of the vestibular nerve was 4.8 ms. This discrepancy, which cannot be attributed either to the recording temperature (29 °C in both cases) or to the age of the animal (the vestibular system is mature in 25-day postnatal rats and in 200 g guinea pig), remains to be explained. A minor EPSP was sometimes recorded under CNQX and APV perfusion, which implied that some other unknown neurotransmitters are at play at this synapse. In a few neurons, an early and small component of EPSP, resistant to high magnesium–0 calcium-containing Ringer, was suggestive of electrical coupling.

4. Finally, and this is perhaps the most interesting result of our preliminary study, we were able to trigger long plateau potentials (FIG. 4A and B) and bursting activity in some of type B MVNn with a single shock applied to the vestibular nerve. They originated in an all-or-none fashion following the orthodromically evoked action potential, or following the EPSP. These nonlinear responses occurred without any pharmacological manipulation, during recordings at resting membrane potential (plateau potentials) or at slightly hyperpolarized level (burst). This is an argument of some weight to support the hypothesis that at least some of the nonlinear properties of the vestibular neurons described in slices[11,12] may be of functional significance in the behaving animal.

A

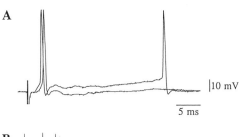

|10 mV

5 ms

B

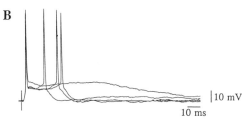

|10 mV

10 ms

FIGURE 4. Spontaneous plateau potentials evoked in two type B medial vestibular nucleus neurons, following stimulation of the ipsilateral vestibular nerve. Monosynaptic excitatory postsynaptic potentials with superimposed action potentials are followed by plateau potentials appearing in an all-or-none fashion.

FUNCTIONAL CONSIDERATIONS RESULTING FROM THE COMBINED *IN VIVO–IN VITRO* APPROACH

Regular versus Irregular MVNn

As stated above, we can now link the discharge regularity and the intrinsic membrane properties of the MVNn (FIG. 3). However, the raison d'être of the segregation of the MVNn in regular and irregular cells remains open to question. To summarize briefly the literature, three hypotheses have been put forward.

First, two main classes of second-order vestibular neurons have been described *in vivo,* [21,22] tonic and kinetic neurons. Kinetic neurons have more irregular resting discharges and higher sensitivity to acceleration than do tonic neurons. Therefore, our results in the IWB tend to demonstrate that type A and B MVNn might correspond to tonic and kinetic neurons, respectively. That would lead to the conclusion that the segregation of the networks controlling gaze and posture in frequency-tuned channels[23] could partially rely on the heterogeneous intrinsic membrane properties of neurons having the same connectivity, as already proposed by other authors.[24,25] One could object that there is a continuum of cells in MVN from the very irregular to very regular *in vivo,* while we have described only three main types of neurons on slices and in the IWB. This would be a misinterpretation of our results because the resting discharges of type B MVNn in the IWB display a wide range of variation coefficients.

Second, a complementary hypothesis would be that, due to different biomechanical properties of the eyes compared to the other mobile segments of the body (neck, trunk, legs), the tonic, regular, putative type A MVNn could mainly be restricted to the oculomotor system, while the kinetic, irregular, putative type B MVNn could be involved in neck, trunk, and leg stabilization.[26]

Third, an alternative view would be that the kinetic, irregular, putative type B MVNn input the velocity storage integrator.[27] This hypothesis fits nicely with a particularity of these neurons, i.e., their subthreshold persistent sodium conductance.[12] This conductance can produce long plateau potentials, even in response to a single shock of the vestibular nerve in the IWB (FIG. 4), an adequate feature for an integrator. Finally, if one admits that some of type B MVNn are involved in oculomotor control, the frequency-tuned channel hypothesis and the velocity storage integrator hypothesis are not mutually exclusive.

It should be mentioned that, in a previous study performed both in slices and in the guinea-pig IWB, we found the same segregation in type A and type B neurons (but without type B + LTS cells) in a nucleus functionally related to the vestibular system, the gigantocellular reticular nucleus of the medulla.[28] This would reinforce the idea that there is indeed a segregation of the sensorimotor networks in channels, which is based on the neuronal membrane properties, whatever the functional meaning of these channels.

Synaptic Transmission between the First- and Second-order Vestibular Neurons

Our results confirm the glutamatergic nature of the synaptic transmission between the first- and second-order vestibular neurons[9] and the existence of electrical coupling at this synapse.[9,29,30] The involvement of NMDA receptors opens the possibility of induction of long-term potentiation. Despite some promising reports from two other groups of investigators,[31,32] our preliminary attempts have not led us to very convincing results on that issue.

On the other hand, taking into account the presence of NMDA receptors carried by second-order MVNn, one can propose a mechanism of regulation of the synaptic transmission between the first- and second-order vestibular neurons via the glycinergic, strychnine-insensitive, modulatory sites of these receptors. Several arguments nicely fit such a hypothesis:

- Glycine is colocalized with glutamate at the level of some primary vestibular afferent terminals.[33]
- MVNn neurons indeed carry functional[34] NMDA receptors,[10] which can be modulated in slices through their glycinergic, strychnine-insensitive sites.[35]
- The VOR gain can either be increased or decreased in the alert guinea pig by perfusing the vestibular complex with specific agonist and antagonist, respectively, of the glycinergic, strychnine-insensitive sites of NMDA receptors.[35]

A regulation of the synaptic transmission between the first- and second-order vestibular neurons by substance P can be also envisaged: Substance P is colocalized with glutamate at the level of the primary vestibular afferent terminals.[9] We have demonstrated, on slices, that substance P receptors are present at the MVNn membrane level.[36]

CONCLUSION

Our studies in the past year show that the combination, in the guinea pig, of recordings in the alert and *in vitro* preparations, together with the use of *in situ* hybridization methods, was rewarding. Our strategy was based on the idea that the IWB would be useful to bridge the gap between the results obtained *in vivo* and on slices. Ongoing studies on that preparation partially fulfill our expectation. It should be also reminded that IWB preparation was successfully used in other species to link the results of *in vivo* and *in vitro* investigations on gaze control. Such studies in the frog and lamprey brought fascinating data in recent years. Hence, to answer the question posed in the title of this paper, *in vivo–in vitro* correlations in the central vestibular system may be a bridge not too far.

REFERENCES

1. LLINAS, R. R. 1988. The intrinsic electrophysiological properties of mammalian neurons: Insights into central nervous system function. Science **242:** 1654–1663.
2. KUNKEL, A. W. & N. DIERINGER. 1994. Morphological and electrophysiological consequences of unilateral pre- versus postganglionic vestibular lesions in the frog. J. Comp. Physiol. A **174:** 621–632.
3. BUSSIERES, N. & R. DUBUC. 1992. Phasic modulation of vestibulospinal neuron activity during fictive locomotion in lampreys. Brain Res. **575:** 174–179.
4. BUSSIERES, N. & R. DUBUC. 1992. Phasic modulation of transmission from vestibular inputs to reticulospinal neurons during fictive locomotion in lampreys. Brain Res. **582:** 147–153.
5. ORLOVSKY, G. N., T. G. DELIAGINA & P. WALLEN. 1992. Vestibular control of swimming in lamprey. I. Responses of reticulospinal neurons to roll and pitch. Exp. Brain Res. **90:** 479–488.

6. DELIAGINA, T. G., G. N. ORLOVSKY, S. GRILLNER & P. WALLEN. 1992. Vestibular control of swimming in lamprey. II. Characteristics of spatial sensitivity of reticulospinal neurons. Exp. Brain Res. **90:** 489–498.
7. DELIAGINA, T. G., G. N. ORLOVSKY, S. GRILLNER & P. WALLEN. 1992. Vestibular control of swimming in lamprey. III. Activity of vestibular afferents: Convergence of vestibular inputs on reticulospinal neurons. Exp. Brain Res. **90:** 499–507.
8. MÜHLETHALER, M., M. DE CURTIS, K. WALTON & R. LLINAS. 1993. The isolated and perfused brain of the guinea-pig in vitro. Eur. J. Neurosci. **5:** 915–926.
9. DE WAELE, C., M. MÜHLETHALER & P. P. VIDAL. 1995. Neurochemistry of the central vestibular pathways. Brain Res. Rev. **20:** 24–46.
10. DE WAELE, C., M. ABITBOL, M. CHAT, C. MENINI, J. MALLET & P. P. VIDAL. 1994. Distribution of glutamatergic receptors and GAD messenger RNA-containing neurons in the vestibular nuclei of normal and hemilabyrinthectomized rats. Eur. J. Neurosci. **6:** 565–576.
11. SERAFIN, M., C. DE WAELE, A. KHATEB, P. P. VIDAL & M. MÜHLETHALER. 1991. Medial vestibular nucleus in the guinea pig. I. Intrinsic membrane properties in brainstem slices. Exp. Brain Res. **84:** 417–425.
12. SERAFIN, M., C. DE WAELE, A. KHATEB, P. P. VIDAL & M. MÜHLETHALER. 1991. Medical vestibular nucleus in the guinea pig. II. Ionic basis of the intrinsic membrane properties in brainstem slices. Exp. Brain Res. **84:** 426–433.
13. SERAFIN, M., A. KHATEB, C. DE WAELE, P. P. VIDAL & M. MÜHLETHALER. 1990. Low threshold calcium spikes in vestibular nuclei neurones in vitro: A role in the generation of the vestibular nystagmus quick phase in vivo? Exp. Brain Res. **82:** 187–190.
14. SERAFIN, M., A. KHATEB, C. DE WAELE, P. P. VIDAL & M. MÜHLETHALER. 1992. Medial vestibular nucleus in the guinea pig: NMDA-induced oscillations. Exp. Brain Res. **88:** 187–192.
15. DE WAELE, C., M. SERAFIN, A. KHATEB, T. YABE, P. P. VIDAL & M. MÜHLETHALER. 1993. Medial vestibular nucleus in the guinea-pig: Apamin-induced rhythmic burst firing—an in vitro and in vivo study. Exp. Brain Res. **95:** 213–222.
16. SERAFIN, M., M. MÜHLETHALER & P. P. VIDAL. 1995. Second-order type I medial vestibular neurones in the head-fixed guinea-pig during alertness and following adaptation. *In* Information Processing Underlying Gaze Control. J. M. Delgado Garcia, E. Godaux & P. P. Vidal, Eds.: 175–186. Pergamon Press. New York.
17. ESCUDERO, M. & P. P. VIDAL. 1992. Eye movements during paradoxical sleep in guinea pig. 22th Annual Meeting of the Society for Neuroscience. Abstr. 92.8.
18. MARLINSKY, V. V. 1992. Activity of lateral vestibular nucleus neurons during locomotion in the decerebrate guinea pig. Exp. Brain Res. **90:** 583–588.
19. ORLOVSKY, G. N. 1972. Activity of vestibulospinal neurons during locomotion. Brain Res. **46:** 85–98.
20. KINNEY, G. A., B. W. PETERSON & N. T. SLATER. 1994. The synaptic activation of N-methyl-D-aspartate receptors in the rat medial vestibular nucleus. J. Neurophysiol. **72:** 1588–1595.
21. SHIMAZU, H. & W. PRECHT. 1965. Tonic and kinetic responses of cat's vestibular neurons to horizontal angular acceleration. J. Neurophysiol. **28:** 991–1013.
22. MAEDA, M., H. SHIMAZU & Y. SHINODA. 1972. Nature of synaptic events in cat abducens motoneurons at slow and quick phase of vestibular nystagmus. J. Neurophysiol. **35:** 279–296.
23. BAKER, R., C. EVINGER & R. A. MCCREA. 1981. Some thoughts about the three neurons in the vestibulo-ocular reflex. Ann. N. Y. Acad. Sci. **374:** 171–188.
24. GOLDBERG, J. M., S. M. HIGHSTEIN, A. K. MOSCHOVAKIS & C. FERNANDEZ. 1987. Inputs from regularly and irregularly discharging vestibular nerve afferents to secondary neurons in the vestibular nuclei of the squirrel monkey. I. An electrophysiological analysis. J. Neurophysiol. **58:** 700–718.
25. BOYLE, R., J. M. GOLDBERG & S. M. HIGHSTEIN. 1992. Inputs from regularly and irregularly discharging vestibular nerve afferents to secondary neurons in the vestibular nuclei of the squirrel monkey. III. Correlation with vestibulospinal and vestibuloocular output pathways. J. Neurophysiol. **68:** 471–484.

26. IWAMOTO, Y., T. KITAMA & K. YOSHIDA. 1990. Vertical eye movement-related secondary vestibular neurons ascending in medial longitudinal fasciculus in cat. I. Firing properties and projection pathways. J. Neurophysiol. **63:** 902–917.

27. ANGELAKI, D. E. & A. A. PERACHIO. 1993. Contribution of irregular semicircular canal afferents to the horizontal vestibuloocular response during constant velocity rotation. J. Neurophysiol. **69:** 996–999.

28. SERAFIN, M., P. P. VIDAL & M. MÜHLETHALER. 1987. Electrophysiological and pharmacological properties of reticular neurons in nucleus gigantocellularis: A study in brainstem slices and isolated whole brain of guinea pig. 17th Annual Meeting of the Society for Neuroscience. Abstr. 239-6.

29. BABALIAN, A. L. & A. I. SHAPOVALOV. 1984. Mode of synaptic transmission between vestibular afferents and neurons of the vestibular nucleus in the frog. Brain Res. **309:** 163–167.

30. PEUSNER, K. D. & C. GIAUME. 1994. The first developing "mixed" synapses between vestibular sensory neurons mediate glutamate chemical transmission. Neuroscience **58:** 99–113.

31. RACINE, R. J., D. A. WILSON, R. GINGELL & D. SUNDERLAND. 1986. Long-term potentiation in the interpositus and vestibular nuclei in the rat. Exp. Brain Res. **63:** 158–162.

32. CAPOCCHI, G., G. DELLA TORRE, S. GRASSI, V. E. PETTOROSSI & M. ZAMPOLINI. 1992. NMDA receptor-mediated long-term modulation of electrically evoked field potentials in the rat medial vestibular nuclei. Exp. Brain Res. **90:** 546–550.

33. REICHENBERGER, I. & N. DIERINGER. 1994. Site-related colocalization of glycine- and glutamate-immunoreactivity in frog and rat vestibular afferents. J. Comp. Neurol. **347:** 1–12.

34. DE WAELE, C., N. VIBERT, M. BAUDRIMONT & P. P. VIDAL. 1990. NMDA receptors contribute to the resting discharge of vestibular neurons in the normal and hemilabyrinthectomized guinea pig. Exp. Brain Res. **81:** 125–133.

35. BENAZET, M., M. SERAFIN, C. DE WAELE, M. CHAT, P. LAPEYRE & P. P. VIDAL. 1993. In vivo modulation of the NMDA receptors by its glycinergic site in the guinea pig vestibular nuclei. 23rd Annual Meeting of the Society for Neuroscience. Abstr. 59-7.

36. VIBERT, N., M. SERAFIN, P. P. VIDAL & M. MÜHLETHALER. 1995. Effects of substance P on guinea-pig's medial vestibular neurones in brainstem slices. Eur. J. Neurosci. In press.

Activation of Immediate Early Genes by Vestibular Stimulation

GALEN D. KAUFMAN[a]

Department of Otolaryngology
University of Texas Medical Branch
Galveston, Texas 77555-1063

INTRODUCTION

The intent of this presentation is to bring those unfamiliar with the field of immediate early genes (IEGs) up to date with a contemporary understanding of these systems and, further, to apply this information to studies of vestibular-related systems. I begin with a review of the field of IEGs, describing the mechanisms associated with rapid response genes and how they are detected *in situ*. Next, previous and recent studies that have used IEGs in the study of vestibular phenomena, such as compensation to a unilateral labyrinth deficit, or adaptation to a change in the gravitational force, will be described. Finally, techniques and avenues for further research will be suggested.

In a broad sense this discussion deals with a subset of cellular homeostasis mechanisms, those employing transcription factors (TFs), or proteins, that play a role in the control and expression of the genes of a cell. One of the remarkable findings associated with these systems is how highly conserved the mechanisms and structures are throughout phylogeny, from yeast to humans. These proteins utilize three basic mechanisms for the control of genetic expression. The first is phosphorylation, where second-messenger cascades result in the addition of a phosphate group to the TF that alters its activity with respect to DNA interaction. The second is ligand-receptor interaction, typical of the steroid family of receptors, where a bound receptor translocates to the cell nucleus to affect transcription of genes. Finally, the mechanism we are interested in here is rapid transcription, where second-messenger cascades cause the rapid transcription and translation of a TF gene whose protein production results in the subsequent control of other genes. It is this form of control that is characterized as "immediate early genes," third messengers, or proto-oncogenes. Some TFs use a combination of these mechanisms.

The IEG TFs have been catagorized into several classes based on the structural motif that interacts with the DNA strand. The best understood form is the leucine zipper, where an α-helix region of the protein repeats hydrophobic leucine residues on one side which "zip up" with a similar molecule into a dimer. Proteins in the Fos and Jun families share this structure, as well as others. Another class is the zinc finger: this cassette uses many proline, cysteine, and histidine residues to bend around a zinc ion and form a finger-like structure capable of fitting into the grooves on a strand of DNA in a base-specific manner. Zif268 (also known as Erg1, Krox24, TIS8, NGF1-A, or ZENK) is an example. The helix-loop-helix motif, for example in the Myc TF, is another functional cassette type with DNA binding properties. Finally, steroid receptor proteins constitute another class of TFs. Many TFs also contain more than one of these functional domains in their structure. The prolifera-

[a] E-mail: gkaufman@marlin·utmb·edu

tion of pseudonyms for some of these TFs is a result of the independent discovery and development of these proteins in different animal and cell models, and is another example of their conservation across species. Some of the genes which these TFs likely control are listed here: prodynorphin, proenkephalin, oxytocin, vasopressin, corticotropin releasing factor, cholecystokinin, galanin, neuropeptide Y, glutamic acid decarboxylase, somatostatin, interleukins, heat shock protein 70, nitric oxide synthase, and calcitonin gene-related peptide.[1] This information has been gathered partly from *in vitro* induction studies, but also from correlative *in vivo* studies. Little solid evidence exists for which genes are affected by which TF; this is partly due to the complexity of the systems in question, which will be illustrated. One solid demonstration of direct control is the up-regulation of prodynorphin by Fos. Molecular biologists are increasing the known genetic targets for these TFs with time. This is an important development in the interpretation of IEG research.

IMMEDIATE EARLY GENE MECHANISMS AND TECHNIQUES

A general overview of IEG mechanisms using the Fos and Jun TFs as a model follows. In response to a cascade of events from the cell membrane, including calcium release, phosphorylation via protein kinase C, and redox regulation,[2] TFs for the c-fos gene activate or disinhibit portions of the promoter region of the gene. This activity, which does not require *de novo* translation, is available within seconds to minutes of the membrane stimulus. Four regulatory elements for the c-fos gene have been identified, including the cyclic AMP response element (CRE), serum response element (SRE), and the activator protein one site (AP-1). Once activated, the machinery for transcription assembles along the DNA strand, and a c-fos RNA is created, edited, and moved to the cytoplasm for translation. The resulting Fos protein is routed back to the nucleus, where it forms a dimer with a TF in the Jun family using its leucine zipper domain. Hundreds of copies of the Fos protein can be synthesized in a time frame of 15 min. If no further stimulus is presented, Fos is generally removed (degraded) from the cell within 6 to 24 h. This dimer then becomes available to regulate other genes with the AP-1 promoter. The DNA binding domain spans 4 to 5 nucleotides and bends the strand slightly. In addition, the Fos/Jun dimer negatively autoregulates its own synthesis, and has activity on the CRE as well.[3] Many different dimer combinations are possible, but Fos can only dimerize with a member of the Jun family, whereas Jun can autodimerize. Dimerization increases DNA binding affinity of the individual TFs, and different combinations of dimers have variable effects on different regulatory elements. Each TF has its own temporal expression properties; for example, the proteins in the Jun family tend to be present all the time, or be regulated more slowly, than the more rapid synthesis and degradation of Fos. Even with these simple examples, the combinatorial possibility for control of specific genes is great. The actual host of mechanisms inside the cell is certainly more complex, but a useful analogy is to view the system as a dynamic biochemical equilibrium, with changes in the input creating different stable states of genetic activation; that is, different patterns of regulation whose sum effect is a cellular phenotype appropriate for its current environment or functional role.

Two techniques are commonly employed to detect IEGs *in situ*. Both have their own unique benefits and drawbacks. The most popular immunohistochemistry protocols employ polyclonal antibodies to detect the TF protein and a layered avidin-biotin, peroxidase colorimetric reaction to visualize the antigen in fixed tissue. Standard problems with specificity of the reaction must be addressed. Fortunately, several good commercial antibody sources for Fos, Jun, Zif268, and others exist, which also account somewhat for the prevalence of reports on these proteins. For the detection of the messenger RNA level of a specific TF transcript, *in situ* hybridization histochemistry (ISHH) is often used. In this technique, a radiolabeled or fluorescently tagged oligonucleotide whose sequence is complementary to a portion of the mRNA of interest is applied to post-fixed tissue sections. Each technique gives a unique temporal and spatial snapshot of TF activity, and, used together and with appropriately placed time points, some of the mechanistic characteristics of a particular TF system can be elucidated.

IEG mechanisms and the techniques to detect them must be framed within the basic sequence of gene product synthesis—that of transcription of the message, editing the introns for expression, translation to protein, and the degradation of the message. Each step is a potential control site, underscoring the need for detection of both the protein and mRNA for a complete picture of a particular TFs activity.

Issues and interpretation regarding the results of *in vivo* IEG studies must include the following: The presence of, or time elapsed since, an anesthetic drug was used in the experimental animal is of critical importance to the results. Although the brief few minutes from a lethal dose of anesthetic that is used for humane sacrifice and tissue collection will not affect the expression patterns of IEGs, any time frame longer than 15 min will most certainly have an effect on neuronal IEG expression. Each drug has its own pattern of central nervous system IEG activation.[4] For example, urethane causes intense solitary nucleus and area postrema Fos immunolabeling, but spares the vestibular nuclei, whereas pentobarbital creates a broad activation of vestibular-related systems. Ketamine can cause strong Fos expression in the inferior olivary beta subnucleus. The volatile inhalant anesthetics have the least effect on IEG expression, especially for short time intervals. Studies performed under anesthesia might mask physiological mechanisms of IEG activity in the alert animal under identical stimulus conditions. The elimination kinetics of a particular drug should be understood in order to interpret the results of IEG expression. IEG research should avoid anesthetic contamination.

Detection nonspecificity must be addressed with antibody or oligo control studies. Is the antibody mono- or polyclonal, and what is the cross-reactivity? Preliminary experiments must determine that the stimulus for IEG activation is adequate, and for vestibular studies, that it originates from the labyrinth. Likewise, it should be shown that an observed expression pattern is consistent with the known function, connectivity, or known pharmacology of the neurons in question, and the expression kinetics of the IEG being measured. Appropriate time points for tissue fixation in relation to the stimulus must be used. A single stimulus evoking Fos expression should be measured within 6 h of the event, whereas ongoing processes like compensation or adaptation can recruit other TFs in longer time frames, for example, Jun B in cell differentiation. Specific patterns of input to a cell, and not necessarily average activity, are sufficient to differentially regulate TF expression.[5] Ideally, all of these factors can be accounted for with careful controls, comparing IEG expression patterns between groups and assigning specific immunolabeling patterns to the different variables.

VESTIBULAR STUDIES

Research involving the vestibular system that uses IEG detection has primarily fallen into three areas to date: compensation to hemilabyrinthectomy, adaptation to a hypergravity stimulus, and the location and mechanism of motion sickness. A brief summary of each area follows.

For the initial compensation studies, a chemical hemilabyrinthectomy (UL) was used to induce compensation in the pigmented rat.[6] Twenty-four hours after application of the toxin to the middle and inner ear, in the acute phase of compensation, the data showed that several areas of the brain stem recruited the Fos IEG. Most notably, and contrary to single unit activity studies, the ipsilateral medial (MVe) and descending vestibular nuclei had a greater expression of Fos than the contralateral nuclei. In addition, the contralateral prepositus hypoglossi (PrH), inferior olivary beta subnucleus (IOβ), and the ipsilateral dorsolateral periaqueductal gray, showed increases in Fos expression above the opposite side. Fos labeling has not been observed under any condition in primary afferent neurons. Most of the expression is gone after two weeks of compensation, although some Fos labeling remains in the PrH and MVe. This work has been verified and expanded by Cirelli et al.[7]

Recently, galvanic DC current of the labyrinth has been found to duplicate the Fos expression patterns seen after hemilabyrinthectomy.[4] Reversing the polarity of the stimulus reversed the symmetry of the expression in the MVe, PrH, and IOβ. Differential brain-stem expression of Fos and Zif268 could also be achieved by varying the location of the stimulating electrode relative to different labyrinth end-organs.

The hypergravity studies were an effort to map adaptive areas of the brain involved in a change of the gravity reference, as in microgravity. The original experiments used pigmented rats exposed to 2 G centripetal acceleration for 90 min, followed by sacrifice and Fos detection.[8,9] Controls used were on-axis animals essentially only experiencing the stress and angular components of the stimulus, and surgery and restraint controls.

The inferior olivary dorsomedial cell column (dmcc) receives vestibular and oculomotor-related inputs and projects to the nodulus and uvula primarily. The on-axis animals showed no immunolabeling. A striking Fos expression in the dmcc was observed only in the animals experiencing hypergravity. This was essentially an all-or-none expression among the neurons in this nucleus.

Other nuclei with hypergravity-dependent Fos immunolabeling were the IOβ, PrH, MVe, descending, y, and x vestibular nuclei; dorsolateral central gray, the interstitial nucleus of Cajal, and the Darkschewitsch's nucleus. Expression amounts did vary with restraint stress and on-axis stimulation in other areas of the brain, and the vestibular-related immunolabeling varied slightly between those animals whose heads were free to move during the stimulus, and those whose heads were fixed in place with a skull cap during the spin.

Although some asymmetries were present depending on the vector of centripetal acceleration across the head, to better dissect this component we combined chronic UL animals with the hypergravity stimulus so that the vector influence of one set of maculae could be observed. In the earth horizontal rotation model, it was assumed that the utricle would be primarily responsible for the hypergravity input. Recent data suggest that the primary input for this expression might be the saccule (Marshburn et al., in preparation).

Fos expression in these animals depended strongly on the orientation of the centripetal vector across the head.[10] Labeling occurred in the dmcc, or strongly occurred in other vestibular-related nuclei, only in the animals that were positioned so that their lesioned ear was toward the axis of rotation during the spin.

Furthermore, in the inferior olivary nucleus, when we looked at other position vectors, the Fos patterns around the dmcc shifted, indicating a possible topography mapped onto these cells from the utricle or saccule.

These findings show the usefulness of IEG studies in demarcating novel functional cell groups responding to a particular vestibular challenge, and can begin to help define the temporal and anatomical characteristics of the mechanisms behind behavioral changes associated with these challenges. Miller and Ruggiero[11] have recently used the Fos protein to map activity within the chemical emetic areas of the cat brain stem. Although no new functional group was identified in this study, the breadth of the areas involved could be appreciated. Finally, these types of experiments can begin to address, on a single-cell basis, the pharmacology of molecular mechanisms *in vivo*. For example, ketamine blocks hypergravity-induced Fos expression in the dmcc (unpublished data). One possibility is that neurons there use NMDA receptors to initiate the Fos cascade. Thus a potential molecular target for gravity-adaptive mechanisms has been defined.

DIRECTIONS

The directions in which *in vivo* studies using IEG markers can take are many, but will likely involve these strategies: Polymerase chain reaction (PCR) amplification and subtractive hybridization of regulated tissue-specific mRNA to reveal up- and down-regulation of specific genes; transgenic expression studies to isolate a single gene's function or relation to a disease or pathology and circumvent the nonspecificity of polyclonal antibody techniques; oligonucleotide probes to block or enhance genetic mechanisms; and a spectrum of correlative studies utilizing the armament of contemporary neuroscience imaging and single-unit techniques to fit IEG expression patterns into a particular mechanistic picture. An example of a subtractive hybridization experiment is isolating and growing mRNA libraries from fixed dmcc neurons of control and hypergravity-adapted animals, and then identifying up- and down-regulated mRNA from the cross subtractions.

Eventually it will be necessary to merge the results of molecular IEG studies with other measures. One strategy to relate a particular group of neurons to a behavioral measure will be to use anti-sense oligonucleotides as a specific blocker of TF activity. For example, it has been shown that 2 G hypergravity-adapted rats have a VOR with increased torsional and vertical components during a horizontal angular sinusoid.[12] A small injection of anti-Fos oligonucleotide around the dmcc prior to the adaptive stimulus might prevent the VOR change, linking the expression of Fos in those neurons with the behavioral adaptation. Single- or multiunit recordings of neurons before and after IEG expression could reveal characteristics of a cell's output that change with the state of TFs present. Pharmacological studies can also use information from IEG measures. Promethazine, an anti-motion sickness remedy, decreases Fos expression in the dmcc of gerbils and rats exposed to hypergravity (Marshburn *et al.,* in preparation), and might therefore slow or prevent adaptation. Finally, the cellular resolution of IEG detection would be a powerful adjunct to contemporary functional brain imaging techniques in animals, like positron emission tomography (PET), magnetic resonance imaging (MRI), and magneto- and electroencephalograms (MEG, EEG).

Those unfamiliar with the IEG literature often ask, "So what does it really mean?" regarding the usefulness of IEG detection. Although it is true that in many cases the exact sequelae of a particular TFs expression is not yet known, these probes are identifying new functional groups, and, more importantly, mechanisms that are function-specific and not simply a measure of metabolic activity. For example, animals undergoing compensation or adaptation to hypergravity both use Fos expression in the vestibular system, but the pattern and distribution of that expression is different. We are now at a point where these data can begin to be merged with other functional measures in a synthesis of understanding that bridges molecules to behavior.

REFERENCES

1. HUGHES, P. & M. DRAGUNOW. 1995. Induction of immediate-early genes and the control of neurotransmitter-regulated gene expression within the nervous system. Pharmacol. Rev. **47(1):** 133–178.
2. ABATE, C. *et al.* 1990. Redox regulation of Fos and Jun DNA-binding activity in vitro. Science **249:** 1157–1161.
3. LUCIBELLO, F. C. *et al.* 1989. Trans-repression of the mouse c-fos promoter: A novel mechanism of Fos-mediated trans-regulation. Cell **59:** 999–1007.
4. KAUFMAN, G. D. & A. A. PERACHIO. 1994. Translabyrinth electrical stimulation for the induction of immediate early genes in the gerbil brainstem. Brain Res. **646:** 345-350.
5. SHENG, H. Z., R. D. FIELDS & P. G. NELSON. 1993. Specific regulation of immediate early genes by patterned neuronal activity. J. Neurosci. Res. **35(5):** 459–467.
6. KAUFMAN, G. D., J. H. ANDERSON & A. J. BEITZ. 1992. Brainstem Fos expression following unilateral labyrinthectomy in the rat. Neuroreport **3(10):** 829–832.
7. CIRELLI, C. *et al.* 1993. Early c-fos expression in the rat vestibular and olivocerebellar systems after unilateral labyrinthectomy. Arch. Ital. Biol. **131(1):** 71–74.
8. KAUFMAN, G. D., J. H. ANDERSON & A. BEITZ. 1991. Activation of a specific vestibulo-olivary pathway by centripetal acceleration in rat. Brain Res. **562(2):** 311–317.
9. KAUFMAN, G. D., J. H. ANDERSON & A. J. BEITZ. 1992. Fos-defined activity in rat brainstem following centripetal acceleration. J. Neurosci. **12(11):** 4489–4500.
10. KAUFMAN, G. D., J. H. ANDERSON & A. J. BEITZ. 1993. Otolith-brain stem connectivity— Evidence for differential neural activation by vestibular hair cells based on quantification of FOS expression in unilateral labyrinthectomized rats. J. Neurophysiol. **70(1):** 117–127.
11. MILLER, A. D. & D. A. RUGGIERO. 1994. Emetic reflexes are revealed by expression of the immediate-early gene c-fos in the cat. J. Neurosci. **14(2):** 871–888.
12. KAUFMAN, G. D., J. H. ANDERSON & A. J. BEITZ. 1995. A torsional component in the horizontal VOR after centripetal acceleration. In preparation.

GABAergic Neurons in the Primate Vestibular Nuclei[a]

GAY R. HOLSTEIN,[b,c] GIORGIO P. MARTINELLI,[d]
JEFFREY W. DEGEN,[b] AND BERNARD COHEN[b,e]

Departments of Neurology,[b] Anatomy/Cell Biology,[c]
Surgery,[d] and Physiology/Biophysics[e]
Mount Sinai Medical Center
One Gustave Levy Place
New York, New York 10029

INTRODUCTION

γ-Aminobutyric acid (GABA) is one of the primary inhibitory neurotransmitters of the vertebrate central nervous system. The concentration of this amino acid is greatest in telencephalic and diencephalic regions, and generally decreases caudally. The central vestibular system, however, is a lower brainstem region that contains a relatively high concentration of GABA. Initial data suggesting the existence of GABAergic neurotransmission in the vestibular nuclear complex (VNC) were obtained from electrophysiological[1] and biochemical[2] experiments. Subsequently, immunocytochemical studies with antibodies against glutamic acid decarboxylase (GAD) or GABA revealed immunostained neurons in the vestibular nuclei of mouse,[3] guinea pig,[4,5] rat,[6–8] rabbit,[9] cat,[10–12] and monkey.[13]

Four general categories of GABAergic neurons have been described anatomically or implicated electrophysiologically in one or more parts of the VNC. These include cells with projections to extraocular motor neuron pools, neurons mediating disynaptic commissural inhibition, cells with descending projections to structures including the inferior olivary complex and spinal cord, and local circuit neurons. In addition, GABA- or GAD-immunolabeled fibers, usually beaded and of variable diameter, course through the VNC.[5–8] In the medial vestibular nucleus (MVN), most of the largest caliber stained fibers project medially toward the nuclei prepositus hypoglossi (NPH). Large diameter GAD-immunoreactive fibers are apparent in the lateral vestibular nucleus (LVN) as well, with a higher density of such processes observed in the dorsal subregion.[8,12] These fibers are often seen in close proximity to the somata of Deiters' neurons.

GABA-immunoreactive puncta are apparent throughout the vestibular nuclei, often in close association with the proximal dendrites and somata of vestibular cells.[5–9] Many of these puncta are attributable to GABAergic commissural and intra-VNC connections, as well as to long-axon VNC projection neurons that provide local axon collaterals within the nucleus of origin. Most extrinsic GABAergic terminals are undoubtedly derived from cerebellar Purkinje cells.[6,14] In LVN, a somewhat greater density of labeled puncta is present in the ventral region.[12] This observation, together with the fiber density distribution, suggests that GABAergic

[a] This work was supported in part by research grant No. 5 RO1 01705-04 from the National Institute on Deafness and Other Communication Disorders, and No. NS 00294 from the National Institute of Neurological Disorders and Stroke, National Institutes of Health.

Purkinje cell afferents may course through the dorsal portion of LVN to terminate in the ventral subnucleus.

We have produced and characterized a monoclonal antibody directed against a GABA-glutaraldehyde conjugate. In the present study, we used this antibody to analyze the synaptic interactions of GABA-immunoreactive elements in MVN. This is part of a long-term effort to understand the synaptology of neurotransmitter-defined circuits in the central vestibular system of the primate. We have found that most GABAergic cells in MVN exhibit a common set of ultrastructural characteristics. In contrast, two different types of GABA-immunoreactive axon terminals were observed frequently in our material, and a third type was present but far less common.

METHODS

Monoclonal antibody production and specificity. Anti-GABA antibodies were induced by immunizing BALB/c mice with GABA conjugated to the protein-carrier keyhole limpet hemocyanin (KLH; Calbiochem, La Jolla, CA) using glutaraldehyde as a linking agent. Once antibody titers reached satisfactory levels (after the third boost), spleen cells were harvested from several mice and fused with myeloma cells (P3×63-Ag8. 653) according to established protocols. Screening for hybrid clones producing anti-GABA antibodies was initially performed by enzyme-linked immunosorbent assay (ELISA) using GABA conjugated to bovine serum albumin (BSA). Hybridomas from positive wells were pick-cloned. Antibodies produced by such clones were subsequently screened by ELISA for cross-reactivity with other amino acid– and neurotransmitter-BSA conjugates as follows: Triplicate volumes (100 μL) of hybridoma supernatant were incubated for 60 min at 37 °C in wells of ELISA plates precoated with glutaraldehyde conjugates of amino acids and neurotransmitters to BSA. Wells were washed and then reacted for 60 min at 37 °C with goat anti-mouse IgG antibodies conjugated to alkaline phosphatase. After washing, the presence of bound monoclonal antibody was revealed by adding a solution of *p*-nitrophenyl phosphate to the wells for 20 min at 37 °C. Reactions were then analyzed at 406 nm in an ELISA reader. Among the positive hybridomas, GABA-93 was the only clone that secreted an antibody exhibiting no cross-reactivity with other amino acid or neurotransmitter molecules (FIG. 1).

Immunocytochemistry. To use this antibody for immunocytochemistry, animals were sacrificed by perfusion with physiological saline, followed by 4% formaldehyde/0.35% glutaraldehyde in 0.1M phosphate buffer (PB) at pH 7.3. Tissue immunocytochemistry tests were conducted in Sprague Dawley rats; vestibular system ultrastructural studies were conducted in one rhesus and two cynomolgus monkeys. Blocks of tissue were cut by stereotaxic instrument, placed in a graded series of sucrose solutions in PB and left in 20% sucrose overnight at 4 °C. The blocks in 20% sucrose were frozen in an isopentane bath cooled by dry ice in acetone, and thawed to room temperature. Vibratome sections cut from blocks containing the vestibular nuclei and cerebellum were rinsed in phosphate buffered saline (PBS) and pretreated with 20% normal goat serum (NGS) in PBS for 60 min. Sections were then incubated for 16 h at 4 °C with appropriate dilutions of the monoclonal anti-GABA (GABA-93) or a commercial polyclonal anti-GABA antibody (Arnel) in 10% NGS in PBS. The sections were subsequently processed using Vectastain ABC Elite kits, and the reaction product visualized using 0.05% diaminobenzidine (DAB) with 0.01% H_2O_2. The incubation steps alternated with five PBS rinses; washes before and after the DAB reaction were with Tris-buffered saline (TBS). Sections for light microscopy were lightly osmicated, rinsed with PBS, dry-mounted on glass slides, and analyzed and photographed using a Zeiss Axiophot microscope system with Nomarski differential interference optics. Material for electron microscopy was dissected, osmicated, dehydrated, infiltrated, and embedded in Epon-Araldite between plastic coverslips. These sections were photographed using a Wild Photomacroscope, traced using a Trisimplex projector, dissected, and serial thin-sectioned onto formvar-coated slot grids. No postmicrotomy staining was performed.

RESULTS

To assess the usefulness of the GABA-93 monoclonal antibody for tissue immunocytochemistry, the extent and specificity of staining were evaluated in known GABAergic neuronal elements. For these studies, Vibratome sections through the

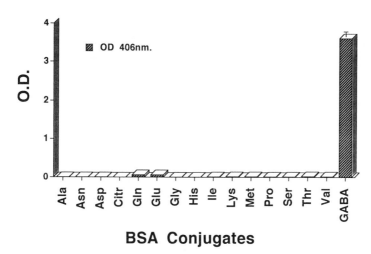

BSA Conjugates

FIGURE 1. Cross-reactivity of monoclonal antibody (mAb) GABA-93 assayed by enzyme linked immunosorbent assay (ELISA). GABA-93 shows negligible cross-reactivity with conjugates of the amino acids, indicated on the abscissa, as well as other neurotransmitter molecules including serotonin, epinephrine, norepinephrine, and histamine (not shown). O.D.: Optical density of *p*-nitrophenyl phosphate reaction product detected through a 406-nm filter.

rat and monkey cerebellar cortex were reacted using serial primary antibody dilutions. As shown in FIGURE 2, the interneurons of cerebellar cortex were stained, as were the baskets surrounding the Purkinje cell somata. The Purkinje cell bodies themselves were not immunoreactive, but the dendritic tree and supraganglionic plexus were labeled. This staining pattern was consistent with the findings obtained using other commercial and private antibody sources.

In the vestibular nuclei, small- and medium-sized GABAergic neurons were distributed throughout the region. Many of these cells were multipolar with round or oval somata (FIG. 3), although a substantial population of fusiform-shaped immunoreactive cells was observed as well (FIG. 4). Stained cells were more numerous in MVN and the superior vestibular nucleus (SVN) than in the other VNC nuclei. In

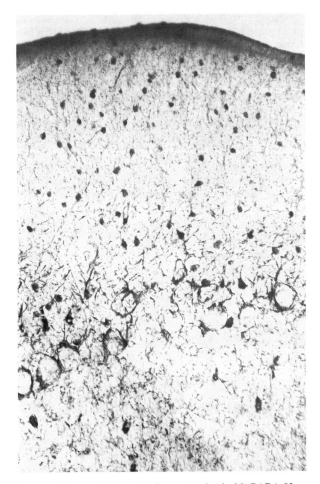

FIGURE 2. Rhesus monkey cerebellar cortex immunostained with GABA-93 supernatant. The pia mater is located at the top of the illustration, and the granular layer at the bottom. The stellate, basket and Golgi cell bodies are immunostained, as well as the baskets surrounding the Purkinje cell bodies, the supraganglionic plexus of Purkinje cell processes, and some of the fibers of the white matter. Nomarski differential interference optics. (Magnification: 175×.)

MVN, the density of immunostained somata appeared to be greatest rostrally and least caudally; at all levels these neurons were more prevalent in the central region of the nucleus. The periventricular zone and the medial aspect of MVN contained few GABAergic neurons. However, immunoreactive fiber processes coursed throughout MVN, including the periventricular and medial regions, and in fact many of the stained axons appeared to be directed toward the midline.

At the ultrastructural level, most of the GABA-immunoreactive cell bodies present in MVN contained large numbers of small dark mitochondria, and a dense cytoplasmic matrix full of large vacuolated cisterns (FIG. 5). At least a portion of these neurons had somal spines, some of which displayed the subcellular features of the parent perikarya. Axosomatic synapses onto the body or spines were common. In FIGURE 5, the neuron received a synapse from a non-GABAergic terminal onto the perikaryal membrane adjacent to the spine (arrows), rather than directly onto the spine itself. Many GABA-immunostained dendrites also appeared to contain numerous small dark mitochondria and a system of large cisternae (FIG. 6A).

Two general types of GABA-immunoreactive axon terminals were prevalent in the primate MVN. One type contained many large cisterns and small dark mitochondria scattered throughout the profile, as well as a moderate density of synaptic vesicles that had variable round and oval shapes (FIG. 6B). A second prevalent type of immunostained axon contained very densely packed spherical synaptic vesicles and several small mitochondria that tended to cluster near the plasma membrane in one region of the profile (FIG. 7).

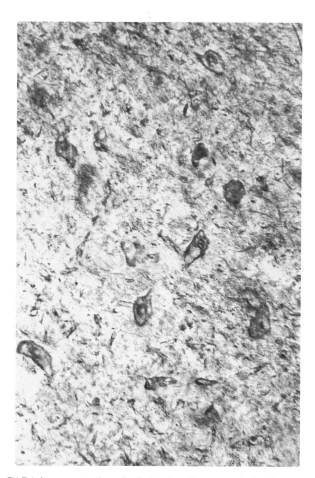

FIGURE 3. GABA-immunoreactive spherical and ovoid neurons in the rhesus monkey medial vestibular nucleus. The immunoreactive cells are scattered in a matrix of GABAergic fibers as well as non-immunostained cells and processes. Nomarski differential interference optics. (Magnification: 350×.)

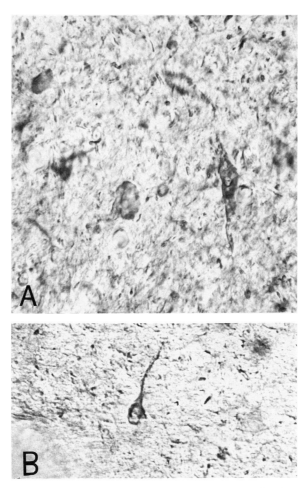

FIGURE 4. Examples of GABA-immunostained fusiform neurons in the monkey medial vestibular nucleus. Nomarski differential interference optics. (Magnification: **(A)** 350× and **(B)** 600×.)

GABAergic axons formed symmetric synapses with different types of postsynaptic targets, most frequently with unstained dendrites (FIG. 8A) and axons (FIG. 8B). For some of these axoaxonic contacts, the polarity of the synapse was difficult to establish with certainty because the peroxidase immunostain tended to obscure the membrane densities. However, it was usually possible to visualize the element that contained synaptic vesicles clustered at, and adherent to, the membrane at the region of the synaptic cleft. This is identified by the arrows in FIGURES 8A and B that point to the postsynaptic membrane specializations. In both examples, the postsynaptic axon terminal contained pale mitochondria with wide intercrestal spaces and small ellipsoid synaptic vesicles that clustered at a distance from the synaptic specializations. In general, as in these figures, the ultrastructure of the pre- and postsynaptic axons were markedly different (FIGS. 8B and 9). In the example shown in FIGURE 9, a GABA-immunoreactive axon terminal, containing cisterns, scattered small dark mitochondria, and a moderate density of pleomorphic synaptic vesicles, formed a synaptic contact (at arrows) with a non-GABAergic axon terminal. This unstained profile contained ellipsoid vesicles and large pale mitochondria dispersed throughout a cytoplasmic matrix that lacked elaborate cisterns. We have not observed any examples of direct synaptic contacts between two GABA-immunoreactive axon terminals.

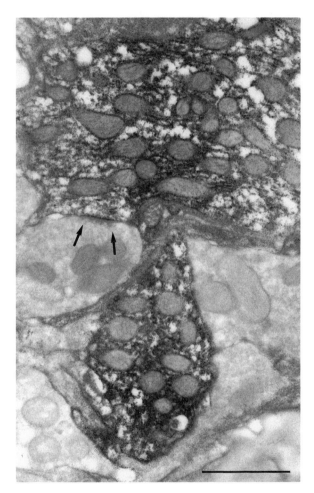

FIGURE 5. A GABA-immunoreactive cell body in the MVN containing numerous small dark mitochondria and many large cisternae. This neuron receives a synapse (*arrows*) from a non-GABAergic terminal that contains presynaptic dense projections. The contact is formed with the perikaryal membrane adjacent to the somal spine, rather than directly onto the spine itself. Scale bar: 1 μm.

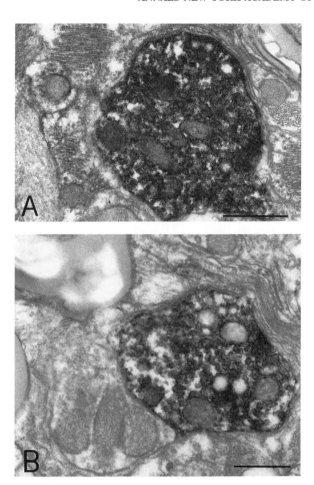

FIGURE 6. A GABA-immunoreactive dendrite (**A**) and axon (**B**) with similar morphologic features in MVN. Both elements contain a few small dark mitochondria and cisternae distributed throughout the cytoplasm. The axon also contains a medium packing density of pleomorphic synaptic vesicles. Scale bars: 0.5 μm.

DISCUSSION

Ultrastructure of GABAergic Vestibular Neurons

At the ultrastructural level, the MVN appeared to be a heterogeneous mixture of myelinated axons, blood vessels, neuronal perikarya, and glial cells and processes. The neuropil constituents were located in small pockets, seemingly squeezed by the larger non-neuropil elements of the region. GABAergic neurons were distributed throughout this matrix, and appeared to have rather uniform ultrastructural characteristics. Most notably, the somal cytoplasm contained numerous small dark mitochondria and an extensive system of large vacuolated cisterns. This uniform ultrastructural appearance of the GABA-immunostained cells in MVN stands in contrast to the variety of cell sizes and shapes seen at the light microscopic level, and with the known differences in connectivity of GABAergic MVN neurons.[13] It is likely, therefore, that differences among GABAergic cells will be reflected in synaptologic features such as differences in the distributions of afferent inputs, of axosomatic, axodendritic, axospinous, and axoaxonic synapses, and of pre- and postsynaptic receptor populations. We are currently pursuing this hypothesis in further studies of GABA in the primate MVN.

Our findings in the primate VNC are similar to the immunocytochemical observations of GABA-related compounds in other species. In the mouse[3] and cat,[12] for example, GABA-immunoreactive neurons were reported to be scattered uniformly through the VNC, although another study in cat[11] found GABA-immunostained neurons in all vestibular nuclei except LVN. In this latter report, labeled neurons were observed throughout the rostro-caudal extent of MVN and the descending vestibular nucleus (DVN), whereas immunopositive cells in SVN were located primarily in the central region of the nucleus, in an area that was also rich in GABAergic axons. Intraventricular colchicine injections before either polyclonal anti-GABA immunohistochemistry in guinea pig,[5] or GAD-immunostaining in rat,[7] resulted in higher concentrations of labeled cells in MVN and possibly DVN than in the other vestibular nuclei. However, this distinction might have been due to the local effects of the injection on cells near the ventricular wall, rather than to actual subregional differences in neurotransmitter complement.

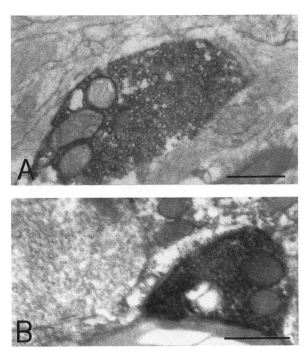

FIGURE 7. A second type of GABAergic terminal in the primate MVN. These profiles contain a high packing density of spherical synaptic vesicles, and several mitochondria that tend to aggregate in one area of the terminal. Scale bars: 0.5 μm.

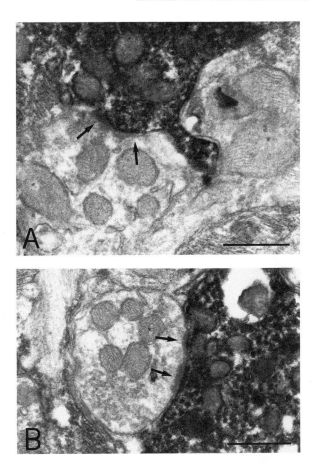

FIGURE 8. Two examples of GABA-immunostained axons forming synapses with unlabeled elements in the MVN. (**A**) An axodendritic symmetric synapse involving a GABAergic terminal with numerous small dark mitochondria and moderately packed round/pleomorphic synaptic vesicles. (**B**) A similar labeled axon terminal forms two symmetric synapses (*arrows*) with an unstained axon of markedly different ultrastructure. The postsynaptic element contains pale mitochondria with wide intercrestal spaces, and small ellipsoid synaptic vesicles that cluster at a distance from the synaptic specializations. Scale bars: 0.5 μm.

In the rat, small round neurons were the predominant GAD-positive cell type in MVN, whereas small- to medium-sized triangular or pear-shaped labeled neurons were scattered throughout DVN.[8] In the guinea pig,[5] GABA-like immunoreactivity was localized in small round, oval, or fusiform vestibular cells. Similarly, *in situ* hybridization studies in rat provided histochemical evidence for the presence of GAD mRNA in many small- to medium-sized MVN neurons, but not in large diameter cells.[15,16] These findings are similar to our observations of small- and medium-sized round, oval and fusiform GABAergic neurons in MVN. One study in the guinea pig has reported GABA immunostaining of Deiters' neurons in LVN.[4] In most studies, however, the giant Deiters' neurons in LVN were not themselves immunoreactive, although labeled puncta surrounded these somata, sometimes so densely as to give the appearance of perikaryal staining.[6] Such an interpretation has been supported by classical degeneration studies that showed Purkinje cell axons forming synapses with the cell bodies and proximal dendrites of dorsal LVN (DLVN) neurons.[17] In addition, physiological studies indicated that the major efferent projection pathway of these cells, the lateral vestibulospinal tract, is excitatory, and immunocytochemical observations suggested that the pathway is glutamatergic.[12]

GABAergic neurons have been conservatively estimated to represent less than 10% of the total cell population in each of the four vestibular nuclei in cat.[12] More recently, a [³⁵S]-labeled GAD 67 oligonucleotide probe has been used to visualize mRNA in autoradiographs of the rat brain.[18] With this approach, as with most of the immunocytochemical studies, more intense labeling is obtained in nucleus prepositus

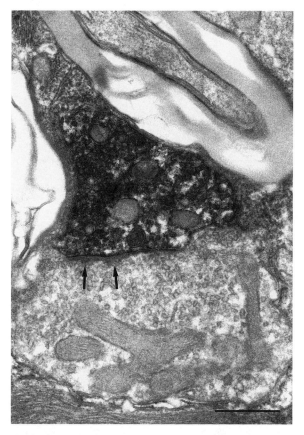

FIGURE 9. A GABA-immunoreactive axon terminal containing cisternae, scattered small dark mitochondria, and a moderate density of pleomorphic synaptic vesicles, in synaptic contact (*at arrows*) with a non-GABAergic axon terminal. Although the polarity of this contact is not certain, the presence of clustered synaptic vesicles adherent to the membrane of the unstained axon suggests that this non-GABAergic terminal is the presynaptic element in a symmetric synapse with the GABAergic bouton. Scale bar: 0.5 μm.

hypoglossi (NPH), MVN, and SVN than in LVN or DVN. In particular, the GAD mRNA-containing cells in MVN and SVN are uniformly distributed throughout the nucleus, and comprise an estimated 33–43% of the total cell population. In contrast, 9–31% of LVN cells are labeled, and none of these are the large Deiters' neurons. Although quantitative information is difficult to glean from pre-embedding immuno-cytochemistry techniques, our large sample of stained sections supports estimates of approximately 30% of neurons showing GABA immunoreactivity.

GABAergic Axon Terminals in the Medial Vestibular Nucleus

Two prevalent types of GABA-immunoreactive axon terminals were observed in the primate MVN. One type shared the ultrastructural features of the neuronal perikarya and dendritic cytoplasm in our material, and also contained a medium packing density of pleomorphic, mostly oval, synaptic vesicles. A second type of GABAergic axon terminal displayed distinctly different cytoplasmic features, including very densely packed, uniformly spherical synaptic vesicles and mitochondria that clustered in one side of the profile. In general, these latter elements were substantially smaller in cross-sectional area than the previously described terminals, and were observed somewhat less frequently.

The two types of GABA-immunoreactive terminals present in the primate MVN can be compared with similar synaptic boutons observed in the cat SVN.[19] In this study, the terminals were subdivided into three types based on the size and shape of the synaptic vesicles. Large round (LR) boutons had large (40 nm diameter) round vesicles and contacted the somata and proximal dendrites of SVN cells at synapses associated with prominent postsynaptic densities. Based on degeneration after vestibular neurectomy, these elements were interpreted as primary afferent terminals. In addition, small round (SR) boutons had smaller round vesicles and prominent postsynaptic densities, whereas other elements (termed "PL") had smaller pleomorphic vesicles and lacked prominent postsynaptic densities. The cells of origin of SR and PL terminals have not been identified.

The SR boutons of the cat closely resemble the ultrastructural appearance of the GABA-immunostained terminals with densely packed spherical vesicles present in our material. In addition, the PL profiles correspond well with the GABAergic terminals containing small dark mitochondria and large cisterns that are prevalent in the primate MVN. The marked similarity in ultrastructural appearance of these terminals with the immunolabeled perikarya and dendrites suggests that these stained profiles are sections through different compartments of the same type of neuron. If so, then the GABAergic terminals with small dark mitochondria, large cisterns, and a moderate density of oval/pleomorphic synaptic vesicles are derived from vestibular neurons, rather than extrinsic afferent sources.

Synaptology of GABAergic Boutons in the Medial Vestibular Nucleus

Occasional axo-axonic synapses have previously been illustrated or reported in the cat[20] and rat[21] LVN, cat SVN[19] and monkey MVN.[22,23] In general, these contacts have been described involving boutons with spherical vesicles presynaptic to those with elongated vesicles. In the present study, we found numerous examples of axoaxonic synapses in which the presynaptic element was a GABAergic terminal with small dark mitochondria, large cisterns, and a moderate density of oval/ pleomorphic synaptic vesicles. The postsynaptic terminal was never immunostained, and usually contained larger, pale mitochondria, a cluster of ellipsoid vesicles, and a prominent postsynaptic density. This synaptology represents a morphologic basis for presynaptic inhibition in MVN. Inasmuch as the markedly ellipsoid synaptic vesicles are likely to contain inhibitory neurotransmitter molecules,[24] but are not GABA-immunoreactive, the postsynaptic terminals containing these vesicles may be the glycinergic afferents that have been implicated to exist in MVN.[25] If so, then the axoaxonic contacts involving GABAergic terminals presynaptic to glycinergic boutons would represent the structural basis for disinhibition in MVN. We are currently conducting studies to test this possibility. Finally, because no synapses between two GABA-immunoreactive profiles have been observed, it is unlikely that disinhibition of GABAergic projection neurons occurs in MVN.

It is possible that some of the GABA-immunostained neurons visualized in the primate MVN also contain other neurotransmitters and/or modulators. Electrophysiological data suggest that vestibular type I neurons may be controlled by both GABA and glycine.[25] Extensive colocalization of GABA and glycine in the rabbit VNC is reported in LVN neurons, and in some axons and boutons of MVN and DVN.[26] In general, most glycinergic cells and myelinated axons appear to colocalize GABA,[12] and conversely, few glycine-immunostained profiles are GABA-immuno-negative.[26] In contrast, GABA immunolabeled fibers of all sizes, and most of the GABA-immunoreactive perisomatic puncta in LVN, are not glycinergic. Coexistence of GABA and glycine is observed less frequently in DVN, where glycine-only neuronal elements are common. Lastly, although GABA apparently does not coexist with glutamate or aspartate in the neurotransmitter pool, some glycinergic cells of DVN also show aspartate and glutamate immunoreactivity.[26] However, because glycine, aspartate, and glutamate are all present as metabolites in neurons, these observations must be viewed with some caution. In addition, despite the colocalization of GABA and glycine in single vestibular neurons, the ultimate impact of synaptic neurotransmission is dependent on the presence and localization of specific postsynaptic receptor sites.

In summary, we have produced a monoclonal antibody directed against a GABA-glutaraldehyde conjugate. This antibody was used to analyze synaptic interactions involving GABA-immunoreactive elements in the rhesus monkey MVN. We found that approximately 30% of the neurons in MVN were immunostained, including multipolar cells with round or oval somata and fusiform neurons. The stained cells were more prevalent in rostral MVN and SVN than in other regions of the VNC. Many stained axons from MVN cells were directed toward the midline, presumably constituting part of the commissural system. The GABAergic neurons had rather uniform ultrastructural characteristics. Cell bodies contained small dark mitochondria and a dense cytoplasmic matrix with large vacuolated cisterns. Many of these neurons had somal spines. Two types of GABA-immunostained axon terminals were prevalent. One type contained large cisterns, small scattered dark mitochondria, and a moderate density of pleomorphic round/oval synaptic vesicles. A second type contained densely packed spherical synaptic vesicles and pale mitochondria that tended to cluster in one region of the terminal. Although axoaxonic contacts were observed frequently, synapses between two GABAergic elements were not found. Therefore, the GABAergic neurons of the commissural system are not likely to exert their effects via direct GABA–GABA neuronal interactions.

ACKNOWLEDGMENTS

The authors wish to thank Rosemary Lang and Victor Rodriguez for expert technical assistance with various aspects of the work.

REFERENCES

1. OBATA, K., M. ITO, R. OCHI & N. SATO. 1967. Pharmacological properties of the postsynaptic inhibition by Purkinje cell axons and the action of γ-aminobutyric acid on Deiters' neurones. Exp. Brain Res. **4:** 43–57.
2. OTSUKA, M., K. OBATA, Y. MIYATA & Y. TANAKA. 1971. Measurement of γ-aminobutyric acid in isolated nerve cells of cat central nervous system. J. Neurochem. **18:** 287–295.
3. OTTERSEN, O. P. & J. STORM-MATHISEN. 1984. Neurons containing or accumulating transmitter amino acids. In Handbook of Chemical Neuroanatomy, vol. 3. Classical Transmitters and Transmitter Receptors in the CNS, part II. A. Björklund, T. Hökfelt & M. J. Kuhar, Eds.: 141–246. Elsevier. Amsterdam.
4. DUPONT, J., M. GEFFARD, A. CALAS & J.-M. ARAN. 1990. Immunohistochemical evidence for GABAergic cell bodies in the medial nucleus of the trapezoid body and in the lateral vestibular nucleus in the guinea pig brainstem. Neurosci. Lett. **111:** 263–268.
5. KUMOI, K., N. SAITO & C. TANAKA. 1987. Immunohistochemical localization of γ-amino-butyric acid– and aspartate-containing neurons in the guinea pig vestibular nuclei. Brain Res. **416:** 22–33.
6. HOUSER, C. R., R. P. BARBER & J. E. VAUGHN. 1984. Immunocytochemical localization of glutamic acid decarboxylase in the dorsal lateral vestibular nucleus: Evidence for an intrinsic and extrinsic GABAergic innervation. Neurosci. Lett. **47:** 413–420.
7. MUGNAINI, E. & W. H. OERTEL. 1985. An atlas of the distribution of GABAergic neurons and terminals in the rat CNS as revealed by GAD immunohistochemistry. In Handbook of Chemical Neuroanatomy. A. Bjorklund & T. Hokfelt, Eds.: 436–622. Elsevier/North Holland. Amsterdam.
8. NOMURA, I. et al. 1984. Neuropeptides and γ-aminobutyric acid in the vestibular nuclei of the rat: An immunocytochemical analysis. I. Distribution. Brain Res. **311:** 109–118.
9. BLESSING, W. W., S. C. HEDGER & W. H. OERTEL. 1987. Vestibulospinal pathway in rabbit includes GABA-synthesizing neurons. Neurosci. Lett. **80:** 158–162.
10. SPENCER, R. F., R. J. WENTHOLD & R. BAKER. 1989. Evidence for glycine as an inhibitory neurotransmitter of vestibular, reticular, and prepositus hypoglossi neurons that project to the cat abducens nucleus. J. Neurosci. **9:** 2718–2736.
11. SPENCER, R. F. & R. BAKER. 1992. GABA and glycine as inhibitory neurotransmitters in the vestibulo-ocular reflex. Ann. N. Y. Acad. Sci. **656:** 602–611.
12. WALBERG, F., O. P. OTTERSEN & E. RINVIK. 1990. GABA, glycine, aspartate, glutamate and taurine in the vestibular nuclei: An immunocytochemical investigation in the cat. Exp. Brain Res. **79:** 547–563.
13. HOLSTEIN, G. R. 1996. Inhibitory amino acid transmitters in the vestibular nuclei. In Neurochemistry of the Vestibular System. J. H. Anderson & A. J. Beitz, Eds. CRC Press. Boca Raton, FL.
14. FONNUM, F., J. STORM-MATHISEN & F. WALBERG. 1970. Glutamate decarboxylase in inhibitory neurons. A study of the enzyme in Purkinje cell axons and boutons in the cat. Brain Res. **20:** 259–275.
15. NAJLERAHIM, A., P. J. HARRISON, A. J. L. BARTON, J. HEFFERNAN & R. C. A. PEARSON. 1990. Distribution of messenger RNAs encoding the enzymes glutaminase, aspartate aminotransferase and glutamic acid decarboxylase in rat brain. Mol. Brain Res. **7:** 17–33.
16. FERRAGUTI, F. et al. 1990. Distribution of glutamic acid decarboxylase messenger RNA-containing nerve cell populations of the male rat brain. J. Chem. Neuroanat. **3:** 377–396.

17. MUGNAINI, E. & F. WALBERG. 1967. An experimental electron microscopical study on the mode of termination of cerebellar cortico-vestibular fibers in the cat lateral vestibular nucleus (Deiters' nucleus). Exp. Brain Res. **4:** 212–236.
18. DEWAELE, C. *et al.* 1994. Distribution of glutamatergic receptors and GAD mRNA-containing neurons in the vestibular nuclei of normal and hemilabyrinthectomized rats. Eur. J. Neurosci. **6:** 565–576.
19. KORTE, G. E. & V. L. J. FRIEDRICH. 1979. The fine structure of the feline superior vestibular nucleus: Identification and synaptology of the primary vestibular afferents. Brain Res. **176:** 3–32.
20. EAGER, R. 1967. Cerebellar projection to the vestibular nuclei. *In* Third Symposium on the Role of the Vestibular Organs in Space Exploration. NASA, Ed.: 225–237. U.S. Government Printing Office. Washington, D.C.
21. SOTELO, C. & S. PALAY. 1970. The fine structure of the lateral vestibular nucleus in the rat. II. Synaptic organization. Brain Res. **18:** 93–115.
22. HOLSTEIN, G. R., G. P. MARTINELLI & B. COHEN. 1992. Immunocytochemical visualization of L-baclofen-sensitive GABA$_B$ binding sites in the medial vestibular nucleus. Ann. N. Y. Acad. Sci. **656:** 933–936.
23. HOLSTEIN, G. R., G. P. MARTINELLI & B. COHEN. 1992. L-Baclofen-sensitive GABA$_B$ binding sites in the medial vestibular nucleus localized by immunocytochemistry. Brain Res. **581:** 175–180.
24. PETERS, A., S. L. PALAY & H. D. WEBSTER. 1976. The Fine Structure of the Nervous System. W. B. Saunders Company. Philadelphia, PA.
25. FURUYA, N., T. YABE & T. KOIZUMI. 1991. Neurotransmitters regulating the activity of the vestibular commissural inhibition in the cat. Ann. N. Y. Acad. Sci. **656:** 594–601.
26. WENTZEL, P. R., C. I. DEZEEUW, J. C. HOLSTEGE & N. M. GERRITS. 1993. Colocalization of GABA and glycine in the rabbit oculomotor nucleus. Neurosci. Lett. **164:** 25–29.

Vestibular Influences on the Autonomic Nervous System[a]

BILL J. YATES[b]

Departments of Otolaryngology and Neuroscience
University of Pittsburgh
EEINS Building, Room 106
203 Lothrop Street
Pittsburgh, Pennsylvania 15213

INTRODUCTION

Traditionally, the influences of the vestibular system have been considered to be mainly confined to those brain-stem and spinal neurons that regulate eye position, head position, and balance. However, for decades clinical evidence has been available that suggests connections between the vestibular system and the autonomic nervous system. For example, one classically appreciated result of vestibular dysfunction is nausea and vomiting.[1] The role of the vestibular system in producing the myriad of autonomic symptoms (ranging from pallor to emesis) during motion sickness is also well established.[2,3]

More recent evidence suggests that the vestibular system participates in producing rapid adjustments in circulation and respiration that are necessary to maintain homeostasis. This evidence will be reviewed here, as will the current knowledge about neural pathways that link the vestibular nuclei with brain-stem areas that regulate blood pressure and breathing. Readers who are interested in the influences of the vestibular system on nausea and vomiting are referred to a recent volume on vestibular autonomic regulation.[4]

CHALLENGES TO CIRCULATION AND RESPIRATION DURING MOVEMENT AND CHANGES IN POSTURE

One of the most profound challenges to the circulatory system in man occurs during the change to standing from a supine position, which results in an over sixfold increase in the height of the orthostatic column that must be overcome for blood to return to the heart from the legs.[5] Smaller, yet considerable, cardiovascular challenges also occur during the change to standing from a sitting or squatting position. If rapid adjustments do not take place in the circulation during these postural changes, cardiac return decreases, thereby producing reduced cardiac output and reduced brain perfusion, which can result in lightheadedness and even syncope.[6] Posturally related hypotension can also occur in quadrupeds during movements such as vertical climbing or rearing that place the animal's long longitudinal axis against the force of gravity. Of course, the resulting stress to the cardiovascular system is dependent on

[a]This work is supported by the National Institute on Deafness and Other Communication Disorders (grants R01 DC00693 and R01 DC02644).
[b]E-mail: byates@pop.pitt.edu

the length of the body, and would be much more severe, for example, in the cat than in the rat.

Movement and changes in posture can also place constraints on the process of respiration. Assuming a head-up posture (by standing in man or nose-up pitch in quadrupeds) results in the diaphragm descending into the abdominal cavity, due to the force of gravity and the fact that this muscle is no longer as well supported by the abdominal viscera. As a result, the resting length of the diaphragm is altered considerably,[7,8] which must be rapidly corrected for (through changes in the activity of all respiratory muscles) if alveolar ventilation is to remain relatively constant. Furthermore, a number of respiratory muscles, including the abdominal muscles (the principal expiratory muscles), intercostal muscles (which have both inspiratory and expiratory roles), and even the diaphragm (the major inspiratory muscle), are involved in producing certain movements and maintaining certain postures;[9–11] thus, their activity must be rapidly adjusted during changes in body position.

WHY SHOULD THE VESTIBULAR SYSTEM INFLUENCE THE CONTROL OF BLOOD PRESSURE AND RESPIRATION?

A number of inputs signal a significant decrease in blood pressure and the occurrence of orthostatic hypotension, including those from baroreceptors[12] and stretch receptors in the walls of limb veins.[13,14] However, orthostatic hypotension only rarely occurs during movement, suggesting that correction for posturally related effects on the circulatory system begin *before* blood pressure changes appreciably. Thus, an open-loop (feedforward) neural mechanism must participate with the closed-loop (feedback) mechanisms described above in maintaining stable blood pressure during changes in posture.

Correction for changes in the resting length of the diaphragm during movement also begin immediately after a postural change (even before the next breath is taken), suggesting that these adjustments are independent of blood oxygenation.[15,16] It might be presumed that inputs from muscle spindles in the diaphragm are chiefly involved in adjusting its resting length. However, the diaphragm is relatively devoid of spindles, suggesting that stretch reflexes are weak in this muscle.[17] Thus, other receptors must also play a role in the control of breathing.

It seems practical for vestibular inputs that are elicited during standing in man or nose-up pitch in quadrupeds to participate in making necessary adjustments in respiration and circulation. It is noteworthy, however, that somewhat different vestibular receptors are likely to be involved in producing autonomic effects in quadrupeds and humans. In quadrupeds, utricular receptors that respond to nose-up pitch would be stimulated when the animal's long axis is exposed to the force of gravity (and orthostatic hypotension as well as disturbances in respiration are likely to occur). In quadrupedal animals, therefore, it might be postulated that vestibular nucleus neurons which receive pitch-related otolith inputs are linked simply and directly with brain-stem autonomic centers. However, standing in man is more complicated and incorporates both an upward linear acceleration and pitch. It could be imagined that an integrative mechanism in the brain stem that detects the pattern of vestibular inputs which occurs during standing would be involved in producing vestibulo-autonomic responses. Thus, the neural circuitry underlying these responses may be more complicated in man than in animals.

EVIDENCE THAT THE VESTIBULAR SYSTEM INFLUENCES THE REGULATION OF BLOOD PRESSURE AND RESPIRATION

The first definitive evidence suggesting that the vestibular system participates in the regulation of blood pressure was published by Doba and Reis.[18] As illustrated in FIGURE 1, these investigators demonstrated that bilateral transection of the vestibular nerves significantly compromised the ability of an anesthetized and paralyzed cat to compensate for orthostatic hypotension produced by 30° or 60° nose-up tilt. Furthermore, a number of studies have shown that electrical stimulation of the vestibular nerve has effects on the activity of sympathetic nerves (see ref. 19 for review), whose principal function is to increase blood pressure by augmenting heart rate and the constriction of smooth muscle in arterioles.[20] An example of a response recorded from the splanchnic nerve (a sympathetic nerve that influences blood vessels in the abdominal viscera) following a 5-shock train delivered to the vestibular nerve is shown in the bottom panel of FIGURE 2.

Sympathetic outflow is also affected by natural vestibular stimulation. A recent study showed that sinusoidal rotations of the head in vertical planes produce sinusoidal modulation of sympathetic nerve activity.[21] These experiments were performed on cats whose upper cervical dorsal roots were transected to remove influences from neck afferents so that the only sensory inputs elicited by the head rotations came from the vestibular system. FIGURE 3A indicates the best direction of vertical tilt for producing increased sympathetic outflow; the response vector orientation was near nose-up pitch in both cerebellectomized and cerebellum-intact animals. FIGURE 3B is an average Bode plot indicating the temporal properties of the vestibulo-sympathetic reflex. The response gain is flat across stimulus frequencies,

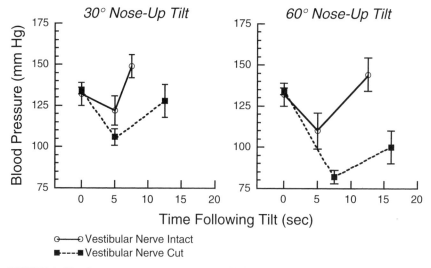

FIGURE 1. Blood pressure response to nose-up tilt in chloralose-anesthetized and paralyzed cats before and after transection of the VIIIth cranial nerve. Data points are average blood pressure measurements in eight animals. Bars indicate SEM. Removal of vestibular inputs to the brain stem significantly compromised the animals' ability to compensate for posturally-related hypotension. Based on data from ref. 18.

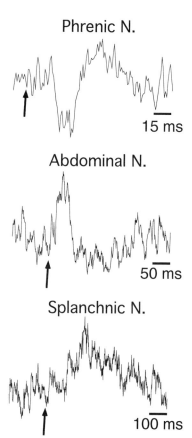

FIGURE 2. Potentials elicited in the phrenic (inspiratory), abdominal (expiratory), and splanchnic (sympathetic) nerves following vestibular nerve stimulation in a decerebrate and paralyzed cat. The traces represent the average of 100 or more sweeps, and were evoked by a train of five shocks (3-ms interpulse interval) at an intensity of 100–300 μA. The threshold for stimulus spread to non-target nerves was considerably higher. The time of occurrence of the first shock of the train is indicated by an arrow. Note that different time bases are used for different waveforms.

and the response phase is near stimulus position. Thus, the response properties of the vestibulo-sympathetic reflex are similar to those of otolith afferents,[22] and are appropriate for tonically bolstering blood pressure during movements involving nose-up rotations that are likely to produce orthostatic hypotension.

Similar approaches have been used to document vestibular influences on respiration. Electrical stimulation of the vestibular nerve evokes large changes in activity of nerves innervating the "pump" muscles that are responsible for the major forces underlying breathing, including the phrenic nerve (which innervates the diaphragm), abdominal nerves, and intercostal nerves;[23] examples are shown in FIGURE 2. Furthermore, vestibular-elicited responses can be recorded from nerves innervating the "valve" muscles that control the resistance of the upper airway, including the tongue, pharyngeal muscles, and laryngeal muscles.[24] Natural vestibular stimulation in vertical planes also produces modulation in the activity of at least some respiratory nerves. FIGURE 4A shows responses recorded from an abdominal nerve during sinusoidal pitch rotations. The activity in the nerve is powerfully affected by these movements, and is maximal during nose-up tilt. FIGURE 4B is a Bode plot illustrating the gain and phase of the abdominal nerve response to pitch. The response gain is flat across stimulus frequencies and the response phase is near stimulus position, suggesting that inputs from otolith receptors are responsible for the effects.[22]

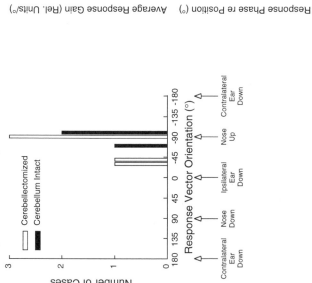

FIGURE 3. Properties of vestibulo-sympathetic responses elicited by natural vestibular stimulation and recorded from the splanchnic nerve in decerebrate and paralyzed cats. Stimuli were sinusoidal vertical rotations that incorporated roll (ear-down tilt) and pitch (nose-up or nose-down tilt). **(A)** Best direction of vertical vestibular stimulation for increasing sympathetic outflow. The response vector orientation was near nose-up pitch in both cerebellectomized and cerebellum-intact animals. **(B)** Gain and phase (relative to stimulus position) of sympathetic nerve responses to sinusoidal rotations in a plane at or near pitch. Data points are the average of standardized gains and phases recorded from eight animals; bars indicate SEM. The response gain was flat across stimulus frequencies, and the phase was near stimulus position. Based on data from ref. 21.

NEURAL SUBSTRATE OF VESTIBULO-SYMPATHETIC REFLEXES

Vestibular Nuclei

Several studies have shown that electrolytic lesions placed in regions of the medial vestibular nucleus just caudal to Deiters' nucleus abolish vestibular-elicited activity in sympathetic nerves.[25–27] Recently, these results have been verified through the use of chemical lesions of the vestibular nuclei.[21,23] FIGURE 5 illustrates the

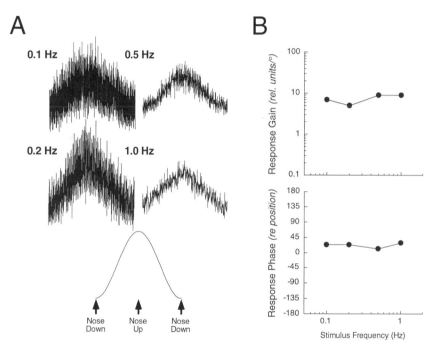

FIGURE 4. Responses of a nerve innervating abdominal (expiratory) muscles to natural vestibular stimulation. (**A**) Responses to sinusoidal pitch rotations at 0.1–1.0 Hz. Nerve activity was full-wave rectified and sampled at 500 Hz. The traces represent the average of 70 (in 0.1 Hz) to 250 (at 1 Hz) responses. (**B**) Gain and phase (relative to stimulus position) of abdominal nerve responses to pitch rotations. The gain remained flat across stimulus frequencies, whereas the phase was consistently near stimulus position.

location of kainic acid injections (based on the location of dye that was dissolved in the injection solution) that abolished sympathetic nerve responses to natural or electrical vestibular stimulation. All of the injections affected the medial vestibular nucleus and the adjacent inferior nucleus between 1–2 mm caudal to Deiters' nucleus. Kainic acid injections into other regions of the vestibular nuclei had little effect on vestibulo-sympathetic responses, indicating that these effects are mediated by a restricted portion of the vestibular nuclear complex.

Studies of the response properties of vestibular nucleus neurons support the results of lesion experiments. In many regions of the vestibular nuclei of the cat,

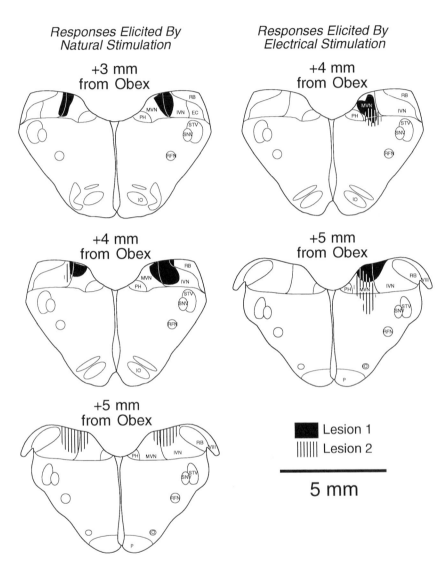

FIGURE 5. Locations of injections of the neurotoxin kainic acid (estimated from the location of dye that was dissolved in the injection solution) that abolished vestibulo-sympathetic responses. Two different sets of kainic acid injections are indicated in each column. **Left panel:** Bilateral kainic acid injections that abolished responses to pitch rotations. **Right panel:** Two different injections that abolished responses to electrical stimulation of the vestibular nerve; the injections were made only on the side ipsilateral to the stimulated nerve. IO, inferior olivary nucleus; IVN, inferior vestibular nucleus; MVN, medial vestibular nucleus; P, pyramid; PH, prepositus hypoglossi; RB, restiform body; RFN, retrofacial nucleus; SNV, spinal nucleus of the Vth cranial nerve; STV, spinal tract of the Vth cranial nerve; VIII, vestibulocochlear nerve. Data from refs. 21 and 23.

including both Deiters' nucleus and the caudal aspect of the medial and inferior vestibular nuclei, most neurons with otolith inputs are better activated by roll than by pitch rotations.[28–30] However, regions of the medial and inferior vestibular nuclei immediately caudal to Deiters' nucleus contain many neurons with pitch-related otolith inputs[28,29,31]—the signals that elicit changes in sympathetic outflow.

Bulbospinal Projections

A number of studies have explored which bulbospinal pathways convey vestibular signals to sympathetic preganglionic neurons located in the thoracic spinal cord. Two groups of neurons in the cat have been identified that (1) are known to regulate cardiovascular function, (2) have direct projections to sympathetic preganglionic neurons, and (3) receive vestibular input. These cells are located in the reticular formation of the rostral ventrolateral medulla (RVLM) and the caudal medullary raphe nuclei.[32–35] The vestibular inputs to these two populations are prominent: over two-thirds of the neurons in each region that presumably influence cardiovascular regulation respond to vestibular nerve stimulation.[32,33] The characteristics of the responses of cells in the RVLM and caudal meduallary raphe nuclei to vertical vestibular stimulation are similar to those of the vestibulo-sympathetic reflex: most neurons in these areas show a more robust response to pitch than to roll rotations, and their response dynamics resemble those of otolith afferents.[34,35] The strength of otolith inputs to raphe and RVLM neurons is considerable: the response gains are only slightly lower than for neurons in the vestibular nuclei.[28–30]

Studies utilizing selective chemical lesions of the RVLM and caudal medullary raphe nuclei have shown that only the former region is necessary for producing vestibulo-sympathetic responses;[36] in fact, lesions of the raphe nuclei have little effect on the amplitude or pattern of potentials recorded from sympathetic nerves following electrical stimulation of the vestibular nerve. Because many raphe-spinal neurons that affect cardiovascular control are believed to be serotonergic[37] and serotonin produces long-lasting *modulatory* actions on its targets,[38,39] it is possible that raphe-spinal neurons with vestibular inputs only serve to regulate the background excitability of sympathetic preganglionic neurons. If this is the case, then it is not unexpected that responses elicited by strong synchronous electrical stimulation of the vestibular nerve are not dependent on the presence of the raphe nuclei. It is possible, however, that the raphe nuclei play a role in regulating the gain of vestibulo-sympathetic responses in awake, behaving animals.

Brain-stem Interneurons

Raphe- and RVLM-spinal neurons respond to stimulation of the vestibular nerve at relatively long latencies ranging from 4 to over 30 ms.[32,33] Thus, it seems unlikely that these bulbospinal neurons receive the bulk of their labyrinthine inputs directly from the vestibular nuclei; one or more interneurons must be interposed in the pathway. This assumption is confirmed by the fact that injections of retrograde neuroanatomical tracers into the RVLM produce little labeling of cell bodies in the vestibular nuclei.[40]

The question of which groups of brain-stem cardiovascular-regulatory interneurons mediate vestibulo-sympathetic responses has been explored using neuroanatomical, lesion, and electrophysiological approaches. Injections of the anterograde tracer *Phaseolus vulgaris* leukoagglutinin (PHA-L) into regions of the medial and inferior vestibular nuclei of the cat that mediate vestibulo-sympathetic responses result in labeled terminals in several areas of the brain stem that contain cardiovascular-regulatory interneurons, including nucleus tractus solitarius (NTS) and the lateral reticular formation near the obex.[41,42] The projection from the medial and inferior vestibular nuclei to NTS has also been demonstrated in the rat[43] and rabbit.[44] However, NTS is a multifunctional nucleus and is involved in relaying several types of visceral signals (including those from the respiratory, cardiovascular, and digestive systems) to many different brain-stem regions.[45] At least in the cat, only a few (< 20%) NTS neurons that receive baroreceptor inputs and are likely to participate in cardiovascular regulation respond to vestibular nerve stimulation, and the inputs to these cells are weak.[41] Furthermore, lesions of NTS do not appreciably alter vestibulo-sympathetic reflexes.[46] Thus, the major function of the vestibulo-solitarius projection in the cat does not seem to be related to adjustment of blood pressure. One possibility is that vestibular inputs to NTS play a role in the generation of vestibular-elicited vomiting and motion sickness, because one-fourth of NTS neurons that receive inputs from the gastrointestinal system (and are likely to provide signals to the brain-stem cells that mediate emesis) respond to vestibular stimulation.[41,47]

Vestibular nucleus projections to the lateral reticular formation of the cat appear to be much more important than those to NTS in influencing cardiovascular control. Lesions of portions of the lateral reticular formation caudal to the obex abolish vestibulo-sympathetic responses[46] (see Steinbacher and Yates, this volume). The caudal and lateral reticular formation (CLRF) does *not* have direct projections to sympathetic preganglionic neurons; however, it influences cardiovascular control through ascending projections to the RVLM.[48–50] In a recent series of experiments, we found that although many CLRF neurons receive labyrinthine inputs, cells that project directly from this region to the RVLM fail to respond to vestibular nerve stimulation.[51] Thus, an indirect pathway must transmit vestibular signals between the two regions. One possiblity is that connections between the CLRF and the lateral reticular formation spanning 1–4 mm *rostral* to the obex are fundamental in producing vestibulo-sympathetic responses, because cells in the latter region play an important role in cardiovascular control[51–54] and receive vestibular inputs at slightly longer latency than do cells in the CLRF.[42] Furthermore, about one-third of the cells in the more rostral portion of the lateral medullary reticular formation that can be antidromically activated from the RVLM respond to vestibular nerve stimulation.[42] However, it is yet to be demonstrated conclusively that vestibular signals are relayed from the caudal to rostral parts of the lateral reticular formation before reaching bulbospinal neurons in the RVLM.

Cerebellum

Regions of the cerebellum that process vestibular inputs, including the nodulus, uvula, anterior lobe, and fastigial nucleus, have been reported to participate in cardiovascular control (see ref. 55 for review). Thus, it is likely that these regions influence vestibulo-sympathetic reflexes. This inference is supported by the fact that cerebellectomy increases the duration of excitatory components but shortens inhibitory components of sympathetic nerve responses to electrical stimulation of the vestibular nerve.[56] However, most aspects of the response elicited by electrical stimulation remain substantially unaffected following cerebellectomy, and aspiration of the medial and intermediate cerebellum does not significantly alter the spatial or temporal properties of the vestibulo-sympathetic reflex elicited by natural stimulation.[21] Thus, the cerebellum is not an essential part of the pathway that links the vestibular nuclei with sympathetic preganglionic neurons, although it may influence the processing of vestibular signals by the cardiovascular-regulatory circuitry.

Higher Centers

Because both electrical and natural vestibular stimulation elicit changes in sympathetic outflow in decerebrate animals, regions rostral to the brain stem are not necessary for the production of vestibulo-sympathetic reflexes.[21,23] Even transection of the brain stem through the rostral part of the superior vestibular nucleus has little effect on the vestibulo-sympathetic reflex elicited by electrical stimulation of the vestibular nerve,[46] indicating that the essential neural circuitry is confined to the pons and medulla. However, a number of higher centers are likely to modulate vestibulo-sympathetic reflexes. Several parts of the hypothalamus that play a role in cardiovascular regulation receive vestibular inputs,[57,58] although the nature of their influences on vestibulo-sympathetic responses is yet to be determined. It also seems plausible that the "intention" to move or change posture as reflected by corollary discharge from regions of motor cortex could alter the processing of vestibular signals by brain stem cardiovascular-regulatory circuitry. This hypothesis remains to be tested.

A Model of the Neural Circuitry That Produces Vestibulo-Sympathetic Reflexes

FIGURE 6 is a model that reflects all current information concerning the minimal neural circuitry that is *essential* for producing vestibulo-sympathetic reflexes in cats. These responses are elicited by otolith receptors that are sensitive to nose-up pitch, and are mediated by a small region of the medial and inferior vestibular nuclei just caudal to Deiters' nucleus, interneuronal relays through the lateral medullary reticular formation, and projections from the rostral ventrolateral medulla to sympathetic preganglionic neurons in the thoracic spinal cord. Undoubtedly, other brain regions also influence vestibular effects on the cardiovascular system, although they are not critical for the production of vestibulo-sympathetic responses. These additional areas include the cerebellum, caudal medullary raphe nuclei, and perhaps regions rostral to the brain stem including the hypothalamus.

NEURAL SUBSTRATE OF VESTIBULO-RESPIRATORY REFLEXES

Vestibular Nuclei

Lesions of the same portions of the inferior and medial vestibular nuclei caudal to Deiters' nucleus that abolish vestibulo-sympathetic responses also eliminate effects of electrical vestibular stimulation on activity of the abdominal and phrenic nerves.[23] The partial specialization of one portion of the vestibular nuclear complex in mediating both vestibulo-sympathetic and vestibulo-respiratory reflexes may simply reflect that common labyrinthine signals—pitch-related otolith inputs—are critical for producing the responses. Furthermore, inasmuch as neurons that regulate circulation and respiration are located in similar parts of the medulla, mainly in or near NTS and the lateral reticular formation,[48–50,52–54,59] it seems practical for one region of the vestibular nucleus to be specialized for relaying similar vestibular signals to these regions.

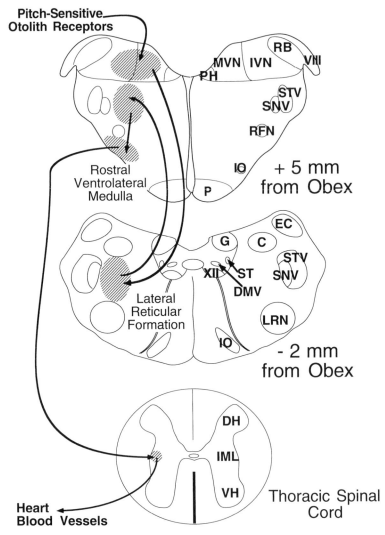

FIGURE 6. A model of the critical neuronal circuitry that mediates vestibulo-sympathetic reflexes. These responses are elicited by stimulation of pitch-sensitive otolith receptors, and are mediated by portions of the medial and inferior vestibular nuclei, the caudalmost portions of the lateral medullary reticular formation, a relay to more rostrally located neurons in the lateral reticular formation, and projections from the rostral ventrolateral medullary reticular formation to the spinal cord. C, cuneate nucleus; DH, dorsal horn of spinal cord; DMV, dorsal motor nucleus of the vagus nerve; EC, external cuneate nucleus; G, gracile nucleus; IML, intermediolateral cell column; IO, inferior olivary nucleus; IVN, inferior vestibular nucleus; LRN, lateral reticular nucleus; MVN, medial vestibular nucleus; P, pyramid; PH, prepositus hypoglossi; RB, restiform body; RFN, retrofacial nucleus; SNV, spinal nucleus of the Vth cranial nerve; ST, solitary tract; STV, spinal tract of the Vth cranial nerve; VH, ventral horn of spinal cord; VIII, vestibulocochlear nerve; XII, hypoglossal nucleus.

Bulbospinal Pathways

Respiratory muscles contract in a highly coordinated manner to produce breathing. The signals that produce patterned discharges of respiratory muscles are relayed to the spinal cord via two groups of reticulospinal neurons: the dorsal respiratory group, located in and near ventrolateral NTS, and the ventral respiratory group in the ventrolateral medualla.[59] Both of these populations have been tested for vestibular inputs. The dorsal respiratory group receives only a paucity of vestibular signals,[41] and lesions of this region have no effect on phrenic nerve responses to vestibular stimulation.[36] In contrast, almost one-half of the bulbospinal neurons in the ventral respiratory group that relay motor commands to inspiratory motoneurons respond to vestibular nerve stimulation,[60] although lesions of the ventral respiratory group do not appreciably alter vestibulo-respiratory reflexes recorded from the phrenic nerve.[36] Thus, other bulbospinal pathways must also participate in generating the responses. Candidates include medial reticulospinal and vestibulospinal neurons, because injections of retrograde tracers into the *vicinity* of phrenic, intercostal, and abdominal motoneurons result in labeling in the vestibular nuclei and medial reticular formation.[61–65] However, since respiratory motoneurons are located near other motoneurons (e.g., the phrenic motoneuron pool is located adjacent to motoneurons that innervate shoulder muscles),[66] these studies are equivocal. It is hopeful that recently developed transneuronal tracing techniques can be used to determine which bulbospinal pathways relay signals to respiratory motoneurons, because this information will be useful in guiding future studies of the neural substrate of vestibulo-respiratory responses. Transneuronal transport of α-herpes viruses in the rat has revealed no evidence to suggest that vestibulospinal and medial reticulospinal pathways make connections with phrenic motoneurons.[67] However, since vestibulo-respiratory responses have not yet been demonstrated in rats, the existence of vestibular nucleus or medial reticular formation projections to inspiratory motoneurons in other species cannot be ruled out.

Vestibular Inputs to Upper Airway Motoneurons

The pathways that relay signals from the vestibular nuclei to upper airway (tongue, pharyngeal, laryngeal) motoneurons have been explored only rudimentarily. Injections of the anterograde tracer PHA-L into the medial and inferior vestibular nuclei produce labeled terminals near nucleus ambiguus,[42] where upper airway motoneurons are located.[59] However, definitive evidence of monosynaptic contracts between axons of vestibular nucleus neurons and these motoneurons is yet to be obtained.

SUMMARY

Considerable evidence exists to suggest that both sympathetic and respiratory outflow from the central nervous system are influenced by the vestibular system. Otolith organs that respond to pitch rotations seem to play a predominant role in producing vestibulo-sympathetic and vestibulo-respiratory responses in cats. Because postural changes involving nose-up pitch challenge the maintenance of stable blood pressure and blood oxygenation in this species, vestibular effects on the sympathetic and respiratory systems are appropriate to participate in maintaining homeostasis during movement. Vestibular influences on respiration and circulation are mediated by a relatively small portion of the vestibular nuclear complex comprising regions in the medial and inferior vestibular nuclei just caudal to Deiters' nucleus. Vestibular signals are transmitted to sympathetic preganglionic neurons in the spinal cord through pathways that typically regulate the cardiovascular system. In contrast, vestibular effects on respiratory motoneurons are mediated in part by neural circuits that are not typically involved in the generation of breathing.

ACKNOWLEDGMENTS

A number of investigators have collaborated with me in studies of vestibulo-autonomic responses described in this paper. My principal collaborator, particularly on investigations of vestibulo-respiratory responses, has been Dr. Alan Miller. Other collaborators include P. S. Bolton, K. Endo, T. Goto, L. Grélot, J. Jakuš, I. A. Kerman, C. Rossiter, R. H. Schor, M. S. Siniaia, B. C. Steinbacher, Y. Yamagata, and T. Yamaguchi. I am also grateful to Joseph Furman, Alan Miller, Robert Schor, Ilan Kerman, and Bernard Steinbacher for helpful comments on earlier versions of this paper.

REFERENCES

1. BALOH, R. W. & V. HONRUBIA. 1990. Clinical Neurophysiology of the Vestibular System. 2nd edit. F. A. Davis Company. Philadelphia, PA.
2. MONEY, K. E., J. R. LACKNER & R. S. K. CHEUNG. 1996. The autonomic nervous system and motion sickness. In Vestibular Autonomic Regulation. B. J. Yates & A. D. Miller, Eds.: 147–173. CRC Press. Boca Raton, FL.
3. MONEY, K. 1970. Motion sickness. Physiol. Rev. **50:** 1–39.
4. YATES, B. J. & A. D. MILLER, Eds. 1996. Vestibular Autonomic Regulation. CRC Press. Boca Raton, FL.
5. SJOSTRAND, T. 1953. Volume and distribution of blood and their significance in regulating the circulation. Physiol. Rev. **33:** 202–228.
6. RUSHMER, R. F. 1976. Cardiovascular Dynamics. 4th edit. Saunders. Philadelphia, PA.
7. LEEVERS, A. M. & J. D. ROAD. 1991. Effect of lung inflation and upright posture on diaphragmatic shortening in dogs. Respir. Physiol. **85:** 29–40.
8. VAN LUNTEREN, E., M. A. HAXHIU, N. S. CHERNIACK & M. D. GOLDMAN. 1985. Differential costal and crural diaphragm compensation for posture changes. J. Appl. Physiol. **58:** 1895–1900.
9. DE TROYER, A. 1983. Mechanical role of the abdominal muscles in relation to posture. Respir. Physiol. **53:** 341–353.
10. GRILLNER, S., J. NILSSON & A. THORSTENSSON. 1978. Intra-abdominal pressure changes during natural movements in man. Acta Physiol. Scand. **103:** 275–283.
11. WHITELAW, W. A., G. T. FORD, K. P. RIMMER & A. DE TROYER. 1992. Intercostal muscles are used during rotation of the thorax in humans. J. Appl. Physiol. **72:** 1940–1944.
12. PAINTAL, A. S. 1972. Cardiovascular receptors. In Handbook of Sensory Physiology. Vol. III/1. Enteroceptors. E. Neil, Ed.: 1–45. Springer-Verlag. Berlin.
13. THOMPSON, F. J., B. J. YATES, O. FRANZEN & J. R. WALD. 1983. Lumbar spinal cord responses to limb vein distention. J. Autonom. Nerv. Syst. **9:** 531–546.
14. YATES, B. J., J. P. MICKLE, W. J. HEDDEN & F. J. THOMPSON. 1987. Tracing of afferent pathways from the femoral-saphenous vein to the dorsal root ganglia using transport of horseradish peroxidase. J. Autonom. Nerv. Syst. **20:** 1–11.
15. BANZETT, R. B., G. F. INBAR, R. BROWN, M. GOLDMAN, A. ROSSIER & J. MEAD. 1981. Diaphragm electrical activity during negative lower torso pressure in quadriplegic men. J. Appl. Physiol. **51:** 654–659.

16. GREEN, M., J. MEAD & T. A. SEARS. 1978. Muscle activity during chest wall restriction and positive pressure breathing in man. Respir. Physiol. **35**: 283–300.
17. CORDA, M., C. VON EULER & G. LENNERSTRANDT. 1965. Proprioceptive innervation of the diaphragm. J. Physiol. **178**: 161–177.
18. DOBA, N. & D. J. REIS. 1974. Role of the cerebellum and vestibular apparatus in regulation of orthostatic reflexes in the cat. Circ. Res. **34**: 9–18.
19. YATES, B. J. 1992. Vestibular influences on the sympathetic nervous system. Brain Res. Rev. **17**: 51–59.
20. LOEWY, A. D. & K. M. SPYER, Eds. 1990. Central Regulation of Autonomic Functions. Oxford University Press. New York.
21. YATES, B. J. & A. D. MILLER. 1994. Properties of sympathetic reflexes elicited by natural vestibular stimulation: Implications for cardiovascular control. J. Neurophysiol. **71**: 2087–2092.
22. FERNÁNDEZ, C. & J. M. GOLDBERG. 1976. Physiology of peripheral neurons innervating otolith organs of the squirrel monkey. III. Response dynamics. J. Neurophysiol. **39**: 996–1008.
23. YATES, B. J., J. JAKUS & A. D. MILLER. 1993. Vestibular effects on respiratory outflow in the decerebrate cat. Brain Res. **629**: 209–217.
24. MILLER, A. D. & M. S. SINIAIA. 1995. Vestibular effects on the upper airway. Soc. Neurosci. Abstr. **21**: 1887.
25. PAN, P. S., Y. S. ZHANG & Y. Z. CHEN. 1991. Role of nucleus vestibularis medialis in vestibulo-sympathetic response in rats. Acta Physiol. Sin. **43**: 184–188.
26. SPIEGEL, E. A. 1946. Effect of labyrinthine reflexes on the vegetative nervous system. Arch. Otolaryngol. **44**: 61–72.
27. UCHINO, Y., N. KUDO, K. TSUDA & Y. IWAMURA. 1970. Vestibular inhibition of sympathetic nerve activities. Brain Res. **22**: 195–206.
28. KASPER, J., R. H. SCHOR & V. J. WILSON. 1988. Response of vestibular neurons to head rotations in vertical planes. I. Response to vestibular stimulation. J. Neurophysiol. **60**: 1753–1764.
29. WILSON, V. J., Y. YAMAGATA, B. J. YATES, R. H. SCHOR & S. NONAKA. 1990. Response of vestibular neurons to head rotations in vertical planes. III. Response of vestibulocollic neurons to vestibular and neck stimulation. J. Neurophysiol. **64**: 1695–1703.
30. ENDO, K., D. B. THOMSON, V. J. WILSON, Y. YAMAGUCHI & B. J. YATES. 1995. Vertical vestibular input to and projections from the caudal parts of the vestibular nuclei of the decerebrate cat. J. Neurophysiol. **74**: 428–436.
31. SCHOR, R. H., B. C. STEINBACHER & B. J. YATES. 1995. Response of medial vestibular nucleus neurons to horizontal linear and angular stimulation of the decerebrate cat. Soc. Neurosci. Abstr. **21**: 1913.
32. YATES, B. J., T. GOTO & P. S. BOLTON. 1992. Responses of neurons in the caudal medullary raphe nuclei of the cat to stimulation of the vestibular nerve. Exp. Brain Res. **89**: 323–332.
33. YATES, B. J., Y. YAMAGATA & P. S. BOLTON. 1991. The ventrolateral medulla of the cat mediates vestibulosympathetic reflexes. Brain Res. **552**: 265–272.
34. YATES, B. J., T. GOTO & P. S. BOLTON. 1993. Responses of neurons in the rostral ventrolateral medulla of the cat to natural vestibular stimulation. Brain Res. **601**: 255–264.
35. YATES, B. J., T. GOTO, I. KERMAN & P. S. BOLTON. 1993. Responses of caudal medullary raphe neurons to natural vestibular stimulation. J. Neurophysiol. **70**: 938–946.
36. YATES, B. J., M. S. SINIAIA & A. D. MILLER. 1995. Descending pathways necessary for vestibular influences on sympathetic and inspiratory outflow. Am. J. Physiol. **268**: R1381–R1385.
37. LASKEY, W. & C. POLOSA. 1988. Characteristics of the sympathetic preganglionic neuron and its synaptic input. Prog. Neurobiol. **31**: 47–84.
38. ZHANG, L. 1991. Effects of 5-hydroxytryptamine on cat spinal motoneurons. Can. J. Physiol. Pharmacol. **69**: 154–163.
39. WHITE, S. R. & R. S. NEUMAN. 1980. Facilitation of spinal motoneurone excitability of 5-hydroxytryptamine and noradrenaline. Brain Res. **188**: 119–127.

40. DAMPNEY, R. A. L., J. CZACHURSKI, K. DEMBOWSKY, A. K. GOODCHILD & H. SELLER. 1987. Afferent connections and spinal projections of the pressor region in the rostral ventrolateral medulla of the cat. J. Autonom. Nerv. Syst. **30:** 73–86.

41. YATES, B. J., L. GRÉLOT, I. A. KERMAN, C. D. BALABAN, J. JAKUS & A. D. MILLER. 1994. Organization of vestibular inputs to nucleus tractus solitarius and adjacent structures in cat brain stem. Am. J. Physiol. **36:** R974–R983.

42. YATES, B. J., C. D. BALABAN, A. D. MILLER, K. ENDO & Y. YAMAGUCHI. 1995. Vestibular inputs to the lateral tegmental field of the cat: Potential role in autonomic control. Brain Res. **689:** 197–206.

43. PORTER, J. D. & C. D. BALABAN. 1995. Connections between medial and spinal vestibular nuclei with brain stem regions that mediate autonomic function in the rat. Assoc. Res. Otolaryngol. Abstr. **18:** 101.

44. BALABAN, C. D. & G. BERYOZKIN. 1994. Vestibular nucleus projections to nucleus tractus solitarius and the dorsal motor nucleus of the vagus nerve: Potential substrates for vestibulo-autonomic interactions. Exp. Brain Res. **98:** 200–212.

45. BARRACO, I. R. A., Ed. 1994. Nucleus of the Solitary Tract. CRC Press. Boca Raton, FL.

46. STEINBACHER, B. C. & B. J. YATES. Brainstem interneurons necessary for vestibular influences on sympathetic outflow. Brain Res. In press.

47. MILLER, A. D. & L. GRÉLOT. 1996. The neural basis of nausea and vomiting. In Vestibular Autonomic Regulation. B. J. Yates & A. D. Miller, Eds.: 85–94. CRC Press. Boca Raton, FL.

48. AGARWAL, A. J., A. J. GELSEMA & F. R. CALARESU. 1990. Inhibition of rostral VLM by baroreceptor activation is relayed through caudal VLM. Am. J. Physiol. **258:** R1271–R1278.

49. LI, Y.-W., Z. J. GIEROBA, R. M. MCALLEN & W. W. BLESSING. 1991. Neurons in rabbit caudal ventrolateral medulla inhibit bulbospinal barosensitive neurons in rostral medulla. Am. J. Physiol. **261:** R44–R51.

50. JESKE, I., S. F. MORRISON, S. L. CRAVO & D. J. REIS. 1993. Identification of baroreceptor reflex interneurons in the caudal ventrolateral medulla. Am. J. Physiol. **264:** R169–R178.

51. YATES, B. J. & B. C. STEINBACHER. 1995. Processing of vestibular, hindlimb, and baroreceptor inputs by neurons in the caudal ventrolateral meducalla (CVLM). Soc. Neurosci. Abstr. **21:** 892.

52. BARMAN, S. M. & G. L. GEBBER. 1983. Sequence of activation of ventrolateral and dorsal medullary sympathetic neurons. Am. J. Physiol. **245:** R438–R477.

53. BARMAN, S. M. & G. L. GEBBER. 1987. Lateral tegmental field neurons of the cat medulla: a source of basal activity of ventrolateral medullospinal sympathoexcitatory neurons. J. Neurophysiol. **57:** 1410–1424.

54. GEBBER, G. L. & S. M. BARMAN. 1985. Lateral tegmental field neurons of cat medulla: A potential source of basal sympathetic nerve discharge. J. Neurophysiol. **54:** 1498–1512.

55. BALABAN, C. D. 1996. The role of the cerebellum in vestibular autonomic function. In Vestibular Autonomic Regulation. B. J. Yates & A. D. Miller, Eds.: 127–144. CRC Press. Boca Raton, FL.

56. MIYAZAWA, T. & T. ISHIKAWA. 1983. Cerebellar inhibitory action on vestibulo-sympathetic responses. J. Autonom. Nerv. Syst. **7:** 185–189.

57. KATAFUCHI, T., K. P. PUTHURAYA, H. YOSHIMATSU & Y. OOMURA. 1987. Responses of rat lateral hypothalamic neuron activity to vestibular nuclei stimulation. Brain Res. **400:** 652–69.

58. INOKUCHI, A., F. LIU & S. KOMIYAMA. 1994. Effects of vestibular stimulations on guinea pig posterior hypothalamic neuron activity. Otol. Fukuoka **40:** 885–892.

59. BIANCHI, A. L., M. DENAVITSAUBIE & J. CHAMPAGNAT. 1995. Central control of breathing in mammals: Neuronal circuitry, membrane properties, and neurotransmitters. Physiol. Rev. **75:** 1–45.

60. MILLER, A. D., T. YAMAGUCHI, M. S. SINIAIA & B. J. YATES. 1995. Ventral respiratory group bulbospinal inspiratory neurons participate in vestibular-respiratory reflexes. J. Neurophysiol. **73:** 1303–1307.

61. RIKARD-BELL, G. C., E. K. BYSTRZYCKA & B. S. NAIL. 1984. Brainstem projections to the phrenic nucleus: A HRP study in the cat. Brain Res. Bull. **12:** 469–477.
62. ELLENBERGER, H. H., P. L. VERA, J. R. HASELTON, C. L. HASELTON & N. SCHNEIDERMAN. 1990. Brainstem projections to the phrenic nucleus: an anterograde and retrograde HRP study in the rabbit. Brain Res. Bull. **24:** 163–174.
63. ONAI, T., M. SAJI & M. MIURA. 1987. Projections of supraspinal structures to the phrenic motor nucleus in rats studied by a horseradish peroxidase microinjection method. J. Autonom. Nerv. Syst. **21:** 233–239.
64. ONAI, T. & M. MIURA. 1986. Projections of supraspinal structures to the phrenic motor nucleus in cats studied by a horseradish peroxidase microinjection method. J. Autonom. Nerv. Syst. **16:** 61–77.
65. RIKARD-BELL, G. C., E. K. BYSTRAZYCKA & B. S. NAIL. 1985. The identification of brainstem neurones projecting to thoracic respiratory motoneurones in the cat as demonstrated by retrograde transport of HRP. Brain Res. Bull. **14:** 25–37.
66. HORNER, M. & H. KUMMEL. 1993. Topographical representation of shoulder motor nuclei in the cat spinal cord as revealed by retrograde fluorochrome tracers. J. Comp. Neurol. **335:** 309–319.
67. DOBBINS, E. G. & J. L. FELDMAN. 1994. Brainstem network controlling descending drive to phrenic motoneurons in rat. J. Comp. Neurol. **347:** 64–86.

Transmission between the Type I Hair Cell and Its Calyx Ending[a]

JAY M. GOLDBERG

Department of Pharmacological and Physiological Sciences
University of Chicago
947 East 58th Street
Chicago, Illinois 60637

INTRODUCTION

The vestibular organs of reptiles, birds, and mammals contain two kinds of hair cells.[1-3] Although type II hair cells are similar to their counterparts in other hair-cell organs, type I hair cells have a peculiar morphology, unlike that seen in nonvestibular organs or in the vestibular organs of fish or amphibians. Much has been learned about the type I hair cell and its calyx ending in the last decade or so. Information has been provided by a re-examination of synaptic relations at an ultrastructural level;[4-7] by morphophysiological studies, which relate the physiology of an afferent with the kinds of hair cells it innervates;[8-10] by whole-cell recordings of solitary hair cells;[11-13] and by intracellular recordings from afferent terminals.[14,15] This paper will review the newer findings with a particular question in mind: Are there novel modes of intercellular communication between the type I hair cell and the calyx ending? In interpreting the findings, use is made of a theoretical analysis, which suggests that, in addition to conventional or quantal transmission, two other modes of intercellular communication are possible.

STRUCTURE OF TYPE I AND TYPE II HAIR CELLS

Type II hair cells are cylindrically shaped and are innervated by several afferent and efferent fibers terminating as boutons near the hair-cell base (FIG. 1, right).[1,2] In contrast, type I hair cells are flask-shaped with a perinuclear cell body connected to a flared apical surface by a thin neck (FIG. 1, left). Perhaps the most extraordinary feature of the type I hair cell is its afferent innervation. A calyx ending, derived from a single afferent fiber, surrounds the hair cell from its base to just underneath its apical surface. Ribbon synapses, which are thought to mediate chemical transmission, are found in both kinds of hair cells. Calyceal invaginations are a peculiar junction found only in type I hair cells. At several places, the calyx ending invaginates into the hair cell, and the width of the intercellular cleft is reduced. Because of the reduction, the invaginations were originally mistaken for electrical synapses. More recent freeze-fracture studies show that they do not have the morphology of such synapses, that is, they are not gap junctions.[16,17]

The unusual morphology of the type I hair cell and the calyx ending has suggested that they are involved in novel forms of intercellular communication. Supporting this notion were reports that type I hair cells contain relatively few ribbon synapses.[16,18]

---

[a] This research was supported by NIH grant DC 02058.

Quantitative electron microscopy shows otherwise. Typically, more than 10 ribbon synapses are found in type I hair cells in mammals[4–6] and in the chick.[7]

CONVENTIONAL SYNAPTIC TRANSMISSION

The large number of ribbon synapses provides evidence that the type I hair cell and the calyx ending use conventional chemical transmission. Physiological evidence exists as well. Intracellular recordings were made from calyx afferents, near their termination in a lizard crista.[14] Small, subthreshold potentials were observed. They had the properties of summed miniature excitatory postsynaptic potentials (mEPSPs). mEPSP frequency depended on external Ca^{2+} concentration, was unaltered by tetrodotoxin (TTX) application, and was modulated by sensory input. When the frequency was reduced, individual mEPSPs were revealed.

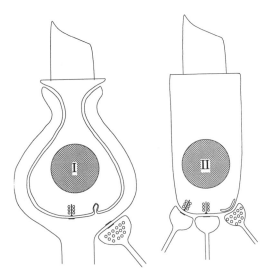

FIGURE 1. Schematic drawings of type I and type II hair cells. The type I hair cell is innervated by a calyx ending; the type II hair cell by several afferent boutons. Ribbon synapses are found in both hair cells, calyceal invaginations only in the type I hair cell. Vesiculated efferent boutons innervate the type II hair cell and the ending surrounding the type I hair cell.

In other systems, mEPSPs are the postsynaptic responses to multimolecular packets of neurotransmitter.[19] Their presence in calyx endings confirms the presence of chemical transmission from the type I hair cell. This raises a question. As pointed out by Bennett,[20] the long, uninterrupted apposition between the type I hair cell and its ending could impede the flow of postsynaptic currents. Two factors are involved. First, the enlarged surface area can lower the input impedance of the ending, which will also lower the postsynaptic voltage produced by a fixed synaptic current. Second, because of the length of the intercellular space, a relatively large intercellular voltage can be present during postsynaptic current flow. Each mEPSP will then consist of an intercellular, as well as an intracellular component. Because only the intracellular component is seen by the outer face of the ending and the parent axon, synaptic transmission is reduced. The situation can be contrasted to one where synapses are made onto afferent boutons. In the latter case, the input impedance is high, and there is no appreciable intercellular voltage.

To analyze conventional synaptic transmission, a system of three simultaneous steady-state cable equations was developed to model the type I hair cell, the intercellular space, and the inner and outer faces of the calyx ending. Solutions are shown in FIGURE 2 where the ending is assumed to have a specific membrane resistance of 150 (upper) or 15,000 ohm · cm^2 (lower). For each resistance value, synaptic inputs are delivered to the base of the calyx. Inner-face (intrinsic) inputs come from the ending's own hair cell (FIG. 2A and C). Outer-face (extrinsic) inputs come from type II hair cells contacting the ending, from other calyx and bouton endings on the terminal tree, and from efferent synapses (FIG. 2B and D). The outer-face voltage, $V_3(0)$, provides a measure of synaptic transmission because it is the voltage delivered to the parent axon. When the membrane resistance is low (FIG. 2A and B), synaptic transmission is reduced to just over 10% of the value that would occur in the absence of the ending. Increasing the membrane resistance 100-fold increases transmission to > 90% (FIG. 2C and D). Large increases in transmission require an increase in the impedances of both faces. Under all conditions, transmission is similar for inner- and outer-face inputs (cf. FIG. 2A and B; FIG. 2C and D).

The findings have implications for afferent physiology. FIGURE 3 shows terminal fields of vestibular-nerve fibers innervating the squirrel-monkey cristae.[21] Three kinds of units are present: calyx units innervate type I hair cells; bouton units innervate type II hair cells; and dimorphic units provide a mixed innervation to both kinds of hair cells. The physiology of the three groups are summarized in FIGURE 4; discharge regularity, measured by a normalized coefficient of variation, is plotted against rotational gain (FIG. 4A) and phase (FIG. 4B) for 125 afferents.[10] Calyx units, which are located in the central zone of the crista, have considerably lower gains than do irregular dimorphs, which are also centrally located. An obvious explanation for the difference is that it reflects the influence of the calyx ending on transmission involving its intrinsic inputs. The theoretical analysis shows that the difference between calyx and dimorphic units cannot be explained in this way because the presence of the ending will have similar effects on all inputs, including the extrinsic inputs from type II hair cells to dimorphic units. A prediction should hold if the calyx ending greatly reduced transmission. Bouton units, as they lack calyx endings, should have larger rotational gains than do dimorphic units. The prediction is not confirmed. Bouton and dimorphic units of similar discharge regularity have similar rotational gains (FIG. 4A). This implies that the presence of calyx endings does not greatly alter transmission. As illustrated in FIGURE 2, a simple way to accomplish this would be to increase the membrane resistances of both faces of the calyx ending.

In discussing the topic of conventional transmission, an additional, obvious function of the calyx ending should be considered. Because the ending makes several synaptic contacts with the type I hair cell, it could function to increase the sensitivity or power of conventional synaptic transmission. As already mentioned, 10 or more ribbons synapses typically contact each calyx ending. In contrast, individual afferent boutons typically make one to a few synaptic contacts with their type II hair cells. Despite these morphological findings, one can doubt that conventional transmission between the type I hair cell and the calyx ending is unusually powerful. One reason for skepticism is related to the low rotational gains of calyx units. In fact, such data have been used to estimate a so-called synaptic gain for calyx and bouton endings.[8,10] The calculations indicate that the synaptic gains for calyx endings are about three times higher than those for afferent boutons. A 3:1 ratio in synaptic gains is considerably smaller than the 100-fold difference in appositional contact areas for the two kinds of endings or the > 10:1 ratio in the number of ribbon synapses contacting them.

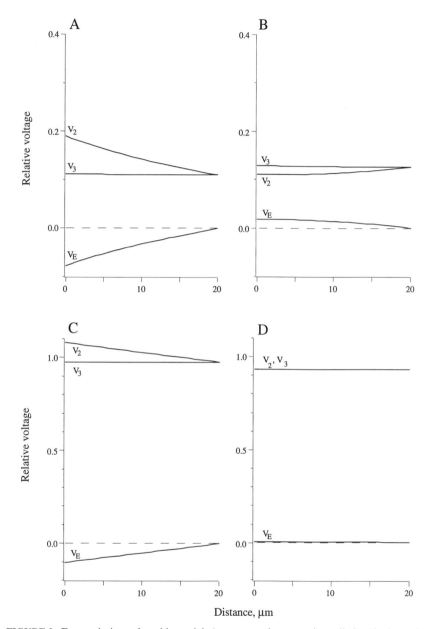

FIGURE 2. Exact solutions of a cable model. A postsynaptic current is applied to the inner (**A** and **C**) or outer face of the calyx ending (**B** and **D**) at the base (x = 0). Both faces of the ending have specific impedances of 150 ohm·cm² (**A** and **B**) or of 15,000 ohm·cm² (**C** and **D**). Voltages of the calyx inner face (V_2), the calyx outer face (V_3), and the intercellular space (V_E) are plotted as a function of the distance along the ending from x = 0 to x = 20 μm (apex) and are expressed relative to the V_3 voltage that would occur if the same current were applied to the parent axon in the absence of a calyx ending.

UNCONVENTIONAL INTERCELLULAR COMMUNICATION

Yamashita and Ohmori,[15] in recordings from calyx afferents in the isolated cristae of 2–5-day-old chicks, obtained evidence for an unconventional mode of intercellular communication that took place in the absence of mEPSPs. Discharge

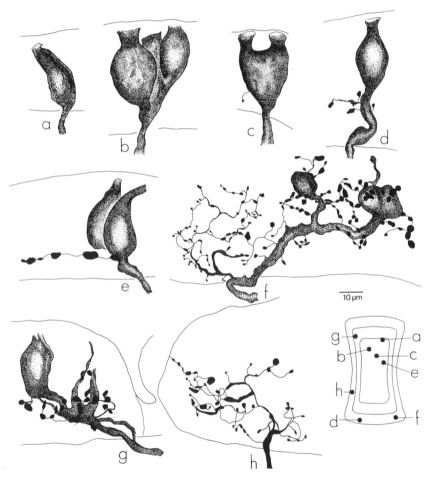

FIGURE 3. Reconstructions of afferent terminals labeled with horseradish peroxidase in the cristae of the squirrel monkey. **a** and **b:** calyx units. **c–g:** dimorphic units. **h:** bouton unit. Locations are indicated on a standard map. (From Fernández *et al.*[21] Reproduced with permission from the *Journal of Neurophysiology.*)

was regular and took a long time to build up and to decay in response to vibratory stimulation. Underlying the unitary response was a slow postsynaptic depolarizing potential on which were superimposed smaller AC responses synchronized to the 250-Hz mechanical stimulus. The results are quite different from those obtained

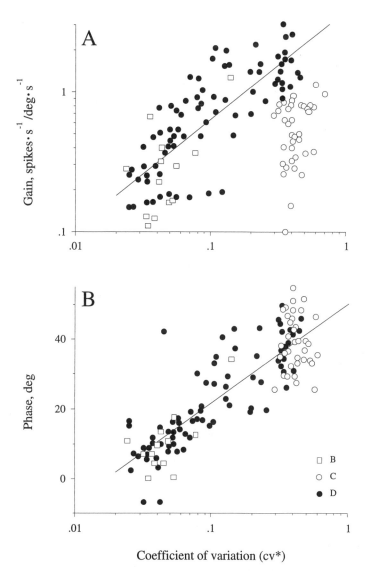

FIGURE 4. Gains (**A**) and phases (**B**) of the responses to 2-Hz sinusoidal head rotations are plotted against a normalized coefficient of variation (cv*), extracellularly recorded semicircular-canal afferents in the squirrel monkey. The units are separated by physiological criteria into three groups. B (bouton) units have antidromic conduction velocities < 13.5 m/s. C (calyx) units are irregularly discharging (cv* > 0.2) and have low rotational gains (< 0.8 spikes · s^{-1}/ deg · s^{-1}). All other units are assigned to the D (dimorphic) category. (From Lysakowski *et al.*[10] Reproduced with permission from the *Journal of Neurophysiology.*)

from calyx afferents in a lizard crista.[14] There, mEPSPs were recorded and discharge was irregular. The differences may be related to differences in the preparations. In the chick experiments, an isolated epithelium was used, temperatures were low compared to normal body temperature, and the tissue was not oxygenated. The labyrinth was intact in the lizard experiments, normal body temperature was maintained, and the animals were artificially respired. Conditions were less physiological in the chick experiments, and this may explain the apparent absence of chemical transmission. Another possibility is that ribbon synapses, even though present in chicks of this age,[7] may be developmentally immature. The regular discharge seen in the chick can be explained by the absence of quantal transmission, which is thought to be a major source of postsynaptic voltage fluctuations and, hence, of discharge irregularity.[22]

What is the basis for the slow postsynaptic depolarizing response? Electrotonic transmission can be ruled as dye-coupling[15] and gap junctions[7] are not found between pre- and postsynaptic elements. Two other possibilities need to be considered.

EPHAPTIC TRANSMISSION

The flow of hair-cell transducer currents will affect the membrane potentials of the calyx ending: the inner face will be hyperpolarized and the outer face will be depolarized. This is an example of ephaptic transmission. The cable model was used to analyze the situation. Of particular interest is the outer-face depolarization. If this were large, it could alter afferent firing and, hence, participate in sensory coding. The outer-face depolarization amounts to $\approx 1.5\%$ of the hair-cell voltage produced by transducer currents. As such, ephaptic transmission is too weak to make more than a minor contribution to the coding process or to be responsible for the slow potential observed by Yamashita and Ohmori.[15] A more likely mechanism for the slow potential will now be considered.

INTERCELLULAR ACCUMULATION OF POTASSIUM IONS

During hair-cell transduction, K^+ ions enter the hair cell through transduction channels located in the stereocilia and leave the basolateral surface predominantly through K^+-selective conductances. Because of the long, uninterrupted apposition between the type I hair cell and the calyx ending, K^+ ions will accumulate in the intercellular space. The accumulation will result in a depolarization of the hair cell and is likely to have the same effect on the calyx ending.

By combining cable theory with the electrodiffusion (Nernst-Planck) equation, it is possible to estimate the accumulation. In FIGURE 5, for example, a transducer current (I_A) of 100 pA is applied to a model hair cell with a relatively low input impedance of 30 MΩ. It is assumed that the basolateral conductance is uniformly distributed. Because of the low impedance, the current results in only a small hair-cell voltage, ≤ 2 mV. The intercellular voltage is even smaller, ≤ 0.5 mV. Despite the small voltages, a substantial increase in the K^+ concentration occurs, from a baseline value of 4 mM at the top of the intercellular space to almost 11 mM at the base. The expected depolarization of the hair cell, due to the K^+ accumulation, can be calculated from the Nernst equation and is also substantial, ≈ 25 mV. The theory predicts that $\Delta[K^+]$, the change in intercellular K^+ concentration, is proportional to I_A. For an intercellular space 20 μm long and 30 nm wide, the proportionality constant is 0.07 mM/pA at the base (x = 0) and declines to zero at the apex (x = 20 μm). Transducer currents have not been measured in type I hair cells. In other hair cells, such currents can reach 600 pA.[23,24] An I_A of this magnitude will result in a Δ[K$^+$] at the base of 42 mM and an expected depolarization of the hair cell (and possibly of the calyx ending) of 60 mV.

The participation of K$^+$ accumulation in vestibular transduction will depend on its kinetics. These were analyzed by deriving the appropriate partial differential

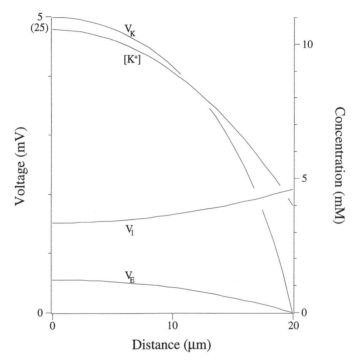

FIGURE 5. Potassium concentration, [K$^+$] (*right ordinate*), is plotted as a function of distance along the intercellular space from the base (0) to the apex (20 μm) (*abscissa*). Transducer current (I_A) of 100 pA; the unapposed input resistance of the hair cell, 30 MΩ. Hair-cell (V_I) and intercellular (V_E) voltages (*left ordinate*, 0–5 mV scale). V_K, expected depolarization of hair cell or calyx ending, calculated from Nernst equation for K$^+$ ions (*left ordinate*, 0–25 mV scale).

equation and determining its rate constants. The slowest rate constant is 12 s^{-1}, which corresponds to a time constant of 80 ms. Because kinetics are dominated by this rate constant, they can be modeled as a low-pass filter with a corner frequency of 2 Hz, near the frequency of normally occurring head movements.[25] Hence, K$^+$ accumulation is sufficiently fast to participate in vestibular transduction. It can do so in two ways: (1) By depolarizing the hair cell, it can increase neurotransmitter release; and (2) by depolarizing the ending, it can increase afferent firing directly. In short, K$^+$ can function as a neurotransmitter.

A Na^+,K^+-ATPase has been localized by immunohistochemistry to parent axons and to calyx endings.[26,27] Active transport out of the intercellular space and into the ending will reduce the calculated K^+ accumulation. No attempt was made to incorporate active transport into the theory because relevant activity levels have not been measured in vestibular organs. Comparison with other tissues suggests that transport rates would be inadequate to eliminate the accumulation. To cite an example, striated muscle, which has among the highest transport rates observed in vertebrate tissues, can pump 4×10^5 K^+ ion/s per μm^2 of membrane under optimal conditions.[28] The rate is 2–10 times lower than needed to eliminate K^+ accumulation from the intercellular space.

Another perspective on active transport is offered by considering a general design feature of hair-cell organs. Sensory transduction is based on the continuous rundown of ionic gradients. To restore the gradients requires a source of energy. In hair-cell organs a partial division of labor exists between the cells responsible for transduction and those responsible for maintaining the gradients. Dark cells located adjacent to the neuroepithelium use active transport to elaborate a K^+-rich endolymph in which the stereocilia and their transducer channels are situated.[29,30] A K^+-rich endolymph allows hair cells to concentrate on transduction. The opening of transducer channels results in an influx of K^+ ions into the hair cell and an efflux of K^+ ions across the basolateral surface. Inasmuch as the apical and basolateral currents are equal, there should be little change in intracellular K^+ concentration, and the energetic requirements of the hair cell are reduced. In addition, the maintenance of K^+ gradients across the basolateral surface can be accomplished by the diffusion of K^+ ions into the rest of the neuroepithelium. The design is so ingrained that a K^+-rich endolymph is found above the neuroepithelium even in the superficial lateral-line neuromasts of freshwater vertebrates.[31] Yet, the type I hair cell and the calyx ending violate an integral feature of the design as the long apposition between these structures impedes diffusion. The situation can be viewed in two ways. First, the type I hair cell has such an important and specialized function to fulfill that it evolved even though a requirement of its presence was that the calyx ending be able to actively transport K^+ ions at rates faster than seen in other cells. The second possibility is that the structures evolved to use K^+ accumulation in the sensory coding process. Evidence is now presented that K^+ accumulation may play an essential role in the vestibular transduction occurring in type I hair cells.

ELECTROPHYSIOLOGY OF HAIR CELLS

The electrophysiology of type I and type II hair cells has been studied by whole-cell methods in a variety of preparations.[11–13,32–34] FIGURE 6 is based on data from hair cells harvested from different regions of the turtle posterior crista. An advantage of the latter preparation is that, as the response characteristics of afferent nerve fibers innervating each of the regions are known,[35] it is possible to correlate the properties of the afferents and the hair cells.

Type II hair cells (FIG. 6A and B) have a variety of inward and outward rectifiers.[32–34] The outward rectifiers usually first become activated near -50 mV. The electrophysiology of type I hair cells is distinctive (FIG. 6C). In many of them, no inward rectifier is evident. There are at least two outward rectifiers. The first, called $g_{K(L)}$ by Rüsch and Eatock[13] and $g_{K(I)}$ by Rennie and Correia,[12] is unusual in that it begins activating at relatively hyperpolarized potentials, in this case near -80 mV. A second outward rectifier is also seen; it has a more typical activation range.

One consequence of the presence of $g_{K(L)}$ is seen in current-clamp records

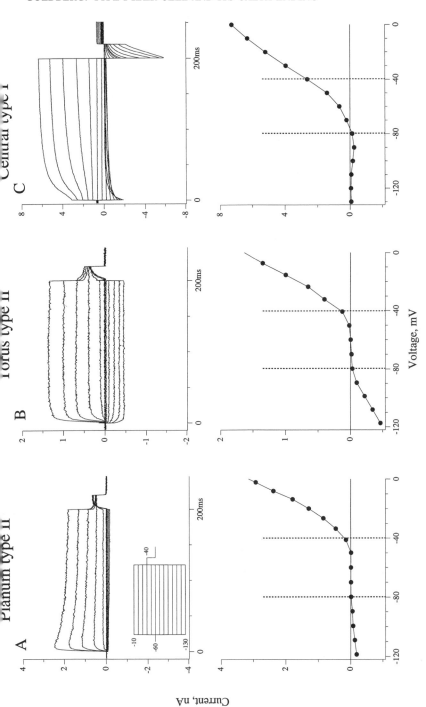

FIGURE 6. Voltage-clamp records from three hair cells harvested from different regions of the turtle posterior crista. Type II hair cells from the peripheral zone near the planum semilunatum (**A**) and near the torus (**B**). A type I hair cell from the central zone (**C**). The corresponding voltage-current (V-I) curves, taken from the end of the 200-ms voltage clamp, are shown below; voltages are corrected for series resistance, but not for a liquid-junction potential of − 5 mV. (Unpublished data of A. M. Brichta, R. A. Eatock, and J. M. Goldberg.)

(FIG. 7), taken from the same type I hair cell illustrated in FIG. 6C. The cell has a zero-current potential of −76 mV. Above this potential, the impedance falls, approaching 10 MΩ at the highest current levels. As a result, even large input currents do not depolarize the cell beyond −60 mV. In most hair cells, Ca^{2+} currents start turning on only above this value.[36,37] Ca^{2+} currents have not been characterized in type I hair cells. Assuming that the situation is similar to that seen in other hair cells, the results imply that, by themselves, transducer currents cannot activate Ca^{2+} currents. Because an influx of Ca^{2+} ions is required for neurotransmitter release, conventional transmission should not be possible. This is where K^+ accumulation may come into play. The expected K^+ depolarization is added to the current-voltage (I-V) curve in FIGURE 7B. Now the hair cell has no trouble reaching depolarizations where conventional transmission should work. The results illustrate that, of the two means of depolarizing the hair cell, the one due to K^+ accumulation is potentially more powerful than the one due to the direct effect of transducer currents on the basolateral membrane.

FUNCTIONAL CONSIDERATIONS

Is there any functional advantage in the proposed coupling of transducer currents to a K-induced depolarization? To discuss this or any other functional issue, it is well to consider afferent discharge. In mammals, calyx units have low rotational gains (FIG. 4A). It has been suggested that the reduced gains would allow these afferents to respond in a linear manner to even high-velocity head movements.[8,10] A similar conclusion may hold for calyx-bearing afferents in turtles.[34]

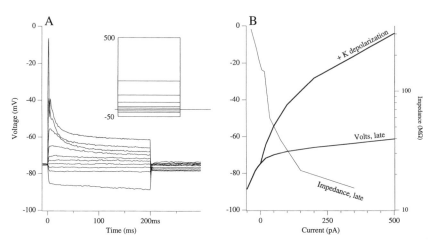

FIGURE 7. (A) Current-clamp records from the same type I hair cell as in FIGURE 6C. **(B)** corresponding current-voltage (I-V) curves (*Volts, late*) taken from the end of the 200-ms current clamp. Also included are the slope impedances (*Impedance, late*) and a curve obtained by adding V_K, the expected depolarization expected from intercellular K^+ accumulation to the I-V curve (*+K⁺ depolarization*); voltages are corrected for series resistance, but not for a liquid-junction potential of − 5 mV. (Unpublished data of A. M. Brichta, R. A. Eatock, and J. M. Goldberg.)

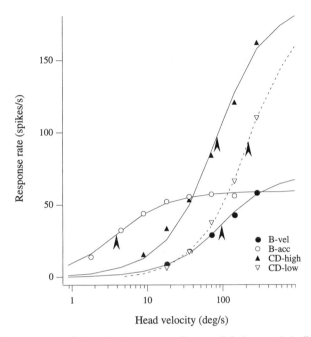

FIGURE 8. Input-output relations for four groups of extracellularly recorded afferents in the turtle posterior crista. Response to the last 0.5 s of a 2-s acceleration step is plotted against the average head velocity during the 0.5-s period. Units were assigned to the groups based on physiological criteria described by Brichta and Goldberg[35] (this volume). B-vel and B-acc are bouton units whose responses to 0.3-Hz sinusoidal head rotations are less than or greater than 45°, respectively. CD-high and CD-low are calyx-bearing afferents with background discharge rates greater than or less than 5 spikes/s, respectively. Points for each group are the mean responses for several units; the curves are empirical fits to the points. Arrowheads mark the inflection points of the curves. (From ref. 35.)

FIGURE 8 shows input-output curves for four groups of afferents innervating the turtle posterior crista. Included are two groups of calyx-bearing (CD) units separated into those with a background discharge higher (CD-high) or lower than 5 spikes/s (CD-low). There are also two groups of bouton (B) afferents distinguished by their rotational phases as encoding nearer angular head velocity (B-vel) or acceleration (B-acc). The stimulus range over which response is linear is indicated by the inflection points in these semilogarithmic plots (arrowheads in FIG. 8). CD units have a relatively broad linear range, extending to nearly 100°/s for CD-high units and to over 200°/s for CD-low units. CD units are distinctive in having maximal rates twice as large as those of B units. CD-low units have low rotational gains, similar to those of calyx units in mammals. A low rotational gain and a high maximal rate combine to give CD-low units a very large linear range.

Each of the several stages in transduction could help to shape the overall input-output function. Too little is known about transduction in any hair-cell system, let alone in type I hair cells, to decide whether the linear range is limited, for example, by a saturation in the relation between hair-bundle displacement and transducer currents, by nonlinear basolateral currents, or by a saturation in the relation between basolateral depolarization and neurotransmitter release. If a definitive analysis of the problem is premature, it can still be suggested that both $g_{K(L)}$ and K^+ accumulation could contribute to linearization. I-V curves for depolarizing currents are nearly linear (FIG. 7B), which reflects the fact that $g_{K(L)}$ is almost fully activated above the zero-current potential. K^+ accumulation could aid in linearization by depolarizing the hair cell and insuring that $g_{K(L)}$ activation was complete. In addition, the K^+-induced depolarization of the calyx ending could partially overcome any saturation in neurotransmitter release. This may explain why CD afferents can reach higher response rates than do B units.

Of the two groups of B afferents shown in FIGURE 8, B-vel and B-acc units are found near the planum and near the torus, respectively. B-vel units have a relatively large linear range, similar to that of CD-high afferents. In this case, an inspection of the corresponding voltage-clamp curves (FIG. 6A), taken from a type II hair cell harvested near the planum, suggests a simple mechanism of linearization. There is a zone of high impedance situated negative to the voltage needed to activate the hair cell's outward rectifier. The impedance is so high than even small transducer currents will displace the membrane potential into the low-impedance zone, where I-V curves should become linear. This is a more straightforward way of achieving linearity than that proposed for the type I hair cell. So the question might be asked: Why would the type I hair cell bother with such a complicated mechanism? A second question relates to B-acc afferents. Their discharge becomes nonlinear for even small head rotations of $< 10°/s$. It is unclear whether the restricted linear range of these units can be explained by the basolateral currents seen in the corresponding type II hair cells (FIG. 6B). These examples illustrate that, despite recent progress, too little is known about the transduction to explain the details of afferent discharge in calyx or noncalyx afferents.

SUMMARY

The long, uninterrupted apposition between the type I hair cell and the calyx ending has implications for the intercellular communication between these structures. Conventional synaptic transmission will be compromised unless the impedance of the ending is made relatively high. The apposition also creates the possibility of ephaptic transmission between the hair cell and the ending. Ephaptic transmission from the hair cell to the outer face of the calyx ending is too weak to make more than a minor contribution to sensory coding. Basolateral currents associated with hair-cell transduction can result in a substantial accumulation of K^+ ions in the intercellular space. The accumulation can alter conventional transmission by depolarizing the hair cell and can alter afferent firing by depolarizing the ending. Reasons were presented suggesting that K^+ accumulation may play an essential role in transduction involving type I hair cells, including the linearization of input-output relations and an increase in the maximal rate of discharge.

ACKNOWLEDGMENTS

The author thanks his colleagues, A. M. Brichta and R. A. Eatock, for allowing him to use unpublished data.

REFERENCES

1. WERSÄLL, J. 1956. Studies on the structure and innervation of the sensory epithelium of the cristae ampullares in the guinea pig. A light and electron microscopic investigation. Acta Oto-Laryngol. Suppl. **126:** 1–85.
2. WERSÄLL, J. & D. BAGGER-SJÖBÄCK. 1974. Morphology of the vestibular sense organ. *In* Handbook of Sensory Physiology. Vol. 6. Vestibular System. Part 1. Basic Mechanisms. H. H. Kornhuber, Ed.: 123–170. Springer-Verlag. Berlin.
3. JØRGENSEN, J. M. 1974. The sensory epithelia of the inner ear of two turtles, *Testudo graeca* and *Psedemys scripta.* Acta Zool. **55:** 289–298.
4. GOLDBERG, J. M., A. LYSAKOWSKI & C. FERNÁNDEZ. 1990. Morphophysiological and ultrastructural studies in the mammalian cristae ampullares. Hear. Res. **49:** 89–102.
5. LYSAKOWSKI, A. & J. M. GOLDBERG. 1989. Regional variations in the synaptic organization of the chinchilla cristae. Abstr. Soc. Neurosci. **15:** 502.
6. LYSAKOWSKI, A. & J. M. GOLDBERG. 1993. Regional variations in synaptic innervation of the squirrel monkey crista. Abstr. Soc. Neurosci. **19:** 1578.
7. YAMASHITA, N. & H. OHMORI. 1991. Synaptic bodies and vesicles in calix type synapse of chicken semicircular canal ampullae. Neurosci. Lett. **129:** 43–46.
8. BAIRD, R. A., G. DESMADRYL, C. FERNÁNDEZ & J. M. GOLDBERG. 1988. The vestibular nerve of the chinchilla. II. Relation between afferent response properties and peripheral innervation patterns in the semicircular canals. J. Neurophysiol. **60:** 182–203.
9. GOLDBERG, J. M., G. DESMADRYL, R. A. BAIRD & C. FERNÁNDEZ. 1990. The vestibular nerve of the chinchilla. V. Relation between afferent discharge properties and peripheral innervation patterns in the utricular macula. J. Neurophysiol. **63:** 791–804.
10. LYSAKOWSKI, A., L. B. MINOR, C. FERNÁNDEZ & J. M. GOLDBERG. 1995. Physiological identification of morphologically distinct afferent classes innervating the cristae ampullares of the squirrel monkey. J. Neurophysiol. **73:** 1270–1281.
11. CORREIA, M. J. & D. G. LANG. 1990. An electrophysiological comparison of solitary type I and type II vestibular hair cells. Neurosci. Lett. **116:** 106–111.
12. RENNIE, K. J. & M. J. CORREIA. 1994. Potassium currents in mammalian and avian isolated semicircular canal hair cells. J. Neurophysiol. **71:** 317–329.
13. RÜSCH, A. & R. A. EATOCK. 1996. Voltage responses of mouse utricular hair cells to injected currents. Ann. N.Y. Acad. Sci. This volume.
14. SCHESSEL, D. A., R. GINZBERG & S. M. HIGHSTEIN. 1991. Morphophysiology of synaptic transmission between type I hair cells and vestibular primary afferents. An intracellular study employing horseradish peroxidase in the lizard, *Calotes versicolor.* Brain Res. **544:** 1–16.
15. YAMASHITA, N. & H. OHMORI. 1990. Synaptic responses to mechanical stimulation in calyceal and bouton type vestibular afferents studied in an isolated preparation of semicircular canal ampullae of the chicken. Exp. Brain Res. **80:** 475–488.
16. GULLEY, R. L. & D. BAGGER-SJÖBÄCK. 1979. Freeze-fracture studies on the synapse between the type I hair cell and the calyceal terminal in the guinea-pig vestibular system. J. Neurocytol. **8:** 591–603.
17. GINZBERG, R. D. 1984. Freeze-fracture morphology of the vestibular hair cell-primary afferent synapse in the chick. J. Neurocytol. **13:** 393–405.
18. FAVRE, D. & A. SANS. 1979. Morphological changes in afferent vestibular hair cell synapses during the postnatal development of the cat. J. Neurocytol. **8:** 765–775.
19. ROSSI, M. L., M. MARTINI, B. PELUCCHI & R. FESCE. 1994. Quantal nature of synaptic transmission at the cytoneural junction in the frog labyrinth. J. Physiol. (Lond.) **478:** 17–35.
20. BENNETT, M. V. L. 1972. A comparison of electrically and chemically mediated transmission. *In* Structure and Function of Synapses. G. D. Pappas & D. P. Purpura, Eds.: 221–256. Raven. New York.
21. FERNÁNDEZ, C., A. LYSAKOWSKI & J. M. GOLDBERG. 1995. Hair-cell counts and afferent innervation patterns in the cristae ampullares of the squirrel monkey with a comparison to the chinchilla. J. Neurophysiol. **73:** 1253–1269.

22. SMITH, C. E. & J. M. GOLDBERG. 1986. A stochastic afterhyperpolarization model of repetitive activity in vestibular afferents. Biol. Cybern. **54:** 41–51.
23. CRAWFORD, A. C., M. G. EVANS & R. FETTIPLACE. 1991. The action of calcium on the mechano-electric transducer of turtle hair cells. J. Physiol. (Lond.) **434:** 369–398.
24. KROS, C. J., A. RÜSCH & G. P. RICHARDSON. 1992. Mechano-electric transducer currents in hair cells of the cultured neonatal mouse cochlea. Proc. R. Soc. Lond. B Biol. Sci. **249:** 185–193.
25. GROSSMAN, G. E., R. J. LEIGH, L. A. ABEL, D. J. LANSKA & S. E. THURSTON. 1988. Frequency and velocity of rotational head perturbations during locomotion. Exp. Brain Res. **70:** 470–476.
26. SPICER, S. S., B. A. SCHULTE & J. C. ADAMS. 1990. Immunolocalization of Na^+,K^+-ATPase and carbonic anhydrase in the gerbil's vestibular system. Hear. Res. **43:** 205–218.
27. ICHIMIYA, I., J. C. ADAMS & R. S. KIMURA. 1994. Immunolocalization of Na^+,K^+-ATPase, Ca^{++}-ATPase, calcium-binding proteins, and carbonic anhydrase in the guinea pig inner ear. Acta Oto-Laryngol. **114:** 167–176.
28. SEJERSTED, O. M. 1988. Maintenance of Na,K-homeostasis by Na,K pumps in striated muscle. In The Na^+,K^+-Pump. Part B. Cellular Aspects. J. C. Skou, J. G. Nørby, A. B. Maunsbach & M. Esmann, Eds.: 195–206. Liss. New York.
29. BERNARD, C., E. FERRARY & O. STERKER. 1986. Production of endolymph in the semicircular canal of the frog. J. Physiol. (Lond.) **371:** 17–28.
30. MARCUS, D. C. & Z. SHEN. 1994. Slowly activating voltage-dependent K^+ conductance is apical pathway for K^+ secretion in vestibular dark cells. Am. J. Physiol. **267:** C857–C864.
31. RUSSELL, I. J. & P. M. SELLICK. 1976. Measurement of potassium and chloride ion concentrations in the cupulae of the lateral lines of Xenopus laevis. J. Physiol. (Lond.) **257:** 245–255.
32. OHMORI, H. 1984. Studies of ionic currents in the isolated vestibular hair cell of the chick. J. Physiol. (Lond.) **350:** 561–581.
33. LANG, D. G. & M. J. CORREIA. 1989. Studies of solitary semicircular canal hair cells in the adult pigeon. II. Voltage-dependent ionic conductances. J. Neurophysiol. **62:** 935–945.
34. MASETTO, S., G. RUSSO & I. PRIGIONI. 1994. Differential expression of potassium currents by hair cells in thin slices of frog crista ampullaris. J. Neurophysiol. **72:** 443–455.
35. BRICHTA, A. M. & J. M. GOLDBERG. 1996. Afferent and efferent responses from morphological fiber classes in the turtle posterior crista. Ann. N.Y. Acad. Sci. This volume.
36. FUCHS, P. A. 1992. Ionic currents in cochlear hair cells. Prog. Neurobiol. **39:** 493–505.
37. PRIGIONI, I., S. MASETTO, G. RUSSO & V. TAGLIETTI. 1992. Calcium currents in solitary hair cells isolated from frog crista ampullaris. J. Vestib. Res. **2:** 31–39.

Candidate Cellular Mechanisms of Vestibulo-Ocular Reflex Plasticity[a]

SASCHA DU LAC[b]

Department of Physiology and
William Keck Foundation Center for Integrative Neuroscience
University of California, San Francisco
San Francisco, California 94143

INTRODUCTION

The vestibulo-ocular reflex (VOR) provides an excellent opportunity for understanding the neural basis of behavioral plasticity in vertebrate animals. The VOR stabilizes images on the retina during head movements by producing compensatory eye movements that are equal in amplitude and opposite in direction to head turns. This simple reflex behavior is subject to many forms of modulation over both short and long time scales. An example of short-term modulation of the VOR occurs during vergence eye movements in which the gain of the VOR (eye speed/head speed) is modulated by vergence angle.[1] Longer-term changes in VOR gain and dynamics occur whenever subjects experience persistent image motion during head movements.[2–8] Extensive anatomical studies and physiological recordings of neurons in awake behaving animals have elucidated the circuitry for the VOR and the functional significance of firing in identified populations of neurons in the VOR circuit. These studies, in combination with brain slice preparations of the vestibular brain stem,[9–14] have set the stage for investigating the cellular mechanisms of short- and long-term plasticity in the VOR.

This paper discusses candidate cellular mechanisms for behavioral plasticity in the VOR and focuses on neurons in the medial vestibular nucleus (MVN). The MVN is an attractive locus for studying the cellular changes that underlie behavioral modulation in the VOR because a subset of MVN neurons have been implicated in mediating plastic changes in the VOR and because MVN neurons have been studied extensively during vestibulo-ocular behavior.[15–27] The MVN receives head movement information from vestibular nerve afferents,[28–30] and some MVN neurons project monosynaptically to the abducens nucleus, which mediates horizontal eye movements.[19,23,31]

In considering plausible cellular mechanisms for behavioral plasticity in the VOR, it is important to keep in mind that almost all neurons in VOR pathways fire spontaneously at high rates: information appears to be encoded in modulations in firing rate. This implies that adaptive changes in the VOR must be mediated by changes in the way neurons modulate their firing rate in response to the firing of their inputs. The transformation from the firing of presynaptic neurons into the firing of postsynaptic neurons can be decomposed into three stages, as illustrated in FIGURE 1. In the first stage, the synaptic apparatus transforms firing in the presynaptic neuron into current at the postsynaptic dendrites. In the second stage, this synaptic

[a]This work was supported by NIH grant EY 11027.

[b]Address correspondence to: Sascha du Lac, Department of Physiology, Box 0444, UCSF, San Francisco, CA 94143-0444. E-mail: sascha@phy.ucsf.edu

current is filtered by the dendrites as it travels toward the soma and axon hillock. In the third and final stage, current that reaches the soma and axon hillock gets transformed into temporal patterns of firing via a process called spike generation.

Each of the stages depicted in FIGURE 1 is critical for determining how a neuron responds to the firing of its inputs, yet studies of the cellular mechanisms of learning have focused almost exclusively on the first stage, that of synaptic transmission. However, changes at other stages, in particular in spike generation, could also underlie behavioral learning. The spike generator in all neurons studied comprises a number of ionic channels in addition to the classic sodium and delayed rectifier potassium channels.[32] The conductances of many of the channels that contribute to spike generation can be modified by mechanisms that are thought to modify synaptic channels, such as phosphorylation (e.g. ref. 33). Consequently, it is important to consider whether and how modulations of spike generation contribute to long- and short-term modulations of behavior.

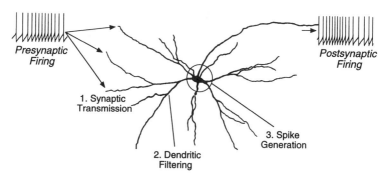

FIGURE 1. Neuronal signal transformations. Three stages in the transformation from the firing of the presynaptic neuron into the firing of the postsynaptic neuron are depicted schematically. See text for further description.

The goal of the studies described here is to explore how modulations of membrane channels in MVN neurons could underlie behavioral plasticity in the VOR. Because the gain and dynamics of the VOR are modifiable, I have focused on the control of the gain and dynamics of spike generation. The studies were performed in brain slices of the MVN in chicks. This animal was chosen because (1) its accessibility and small head make it amenable to the brain-slice technique, (2) the VOR in chicks undergoes the same sort of adaptive changes as does the VOR in primates,[7] and (3) pathways that control adaptive changes in the VOR are similar in chicks and in mammals.[34]

PROPERTIES OF THE MEDIAL VESTIBULAR NUCLEUS SPIKE GENERATOR

To investigate the normal properties of the MVN spike generator, firing rate responses to steps of intracellularly injected current were recorded from MVN neurons in brain slices, as depicted in FIGURE 2. The methods are described fully in reference 9. FIGURE 3 summarizes the normal properties of the avian MVN spike generator. MVN neurons are spontaneously active in the slice, firing at rates between about 10 and 60 spikes/s. FIGURE 3A shows an example of spontaneous

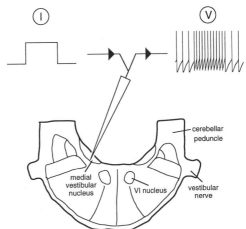

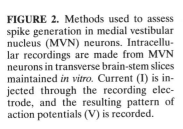

FIGURE 2. Methods used to assess spike generation in medial vestibular nucleus (MVN) neurons. Intracellular recordings are made from MVN neurons in transverse brain-stem slices maintained *in vitro*. Current (I) is injected through the recording electrode, and the resulting pattern of action potentials (V) is recorded.

firing in an MVN neuron; the regular firing pattern evident in FIGURE 3A is typical of MVN neurons. Action potentials are typically followed by a rapid after-hyperpolarization. The trajectory of the membrane potential between spikes varies among neurons and across firing rates, but the input-output properties of the MVN spike

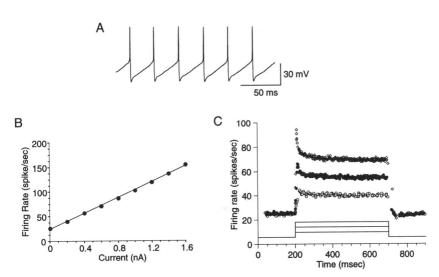

FIGURE 3. Normal properties of spike generation in medial vestibular nucleus (MVN) neurons. (A) Spontaneous firing rate of a typical MVN neuron, plotted as membrane potential as a function of time. (B) Mean firing rate attained during 500-ms steps of input current as a function of the current step amplitude. The line indicates the best linear fit to the data. (C) Instantaneous firing rate as a function of time in response to injection of current steps of 200 pA (*open circles*), 400 pA (*filled circles*), and 600 pA (*diamonds*); the data plotted are the responses to six current steps of each amplitude. Current traces are plotted below as the solid lines. No current was injected between 0 and 200 ms and between 700 and 1000 ms. Data in A, B, and C were taken from the same neuron.

generator are qualitatively similar both across avian MVN neurons and across species.[9]

The MVN spike generator transforms input current into firing rate in a remarkably linear fashion. In FIGURE 3B, the mean firing rate during current steps is plotted as a function of current amplitude; the line indicates the best linear fit to the data. In most MVN neurons, the relationship between current and mean firing rate is linear up to firing rates of about 200 spikes/s. Thus, spike generation in MVN neurons is linear over the approximate normal range of firing rates that have been measured in awake behaving animals. Spike generation is also linear over the approximate range of head movement frequencies typically experienced by animals (0.1 to 10 Hz): responses to current steps can be predicted from the Fourier synthesis of the responses to sinusoidal current inputs.[35]

The dynamics of the MVN spike generator are highly stereotypic and reproducible. FIGURE 3C shows instantaneous firing rate as a function of time in response to six repetitions of current steps at three different amplitudes. The neuron in FIGURE 3C fired spontaneously at 25 spikes/s. In response to a depolarizing current step of 200 pA (small step), the firing rate increased rapidly to a peak of 44 spikes/s and then settled within less than 200 ms to a stable rate of 40 spikes/s. When the current step was turned off, the firing rate returned to the spontaneous level. Firing rate responses to larger amplitude inputs had similar dynamics, exhibiting little adaptation in spike rate during the current step. The lack of pronounced spike rate adaptation is consistent with the broad-band filtering properties of MVN neurons evident in their responses to sinusoidal current injection.[35] The tight clustering of responses to each current step amplitude indicates that the MVN spike generator transforms its inputs into firing rate in a highly reproducible fashion.

In summary, the MVN spike generator can be characterized as a highly reliable linear filter: it transforms input current in modulations of firing rate in a precise and linear fashion over a wide range of input amplitudes and frequencies. It appears that MVN neurons are well suited for mediating vestibulo-ocular behavior, which itself is linear and precise over a wide range of input amplitudes and frequencies.

CONTROL OF SPIKE GENERATION GAIN AND DYNAMICS BY ION CHANNELS

To investigate how intrinsic membrane channels in MVN neurons control spike generation gain and dynamics, I have assessed the effects of pharmacological channel blockers on the firing rate responses to intracellularly injected current. Because a variety of types of cellular plasticity depend on calcium entry into neurons, this paper addresses how calcium-dependent mechanisms control spike generation in MVN neurons.

Effects of Blocking the Apamin-sensitive Calcium-activated Potassium Channel

Calcium-activated potassium channels have been implicated in the control of spike generation in a variety of cell types. Apamin, a toxin derived from honeybees, is thought to specifically block one of the subtypes of calcium-activated potassium channels (the SK channel). FIGURE 4 shows the effects of apamin on spike generation in MVN neurons. First, apamin (100–200 nM) causes MVN neurons to fire faster. The neuron in FIGURE 4A fired spontaneously at 18 spikes/s. After calcium-activated potassium channels were blocked by apamin, the neuron increased its spontaneous firing rate to 25 spikes/s. In eight neurons tested, apamin caused firing rate to increase to a mean of 135% of the control firing rate (range, 103 to 240%).

More interestingly, blocking calcium-activated potassium channels with apamin caused a specific increase in spike generation gain without affecting linearity or dynamics. FIGURE 4B compares the current–firing rate relationship before and after bath-application of apamin. In control ringer, the relationship between current and firing rate was linear, with a slope of 124 spikes-nA/s. After addition of apamin, the current firing rate relationship remained linear, but the slope of the relationship

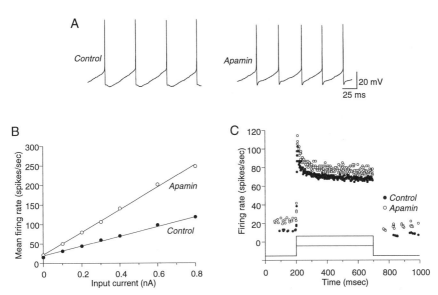

FIGURE 4. Effects of apamin on spike generation. (A) Spontaneous firing rate of medial vestibular nucleus neuron before (Control) and after (Apamin) the addition of 100 nM apamin to the bathing ringer. (B) Mean firing rate during current steps, 500 ms in duration, is plotted as a function of the current step amplitude. *Filled circles* are data from the control neuron; *open circles* are from the same neuron after application of apamin. The lines indicate the best linear fit to the data. (C) Dynamics of spike generation in the presence (*open circles*) and absence (*filled circles*) of apamin. Data plotted indicate instantaneous firing rate as a function of time in response to injection of six repetitions of current steps. The current step used to evoke the control response was 400 pA; the step used to evoke the response in the presence of apamin was 200 pA. Current traces are plotted below as the solid lines. Data in **A**, **B**, and **C** were taken from the same neuron.

increased to 283 spikes-nA/s. In eight neurons tested with apamin, the slope of the current–firing relationship increased by a mean of 167% of the control value (range, 138 to 228%).

Although apamin caused an increase in spike generation gain, the dynamics of spike generation were unaffected by apamin. FIGURE 4C compares instantaneous firing rate during six repetitions of steps of current injected before and after application of apamin. The current step used to evoke the response in apamin was half that used to evoke the control response, but the time course of the firing rate response was unaffected by apamin.

Effects of Blocking Calcium Channels

Calcium-activated potassium channels represent only one of many mechanisms by which calcium entry into neurons could influence spike generation. To investigate whether other calcium-dependent mechanisms play a role in modulating the gain

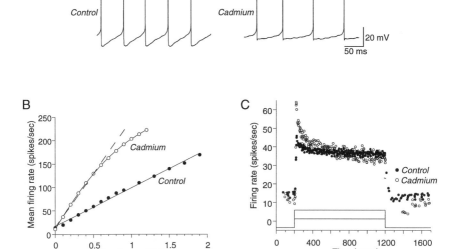

FIGURE 5. Effects of cadmium on spike generation. (**A**) Spontaneous firing rate of a medial vestibular nucleus neuron before (Control) and after (Cadmium) the addition of 100 μM cadmium to the bathing ringer. (**B**) Mean firing rate during current steps, 1000 ms in duration, is plotted as a function of the current step amplitude. *Filled circles* are data from the control neuron; the *open circles* are from the same neuron after application of cadmium. The solid line through the control data indicates the best linear fit to the data. The dashed line through the points obtained in cadmium indicates the best linear fit to the responses to current steps of less than 0.7 nA; the solid line indicates the best third-order polynomial fit to the data. (**C**) Dynamics of spike generation in the presence (*open circles*) and absence (*filled circles*) of cadmium. Data plotted indicate instantaneous firing rate as a function of time in response to injection of six repetitions of current steps. The current step used to evoke the control response was 400 pA; the step used to evoke the response in the presence of cadmium was 200 pA. Current traces are plotted below as the solid lines. Data in **A**, **B**, and **C** were taken from the same neuron.

and dynamics of spike generation, I assessed the effects of cadmium, which blocks all calcium channels. FIGURE 5 shows the effects of cadmium on spike generation in a representative MVN neuron. Cadmium (100 uM) caused the neuron to fire more slowly; its spontaneous firing rate decreased from 20 spikes/s in control ringer to 16 spikes/s in the presence of cadmium. In five neurons tested with cadmium, spontaneous firing rate decreased to a mean of 80% of the control value (range, 22 to 128%).

Calcium conductances that are blocked by cadmium play a role in determining spike generation gain. FIGURE 5B compares the current–firing rate relationship before and after addition of cadmium. In control solution, the neuron responded linearly to steps of current with a slope of 82 spikes-nA/s. In the presence of cadmium, the slope of the current–firing rate relationship increased dramatically, but the relationship deviated from linear at input amplitudes greater than 0.6 nA. In each of the five neurons subjected to cadmium, the current–firing rate relationship deviated from linear at mean firing rates between 100 and 160 spikes/s. The slope of the linear portion of the relationship increased by a mean of 264% (range, 227 to 316%) of that in control ringer.

Spike generation dynamics are also altered when calcium channels are blocked with cadmium. FIGURE 5C compares instantaneous firing rate during six repetitions of current steps before and after cadmium application. To facilitate the comparison, the current step used to evoke the control response was half the size of that in the presence of cadmium. Note that although the steady-state firing rate was approximately equal in cadmium and control ringer, firing rate during the first 200 ms of the response was significantly greater in cadmium. A similar change in spike generation dynamics was evident in each of the other four neurons tested.

Multiple Calcium-dependent Mechanisms for Controlling Spike Generation

The effects of blocking calcium channels on spike generation must be partially due to the lack of calcium available to calcium-activated potassium channels. However, comparison of the effects of apamin and cadmium suggests that calcium entry into MVN neurons affects spike generation via at least two separate mechanisms, only one of which relies on apamin-sensitive calcium-activated potassium conductances. When calcium-activated potassium channels are blocked with high concentrations of apamin (presumably in the suprasaturating range), spike generation gain increases, but dynamics are unaffected. In contrast, blocking calcium channels causes a larger increase in spike generation gain as well as a small change in dynamics. These results indicate that calcium-dependent processes control spike generation in MVN neurons via at least two separate mechanisms. Because cadmium blocks all types of neuronal calcium channels,[36] it remains unknown whether the additional effects of cadmium (on gain, dynamics, and spontaneous firing rate) depend on blocking a single type or multiple types of calcium channels.

Cellular Mechanisms of Behavioral Plasticity in the Vestibulo-Ocular Reflex

Given that MVN neurons play a critical role in transforming head movement inputs into oculomotor commands, the gain and dynamics of spike generation in these neurons should affect the gain and dynamics of the vestibulo-ocular reflex. Consequently, modifications of spike generation in MVN neurons could underlie plastic changes in the VOR. Calcium and calcium-activated potassium conductances can be regulated both in a short-term fashion with neurotransmitters[37] and in a longer-term manner by enzymatic processes such as phosphorylation (e.g. ref. 33). The findings that these conductances control spike generation in MVN neurons raises the possibility that the VOR could be adaptively controlled by modulation of calcium or calcium-activated potassium channels.

The gain of the VOR can be controlled in a frequency-selective fashion under conditions in which subjects experience different amounts of image motion during different frequencies of head movement.[5,7,8,38–42] Changes in VOR gain can therefore be accompanied by changes in dynamics. It is conceivable that regulation of the calcium channels that cause changes in both gain and dynamics of spike generation could underlie frequency-selective changes in VOR gain. In contrast, regulation of calcium-activated potassium channels could underlie frequency-independent forms of VOR gain changes.

ACKNOWLEDGMENT

I thank Jennifer Raymond for critically reviewing the manuscript.

REFERENCES

1. SNYDER, L. H. & W. M. KING. 1992. Effect of viewing distance and location on the axis of head rotation on the monkey's vestibuloocular reflex. I. Eye movement responses. J. Neurophysiol. **67(4):** 861–874.
2. ITO, M., T. SHIIDA, N. YAGI & M. YAMAMOTO. 1974. The cerebellar modification of rabbit's horizontal vestibulo-ocular reflex induced by sustained head rotation combined with visual stimulation. Proc. Jpn. Acad. **50:** 85–89.
3. GONSHOR, A. & G. MELVILL-JONES. 1976. Extreme vestibulo-ocular adaptation induced by prolonged optical reversal of vision. J. Physiol. (Lond.) **256:** 381–414.
4. MELVILL-JONES, G. 1977. Plasticity in the adult vestibulo-ocular reflex arc. Philos. Trans. R. Soc. Lond. Ser. B **278:** 319–334.
5. COLLEWIJN, H. & A. F. GROOTENDORST. 1978. Adaptation of the rabbit's vestibulo-ocular reflex to modified visual input: Importance of stimulus conditions. Arch. Ital. Biol. **116:** 273–280.
6. MILES, F. A. & B. B. EIGHMY. 1980. Long-term adaptive changes in primate vestibulo-ocular reflex. I. Behavioral observations. J. Neurophysiol. **43:** 1406–1425.
7. WALLMAN, J., J. VELEZ, B. WEINSTEIN & A. GREEN. 1982. Avian vestibulo-ocular reflex: Adaptive plasticity and developmental changes. J. Neurophysiol. **48:** 952–967.
8. SCHAIRER, J. O. & M. V. L. BENNETT. 1986. Changes in the gain of the vestibulo-ocular reflex by combined visual and vestibular simulation in goldfish. Brain Res. **373:** 164–176.
9. DU LAC, S. & S. G. LISBERGER. 1995. Membrane and firing properties of avian medial vestibular nucleus neurons *in vitro.* J. Comp. Physiol. A **176:** 641–651.
10. GALLAGHER, J. P., K. D. PHELAN & P. SHINNICK-GALLAGHER. 1992. Modulation of excitatory transmission at the rat medial vestibular nucleus synapse. Ann. N. Y. Acad. Sci. **656:** 630–644.
11. LEWIS, M. R., J. P. GALLAGHER & P. SHINNICK-GALLAGHER. 1987. An *in vitro* brain slice preparation to study the pharmacology of central vestibular neurons. J. Pharmacol. Methods **18:** 267–273.
12. SERAFIN, M., C. D. WAELE, A. KHATEB, P. P. VIDAL & M. MUHLETHALER. 1991. Medial vestibular nucleus in the guinea-pig. I. Intrinsic membrane properties in brainstem slices. Exp. Brain Res. **84:** 417–425.
13. JOHNSTON, A. R., N. K. MACLEOD & M. B. DUTIA. 1994. Ionic conductances contributing to spike repolarization and after-potentials in rat medial vestibular nucleus neurones. J. Physiol. **481:** 61–77.
14. KINNEY, G. A., B. W. PETERSON & N. T. SLATER. 1994. The synaptic activation of N-methyl-D-aspartate receptors in the rat medial vestibular nucleus. J. Neurophysiol. **72:** 1588–1595.
15. FUCHS, A. F. & J. KIMM. 1975. Unit activity in the vestibular nucleus of the alert monkey

during horizontal angular acceleration and eye movement. J. Neurophysiol. **38:** 1140–1161.

16. LISBERGER, S. G. & F. A. MILES. 1980. Role of primate medial vestibular nucleus in adaptive plasticity of vestibulo-ocular reflex. J. Neurophysiol. **43:** 1725–1745.
17. CHUBB, M. C., A. F. FUCHS & C. A. SCUDDER. 1984. Neuronal activity in monkey vestibular nuclei during vertical vestibular stimulation and eye movements. J. Neurophysiol. **52:** 724–742.
18. TOMLINSON, R. D. & D. A. ROBINSON. 1984. Signals in vestibular nucleus mediating vertical eye movements in the monkey. J. Neurophysiol. **51:** 1121–1136.
19. MCCREA, R. A., A. STRASSMAN, E. MAY & S. M. HIGHSTEIN. 1987. Anatomical and physiological characteristics of vestibular neurons mediating the horizontal vestibulo-ocular reflex of the squirrel monkey. J. Comp. Neurol. **264:** 547–570.
20. MCCREA, R. A., A. STRASSMAN, E. MAY & S. M. HIGHSTEIN. 1987. Anatomical and physiological characteristics of vestibular neurons mediating the vertical vestibulo-ocular reflex of the squirrel monkey. J. Comp. Neurol. **264:** 571–594.
21. OHGAKI, T., I. S. CURTHOYS & C. H. MARKHAM. 1988. Morphology of physiologically identified second-order vestibular neurons in cat, with intracellular injected HRP. J. Comp. Neurol. **276:** 387–411.
22. MCFARLAND, J. L. & A. F. FUCHS. 1992. Discharge patterns of the nucleus prepositus and adjacent medial vestibular nucleus during horizontal eye movements in behaving monkeys. J. Neurophysiol. **68:** 319–332.
23. SCUDDER, C. A. & A. F. FUCHS. 1992. Physiological and behavioral identification of vestibular nucleus neurons mediating the horizontal vestibuloocular reflex in trained rhesus monkeys. J. Neurophysiol. **68(1):** 244–264.
24. CULLEN, K. E., C. CHEN-HUANG & R. A. MCCREA. 1993. Firing behavior of brain stem neurons during voluntary cancellation of the horizontal vestibuloocular reflex. II. Eye movement related neurons. J. Neurophysiol. **70:** 844–856.
25. CULLEN, K. E. & R. A. MCCREA. 1993. Firing behavior of brain stem neurons during voluntary cancellation of the horizontal vestibuloocular reflex. I. Secondary vestibular neurons. J. Neurophysiol. **70:** 828–843.
26. LISBERGER, S. G., T. A. PAVELKO & D. M. BROUSSARD. 1994. Neural basis for motor learning in the vestibulo-ocular reflex of primates. I. Changes in the responses of brainstem neurons. J. Neurophysiol. **72:** 928–953.
27. LISBERGER, S. G., T. A. PAVELKO & D. M. BROUSSARD. 1994. Responses during eye movements of brainstem neurons that receive monosynaptic inhibition from the flocculus and ventral paraflocculus in monkeys. J. Neurophysiol. **72:** 909–928.
28. FERNANDEZ, C. & J. GOLDBERG. 1971. Physiology of peripheral neurons innervating semicircular canals of the squirrel monkey. II. Response to sinusoidal stimulation and dynamics of peripheral vestibular system. J. Neurophysiol. **34:** 661–675.
29. WOLD, J. E. 1975. The vestibular nuclei in the domestic hen (*Gallus domesticus*). II. Primary afferents. Brain Res. **95:** 531–543.
30. COX, R. & K. PEUSNER. 1990. Horseradish peroxidase labelling of the central pathways in the medulla of the ampullary nerves in the chicken, *Gallus gallus.* J. Comp. Neurol. **297:** 564–585.
31. LABANDEIRA-GARCIA, J. L., M. J. GUERRA-SEIJAS, J. A. LABANDEIRA-GARCIA & J. M. SUAREZ-NUNEZ. 1989. Afferent connections of the oculomotor nucleus in the chick. J. Comp. Neurol. **282:** 523–534.
32. HILLE, B. 1992. Ionic channels of excitable membranes. Sinauer Associates. Sunderland, MA.
33. REINHART, P. H., S. CHUNG, B. L. MARTIN, D. L. BRAUTIGAN & I. B. LEVITAN. 1991. Modulation of calcium-activated potassium channels from rat brain by protein kinase A and phosphatase 2A. J. Neurosci. **11:** 1627–1635.
34. DU LAC, S. & S. G. LISBERGER. 1992. Eye movements and brainstem neuronal responses evoked by cerebellar and vestibular stimulation in chicks. J. Comp. Physiol. A **171:** 629–638.
35. DU LAC, S. & S. G. LISBERGER. 1995. Cellular processing of temporal information in medial vestibular nucleus neurons. J. Neurosci. **15:** 8000–8010.

36. TSIEN, R. W., D. LIPSCOMBE, D. V. MADISON, K. R. BLEY & A. P. FOX. 1988. Multiple types of neuronal calcium channels and their selective modulation. Trends Neurosci. **11:** 820–824.
37. NICOLL, R. A., R. C. MALENKA & J. A. KAUER. 1990. Functional comparison of neurotransmitter receptor subtypes in mammalian central nervous system. Physiol. Rev. **70(2):** 513–565.
38. PASTOR, A. M., R. R. D. L. CRUZ & R. BAKER. 1992. Characterization and adaptive modification of the goldfish vestibuloocular reflex by sinusoidal and velocity step vestibular stimulation. J. Neurophysiol. **68:** 2003–2015.
39. GODAUX, E., J. HALLEUS & C. GOBERT. 1983. Adaptive change of the vestibulo-ocular reflex in the cat: The effects of a long-term frequency-selective procedure. Exp. Brain Res. **49:** 28–34.
40. LISBERGER, S. G., F. A. MILES & L. M. OPTICAN. 1983. Frequency-selective adaptation: Evidence for channels in the vestibulo-ocular reflex? J. Neurosci. **3(6):** 1234–1244.
41. PAIGE, G. D. 1983. Vestibuloocular reflex and its interactions with visual following mechanisms in the squirrel monkey. II. Response characteristics and plasticity following unilateral inactivation of horizontal canal. J. Neurophysiol. **49:** 152–168.
42. POWELL, K. D., K. J. QUINN, S. A. RUDE, B. W. PETERSON & J. F. BAKER. 1991. Frequency dependence of cat vestibulo-ocular reflex direction adaptation: Single frequency and multifrequency rotations. Brain Res. **550:** 137–141.

Potential Mechanisms of Plastic Adaptive Changes in the Vestibulo-Ocular Reflex[a]

B. W. PETERSON, G. A. KINNEY, K. J. QUINN,
AND N. T. SLATER

Northwestern University Medical School
303 East Chicago Avenue
Chicago, Illinois 60611

INTRODUCTION

Because the vestibulo-ocular reflex (VOR) functions in an open-loop fashion, where the eye movements it generates are not sensed by the vestibular end organs that provide its input, its accuracy depends upon plastic, adaptive adjustments in its gain, dynamics, and spatial properties. These learned adaptive changes can be easily induced by altering the visual feedback that accompanies head rotation by placing reversing prisms[1-3] or magnifying or reducing lenses[3-5] in front of the eyes, or by pairing body rotation with motion of an optokinetic pattern in the same[6] or orthogonal[7-9] directions. The adaptive changes that are observed are tuned to the frequency of the applied body rotation[8,10] and can selectively alter VOR phase when out-of-phase body and optokinetic pattern motions are applied.[11] These findings, together with reports that adaptive changes in the VOR can alter the properties of saccadic or optokinetic eye movements,[12,13] (but see ref. 14) suggest that the neural changes underlying these adaptive responses occur at multiple points in the vestibulo-oculomotor circuitry.

Although adaptive changes in the VOR may occur at multiple sites, interest has been focused especially upon the site of the neural changes responsible for the shortest latency changes in vestibulo-ocular eye movements evoked by a sudden stimulation of semicircular canal afferent fibers. Lisberger[15] applied an abrupt, $600°/s^2$ horizontal angular acceleration to the head and body of rhesus monkeys whose VOR gains had been increased or decreased by prolonged wearing of magnifying or reducing lenses. He found that the initial portion of the horizontal VOR produced by this acceleration, which began at 13 ms, was unaltered, whereas the amplitude of movements beginning 19 or more ms after the stimulus was changed by wearing the lenses. This observation made it unlikely (but not impossible) that cerebellar Purkinje cells, which begin to respond 6 ms after the stimulus,[16] could contribute to the shortest latency changes in the VOR. Thus the site of the earliest adaptive changes is likely within brain-stem VOR circuits. To pinpoint this site more precisely, Khater et al.[17] induced adaptive changes in the VOR in cats by having them wear magnifying or reducing lenses or by exposing them to 0.25-Hz sinusoidal horizontal body rotations coupled with vertical optokinetic pattern motions. Their VOR responses to $4000°/s^2$ horizontal head velocity transitions were then tested. This strong stimulus elicited normal horizontal VOR eye velocity changes at 13.0 ± 0.3 (mean $\pm$ SE) ms. Increases or decreases in VOR responses induced by prolonged

[a] This work was supported in part by grants EY 06485 and NS 31805 from the NIH and grant ONR 14-941265 from the Office of Naval Research.

wearing of magnifying or reducing lenses had an initial component with a latency of 12.5 ± 0.4 ms and a second component at 68 ± 1 ms. Cross-axis responses induced by 2-h pairing of horizontal head rotation with vertical image motion had an initial component with a latency of 15.2 ± 1.1 ms and a second component at 77 ± 2 ms. No significant difference was found between latencies of the normal horizontal VOR and the adaptively generated changes, indicating that the latter are produced by changes in the three-neuron VOR arc. Broussard and Lisberger[18] reached similar conclusions based on observations of eye movements elicited by less physiological but more precisely timed electrical stimulation of semicircular canal afferents in monkeys. Even the earliest portions of the horizontal eye movements induced by these stimuli were increased or decreased by prior wearing of magnifying or reducing lenses.

Thus it is clear that adaptive changes in the VOR involve changes in the most rapid, three-neuron arcs of the VOR. Further, these changes are unlikely to involve alteration of transmission at the final synapse in these arcs—between second-order vestibulo-ocular relay neurons (VORNs) and extraocular motoneurons—because, in addition to vestibular head velocity signals, VORNs carry eye position and smooth pursuit eye movement signals, whose action on motoneurons is usually not altered by adaptive changes in the VOR. Miles and Braitman[19] showed that vestibular afferent input does not change during adaptive changes in the VOR. Thus, the earliest adaptive changes must involve a change in the response of VORNs to activation of vestibular afferent fibers. It is curious, then, that adaptive changes in the VOR in mammals require the presence of an intact cerebellum.[2,20,21] Somehow neural circuits involving the cerebellum must play a role in inducing changes at a site outside the cerebellum.

MODEL SIMULATIONS

To investigate potential mechanisms involved in altering the response of VORNs to activation of vestibular afferent fibers during adaptive changes in VOR gain or direction, we performed computer simulations of vestibulo-cerebellar circuits to test hypotheses about how signals within cerebellar-vestibular circuits could interact to generate plastic adaptive changes.[22] FIGURE 1 shows the neural network, based on the vestibulo-cerebellar model of Miles et al.,[23] that was used to run simulations of VOR adaptation. The model incorporates a basic three-neuron VOR arc consisting of a semicircular canal (SCC) afferent fiber (VN1) and second-order VORN (VN2) that projects to contralateral extraocular motoneurons. (The "-1" in the diagram is a shorthand to reflect the processing resulting in an eye-velocity signal in a direction opposite to the original head movement; numbers in other boxes represent time delays.) The model also incorporates a gaze-velocity Purkinje (GVP) cell that receives head and eye velocity inputs[24] and inhibits VN2 and an accessory optic system (AOS) that carries retinal slip velocity signals to VN2 and GVP.[25]

The initial state of the network, configured to have a VOR gain = 1.0 was determined using the global optimization method described by Bremermann.[26] This technique is less prone to getting trapped in local minima than standard gradient descent algorithms (see ref. 27). After determination of the weight set that yielded a low error solution, we applied a series of different types of learning algorithms described below, which adjusted selected weights in the network in order to raise (to 2.0) or lower (to 0.5) the gain of the VOR. Whereas the optimization technique used to initially configure the network was not meant to have any physiological basis, the learning algorithms we used were constrained to use signals present in the network and in the actual nervous system which were reasonable for the task that we studied.

We first examined the effect of using the simple spike discharge of the GVP as a "teacher signal" that would cause adaptive changes to occur in brain-stem pathways. Miles and Lisberger[28] had suggested that this signal could be used to adjust the strength of action of vestibular afferents on all of their target neurons within the model. We modeled this by allowing GVP activity to adjust weight F in FIGURE 1 according to an associative learning rule where $\Delta F = k * (1 - |F|) * N_j * N_Z$, where k is a learning rate constant, N_Z is the output of the GVP cell, and N_j is the output of the vestibular afferents. The dashed line in FIGURE 2A shows that this mechanism

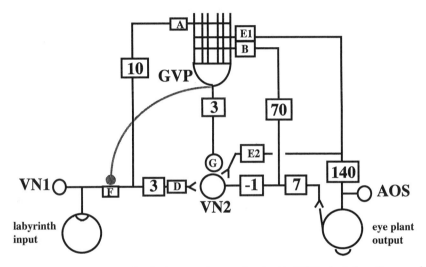

FIGURE 1. Model of cerebellar/brain-stem elements involved in VOR adaptation; diagram of neural circuit used for computer simulations. Synaptic weights are indicated by letters in boxes or circles. Positive numbers in larger boxes indicate time delays in ms. The -1 indicates the processing resulting in an eye velocity signal in a direction opposite to the original head movement. VN1 is a vestibular afferent fiber; VN2 is a second-order VORN; GVP is a gaze velocity Purkinje cell; and AOS indicates the accessory optic system.

leads to well-behaved changes in VOR gain. A possible neural substrate for such an adaptive mechanism is the $GABA_B$ receptor-mediated long-term depression (LTD) of transmission between vestibular afferents and second-order neurons that is described below.

The observation that adaptive changes in the VOR cause especially strong changes in the behavior of those second-order neurons that receive inhibitory synaptic input from GVPs (so-called flocculus target neurons or FTNs[29]) led Lisberger[5] to suggest that GVP discharge might act as a teacher signal that selectively modulates the weight of synaptic action of vestibular afferents on FTNs. The simulation illustrated in FIGURE 2B reveals a problem with this concept. We used GVP discharge to adjust weight D in FIGURE 1 according to an associative learning rule where $\Delta D = k * (1 - |D|) * N_j * N_Z$, where k is a learning rate constant. N_Z is the output of the GVP cell (after passing thorough weight G), and N_j is the output of the vestibular afferents (after passing through weight D). In addition, we used the output of the AOS pathway to modify the strength of weight A, using an analogous learning rule to that described above for weight D. Under these conditions, VOR gain in many cases exhibited unstable oscillations. When the strength of the eye-velocity feedback from VN2 to PK1 was set very high, to optimize the model's ability to generate smooth pursuit eye movements, gain did converge in some cases to the appropriate value, but again such convergence involved nonmonotonic oscilla-

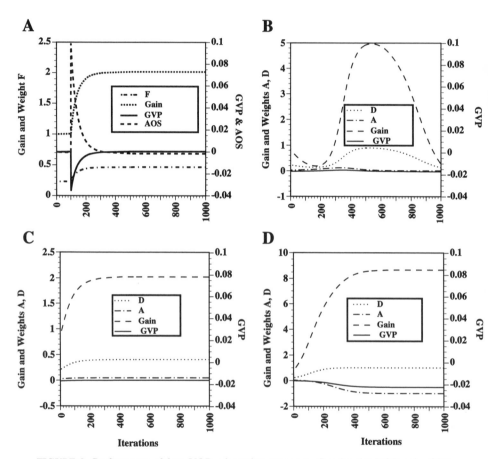

FIGURE 2. Performance of four VOR adaptation processes. Graphs plot VOR gain, GVP, AOS activation, and synaptic weight values after visual feedback generated by head rotation was doubled, requiring 2X VOR gain increase. Each iteration represents a snapshot of network performance after one trial run, which consisted of 5000 time steps (1 time step = 1 ms).

tions of gain, which are not observed physiologically. Thus, within the context of this model circuit, utilizing simple spike discharge of GVPs as a teacher signal to adjust weight D does not appear to generate physiologically realistic adaptive changes.

Simulations were also run in which the retinal slip signal, such as the one carried by the AOS and by climbing fiber afferents to the cerebellar flocculus,[30–32] was used as a teacher signal, for both weights A and D. As shown in FIGURE 2C, well-behaved gain learning occurred when a retinal slip signal directly modulated weight D via an associative learning rule where $\Delta D = k * (1 - |D|) * N_j * N_z$, where k is a learning rate constant, N_z is the retinal slip path activity (after having passed through weight E2), and N_j is the unit activity passing through weight D. How might such a learning mechanism operate within cerebello-vestibular circuits? Retinal slip signals are known to reach vestibular nuclei via collaterals of climbing fibers.[25] Presumably these collaterals synapse upon VORNs. Then, to implement the associative learning rule given above, a mechanism is required whereby synaptic action of AOS fibers on VN2 neurons can be conveyed selectively to VN1-VN2 synaptic terminals. Although such mechanisms exist (e.g., NO diffusion),[33] we sought a simpler process and therefore evaluated a Hebbian learning rule wherein weight D changes according to $\Delta D = k * (1 - |D|) * N_j * N_i$, where N_j represents the input to VN2, and N_i represents the overall activation state of the VN2 unit (here the activation state of VN2 is determined in part by AOS input). As shown by FIGURE 2D, such a rule failed to give accurate learning—rather than increasing to 2.0, gain rose to 9.5 and saturated there. Thus despite its inherent simplicity, the Hebbian learning rule is not effective in situations where precise gain changes must be learned, as discussed by Sutton and Barto.[34]

Another problem with the learning scheme discussed above (in which the AOS pathway regulates both changes at weights A and D) is that it does not readily explain why the cerebellum is required for VOR learning to occur nor why changes occur primarily on FTNs. One could postulate that cerebellectomy causes the pathways carrying retinal slip signals to the vestibular nuclei to degenerate, as might be the case for climbing fiber collaterals, but one would also then have to postulate that these pathways end primarily on FTNs, and this has not been shown. An alternative is to hypothesize that the specific patterns of discharge of GVPs that are elicited by climbing fiber afferents can exert an action upon FTNs that leads to long-term alteration of their responses to vestibular afferent input. It is known that activation of the climbing fiber synapsing with a Purkinje cell leads to a brief burst of action potentials from that cell followed by a 30–40-ms silent period.[35] We will argue below that this pattern of activity might release NMDA transmission at the VN1-VN2 synapse, leading to long-term changes caused by Ca^{2+} influxes.

IN VITRO STUDIES

To discover potential cellular mechanisms for adaptive VOR plasticity, we have undertaken patch-clamp recordings from vestibular neurons in brain-stem slices from 14–16-day-old Sprague-Dawley rats. Coronal slices (250–350 μm thick) were cut from the brain stem at the level of nVIII so that they contained both lateral and medial vestibular nuclei, and the projections to MVN from nVIII and commissural fibers from the contralateral MVN.[36–39] During recording, slices were transferred to a submersion chamber mounted on the stage of an upright microscope and continuously perfused with oxygenated modified Krebs solution at room temperature. Patch-clamp recordings were performed using the "blind patch" method of Blanton *et al.*[40]

Electrical stimulation (100 μs duration) of both the medial longitudinal fasciculus (MLF) or nVIII evoked a fast EPSP in MVN neurons. Pharmacological studies of the nVIII-evoked synaptic response in mammalian MVN neurons *in vitro* have demonstrated that the monosynaptic response is mediated by both AMPA and NMDA subtypes of glutamate receptor.[37,39,41] At low frequencies of stimulation the

EPSP is largely mediated by AMPA receptors,[37] but a prominent NMDA receptor-mediated component is revealed when GABA$_A$ receptors are blocked.[39,41] These studies also revealed the presence of extensive feedforward and recurrent polysynaptic excitation within the MVN.[39] Voltage-clamp studies of the NMDA receptor-mediated excitatory postsynaptic current (EPSC) demonstrated that the time course of the EPSC is similar to that at other "conventional" glutamatergic synapses in the central nervous system[42,43] (but see also Rossi *et al.*[44]) but neither the rise time, nor the decay rate is affected by membrane potential.[39] This indicates that there are differences in the kinetics of NMDA receptor-mediated synaptic currents in the two cell types. During periods of high-frequency activity of primary vestibular afferents, patch-clamp recording and modeling studies of MVN neurons have shown that the nVIII-evoked synaptic current summates as the NMDA component of EPSCs fuse to produce a depolarizing plateau. Furthermore, the efferent output of both type A and type B MVN neurons is sculpted primarily by the kinetics of desensitization of NMDA receptors, rather than by differences in the voltage-gated channels or AMPA receptors in these two cells classes.[45]

In the search for a mechanism by which Purkinje cells might produce long-term changes in vestibular afferent transmission, we rationalized that a potential candidate might be activation of GABA$_B$ receptors on MVN neurons by GABA released from Purkinje terminals or GABAergic interneurons within the MVN. All forms of long-lasting synaptic plasticity studied to date involve intracellular biochemical messenger systems, and GABA$_B$ receptors, but not GABA$_A$ receptors, trigger intracellular messenger cascades.[46,47] Moreover, both pre- and postsynaptic GABA$_B$ receptors have been identified in the MVN using anatomical[48] and electrophysiological[49] techniques, although a role for GABA$_B$ receptors in long-term synaptic plasticity has yet to be described.

To investigate the potential role for GABA$_B$ receptors, the GABA$_B$ agonist $(+/-)$baclofen was applied to slices by bath perfusion at concentrations from 1–10 μM. In the presence of baclofen, a modest membrane hyperpolarization and increased input conductance were observed, consistent with the expected activation of postsynaptic GABA$_B$ receptors.[50] This moderate sensitivity to baclofen resembles that observed in neurons of the nucleus of the solitary tract.[51] A very potent reduction of both the nVIII and MLF-evoked EPSPs was observed (FIG. 3), which may reflect the reversible actions of baclofen on presynaptic GABA$_B$ receptors in the MVN,[49] which could normally be induced by GABA release from synaptic terminals adjacent to the primary afferent terminals.[52] However, following the washout of baclofen, the nVIII-evoked EPSP did not recover to control levels, despite a rapid and complete recovery of all other cell properties, including input resistance and firing properties. This indicates that activation of GABA$_B$ receptors on MVN neurons induces a long-term depression of primary afferent transmission to second-order vestibular neurons. This long-term effect was observed on 17 of 19 neurons studied which displayed a monosynaptic EPSP to nVIII stimulation, the amplitude of the nVIII-evoked EPSP being reduced to 40% of control after 30 min or more of washing the drug from the bath. Moreover, when responses to stimulation of the MLF were compared, the LTD of the nVIII-evoked EPSP was synapse-specific, because although baclofen profoundly reduced both EPSPs, the actions on the MLF-evoked EPSP recovered to control levels, whereas the nVIII-evoked EPSP in these experiments remained depressed, as before (FIG. 3).

In further experiments, we used the GABA$_B$ receptor antagonist 2-hydroxy-saclofen (200 μM[47]) in an attempt to block the baclofen-induced LTD of primary afferent-evoked EPSPs. On the basis of experiments done in other brain regions, this compound would not be expected to have direct actions on MVN neurons, but would

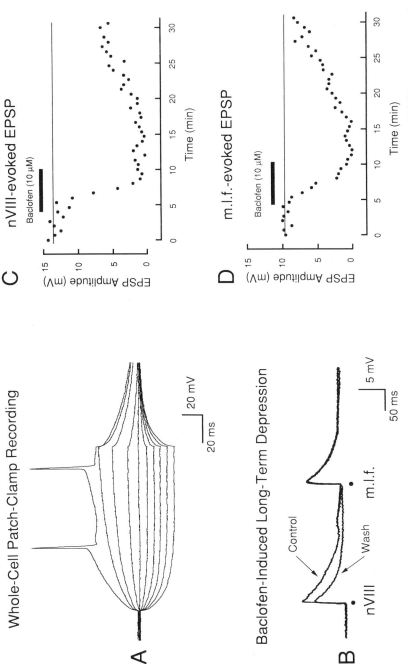

FIGURE 3. Synapse-specific long-term depression of the nVIII-evoked EPSP produced by activation of GABA$_B$ receptors. (**A**) Voltage responses of a patch-clamped MVN neuron to injected current. (**B**) EPSPs evoked by stimulation of the nVIII and the medial longitudinal fasciculus (m.l.f.) before and after bath application of the GABA$_B$ receptor agonist baclofen (10µM). The time course of effects of baclofen on the amplitude of the EPSPs are illustrated in C and **D**.

block the reversible pre- and postsynaptic actions of baclofen. Its effects on baclofen-induced LTD were unknown because this phenomenon had not been previously observed. Although the reversible effects of baclofen were blocked by prior exposure to 2-hydroxy-saclofen, the drug itself directly depressed the EPSPs evoked by either MLF or nVIII stimulation in a reversible manner, but did not block baclofen-induced LTD of the nVIII-evoked EPSP.

These results indicated that activation of $GABA_B$ receptors on MVN neurons produces both short- and long-lasting depression of the efficiency of transmission at the primary afferent second-order vestibular neuron synapse. Recently, a similar form of GABA-induced LTD was reported in hippocampal CA1 neurons that is insensitive to GABA antagonists but blocked by mGluR antagonists.[53] This observation raises the possibility that mGluRs may also contribute to the effects of baclofen in the MVN.

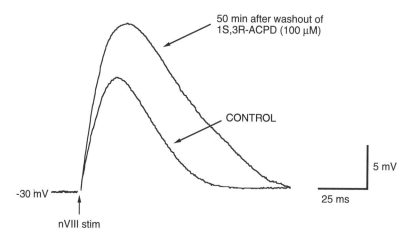

FIGURE 4. Long-term potentiation produced by activation of metabotropic glutamate receptors (mGluRs). This figure illustrates the EPSP evoked by nVIII stimulation recorded at −30 mV. The mGluR agonist 1S,3R-ACPD (100 μM) was bath-applied for 10 min. Traces illustrate the averaged EPSP (n = 6) before (Control) and 50 min after the washout of 1S,3R-ACPD. During the application of 1S,3R-ACPD, a modest depolarization (∼ 6 mV) and acute depression of EPSP amplitude were observed which readily reversed upon washout of the drug to reveal a potentiated reponse.

Subsequent work has revealed other candidate mechanisms for inducing the long-term modulation of vestibular afferent input. Having established a role for NMDA transmission in the MVN, we also examined the action of metabotropic glutamate receptors (mGluRs), which have been proposed to play a critical role in induction and/or maintenance of long-term plasticity in hippocampus[54,55] and cerebellum.[56] Following an initial reversible depression of the nVIII-evoked EPSP during a 10-min bath application of the mGluR agonist 1S,3R-ACPD (100 μM), a long-term potentiation of this EPSP was observed in 9 of the 13 cells examined to date (FIG. 4). This potentiation of the nVIII EPSP was not associated with changes in input resistance, and was observed for as long as stable recordings were maintained after washout of the drug (> 1 h).

CONCLUSIONS

Taken together, our simulations and *in vitro* recordings suggest two ways in which projections of GVPs to the vestibular nuclei could participate in adaptive adjustments of signal transmission between vestibular afferents and second order neurons involved in the VOR. First, simple spike signals related to ipsilateral gaze velocity carried by GABAergic GVP axons could modify the strength of vestibular afferent activation of VORNs and vestibulo-cerebellar projections via the $GABA_B$-induced LTD described above. A possible way for this to work would be via activation of presynaptic $GABA_B$ receptors on vestibular afferent terminals[48] by GABA released from GVP synaptic terminals adjacent to those primary afferent terminals as occurs in the hippocampus.[52] Our simulations indicate that for this to work properly, equal changes should be induced in vestibular actions upon VORNs and vesitbulo-cerebellar neurons. The high prevalence of $GABA_B$-induced LTD in the population of MVN neurons that we recorded suggests that such a combined action is possible, but to date no evidence exists that such changes actually occur *in vivo*. It also should be noted for $GABA_B$-induced LTD to participate in adaptive reductions in VOR gain it would have to function in a use-dependent fashion. LTD should only occur in those vestibular afferent terminals that are activated above their resting level at the same time that GABA release from GVP terminals is above its normal resting level. As of yet no attempt has been made to observe such effects.

The second mechanism by which projections of GVPs to the vestibular nuclei could participate in adaptive adjustments of signal transmission between vestibular afferents and second-order neurons involves their modulation of NMDA-mediated transmission between vestibular afferents and FTNs. If the latter receive most or all of their $GABA_A$ receptor-mediated inhibition from GVPs, the synchronous pause in discharge of those GVPs following activation of their climbing fibers by retinal slip signals could release $GABA_A$ receptor-mediated shunting of NMDA transmission on those neurons, causing an influx of calcium. This could then induce long-term potentiation (LTP) of vestibular afferent synaptic transmission to those neurons by mechanisms analogous to those involved in LTP in the hippocampus.[57] The brief burst of spikes in GVP axons that would precede the climbing fiber–related pause in discharge could further enhance this process by activating $GABA_B$ receptors on inhibitory terminals on the FTNs (cf. ref. 58), causing a further reduction in GABA inhibition during the critical post-climbing fiber discharge interval. A possible problem with the scenario is that NMDA receptor-mediated transmission in the hippocampus exhibits rapid desensitization, and hence is unable to follow rates of afferent activation much in excess of 10 Hz.[59,60] However, we recently observed that the NMDA-mediated component of nVIII activation of some MVN neurons is much more resistant to repetitive stimulation than would be expected from the properties of NMDA transmission in the hippocampus,[45] as shown in FIGURE 5. This may be related to differences in the subunit composition of NMDA receptors in the two cell types. It thus appears that NMDA-mediated transmission could participate in the modulation of transmission of signals by vestibular afferents, which commonly fire at rates of 100 Hz or more. As envisioned here, NMDA-related mechanisms would participate in increasing synaptic strength at afferent-VORN synapse as occurs during increase in VOR gain. It is therefore of interest that work in intact goldfish has shown that increases in VOR gain can be blocked by administration of the NMDA antagonist MK 801, whereas decreases in VOR gain are not affected by this agent.[61]

What might be the role of the mGluR-mediated LTP that we observed *in vitro?*

mGluRs are located at both pre- and postsynaptic sites at glutamatergic synapses.[62] As a consequence of this ultrastructural localization and the relatively low affinity of mGluRs for glutamate, postsynaptic mGluRs would be activated primarily by ambient levels of glutamate escaping from the cleft, and by glutamate diffusing from adjacent synapses. Thus, they would not be activated in the same manner as the ionotropic glutamate receptor subclasses mediating rapid synaptic currents following each presynaptic action potential. Instead, they would serve to "signal average" global activity levels at the synapse, or be activated by temporally coincident activity in glutamatergic afferents to the same microdomain of the dendritic tree, wherein a

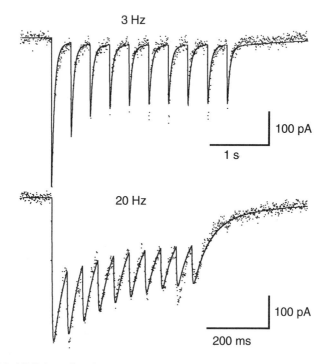

FIGURE 5. NMDA-mediated transmission between nVIII fibers and MVN neurons at two frequencies of afferent stimulation (3 and 20 Hz). Currents were recorded in whole-cell voltage-clamp (-80 mV) in the absence of extracellular magnesium from an MVN neuron using an electrode containing cesium and QX314 to block voltage-dependent conductances. DNQX (10 μM) and bicuculline (10 μM) were added to the bath to block AMPA and GABA$_A$ receptors, respectively. Superimposed upon the digitized EPSCs are fits produced by a kinetic model of NMDA transmission in MVN neurons that is being developed in collaboration with L. Eisenman and J. Houk.[63]

rapid rise of glutamate concentration would be produced. Such a scenario would predict that mGluR-mediated LTP in the MVN could occur both through homosynaptic activation by primary afferent fibers alone, and through heterosynaptic mechanisms. Because primary vestibular afferents normally fire at rates sufficient to induce homosynaptic LTP in other brain regions (> 100 Hz[57]), it would seem unlikely that such a phenomenon occurs in the MVN. Heterosynaptic interactions in which activity of vestibular afferents coincide with glutamatergic inputs from other sources, such as recurrent excitatory projections within the MVN,[39] would, therefore, provide a candidate mechanism by which mGluRs could contribute to vestibular reflex plasticity.

A final caveat is that our model-based analysis of VOR plasticity relies on the assumptions inherent in the gaze-velocity model originally proposed by Miles *et al.*[23] In our simulations, GVP cells respond in a linear fashion to the sum of head velocity and combined eye velocity command signals, and their learning rates are similar to those of VORNs. If GVPs were insensitive to changes in eye velocity produced by their actions on FTNs or if they adapted sufficiently quickly that they continued to signal gaze error regardless of the changes occurring in brain-stem VOR pathways, it is possible that their simple spike discharge could be used as a teacher signal to alter transmission in the latter pathways.

In closing, it must be stressed that these conclusions are very tentative. We are putting them forth here as suggestions for further investigations that we feel represent "new directions in vestibular research." Their primary value at present is to demonstrate the promise of combining systems modeling and cellular electrophysiological approaches in identifying neuronal substrates of learning in the VOR as well as in other sensorimotor systems.

REFERENCES

1. DAVIES, P. & G. MELVILL-JONES. 1976. An adaptive neural model compatible with plastic changes induced in the human vestibulo-ocular reflex by prolonged optical reversal of vision. Brain Res. **103:** 546–550.
2. ROBINSON, D. A. 1976. Adaptive gain control of vestibulo-ocular reflex by the cerebellum. J. Neurophysiol. **39:** 954–969.
3. MILES, F. A. & B. B. EIGHMY. 1980. Long-term adaptive changes in primate vestibulo-ocular reflex. I. Behavorial observations. J. Neurophysiol. **43:** 1406–1425.
4. COLLEWIJN, H., A. J. MARTINS & R. M. STEINMAN. 1983. Compensatory eye movements during active and passive head movements: Fast adaptation to changes in visual magnification. J. Physiol. (Lond.) **340:** 259–286.
5. LISBERGER, S. 1988. The neural basis for the learning of simple motor skills. Science **242:** 728–735.
6. ITO, M., P. J. JASTREBOFF & Y. MIYASHITA. 1979. Adaptive modification of the rabbit's vestibulo-ocular reflex during sustained vestibular and optokinetic stimulation. Exp. Brain Res. **37:** 17–30.
7. SCHULTHEIS, L. W. & D. A. ROBINSON. 1981. Directional plasticity of the vestibulo-ocular reflex in the cat. Ann. N.Y. Acad. Sci. **374:** 504–512.
8. HARRISON, R. E. W., J. F. BAKER, N. ISU, C. R. WICKLAND & B. W. PETERSON. 1986. Dynamics of adaptive change in vestibulo-ocular reflex direction. I. Rotations in the horizontal plane. Brain Res. **371:** 162–165.
9. BAKER, J., R. E. W. HARRISON, N. ISU, C. WICKLAND & B. PETERSON. 1986. Dynamics of adaptive change in vestibulo-ocular reflex direction. II. Sagittal plane rotations. Brain Res. **371:** 166–170.
10. LISBERGER, S., F. A. MILES & L. M. OPTICAN. 1983. Frequency-selective adaptation: Evidence for channels in the vestibulo-ocular reflex? J. Neurosci. **3:** 1234–1244.
11. POWELL, K. D., S. A. RUDE, K. J. QUINN, B. W. PETERSON & J. F. BAKER. 1989. Vestibulo-ocular reflex (VOR) direction adaptation to a phase shifted optokinetic stimulus. Soc. Neurocsci. Abstr. **15:** 211.6.
12. DEMER, J. L. 1981. The variable gain element of the vestibulo-ocular reflex is common to the optokinetic system of the cat. Brain Res. **229:** 1–13.
13. TILIKET, C., M. SHELHAMER, D. ROBERTS & D. S. ZEE. 1994. Short-term vestibulo-ocular reflex adaptation in humans. I. Effect on the ocular motor velocity-to-position neural integrator. Exp. Brain Res. **100:** 316–327.

14. LISBERGER, S., F. A. MILES, L. M. OPTICAN & B. B. EIGHMY. 1981. Optokinetic response in the monkey: Underlying mechanisms and their sensitivity to long-term adaptive changes in vestibulo-ocular reflex. J. Neurophysiol. 45: 869–890.

15. LISBERGER, S. 1984. The latency of pathways containing the site of motor learning in the monkey vestibulo-ocular reflex. Science 225: 74–76.

16. LISBERGER, S.G., T. A. PAVELKO, H. M. BRONTE-STEWART & L. S. STONE. 1994. Neural basis for motor learning in the vestibuloocular reflex of primates. II. Changes in the responses of horizontal gaze velocity Purkinje cells in the cerebellar flocculus and ventral paraflocculus. J. Neurophysiol. 72: 954–973.

17. KHATER, T. T., K. J. QUINN, J. PENA, J. F. BAKER & B. W. PETERSON. 1993. The latency of the cat vestibulo-ocular reflex before and after short and long term adaptation. Exp. Brain Res. 94: 16–32.

18. BROUSSARD, D. M. & S. G. LISBERGER. 1992. Vestibular inputs to brain stem neurons that participate in motor learning in the primate vestibuloocular reflex. J. Neurophysiol. 68: 1906–1909.

19. MILES, F. A., & D. J. BRAITMAN. 1980. Long-term adaptive changes in primate vestibulo-ocular reflex. II. Electrophysiological observations on semicircular canal primary afferents. J. Neurophysiol. 43: 1437–1476.

20. OPTICAN, L. M. & D. A. ROBINSON. 1980. Cerebellar dependent adaptive control of the primate saccadic system. J. Neurophysiol. 44: 1058–1076.

21. ZEE, D. S., Z. YAMAZAKI, P. H. BUTLER & G. GRUCER. 1981. Effects of ablation of flocculus and paraflocculus on eye movements in primate. J. Neurophysiol. 46: 878–899.

22. QUINN, K. J., J. F. BAKER & B. W. PETERSON. 1992. Simulation of cerebellar-vestibular interactions during VOR adaptation. Soc. Neurosci. Abstr. 504.5.

23. MILES, F. A., J. H. FULLER, D. J. BRAITMAN & B. M. DOW. 1980. Long-term adaptive changes in primate vestibuloocular reflex. III. Electrophysiological observations in flocculus of normal monkeys. J. Neurophysiol. 43: 1437–1476.

24. MILES, F. A., D. J. BRAITMAN & B. M. DOW. 1980. Long-term adaptive changes in primate vestibuloocular reflex. IV. Electrophysiological observations in flocculus of adapted monkeys. J. Neurophysiol. 43: 1477–1493.

25. BALABAN, C. D. 1988. Distribution of inferior olivary projections to the vestibular nuclei of albino rabbits. Neuroscience 24: 119–134.

26. BREMERMANN, H. 1970. A method of unrestrained global optimization. Math. Biosci. 9: 1–15.

27. LEVINE, D. S. 1991. Introduction to Neural and Cognitive Modeling. Lawrence Erlbaum Associates, Inc. Hillsdale, NJ.

28. MILES, F. A. & S. G. LISBERGER. 1981. The "error" signals subserving adaptive gain control in the primate vestibulo-ocular reflex. Ann. N.Y. Acad. Sci. 374: 513–525.

29. LISBERGER, S. G., T. A. PAVELKO & D. M. BROUSSARD. 1994. Neural basis for motor learning in the vestibuloocular reflex in primates. I. Changes in the responses of brain stem neurons. J. Neurophysiol. 72(2): 928–953.

30. LEONARD, C. S., J. I. SIMPSON & W. GRAF. 1988. Spatial organization of visual messages of the rabbit's cerebellar flocculus. I. Typology of inferior olive neurons of the dorsal cap of Kooy. J. Neurophysiol. 60: 2073–2090.

31. GRAF, W., J. I. SIMPSON & C. S. LEONARD. 1988. Spatial organization of visual messages of the rabbit's cerebellar flocculus. II. complex and simple spike responses of P cells. J. Neurophysiol. 60: 2091–2021.

32. STONE, L. S. & S. G. LISBERGER. 1990. Visual responses of Purkinje cells in the cerebellar flocculus during smooth-pursuit eye movements in monkeys. I. Complex spikes. J. Neurophysiol. 63: 1262–1275.

33. BREDT, D. S., P. M. HWANG & S. H. SNYDER. 1990. Localization of nitric oxid synthase indicating a neural role for nitric oxide. Nature 347: 768–770.

34. SUTTON, R. S. & A. G. BARTO. 1981. Toward a modern theory of adaptive networks: Expectation and prediction. Psychol. Rev. 88: 135–170.

35. EBNER, T. J. & J. R. BLOEDEL. 1981. Role of climbing fiber afferent input in determining the responsiveness of Purkinje cells to mossy fiber inputs. J. Neurophysiol. 45: 962–971.

36. LEWIS, M. R., P. SHINNICK-GALLAGHER & J. P. GALLAGHER. 1987. An in vitro brain slice

preparation to study the pharmacology of central vestibular neurons. J. Pharmacol. Methods **18:** 267–273.

37. LEWIS, M. R., K. D. PHELAN, P. SHINNICK-GALLAGHER & J. P. GALLAGHER. 1989. Primary afferent excitatory transmission recorded intracellularly *in vitro* from rat medial vestibular neurons. Synapse **3:** 149–153.

38. SERAFIN, M., C. DE WAELE, A. KHATEB, P. P. VIDAL & M. MÜHLTHALER. 1991. Medial vestibular nucleus in the guinea-pig. I. Intrinsic properties in brainstem slices. Exp. Brain Res. **84:** 417–425.

39. KINNEY, G. A., B. W. PETERSON & N. T. SLATER. 1994. The synaptic activation of *N*-methyl-D-aspartate receptors in the rat medial vestibular nucleus. J. Neurophysiol. **72:** 1588–1595.

40. BLANTON, M.G., J. J. LO TURCO & A. R. KRIEGSTEIN. 1989. Whole cell recording from neurons in slices of reptilian and mammalian cerebral cortex. J. Neurosci. Methods **30:** 203–210.

41. TAKAHASHI, Y., T. TSUMOTO & T. KUBO. 1994. *N*-methyl-D-aspartate receptors contribute to afferent synaptic transmission in the medial vestibular nucleus of young rats. Brain Res. **659:** 287–291.

42. MAYER, M. L. & G. L. WESTBROOK. 1987. The physiology of excitatory amino acids in the vertebrate central nervous systems. Prog. Neurobiol. **28:** 197–276.

43. JONAS, P. & N. SPRUTSON. 1994. Mechanisms shaping glutamate-mediated excitatory postsynaptic currents in the CNS. Curr. Opin. Neurobiol. **4:** 366–372.

44. ROSSI, D. J., S. ALFORD, E. MUGNAINI & N. T. SLATER. 1995. Properties of transmission at a giant glutamatergic synapse in cerebellum: The mossy fiber-unipolar brush cell synapse. J. Neurophysiol. **74:** 24–42.

45. SLATER, N. T., L. N. EISENMAN, G. A. KINNEY, B. W. PETERSON & J. C. HOUK. 1996. Glutamergic transmission in the medial vestibular nucleus. *In* Neurochemistry of the Vestibular System. A. J. Beitz & J. H. Anderson, Eds. CRC Press. In press.

46. SIVILOTTI, L. & A. NISTRI. 1991. GABA receptor mechanisms in the central nervous system. Prog. Neurobiol. **36:** 35–92.

47. BOWERY, N. G. 1993. GABA$_B$ receptor pharmacology. Annu. Rev. Pharmacol. Toxicol. **33:** 109–147.

48. HOLSTEIN, G. R., G. P. MARTENELLI & B. COHEN. 1992. Baclofen-sensitive GABA$_B$ binding sites in the medial vestibular nucleus localized by immunocytochemistry. Brain Res. **581:** 175–180.

49. GALLAGHER, J. P., K. D. PHELAN & P. SHINNICK-GALLAGHER. 1992. Modulation of excitatory transmission at the rat medial vestibular nucleus synapse. Ann. N.Y. Acad. Sci. **656:** 630–644.

50. NICOLL, R. A., R. C. MALENKA & J. A. KAUER. 1990. Functional comparison of neurotransmitter receptor subtypes in mammalian central nervous system. Physiol. Rev. **70:** 513–565.

51. BROOKS, P. A., S. R. GLAUM, R. J. MILLER & K. M. SPYER. 1992. The actions of baclofen on neurones and synaptic transmission in the nucleus tractus solitarii of the rate in vitro. J. Physiol. **457:** 115–129.

52. ISAACSON, J. S., J. M. SOLÍS & R. A. NICOLL. 1993. Local and diffuse synaptic actions of GABA in the hippocampus. Neuron **10:** 165–175.

53. YANG, X.-D., J. A. CONNOR & D. S. FABER. 1994. Weak excitation and simultaneous inhibition induce long-term depression in hippocampal CA1 neurons. J. Neurophysiol. **71:** 1586–1590.

54. BASHIR, Z. I., Z. A. BORTOLOTTO, C. H. DAVIES, N. BERRETTA, A. J. IRVING, J. M. HENLEY, D. E. JANE, J. C. WATKINS & G. L. COLLINGRIDGE. 1993. The synaptic activation of glutamate metabotropic receptors is necessary for the induction of LTP in the hippocampus. Nature **363:** 347–350.

55. LIU, Y. -B., J. F. DISTERHOFT & N. T. SLATER. 1993. Activation of metabotropic glutamate receptors induces long-term depression of GABAergic inhibition in hippocampus. J. Neurophysiol. **69:** 1000–1004.

56. LINDEN, D. J. 1994. Long-term synaptic depression in mammalian brain. Neuron **12:** 457–472.

57. BLISS, T. V. P. & G. L. COLLINGRIDGE. 1993. A synaptic model of memory: Long-term potentiation in the hippocampus. Nature **361:** 31–39.
58. DAVIES, C. H. & G. L. COLLINGRIDGE. 1993. The physiological regulation of synaptic inhibition by GABA$_B$ autoreceptors in rat hippocampus. J. Physiol. (Lond.) **472:** 245–265.
59. LESTER, R. A. J. & C. E. JAHR. 1992. NMDA channel behavior depends on agonist affinity. J. Neurosci. **12:** 635–643.
60. LESTER, R. A. J., J. D. CLEMENTS, G. L. WESTBROOK & C. E. JAHR. 1990. Channel kinetics determine the time course of NMDA receptor-mediated synaptic currents. Nature **346:** 565–567.
61. MCELLIGOTT, J. G., T. L. CARTER & R. BAKER. 1991. Effects of MK-801 on adaptive vestibulo-ocular reflex modifications in the goldfish. Soc. Neurosci. Abstr. **17:** 313.
62. PIN, J.-P. & R. DUVOISIN. 1995. The metabotropic glutamate receptors: Structure and function. Neuropharmacology **34:** 1–26.
63. EISENMAN, L. N., G. A. KINNEY, N. T. SLATER, B. W. PETERSON & J. C. HOUK. 1995. Temporal summation of NMDA current in the medial vestibular nucleus of the rat. Soc. Neurosci. Abstr. **21: 82.**

Role of the Y Group of the Vestibular Nuclei in Motor Learning or Plasticity of the Vestibulo-Ocular Reflex in the Squirrel Monkey

A. M. PARTSALIS AND STEPHEN M. HIGHSTEIN[a]

Department of Otolaryngology
Washington University School of Medicine
4566 Scott Avenue, Box 8115
St. Louis, Missouri 63110

INTRODUCTION

Plasticity of the vestibulo-ocular reflex (VOR) has been recognized as a model for motor learning since the first evidence for this adaptive behavior was presented in 1971 by Gonshor and Melvill-Jones.[1] A slow-phase eye movement of vestibular semicircular origin is certainly one of the simplest motor acts possible because no multi-jointed muscles are involved and the elicited movement can be limited to one dimension by controlling the plane of head rotation. Lorente de No[2] and Szent-agothai[3] demonstrated the "three-neuron arc," the main pathway subserving the reflex consisting of the vestibular nerve afferent, the vestibular nucleus relay neuron and the extraocular motoneuron. Subsequently a few more neurons have been included in the pathway; for example, Robinson[4] added the integrator of the VIIIth nerve head velocity signal to produce motoneuronal eye position signals, Scudder and Fuchs[5] and others demonstrated neurons interposed between the VIIIth nerve and the motoneurons carrying head and/or eye velocity signals, and the cerebellar flocculus has also been implicated.[6–9] Thus, there originated a clear and logical premise that changes in the patterns of discharge in these few, identifiable neurons might account for the changes in behavior (adaptation) of the reflex. This expected result has been elusive and the interpretations of experiments designed to prove or disprove the above premise have led to much contention.

Our laboratory continues to believe that adaptation of the VOR is the expression of changes in its underlying neural system and we have therefore chosen to seek these changes. To simplify the neural system test substrate, the vertical VOR and the corresponding vertical (V) zone of the flocculus were chosen for study. A brain-stem site, the Y group of the vestibular complex, a small nucleus situated ventromedially to the dentate nucleus of the cerebellum, was also chosen because it receives a dense projection from the flocculus; additionally, the Y group is activated disynaptically from the VIIIth nerve and provides a powerful excitatory projection to vertical extraocular motoneurons.[10–12]

The signal content conferred by the floccular input onto the Y group was assessed by pharmacological inactivation of the flocculus while recording from Y cells. Results indicate that the flocculus input to Y confers the visual following eye velocity signals normally present in the Y group. Further, results support the existence of a second

[a]Corresponding author. E-mail: highstein@WUMS.WUSTL.EDU

input to the Y group stemming from the vestibular nucleus, namely, a vertical canal head velocity signal. The brain utilizes head velocity information and visual information concerning target position and stability on the retina to compute an internal estimate of head velocity in space to produce the appropriate (i.e., compensatory) eye movement. This situation in the light may be looked upon as a *closed-loop* circumstance inasmuch as the visual system closes the loop between vestibular input and oculomotor output. When an animal is exposed to conflicting information from the visual and vestibular systems (visual-vestibular mismatch), it initially utilizes visually-driven mechanisms to correct its now inappropriate VOR. Such behavior will be called rapid modification of the VOR. Rapid modifications minimize retinal slip produced by the visual-vestibular mismatch; if such conditions persist, however, the *open-loop* gain of the reflex (measured during rotation in darkness) is gradually recalibrated to a new appropriate value, over a period of hours to days: this is the phenomenon of adaptation, or long-term modification of VOR gain.[1,13,14] Because the head velocity sensitivity of the VIIIth nerve does not change in the process of adaptation,[15] the central nervous system reconciles the visual and vestibular system mismatched signals by producing a different (that is, adapted) eye velocity command or output to vestibular stimulation. Experiments described below suggest that the Y group is one node of the vertical VOR system that expresses head velocity sensitivity changes with adaptation. On the other hand, the results also strongly suggest that changes, of probably greater magnitude, also occur in a side-path circuit involving the floccular V zone cortex.

METHODS

Y-group neuronal responses were studied in alert, behaving squirrel monkeys, using standard extracellular recording techniques. Animals were seated on a turntable (FIG. 1), surrounded by an optokinetic drum. Optokinetic (drum) and vestibular (table) stimuli were delivered sinusoidally. Turntable rotation elicited a vertical VOR eye movement, whereas drum motion elicited a visual following eye movement, which, at the frequency used here (0.5 Hz), can be considered closely related to smooth pursuit.[16,17] Combined movement of the turntable and drum resulted in VOR suppression when they were in phase and of equal amplitude, VOR enhancement when they were out of phase, and VOR reversal when the in-phase drum velocity was double that of the turntable. To induce adaptation of the VOR, the animals were fitted with lenses, either magnifying or reducing, and subjected to rotary paradigms and/or prolonged wearing of the lenses in their home cages. A flocculus chamber was placed over the cerebellum posteriorly to aid in the examination of the effects of electrical stimulation and of pharmacological inactivation of the flocculus on Y-group firing. A pair of 21-gauge syringes for muscimol infusion, bearing microelectrodes, was placed into the flocculus. The flocculus was identified by its characteristic discharges related to eye movement, and by the behavioral effects of electrical pulse train stimulation. To inactivate the flocculus, 2% muscimol in saline was injected. A 2% solution of muscimol abolished cell firing in the cerebellar cortex including complex spikes within a sphere of 4 mm approximate diameter centered on the injection site (see Partsalis *et al.*[17,18] for details about methods and experimental paradigms).

RESULTS

Input and Output Signals of Y Cells in the Naive Animal

Physiologically, the Y group is a homogeneous population of cells. In the squirrel monkey, the cells have a characteristic set of responses, very similar to those reported by Chubb and Fuchs[19] for the rhesus monkey. Typical discharge patterns in response to optokinetic, vestibular, and combined stimulation are shown in FIGURE 2. In naive animals, Y cells exhibit a very weak modulation during the VOR in darkness. They fire robustly during visual following, approximately in phase with eye velocity. During rapid modifications of the VOR, Y-group neurons reflect or predict the changes in eye velocity re:head velocity. During VOR suppression and reversal, firing is in

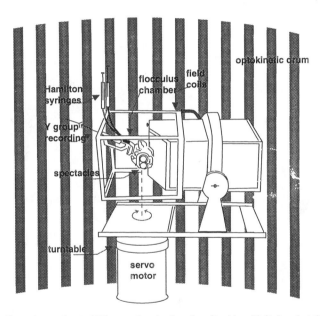

FIGURE 1. Experimental setup. The monkey is placed on its side with its head at the center of rotation. Spectacles are affixed to the head restraint device to cover the entire visual field. A standard metal microelectrode recording chamber is placed over the Y group, and a modified chamber bearing two Hamilton syringes placed over the flocculus.

phase with head velocity. During VOR enhancement, firing is out of phase with head velocity. Responses of 113 Y cells were recorded in five naive animals. Data for 16 cells from one animal, representative of the total population of cells, are presented in FIGURE 3A. In this polar plot the average response of each cell during the various paradigms is plotted with reference to head velocity (phase of 180 deg). It is clear that the phase of Y-cell firing changes from in-phase with head velocity during reversal and suppression of the VOR to out-of-phase during VOR enhancement. In FIGURE 3B the average eye velocity gain during each of the paradigms is plotted against drum velocity as a fraction of head velocity. The slope of the regression line

(0.71) is very close to the eye velocity gain during visual following, thus supporting the notion that visual-following mechanisms are used to modify the gain of the VOR. In FIGURE 3C, the mean gain of all 16 cells during each of the five paradigms is plotted against the corresponding eye velocity gain (eye velocity/head velocity). The slope is an expression of the contribution of the Y group in modulating eye velocity

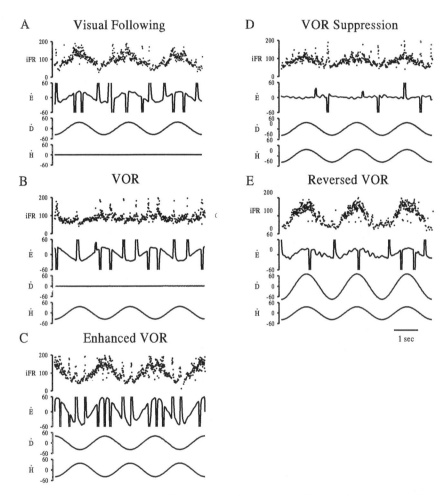

FIGURE 2. Responses of a typical Y-group cell during visual following, the vestibulo-ocular reflex (VOR) in darkness, VOR enhancement, suppression, and reversal. Traces in each panel, from the top down are instantaneous firing rate of the cell, vertical eye velocity, drum velocity, and head velocity.

during visual vestibular interaction. For this specific animal, firing of the Y group at 1.03 spikes/s was related to 1 deg/s of rapid modification of eye velocity during visual-vestibular interaction. The same cells fired at 1.10 spikes/s per deg/s of eye velocity during visual following. The numerical proximity of the two gains, taken

A

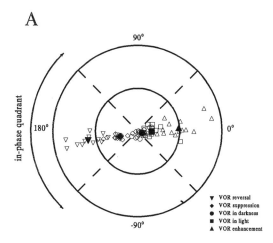

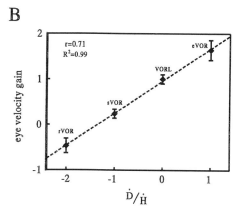

FIGURE 3. (A) Polar plot of responses of 16 Y cells during vestibulo-ocular reflex (VOR) reversal (*inverse triangles*), VOR suppression (*diamonds*), the VOR in darkness and in light (*circles* and *squares,* respectively), and VOR enhancement (*triangles*). Radii of the two circles are 1 and 2 spikes/s/deg/s. Head velocity phase is 180 deg. (B) Mean gain of eye velocity during four paradigms of visual-vestibular interaction plotted against drum velocity as a fraction of head velocity. (C) Mean gain of all 16 cells of FIGURE 2B during each paradigm is plotted against the corresponding eye velocity gain (eye velocity/head velocity; the convention used is that eye velocity in phase with head velocity is negative).

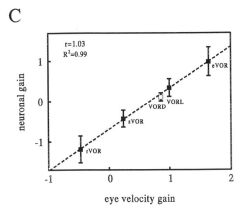

together with behavioral evidence,[16,17] suggests that firing of the Y group during rapid modifications of the VOR represents action of visual-following mechanisms, utilized to modify the outcome of the vestibular command.

The contribution of the flocculus to the signal content of the Y group was examined directly, by comparing the responses of single Y cells, before and after temporary pharmacological inactivation of the ipsilateral cerebellar flocculus. Muscimol, a $GABA_A$ agonist, was used to inactivate the flocculus. Raw data from one such experiment is shown in FIGURE 4, where the left-hand panels are the control

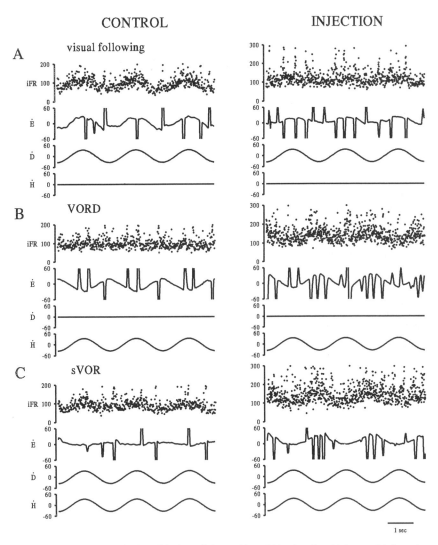

FIGURE 4. Responses of a Y cell before (*left panels*) and 13 min after (*right panels*) flocculus inactivation. Traces as in FIGURE 2.

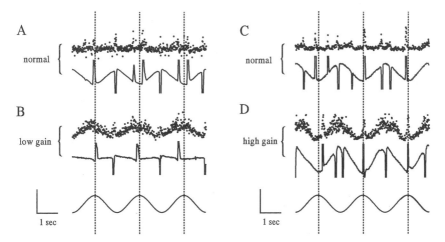

FIGURE 5. Responses of Y cells during the vestibulo-ocular reflex (VOR) in darkness. Panels **A** and **B** are cells recorded from the same animal, in its normal (naive) state (**A**) and after high-gain adaptation of the VOR (**B**). Panels **C** and **D** are cells from a second animal, in its normal state (**C**) and after low-gain adaptation (**D**).

responses of a Y cell and the right-hand panels the responses of the same cell after flocculus inactivation. The cell lost its signal during visual following (FIG. 4A), as well as during VOR suppression (FIG. 4C), while there was a modest increase in modulation during the VOR in darkness (FIG. 4B). Results from five cells in these three naive animals were similar, showing (1) usually minor effects on Y-cell responses during the VOR in darkness, (2) loss of the response during visual following and rapid VOR modifications, and (3) increased dc level of firing.

Three of the five cells retained, or even increased, their modulation during the VOR in darkness following flocculus inactivation. Taking into account that Y cells are activated at a disynaptic latency following electrical stimulation of both labyrinths,[20] we attribute this retained response to an unmasked vestibular input. In other words, the head velocity signal from the vestibular nuclei was revealed by the inactivation of the flocculus input to the Y group. In the absence of the visual-following input from the flocculus, the response of Y cells due to their vestibular input was the same under different visual conditions: Y cells now showed the same modulation during the VOR in darkness as during VOR suppression or enhancement.

Input and Output Signals of Y Cells in the Adapted Animal

Y-cell responses were recorded in three animals whose VORs had been adapted. Comparison with normal (naive) responses from the same three animals revealed dramatic differences in Y-group firing. In animals adapted to high VOR gain, Y cells fire robustly during the VOR in darkness, with a phase roughly opposite to that of head velocity. In animals adapted to low VOR gain, Y cells also show pronounced modulation, but with a phase approximating that of head velocity. FIGURE 5 shows recordings from two animals, before and after VOR adaptation: panels A and C are responses in two normal (naive) animals, and panels B and D are responses after the two animals were adapted to high (D), or low VOR gain (B).

Y cells monosynaptically excite extraocular motoneurons of the superior rectus and inferior oblique muscles. Thus, firing of Y cells out of phase with head velocity acts to augment VOR gain, whereas firing in phase with head velocity diminishes VOR gain, and, accordingly the observed patterns of Y-group firing after adaptation of the VOR are in the "correct" direction to support the behavioral changes.

Therefore, the Y group is one set of premotor cells that express adapted signals. How is this adapted output of the Y group produced? Since the flocculus projects to the Y group, one possibility is that adapted signals are conveyed to the Y group from the flocculus. Alternatively, the adapted signals might be conveyed to the Y group from its vestibular input source. We addressed the question by assessing the contribution of the flocculus to the adapted response of Y cells, using the same technique of pharmacological inactivation of the flocculus described above. The abolition of Y-cell response during visual following was used as the primary index of the efficacy of the injections. Histological verification of the injection sites and reconstruction of the presumed sphere of muscimol spread were also performed. In all cases Y-group cells lost their visual following eye velocity sensitivity, thus indicating that the flocculus projection to the Y group was inactivated.

Two animals were adapted to low, and one to high, VOR gain. As described above, modulation of Y cells during the VOR in darkness is in phase with head velocity in low-gain adaptation, and out of phase with head velocity in high-gain adaptation. A total of 12 cells were studied.

Flocculus inactivation invariably resulted in loss of the adapted responses of the 12 Y cells studied. This loss was complete in one animal (adapted to low gain, 4 cells). In the two other animals, the average loss of the learned response of Y cells amounted to 35% (animal adapted to low gain, 3 cells) and are only estimates of the contribution of the flocculus to the adapted responses of the Y group, because release of Y cells from tonic floccular inhibition and the putative head velocity signal of gaze velocity Purkinje cells might allow the vestibular input to produce a response of greater amplitude than with an intact system.

DISCUSSION

Modification of the gain of the VOR involves the process of the learning of a new VOR gain and the subsequent storage of this learned behavior. It is well known that surgical removal of the flocculus prevents further modification of the VOR, but because surgery is permanent and the brain is thus damaged the nervous system might have time to adjust to its new condition without the flocculus. To assess the effects of *acute* flocculectomy on the adapted VOR gain, a temporary flocculectomy was performed utilizing pharmacological inactivation with muscimole. The learned behavior and the underlying learned neural behavior of Y-group cells were subsequently assayed. Following flocculectomy, in two animals a portion of the behavior and of the neural learning was preserved, whereas in a third animal the behavior and the Y-group firing reverted to their control, pre-learning state. There are two possible explanations or interpretations of these findings. Because temporary flocculectomy modified the learned state, a part of the neural changes underlying adaptation of the VOR might have occurred at the level of the cerebellar cortex, or, alternatively, changes might have occurred in the brain stem and have been relayed via the flocculus to the Y group. Inactivation of the flocculus prevents transmission through this pathway, thereby opening the neural loop or side-path circuit through the flocculus. Because transmission through the cerebellum is interdicted, the present experimental paradigm cannot discriminate between the two possibilities: (1) storage of the learned behavior in the flocculus and (2) transmission of the learned behavior from an outside storage site through the flocculus. To prove that the floccular cortex had actually learned something would require an independent test of the excitability of this part of the VOR circuitry or some other experimental paradigm. This has not yet been done. However, the positive result—that of retention of some of the learning in the firing of Y cells following floccular inactivation—strongly suggests that at least a part of the learning of the neural changes underlying motor learning of the VOR occurs in the brain stem.

That part of the adapted response of Y cells was preserved following flocculus inactivation suggests that this part was independent of the flocculus. We believe that this result reflects changes in the strength of the vestibular input expressed through the Y group. This input was related to upward head velocity in the animal adapted to low gain, and downward head velocity in the animal adapted to high gain. One hypothesis is that the Y group receives input from both upward and downward head velocity neurons of the vestibular nucleus. In the process of adaptation, one of these two inputs may get stronger while the other gets weaker, producing a net input of upward head velocity in low-gain and downward head velocity in high-gain adaptation. Miles and Lisberger[9] have hypothesized that the output signal of the flocculus may serve as a "teacher" signal to correct the inappropriate response of brain-stem neurons to a fixed vestibular input. As shown above, the flocculus provides Y cells with an input signal related to visual following. Visual following is employed by the animal to correct inappropriate VOR gain, and it could guide modifications of the vestibular inputs to the Y group. After completion of the adaptation, floccular input would not be necessary for maintenance of such changes. To support this hypothesis, the next experimental step is to characterize the vestibular nucleus neurons that project to the Y group, and to examine the potency of their projections onto the Y group in normal and adapted animals.

The present study showed that the Y group, one of the cell groups projecting to vertical extraocular motoneurons, carries signals related to adaptation of the VOR. Whether this is true for other, or all, premotoneuronal cell groups is at present unclear. However, some evidence exists relating to this issue. A second class of cells receiving floccular input are the "flocculus target neurons" (FTNs) of the superior vestibular nucleus.[21,22] As discussed above, floccular output changes with adaptation. It is thus highly likely that FTNs also carry adapted signals to the motoneurons. One possible objection is that FTNs receive input from Purkinje cells not involved in adaptation, different from the Purkinje cells projecting to the Y group. However, flocculus inactivation experiments[17,18,21,22] suggest that the signal content of the floccular projections to the Y group and FTNs are quite similar (in naive animals, at least), and Simpson and colleagues[23] have described Purkinje cells in the rabbit flocculus that synapse onto both Y cells and FTNs. We therefore believe that FTNs are also involved in adaptation of the VOR, because they probably relay part of the changed output of the flocculus to the motoneurons. There is no evidence, however, concerning changes occurring at FTNs, as suggested above for Y-group cells, because the synapses carrying head velocity information to the Y group and FTNs are quite different: FTNs receive input from primary afferents, whereas Y cells receive input from vestibular nucleus interneurons.

The Y group contributes to both rapid modifications of the VOR and adaptation of motor learning. We may define an index of the contribution of the Y group to modification of VOR gain, either rapid or adaptive, as the ratio of the difference in neuronal gain (gain during the modification paradigm minus gain during the normal

VOR in darkness) over the difference in behavioral gain. This index of Y-group contribution to behavior increases with VOR adaptation. For instance, in one monkey mean Y response during suppression of the VOR to 0.24 deg/s was 0.43 spikes/s/deg/s. After adaptation gain of the VOR in darkness, gain was 0.27 (very close to suppression in the normal state), but mean Y response gain was 0.70 spikes/s/deg/s. The calculated index of Y-group contribution increased from 0.52 to 1.00 (absolute value), an increase of 94%. The increase was 42 and 81%, respectively,

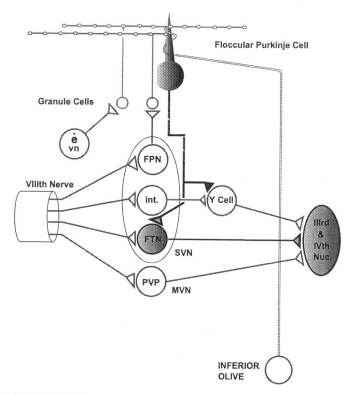

FIGURE 6. Simplified diagram of the system producing the vertical vestibulo-ocular reflex (VOR). We suggest the existence of two modifiable circuits in the double loop involving the Y group, one via the cerebellar cortex and one via the Y group. It is likely that the FPN-flocculus-FTN loop also participates in plasticity. A third pathway to the motor neurons (possibly including PVP cells) is not related to the flocculus and is not directly involved in adaptation of the vertical VOR.

in the other two adapted animals. The fact that the Y group increases its contribution to eye movement with adaptation may be explained by supposing that other pools of premotoneuronal cells do not change their firing patterns with adaptation, and thus the Y group assumes a greater burden. Therefore, indirect evidence suggests that premotoneuronal cells other than the Y group are likely to also contribute to adaptation (the FTNs), while it is also likely that the responses of a different pool of premotoneuronal cells (a candidate might be position vestibular-pause cells) do not change with adaptation.

A simple schematic representation of the VOR circuit is shown in FIGURE 6. Although the vestibular nucleus neurons projecting to the Y group have not yet been identified, we believe it will be proved that they carry head velocity signals, much like FPNs. In fact, as the case is with other types of mossy fibers that send collaterals to the deep cerebellar nuclei, FPNs may project to both flocculus and the Y group.

An obvious question is why should there be multiple mechanisms and brain sites underlying VOR adaptation? A probable answer lies in the consideration of the evolution of the system. In primitive vertebrates there was no visual following or ocular pursuit and therefore no visual following eye velocity signals were found in the brain stem or cerebellum. With the advent of the fovea and the pursuit system, greater complexity of visual vestibular interaction was necessary, and the neural mechanisms responsible for this more complex behavior were superimposed upon the existing brain architecture. Novel mechanisms of plasticity were thus also necessary to keep the system calibrated. The vestibulo-ocular system has several putative mechanisms that it might rely upon, namely, behavioral error or retinal slip on the one hand and constant visually-driven effort to correct inappropriate gain on the other. A process based on error only might deprive an animal of steady vision during the adaptation period. Therefore, a mechanism based on constantly correcting gain may seem more advantageous behaviorally. Visual following or pursuit, on which such a mechanism relies, may occasionally not be sufficient even for rapid VOR modifications. For example, humans wearing spectacles may suffer oscillopsia during the first few days.[24] Another possibility is that long-term changes that such a mechanism may produce (such as the flocculus-independent part of Y group adaptation) might saturate before the completion of adaptation. The central nervous system might then use the ensuing retinal slip to aid in changes expressed via the cerebellar cortex to complete or complement the process of adaptation.

REFERENCES

1. GONSHOR, A. & G. MELVILL-JONES. 1971. Plasticity in the adult human vestibulo-ocular reflex arc. Proc. Can. Fed. Biol. Soc. **14:** 11.
2. LORENTE DE NO, R. 1933. Vestibulo-ocular reflex arc. Arch. Neurol. Psychiatry **30:** 245–291.
3. SZENTAGOTHAI, J. 1950. The elementary vestibulo-ocular reflex arc. J. Neurophysiol. **13:** 395–407.
4. ROBINSON, D. A. 1981. Control of eye movements. *In* The Nervous System, Handbook of Physiology **2(2):** 1275–1320. Williams & Wilkins. Baltimore, MD.
5. SCUDDER, C. A. & A. F. FUCHS. 1992. Physiological and behavioral identification of vestibular nucleus neurons mediating the horizontal vestibuloocular reflex in trained rhesus monkeys. J. Neurophysiol. **68:** 244–264.
6. ITO, M. 1972. Neural design of the cerebellar motor control system. Brain Res. **40:** 81–84.
7. ITO, M. 1982. Cerebellar control of the vestibulo-ocular reflex: Around the flocculus hypothesis. Annu. Rev. Neurosci. **5:** 275–296.
8. ROBINSON, D. A. 1976. Adaptive gain control of vestibulo-ocular reflex by the cerebellum. J. Neurophysiol. **39:** 954–969.
9. MILES, F. A. & S. G. LISBERGER. 1981. Plasticity in the VOR: A new hypothesis. Annu. Rev. Neurosci. **4:** 273–299.
10. HIGHSTEIN, S. M. 1973. The organization of the vestibulo-oculomotor and trochlear reflex pathways in the rabbit. Exp. Brain Res. **17:** 285–300.
11. LANGER, T., A. F. FUCHS, M. C. CHUBB, C. A. SCUDDER & S. G. LISBERGER. 1985. Floccular efferents in the rhesus macaque as revealed by autoradiography and horseradish peroxidase. J. Comp. Neurol. **235:** 26–37.

12. SATO, Y. & T. KAWASAKI. 1987. Target neurons of floccular caudal zone inhibition in Y-group nucleus of vestibular nuclear complex. J. Neurophysiol. **57:** 460–480.
13. ITO, M., T. SHIIDA, N. YAGI & M. YAMAMOTO. 1974. The cerebellar modification of rabbit's horizontal vestibulo-ocular reflex induced by sustained head rotation combined with vestibular stimulation. Proc. Jpn. Acad. **50:** 85–89.
14. MILES, F. A. & B. B. EIGHMY. 1980. Long term adaptive changes in primate VOR. I. Behavioral observations. J. Neurophysiol. **43:** 1406–1425.
15. MILES, F. A., J. H. FULLER, D. J. BRAITMAN & B. M. DOW. 1980. Long term adaptive changes in primate VOR. III. Electrophysiological observations in flocculus of normal monkeys. J. Neurophysiol. **43:** 1437–1476.
16. PAIGE, G. D. 1983. Vestibulo-ocular reflex and its interactions with visual following mechanisms in the squirrel monkey. I. Response characteristics in normal animals. J. Neurophysiol. **49:** 134–151.
17. PARTSALIS, A. M., Y. ZHANG & S. M. HIGHSTEIN. 1995. Dorsal Y group in the squirrel monkey. I. Neuronal responses during rapid and long-term modifications of the VOR. J. Neurophysiol. **73:** 615–631.
18. PARTSALIS, A. M., Y. ZHANG & S. M. HIGHSTEIN. 1995. Dorsal Y group in the squirrel monkey. II. Contribution of the flocculus to neuronal responses in normal and adapted animals. J. Neurophysiol. **73:** 632–650.
19. CHUBB, M. C. & A. F. FUCHS. 1982. Contribution of Y group of vestibular nuclei and dentate nucleus of cerebellum to generation of vertical smooth eye movements. J. Neurophysiol. **48:** 75–99.
20. BLAZQUEZ, P. M., A. M. PARTSALIS & S. M. HIGHSTEIN. 1994. Vestibular inputs to the dorsal Y group nucleus in the squirrel monkey. Neurosci. Abstr. **20:** 1192.
21. ZHANG, Y., A. M. PARTSALIS & S. M. HIGHSTEIN. 1995. Properties of superior vestibular nucleus flocculus target neurons in the squirrel monkey. I. General properties in comparison to flocculus projecting neurons. J. Neurophysiol. **73:** 2261–2278.
22. ZHANG, Y., A. M. PARTSALIS & S. M. HIGHSTEIN. 1995. Properties of superior vestibular nucleus flocculus target neurons in the squirrel monkey. II. Signal components revealed by reversible flocculus inactivation. J. Neurophysiol. **73:** 2279–2292.
23. DE ZEEUW, C. I., D. R. WYLIE, P. L. DIGIORGI & J. I. SIMPSON. 1994. Projections of individual Purkinje cells of identified zones in the flocculus to the vestibular and cerebellar nuclei in the rabbit. J. Comp. Neurol. **349:** 428–447.
24. ZEE, D. S. 1981. The vestibulo-ocular reflex: Clinical concepts. *In* Models of Ocular Motor Behavior and Control. B. Zuber, Ed.: 257–278. CRC Press. Long Beach, CA.

Motor Learning and Memory in the Vestibulo-Ocular Reflex: The Dark Side

STEPHEN G. LISBERGER[a]

*Department of Physiology and W. M. Keck Foundation Center
for Integrative Neuroscience
University of California, San Francisco
San Francisco, California*

Long-term adaptive changes in the vestibulo-ocular reflex (VOR) consist of separate processes that we refer to as "learning" and "memory." Memory refers to the static state measured by the "gain" of the VOR, which is defined as eye speed divided by head speed during passive head turns in the dark. Learning refers to the dynamic process that occurs during head turns in the light and that leads to changes in the gain of the VOR.

We now have a unifying hypothesis that accounts for virtually all available data relevant to the sites of memory in the VOR. A combination of behavioral experiments, single-unit recordings, and computer simulations has led to a model in which long-term adaptive changes in the gain of the VOR are caused by cellular changes in the vestibular pathways through both the brain stem and the cerebellum.[1] One of the strengths of the model is that it reproduces seemingly contradictory data obtained by Watanabe[2] and Miles *et al.*[3] in recordings from the Purkinje cells in the floccular lobe of the cerebellum. A series of recent papers[1,4–7] includes the detailed data on which our current hypothesis is based as well as explanations of all aspects of our model. The present paper will not attempt to summarize those papers. Instead, it will consider what we do not know.

Is Our Understanding of the Function of the Floccular Lobe Incorrect because We Have Failed To Study Groups of Purkinje Cells That Make Fundamental Contributions of Which We Are Not Aware?

One important issue that has come to light recently is the fact that the floccular lobe consists of both the flocculus and the ventral paraflocculus and the question as to which part of the floccular lobe is relevant for the VOR—the ventral paraflocculus, the flocculus, or both.[8] Initial attention to the possible role of the cerebellum in motor learning in the VOR was based on experiments in nonprimates showing connections from the flocculus to the brain-stem VOR pathways (e.g., ref. 9). The most extensive physiological analysis of the role of the floccular lobe in learning has been conducted in primates and has focused heavily, but not extensively, on the ventral paraflocculus. It is possible, as suggested by Nagao,[10] that the flocculus proper plays the most important role in motor learning in the VOR, even in primates, and that we do not have recordings to form a basis for understanding that role. Existing data, including those of Nagao,[10] fail to support or refute this possibility. There is circumstantial evidence that the flocculus and ventral parafloccu-

[a]Address correspondence to Stephen G. Lisberger, Department of Physiology, Box 0444, UCSF, San Francisco, CA 94143. E-mail: sgl@phy.ucsf.edu

lus mediate similar functions (reviewed in ref. 6), but models based heavily on data recorded in the ventral paraflocculus must be tested by analysis of the flocculus proper. Because the flocculus and ventral paraflocculus have similar anatomical inputs and outputs, with the exception of their visual mossy fiber inputs, it seems unlikely to me that the two parts of the floccular lobe mediate fundamentally different functions.

In my opinion, a more serious question concerns a substantial group of Purkinje cells that are found throughout the floccular lobe but have not been analyzed for changes in responses in association with learning in the VOR. Previous studies in trained monkeys have focused on horizontal gaze velocity Purkinje cells (HGVPs), which discharge in relation to eye velocity with respect to the world (defined as "gaze" velocity) under a variety of visual tracking conditions as well as during the VOR in the dark. Little is known about frequently encountered Purkinje cells that discharge primarily in relation to eye movement (rather than gaze movement) when the gain of the VOR is normal[11] (also, J. Raymond and S. G. Lisberger, unpublished observations). In my opinion, data from rabbits suggest that learning will cause changes in the firing rate of primate Purkinje cells that are not HGVPs during the VOR in the dark, and those changes will be similar to the changes already documented in HGVPs. The basis for this assertion is that (1) most of the Purkinje cells recorded in the rabbit flocculus discharge primarily in relation to eye movement[12] and therefore resemble a large group of non-HGVPs in the monkey, and (2) changes in the gain of the VOR have the same effect on Purkinje cell responses measured during the VOR in the dark in rabbits[13] and in monkeys.[2,3,6] Still, experiments need to be done to determine the effects of motor learning on non-HGVPs in both the flocculus and the ventral paraflocculus.

Is It Incorrect to Model the Mechanism of Memory as a Change in the Strength of Synaptic Transmission?

It has been most common to think of the mechanism of memory in the VOR as a cellular volume control. For example, we often think and talk about changes in "synaptic efficacy," which presumably means either changes in the amount of transmitter released or in the amount of synaptic current caused by a given amount of transmitter. Our model, as well as some recent data obtained with electrical stimulation of the vestibular apparatus, argues that this concept is too simple for the mechanism of memory in the VOR. In a simplified model of the VOR, for example, changes in the time course of vestibular transmission through the floccular lobe were the only mechanism that allowed HGVPs to show changes in their responses during the VOR in the dark like those recorded in the monkey.[7] In the model, decreases in the gain of the VOR were produced by decreasing the strength of vestibular transmission through the HGVPs while at the same time making the time course more transient. This had the effect of strengthening transmission early in the response to a head turn (or for high-frequency stimuli) and weakening transmission later in the response (or for low-frequency stimuli). If learning-related changes in the time course of neural signals can be documented in recordings from the brain, then it will be necessary to determine whether changes in time course are direct effects of the cellular mechanisms of plasticity. As an alternative, changes in the time course of signals could result from conventional synaptic potentiation or depression at a site that is embedded within recurrent neural networks.

Recordings of the eye movements evoked by stimulation of the vestibular apparatus with single electrical pulses are not compatible with models in which the mechanism of memory in the VOR is a large change in the strength of vestibular transmission. Quantitative analysis of the effect of changes in the gain of the VOR on these eye movements led Broussard et al.[14] to conclude that learning was expressed in the earliest part of the response and therefore resided in the most direct brain-stem VOR pathways, which are disynaptic. However, the magnitude of those changes was tiny by comparison with the companion changes in the gain of the VOR evoked by head turns in darkness. In contrast, motor learning in the VOR caused changes in the size of the eye movements evoked by electrical stimulation with 100-ms trains of pulses comparable in size to the changes in the gain of the VOR evoked by head turns.[15] It is not clear how to fit these findings with models in which the mechanism of learning is simply long-term potentiation or depression such as those now well studied in the hippocampus or cerebellum. The results of our experiments with electrical stimulation imply that the mechanism of memory in the VOR involves temporal summation and facilitation that works only with multiple pulses. Possible implementations of such a mechanism might include (1) a change in the dynamics of the cellular processing that converts synaptic current into trains of action potentials and (2) small amounts of synaptic potentiation or depression that are amplified gradually by recurrent feedback loops, either within the network that constitutes the "velocity-to-position" integrator in the brain stem, or in the eye velocity positive feedback loop between the brain stem and the floccular lobe.

Is Retinal Slip Required for Learning in the Vestibulo-Ocular Reflex?

To determine the sites of memory for the VOR, the question of the error signals that guide learning is probably of minor importance. To go on, however, to the question of the mechanisms of learning, it will be essential to know the details of the signals that guide learning. This will entail behavioral analysis of the "error" signals that guide learning as well as identification of the central representation of those error signals.

The behavioral learning rule for the VOR is generally thought to be:

Retinal image motion + head turns → learning

If head motion and image motion are in the same direction, then the gain of the VOR is too large and needs to decrease. If head motion and image motion are in opposite directions, then the gain of the VOR is too small and needs to increase. The tacit assumption of such a learning rule is that, in the brain, temporal conjunction of signals related to image motion and head turns causes cellular changes that lead to learning. Miles and Lisberger[16] raised the possibility that retinal slip might not be of primary importance in monkeys and that a central signal related to tracking eye movements might substitute for image motion. They had in mind the "gaze velocity" output from the floccular lobe as a potential error signal to guide learning at the vestibular inputs to the floccular target neurons. In support of this idea, subsequent experiments found that changes in the gain of the VOR occurred when retinal image motion was minimized by having monkeys track small targets in a dark room during passive head turns for several days.[17] If the target moved exactly with the monkey (times zero tracking), then the gain of the VOR decreased. If the target moved opposite to the monkey (times two tracking), then the gain of the VOR increased. However, there were certainly small retinal slips during the tracking conditions, so that this set of experiments reveals only the sufficiency of visual inputs from small targets for learning in the VOR.

The identification of floccular target neurons and the evidence for one site of memory in the vestibular inputs to floccular target neurons renews the question of error signals that might guide learning in the brain stem. Although the gaze velocity output from the floccular lobe is still an attractive candidate to guide learning in floccular target neurons, it has one major drawback. Any ideal error signal should be present under conditions when the gain of the VOR is supposed to change and absent under conditions when the VOR is appropriate. This means that the error signal should be unmodulated during the VOR in the dark, no matter the gain of the VOR. The gaze velocity output from the floccular passes this test when the gain of the VOR is 1.0, but fails after large increases or decreases in the gain of the VOR. For example, after decreases in the gain of the VOR, the gaze velocity output from the floccular lobe remains modulated during the VOR in the dark, and the phase relationship between this signal and head velocity would promote further decreases in the gain of the VOR. This prediction has not been tested directly, but it seems inconceivable that head rotation in darkness would continue to reduce the gain of the VOR in a monkey that already has a lowered VOR gain! I do not have an solution for this problem. I raise it to illustrate the potential complexity of the neural conditions that guide learning, in contrast to the apparent simplicity of the behavioral learning rule.

Are There Sites of Learning for the Vestibulo-Ocular Reflex That Are Not Sites of Memory?

It has been common to use "learning" and "memory" interchangeably and to assume that any site of learning will also be a site of memory. For classical conditioning of the eyelid reflexes, Perrett and Mauk[18] have suggested a plausible scenario that would allow sites of learning where long-term memory would not necessarily be expressed. Transformed into the terminology of the VOR, their suggestion is that learning occurs both in the cerebellar cortex and the brain stem, but that the learning in the cerebellar cortex causes changes in Purkinje cell simple-spike output that are used as error signals to promote learning in the brain stem. Eventually, the memory that starts in the cerebellum would be transferred partially and possibly completely to the brain stem. Depending on the relative rates of learning in the cerebellar cortex and the brain stem, the degree to which memory is found in the two sites would depend on when the measurements were made relative to the time course of adaptation. For example, recordings from the cerebellum after months of adaptation to magnifying or miniaturizing spectacles might fail to reveal any expression of the changes in the gain of the VOR, even though the same experiments have revealed substantial expressions of memory at earlier times.[2,6,11] In a similar vein, experiments that recorded continuously the responses of HGVPs during cancellation of the VOR from the very beginning of learning might reveal that an initial change in vestibular sensitivity in the direction predicted by Ito,[19] followed by changes in the direction found by Miles et al.[3] after days or weeks of learning.

Can Simple Mechanisms of Plasticity, such as Cerebellar Long-Term Depression or Hippocampal Long-Term Potentiation Be Made To Work in a Real Brain?

In the current world of neuroscience, we converse easily in the jargon of cellular mechanisms of plasticity (e.g., "LTP," long-term potentiation, and "LTD," long-term depression) that are studied in vitro, in slices of brain tissue. At the same time, we have only just begun to try to fit the simplified mechanisms studied in dishes into the harsh reality of the intact, functioning brain. Given the highly reduced situations in which candidate cellular mechanisms of learning have been studied, it seems impossible to predict how or if they will work in a real brain. How, for example, might LTP or LTD work in the brain stem or the cerebellar cortex under conditions where neurons are spontaneously active and receive multiple inputs related to head turns, eye movement, and image motion, but where only one of those inputs should be subject to modification? Is it possible to elevate cellular mechanisms of plasticity, as studied *in vitro,* into cellular mechanisms of behavioral learning that operate *in vivo* at specific sites with required specificity given available neural error signals?

Du Lac *et al.*[20] have provided a detailed analysis of this problem for learning in the VOR, both in the cerebellar cortex and the brain stem. They concluded that the existing mechanisms, as understood from *in vitro* experiments, require considerable modification to operate in neurons that are spontaneously active. More importantly, they concluded that the mechanisms of plasticity that have been studied lacked the specificity required to cause changes in vestibular but not eye movement or visual signals at the putative sites of learning for the VOR.

Raymond and Lisberger[21] have shown that the relative timing of visual and vestibular input signals is one major problem that must be addressed in fitting cellular mechanisms of plasticity into neural networks that mediate behavioral learning. Previous hypotheses have suggested that the climbing-fiber input to Purkinje cells would provide an error signal to guide learning in the cerebellar cortex (e.g., ref. 19), whereas the simple-spike firing of the same cells would provide an error signal to guide learning in the brain stem.[11] By comparing the responses of HGVPs in behavioral paradigms that cause increases or decreases in the gain of the VOR, Raymond and Lisberger[21] have revealed the stimulus conditions under which the simple-spike and complex-spike firing of HGVPs would be useful error signals. As expected from earlier recordings, the phase relationship between head velocity and either simple-spike or complex-spike firing provided useful information about whether the gain of the VOR should be increased or decreased when the head and a large visual texture were oscillated sinusoidally at 0.5 Hz. At this frequency, either the simple spikes or the complex spikes would provide a useful error signal. When the head and visual texture moved sinusoidally at 5 Hz, however, the results posed new challenges for thinking about the mechanisms of learning in the VOR. First, the simple-spike modulation of the HGVPs provided little or no useful information about whether to increase or decrease the gain of the VOR. Second, the phase shift between complex-spike firing and head velocity still provided information about whether the gain of the VOR needed to increase or decrease, but according to a different rule from that applied at low frequencies. For oscillation at 0.5 Hz, complex-spike firing was in phase with *contraversive* head rotation when the gain of the VOR needed to decrease. For oscillation at 5 Hz, complex-spike firing was in phase with *ipsiversive* head rotation when the gain of the VOR needed to decrease. The relationship between phase shift and frequency can be easily modeled as a visual input with a 130-ms time delay.

What are the consequences of these data for fitting a mechanism such as cerebellar LTD into motor learning in the VOR? Two possibilities come to mind: (1) the temporal contingencies involved in LTD may compensate for the time delay in visual climbing-fiber inputs, so that the adequate conditions for LTD may be parallel fiber inputs followed about 100-ms later by a complex spike; and (2) complex spikes may play completely different roles in learning depending on the frequency content of the vestibular oscillation. Because LTD exists clearly in cerebellar cortices *in vitro* (e.g., ref. 22), it is tempting to conclude that LTD is the mechanism of cerebellar learning. Evidence also exists, however, for potentiation in the cerebellar cortex under some conditions.[23,24] Under conditions that decrease the gain of the VOR in intact brains, could complex-spike inputs be causing depression of vestibular transmission at low frequencies and potentiation at high frequencies? This idea is compatible with the finding that the phase relationship between complex-spike firing and head velocity is reversed at high versus low frequencies. It would also provide potential mechanisms for obtaining the changes in the time course of vestibular transmission to HGVPs postulated by Lisberger and Sejnowski,[7] as well as the "wrong-way" changes in vestibular sensitivity demonstrated by Miles et al.[3]

CONCLUSION

As we have learned more about the operation of the VOR at the systems level, the neural system has appeared more and more complex, and models of it have become more realistic. It seems inevitable that ongoing analyses of the error signals that guide learning and of the cellular basis for learning and memory in the VOR will encounter this same situation. Simple behavioral learning rules, such as the conjunction of retinal image motion and head turns, seem likely to have complex, distributed representations in the brain. Popular examples of synaptic plasticity, although elegant and simple in tissue culture and brain slices, seem unlikely to work in intact, functioning brains where neurons are spontaneously active and learning must be implemented by selective changes in the responses of neurons to one of their many inputs. As progress is made on current questions of the neural and cellular mechanisms of learning and memory in the VOR, it seems likely that increased complexity will lead to more realistic explanations and models.

REFERENCES

1. LISBERGER, S. G. 1994. Neural basis for motor learning in the vestibulo-ocular reflex in primates. III. Behavioral and computational analysis of the sites of learning. J. Neurophysiol. 72: 954–973.
2. WATANABE, E. 1984. Neuronal events correlated with long-term adaptation of the horizontal vestibulo-ocular reflex in the primate flocculus. Brain Res. 297: 169–174.
3. MILES, F. A., D. J. BRAITMAN & B. M. DOW. 1980. Long-term adaptive changes in primate vestibuloocular reflex. IV. Electrophysiological observations in flocculus of adapted monkeys. J. Neurophysiol. 3(5): 1477–1493.
4. LISBERGER, S. G., T. A. PAVELKO & D. M. BROUSSARD. 1994a. Responses during eye movement of brainstem neurons that receive monosynaptic inhibition from the flocculus and ventral paraflocculus in monkeys. J. Neurophysiol. 72: 909–927.
5. LISBERGER, S. G., T. A. PAVELKO & D. M. BROUSSARD. 1994b. Neural basis for motor learning in the vestibulo-ocular reflex of primates. I. Changes in the responses of brainstem neurons. J. Neurophysiol. 72: 928–953.
6. LISBERGER, S. G., T. A. PAVELKO, H. M. BRONTE-STEWART & L. S. STONE. 1994. Neural basis for motor learning in the vestibulo-ocular reflex in primates. II. Changes in the responses of Purkinje cells in the cerebellar flocculus and ventral paraflocculus. J. Neurophysiol. 72: 974–998.
7. LISBERGER, S. G. & T. J. SEJNOWSKI. 1992. A novel mechanism of motor learning in a recurrent network model based on the vestibulo-ocular reflex. Nature 360: 159–161.
8. GERRITS, N. M. & J. VOOGD. 1989. The topographical organization of climbing and mossy fiber afferents in the flocculus and the ventral paraflocculus in rabbit, cat, and monkey. Exp. Brain Res. Suppl. 17: 26–29.
9. HIGHSTEIN, S. M. 1973. Synaptic linkage in the vestibulo-ocular and cerebello-vestibular pathways to the VIth nucleus in the rabbit. Exp. Brain Res. 17: 301–314.

10. NAGAO, S. 1992. Different roles of flocculus and ventral paraflocculus for oculomotor control in the primate. Neuroreport **3:** 13–16.
11. MILES, F. A., J. H. FULLER, D. J. BRAITMAN & B. M. DOW. 1980. Long-term adaptive changes in primate vestibulo-ocular reflex. III. Electrophysiological observations in flocculus of normal monkey. J. Neurophysiol. **43:** 1437–1476.
12. LEONARD, C. S. 1986. Signal characteristics of cerebellar Purkinje cells in the rabbit flocculus during compensatory eye movements. PhD thesis. New York University. New York.
13. DUFOSSE, M., M. ITO, P. J. JASTREBOFF & Y. MIYASHITA. 1978. A neuronal correlate in rabbit's cerebellum to adaptive modification of the vestibulo-ocular reflex. Brain Res. **150(3):** 611–616.
14. BROUSSARD, D. M., H. M. BRONTE-STEWART & S. G. LISBERGER. 1992. Expression of motor learning in the response of the primate vestibuloocular pathway to electrical stimulation. J. Neurophysiol. **67:** 1493–1508.
15. BRONTË-STEWART, H. M. & S. G. LISBERGER. 1994. Physiological properties of vestibular primary afferents that mediate motor learning and normal performance of the vestibulo-ocular reflex in monkeys. J. Neurosci. **14:** 1290–1308.
16. MILES, F. A. & S. G. LISBERGER. 1981. Plasticity in the vestibulo-ocular reflex: A new hypothesis. Annu. Rev. Neurosci. **4:** 273–299.
17. LISBERGER, S. G., F. A. MILES & D. S. ZEE. 1984. Signals used to compute errors in monkey vestibuloocular reflex: Possible role of flocculus. J. Neurophysiol. **52(6):** 1140–1153.
18. PERRETT, S. P. & M. D. MAUK. 1995. Extinction of conditioned eyelid responses requires the anterior lobe of cerebellar cortex. J. Neurosci. **15(3 Pt. 1):** 2074–2080.
19. ITO, M. 1972. Neural design of the cerebellar motor control system. Brain Res. **40:** 80–84.
20. DU LAC, S., J. L. RAYMOND, T. J. SEJNOWSKI & S. G. LISBERGER. 1995. Learning and memory in the vestibulo-ocular reflex. Annu. Rev. Neurosci. **18:** 409–441.
21. RAYMOND, J. L. & S. G. LISBERGER. 1996. Error signals in horizontal gaze velocity Purkinje cells under stimulus conditions that cause learning in the VOR. Ann. N. Y. Acad. Sci. This volume.
22. LINDEN, D. J., M. H. DICKINSON, M. SMEYNE & J. A. CONNOR. 1991. A long-term depression of AMPA currents in cultured cerebellar Purkinje neurons. Neuron **7:** 81–89.
23. CREPEL, F. & D. JAILLARD. 1991. Pairing of pre- and postsynaptic activities in cerebellum Purkinje cells induces long-term changes in synaptic efficacy in vitro. J. Physiol. **432:** 123–141.
24. SHIBUKI, K. & D. OKADA. 1992. Cerebellar long-term potentiation under suppressed postsynaptic Ca^{2+} activity. Neuroreport **3:** 231–234.

Pathways from Cell Groups
of the Paramedian Tracts
to the Floccular Region[a]

J. A. BÜTTNER-ENNEVER[b] AND A. K. E. HORN

Institute of Neuropathology
University of Munich
Pettenkoferstr. 12
80336 Munich, Germany

INTRODUCTION

The cell groups of the paramedian tracts (PMT-cell groups), lying along the midline of the pons and medulla, provide a more significant input to the floccular region, based on cell numbers alone, than do the vestibular nuclei.[1] However, they have not been the subject of many studies.[2] In this article we will first review the current knowledge on PMT-cell groups, and then present experiments in which we have traced the route taken by the fibers from one group of PMT cells in the mid-medulla oblongata to the floccular region.

Nomenclature of PMT-Cell Groups

The "cell groups of the paramedian tracts" is a collective term used to refer to clusters of neurons scattered along the midline fibers tracts in the pons and medulla, which project to the floccular region.[2–4] The existence of individual cerebellar-projecting subgroups in the midline fiber tracts was known from earlier studies: for example, the accessory division of the paramedian reticular nucleus of Brodal, which lies close to hypoglossal nucleus (XII).[5–7] The first systematic description of a functional continuum came from experiments in which retrograde tracer substances were injected into the cerebellar floccular region (rat,[8] cat,[1,9] monkey[10]). These authors reported numerous aggregations of small, medium, and even some large, retrogradely-filled neurons, scattered in and around the pontine and medullary midline fibers, or paramedian fiber tracts (PMT). These tracts contain axons of the medial longitudinal fasciculus (MLF), reticulo-, tecto-, and interstitio-spinal pathways. The labeled neurons lay immediately lateral to the raphe nuclei and tended to be more chromophilic than those of the raphe nuclei. The floccular-projecting neurons or PMT-cell groups were described as forming a continuum, appearing as a thin layer at some levels, then collecting into significant, sizable cell clusters at others. A different nomenclature for the neurons was adopted in each study. In the rat, the Blanks group[8,9] termed the two major clusters that lay rostral and caudal to

[a]This work was supported by the German Research Council, grant SFB 220/D8.

[b]Address correspondence to Prof. J. A. Büttner-Ennever, c/o Institute of Physiology, University of Munich, Pettenkoferstr. 12, 80336 Munich, Germany. E-mail: U7224aa@sunmail.lrz-muenchen.de

the abducens nucleus, the *intermediate* and the *caudal interstitial nuclei of the MLF,* respectively. In the cat, Sato and colleagues[1] used the terms *accessory group of the paramedian reticular nucleus* for the caudal group and *dorsal nucleus of the raphe* for the rostral group, whereas recently Cheron and co-workers (this volume) chose the name *nucleus incertus* for their PMT-cell group in the cat. Finally, in the monkey Langer's group[10] differentiated between at least seven nuclei, shown as asterisks in FIGURE 1, and called, from rostral to caudal: the dorsal midline pontine group, the

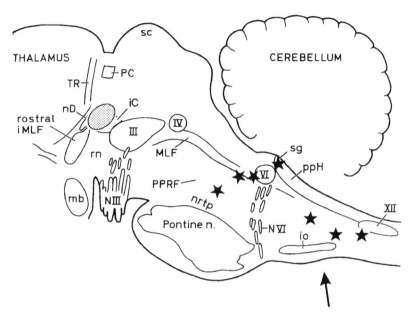

FIGURE 1. Sagittal view of the primate brain stem. The uptake area of a [³H]leucine injection (B46) into the interstitial nucleus of Cajal (iC) is shown rostrally. The asterisks mark the position of the larger aggregations of floccular-projecting neurons lying within the paramedian tracts (PMT-cell groups), and receiving projections from iC. The arrow indicates the orientation of the transverse cross section drawn in FIGURE 4. IV, trochlear nucleus; VI, abducens nucleus; XII, hypoglossal nucleus; io, inferior olive; mb, mammillary body; MLF, medial longitudinal fasciculus; NIII, oculomotor nerve; NVI, abducens nerve; nD, nucleus Darkschewitsch; nrtp, nucleus reticularis tegmenti pontis; PC, posterior commissure; ppH, nucleus prepositus hypoglossi; PPRF, paramedian pontine reticular formation; rn, red nucleus; rostral iMLF, rostral interstitial nucleus of MLF; sc, superior colliculus; sg, nucleus supragenualis; TR, tractus retroflexus.

interfascicular nuclei of the preabducens area, the rostral cap of the abducens nucleus, the nucleus supragenualis, the nucleus pararaphales, the ventral medullary interfascicular nucleus and the dorsal medullary interfascicular nucleus (which is equivalent to Brodal's accessory division of the paramedian reticular nucleus). These cell aggregations can easily be mistaken for the raphe nuclei and, in some cases, certainly have been.[11]

Afferent Connections

In a review of the connectivity of the PMT-cell groups in the monkey, we noticed that the input profile to the PMT-cell groups is very similar to that of the motoneurons of the extraocular eye muscles.[3,4] That is, all known premotor cell groups of the oculomotor system—the excitatory and inhibitory burst neurons in the paramedian pontine reticular formation (PPRF), the rostral interstitial nucleus of the MLF (rostral iMLF), and the interstitial nucleus of Cajal (iC), the vertical and horizontal secondary vestibular neurons, abducens internuclear neurons, and nucleus prepositus hypoglossi—were found to also project, usually via collaterals, to the PMT-cell

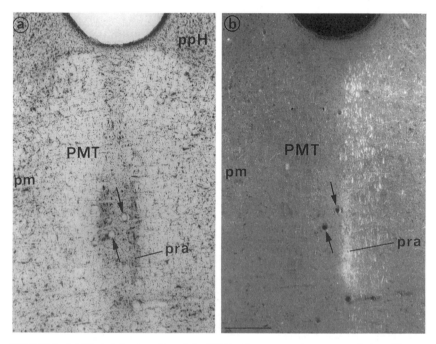

FIGURE 2. (a) Nissl-stained section of the PMT-cell group, nucleus pararaphales of Langer (pra). (b) Dark-field illumination of the same section to show the labeled fibers descending in the ipsilateral paramedian fiber tracts (PMT) after the injection of [³H]leucine into the interstitial nucleus of Cajal (see FIG. 1). Note fine silver-grain deposit indicating axon terminals over the cells of pra. pm, paramedian reticular nucleus; ppH, nucleus prepositus hypoglossi. Arrows indicate blood vessels as points of reference. Calibration = 500 μm.

groups.[2,12–17] For example, injections into the premotor cell groups for vertical eye movements, the rostral iMLF, and the iC labeled the floccular-projecting cell groups in the midline fiber tracts both rostral and caudal to the abducens nucleus (FIG. 2), as well as the motoneuron-like neurons in the rostral cap of the abducens nucleus.[4] Initially the iC projection to the abducens nucleus was surprising because the iC signal contains vertical oculomotor information and the abducens nucleus is associated with purely horizontal eye movement signals. However, the rostral cap of the abducens nucleus was shown to contain only floccular-projecting neurons (i.e., it is a

PMT-cell group), and no abducens internuclear neurons, or abducens motoneu-rons.[18] As a result of these findings, the abducens nucleus must now be considered as containing at least three main cell types: abducens motoneurons, abducens inter-nuclear neurons, and floccular-projecting neurons, some of which carry a vertical oculomotor signal.

Physiological Properties

What signals do the PMT-cell groups transmit? The function of PMT-cell groups is not known, but based on the connectivity described above we proposed that they could provide a motor-feedback signal of extraocular eye muscle activity to the floccular region.[2,4] Nakao et al.[19] showed that floccular-projecting neurons in the region of the dorsal PPRF relay burst-tonic activity, encoding information on the horizontal saccadic burst as well as the horizontal eye position. Cheron et al. (this volume) report similar physiological properties for their nucleus incertus. Burst-tonic information, related to both horizontal and vertical saccades, has in turn been recorded in the floccular region itself.[20,21] The lesion studies of the floccular region showed that deficits in gaze-holding and smooth pursuit occurred after bilateral flocculectomy.[22] Therefore, it is possible that the PMT-cell groups carry the eye position signals essential for gaze stabilization, to the floccular region.

We have begun investigating the efferents of a PMT-cell group in the mid-medullary region of the monkey called the nucleus pararaphales (pra).[10] This PMT-cell group was chosen first, because of its relative isolation from other oculomotor structures, which simplifies the anatomical interpretation. The experi-ments reported here will show that it receives premotor afferents from iC, and will demonstrate the route followed by its efferents to the cerebellum. In addition, these experiments allow us to study the extent of PMT-cell group terminations within the floccular region.

METHODS

The efferents of the iC or midline medullary cell groups were labeled with tritiated leucine. This tracer has the advantage that, unlike any other neuroanatomi-cal tracer, it is not taken up by fibers of passage—an important advantage in the study of cell groups embedded in fiber tracts. In these experiments, injections of concentrated (100 μC/μl) L-[4,5,-^{3}H]leucine (Amersham), with a volume of 0.5 μl, were stereotaxically placed in macaque monkeys. After four days to two weeks survival time the animals were killed with an overdose of Nembutal and perfused through the heart with 4% paraformaldehyde solution in 0.1 M phosphate buffer (pH 7.4). Frozen sections (40 μm or 50 μm) were mounted, de-fatted, and processed for autoradiography, or for immunohistochemistry to visualize serotoninergic cells.[23]

RESULTS

The mid-medullary PMT-cell group in the monkey, nucleus pararaphales,[10] lies approximately halfway between the abducens and the hypoglossal nucleus, and can be identified on the basis of its location and cytoarchitecture alone (FIG. 2); in addition, its cells are not serotoninergic. An injection of [^{3}H]leucine into the premotor region for vertical eye movements, centered on the iC (see FIG. 1, hatched area), labeled afferents that can be seen terminating over the mid-medullary PMT-cell group (FIG. 2, pra).

Injections of anterograde tracer [³H]leucine were placed in and around the PMT-cell group nucleus pararaphales (pra); see FIGURE 4. In cases Z9 and Z18, pra was filled mainly unilaterally. Labeled efferent fibers were traced to the cerebellum, and the results are shown in FIGURE 3: one group of fibers collected on the ventral midline, then turned laterally within the medial lemniscus, past the inferior olive

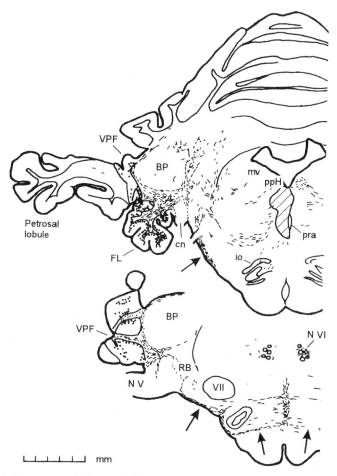

FIGURE 3. The pattern of silver-grain labeling on two transverse sections from case Z18. The [³H]leucine uptake area (*hatched*) involves the PMT-cell group (pra) mainly on one side. In the upper caudal section, labeled efferents (*arrows*) run with the external arcuate fibers[25] along the ventral margin of the medulla and enter the restiform body. Terminal labeling is found in the flocculus and ventral paraflocculus. The projection is equally strong on both sides (not shown). BP, brachium pontis; cn, cochlear nucleus; FL, flocculus; mv, medial vestibular nucleus; NV, trigeminal nerve; NVI, abducens rootlets; ppH, nucleus prepositus hypoglossi; pra, nucleus pararaphales; RB, restiform body (inferior cerebellar peduncle); VPF, ventral paraflocculus; VII, facial nucleus.

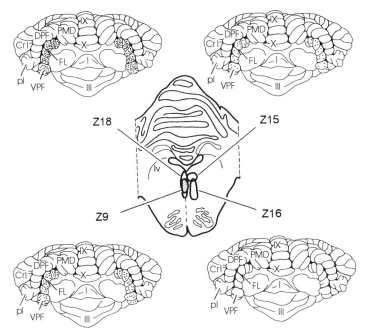

FIGURE 4. A summary of the terminal projections in the floccular complex after four [³H]leucine injections into the medulla oblongata. Note that injection sites involving the midline PMT-cell groups (Z9, Z18, and to a minor extent Z15) label afferents to the flocculus (FL) and ventral paraflocculus (VPF), bilaterally. CrI, crus I; DPF, dorsal paraflocculus; lv, lateral vestibular nucleus; pl, petrosal lobule; PMD, paramedian lobule; IX, uvula; X, nodulus; I and III, anterior lobe.

(io), or along the dorsal margin of the pyramidal tract to the ventral surface of the brain stem (see arrows FIG. 3). They followed the ventral external arcuate pathway dorsally into the restiform body (RB, inferior cerebellar pedunculi), and finally entered the floccular peduncle. Some of the fibers arched around borders of the brachium pontis (BP, medial cerebellar peduncle), but did not penetrate into BP. Rosettes of terminal labeling were found within the granular layer of the flocculus proper of both sides, as well as in the adjacent folia of the ventral paraflocculus. No labeling was found in the dorsal paraflocculus, including the petrosal lobule, but a diffuse group of fibers could be followed into the core of lobule VII in Z9 and Z18 (not shown in FIG. 4).

Control injections, slightly lateral to the midline were centered on the paramedian reticular nucleus (Z15 dorsal and Z16 ventral to pra). In these cases very few fibers entered the floccular peduncle in Z15 to terminate in the ventral paraflocculus and the flocculus, and none at all in Z16 (FIG. 4).[24]

DISCUSSION

The results of the autoradiographic tracing experiments show that fibers from the mid-medullary PMT-cell group, nucleus pararaphales, follow the ventral external arcuate fibers, which run along the ventrolateral surface of the brain stem into the RB of the cerebellum: a pathway first described by Bechterew.[25] The PMT-cell group provides mossy fiber terminals to both the flocculus proper and the ventral paraflocculus, but not to the dorsal paraflocculus. Until now it was not clear from the retrograde injections into the flocculus region, which subdivisions of the floccular complex were supplied by PMT-cell groups. The functional significance of a projection to the flocculus and ventral paraflocculus is uncertain (see Voogd, this volume), but it is clearly separate from the visual pontine inputs which target the dorsal paraflocculus.[26] There has been some confusion over the nomenclature of the folia in the floccular complex of the monkey; we have used the terminology proposed by Larsell in which the posterolateral fissure separates three folia of the flocculus from the ventral paraflocculus (see Voogd, this volume).[27]

The PMT-cell group that we investigated is the nucleus pararaphales, which was named after a cell group of the same name in the human described by Olszewski and Baxter.[10,28] Olszewski and Baxter proposed that their nucleus paparaphales could be considered as a caudal, or displaced, pontine nucleus, and that it was related to the arcuate nuclei, which lie along the midline and around the outer surface of the pyramidal tract. The arcuate efferents follow the same pathway as the PMT-cell groups into the RB.[25,28]

We have shown that the nucleus pararaphales receives afferent terminals from iC and therefore, at least in part, relays vertical eye position signals to the floccular complex. If this information is used by the cerebellum as a motor-feedback signal, then lesions of this PMT-cell group, or its afferent pathways, should, theoretically, lead to disorders in vertical eye position, and result in gaze-evoked nystagmus. Small lesions in the medulla caudal to the vestibular nuclei can cause up-beat nystagmus.[29-31] The demonstration here of the route taken by some PMT-cell group efferents to the flocculus may also help in the analysis of some of these clinical lesions causing gaze deficits. However, before these results can be applied to the analysis of human material, further information on the individual PMT-cell groups must be collected, and the homologue of the PMT-cell groups in man must be clarified.

SUMMARY

A group of cells lying along the midline of the mid-medulla, nucleus pararaphales, is shown to play a role in vertical eye movements. Its efferents project along the midline, then pass laterally to follow the ventral external arcuate fibers around the surface of the medulla into the restiform body. The fibers terminate in the flocculus and ventral paraflocculus. This nucleus is one of the "cell groups of the paramedian tracts," which, based on their connectivity, could provide a motor-feedback signal for eye-head position to the cerebellum. Lesions of these pathways could lead to gaze-evoked nystagmus.

ACKNOWLEDGMENTS

The authors are very grateful to Professor Volker Henn and Dr. Nicolaas Gerrits for their help and advice, and to Ursula Schneider for her technical assistance.

REFERENCES

1. SATO, Y., T. KAWASAKI & K. IKARASHI. 1983. Afferent projections from the brainstem to the three floccular zones in cat. II. Mossy fibre projections. Brain Res. **272:** 37–48.
2. BÜTTNER-ENNEVER, J. A. 1992. Paramedian tract cell groups: A review of connectivity and oculomotor function. *In* Vestibular and Brain Stem Control of Eye-Head and Body Movements. H. Shimazu & Y. Shinoda, Eds.: 323–330. Japan Scientific Societies Press. Tokyo.
3. BÜTTNER-ENNEVER, J. A. & U. BÜTTNER. 1988. The reticular formation. *In* Neuroanatomy of the Oculomotor System. J. A. Büttner-Ennever, Ed.: 119–176. Elsevier Science Publishers B. V. Amsterdam.
4. BÜTTNER-ENNEVER, J. A., A. K. E. HORN & K. SCHMIDTKE. 1989. Cell groups of the medial longitudinal fasciculus and paramedian tracts. Rev. Neurol. (Paris) **145:** 8–9, 533–539.
5. BRODAL, A. 1953. Reticulo-cerebellar connections in the cat. An experimental study. J. Comp. Neurol. **98:** 113–154.
6. BRODAL, A. 1981. Neurological Anatomy. Oxford University Press. Oxford, UK.
7. SOMANA, R. & F. WALBERG. 1978. Cerebellar afferents from the paramedian reticular nucleus studied with retrograde transport of horseradish peroxidase. Anat. Embryol. **154:** 353–368.
8. BLANKS, R. H. I., W. PRECHT & Y. TORIGOE. 1983. Afferent projections to the cerebellar flocculus in the pigmented rat demonstrated by retrograde transport of horseradish peroxidase. Exp. Brain Res. **52:** 293–306.
9. BLANKS, R. H. I. 1990. Afferents to the cerebellar flocculus in cat with special reference to pathways conveying vestibular, visual (optokinetic) and oculomotor signals. J. Neurocytol. **19:** 628–642.
10. LANGER, T., A. F. FUCHS, C. A. SCUDDER & M. C. CHUBB. 1985. Afferents to the flocculus of the cerebellum in the rhesus macaque as revealed by retrograde transport of horseradish peroxidase. J. Comp. Neurol. **235:** 1–25.
11. YAMADA, J. & H. NODA. 1987. Afferent and efferent connections of the oculomotor cerebellar vermis in the macaque monkey. J. Comp. Neurol. **265:** 224–241.
12. BELKNAP, D. B. & R. A. MCCREA. 1988. Anatomical connections of the prepositus and abducens nuclei in the squirrel monkey. J. Comp. Neurol. **268:** 13–28.
13. MCCREA, R. A., A. STRASSMAN & S. M. HIGHSTEIN. 1986. Morphology and physiology of abducens motoneurons and internuclear neurons intracellularly injected with horseradish peroxidase in alert squirrel monkeys. J. Comp. Neurol. **243:** 291–308.
14. MCCREA, R. A., A. STRASSMAN, E. MAY & S. M. HIGHSTEIN. 1987. Anatomical and physiological characteristics of vestibular neurons mediating the horizontal vestibulo-ocular reflex in the squirrel monkey. J. Comp. Neurol. **264:** 547–570.
15. MCCREA, R. A., A. STRASSMAN & S. M. HIGHSTEIN. 1987. Anatomical and physiological characteristics of vestibular neurons mediating the vertical vestibulo-ocular reflex in the squirrel monkey. J. Comp. Neurol. **264:** 571–594.
16. STRASSMAN, A., S. M. HIGHSTEIN & R. A. MCCREA. 1986. Anatomy and physiology of saccadic burst neurons in the alert squirrel monkey. I. Excitatory burst neurons. J. Comp. Neurol. **249:** 337–357.
17. STRASSMAN, A., S. M. HIGHSTEIN & R. A. MCCREA. 1986. Anatomy and physiology of saccadic burst neurons in the alert squirrel monkey. II. Inhibitory burst neurons. J. Comp. Neurol. **249:** 358–380.
18. LANGER, T., C. S. KANEKO, C. A. SCUDDER & A. F. FUCHS. 1986. Afferents to the abducens nucleus in the monkey and cat. J. Comp. Neurol. **245:** 379–400.
19. NAKAO, S., I. S. CURTHOYS & C. H. MARKHAM. 1980. Eye movement related neurons in the cat pontine reticular formation: Projection to the flocculus. Brain Res. **183:** 291–299.
20. MILES, F. A., J. H. FULLER, D. J. BRAITMAN & B. M. DOW. 1980. Long-term adaptive changes in the primate vestibulo-ocular reflex. III. Electrophysiological observations in flocculus of monkeys. J. Neurophysiol. **43:** 1437–1476.

21. NODA, H. & D. A. SUZUKI. 1979. Processing of eye movement signals in the flocculus of the monkey. J. Physiol. **294:** 349–364.
22. ZEE, D. S., A. YAMAZAKI, P. H. BUTLER & G. GÜCER. 1981. Effects of ablation of flocculus and paraflocculus on eye movements in primates. J. Neurophysiol. **46:** 878–899.
23. HORN, A. K., J. A. BÜTTNER-ENNEVER, P. WAHLE & I. REICHENBERGER. 1994. Neurotransmitter profile of saccadic omnipause neurons in nucleus raphe interpositus. J. Neurosci. **14:** 2037–2046.
24. COWIE, R. J., M. K. SMITH & D. L. ROBINSON. 1994. Subcortical contributions to head movements in macaques. 2. Connections of a medial pontomedullary head-movement region. J. Neurophysiol. **72:** 2665–2682.
25. VOOGD, J., H. K. P. FEIERABEND & J. H. R. SCHOEN. 1990. Cerebellum and precerebellar nuclei. *In* The Human Nervous System. G. Paxinos, Ed.: 321–386. Academic Press. San Diego, CA.
26. GLICKSTEIN, M., N. GERRITS, I. KRALJ-HANS, B. MERCIER, J. STEIN & J. VOOGD. 1994. Visual pontocerebellar projections in the macaque. J. Comp. Neurol. **349:** 51–72.
27. VOOGD, J., N. GERRITS & D. T. HESS. 1987. Parasagittal zonastion of the cerebellum in macaques: An analysis based on acetylcholinesterase histochemistry. *In* Cerebellum and Neuronal Plasticity. M. Glickstein, C. Yeo & J. Stein, Eds.: 15–39. Plenum Press. New York.
28. OLSZEWSKI, J. & D. BAXTER. 1954. Cytoarchitecture of the human brainstem. S. Karger. Basel.
29. BALOH, R. W. & R. D. YEE. 1989. Spontaneous vertical nystagmus. Rev. Neurol. (Paris) **145:** 527–532.
30. BRANDT, T. & M. DIETERICH. 1995. Central vestibular syndromes in the roll, pitch, and yaw planes: Topographic diagnosis of the brainstem disorders. Neuro-ophthalmol. **15:** 291–303.
31. BÜTTNER, U., C. HELMCHEN & J. A. BÜTTNER-ENNEVER. 1995. The localizing value of nystagmus in brainstem disorders. Neuro-ophthalmol. **15:** 283–290.

Gabaergic Pathways Convey Vestibular Information to the Beta Nucleus and Dorsomedial Cell Column of the Inferior Olive

NEAL H. BARMACK[a]

R. S. Dow Neurological Sciences Institute
Legacy Good Samaritan Hospital
Portland, Oregon

INTRODUCTION

Although composed of histologically similar cell types,[1] the mammalian inferior olive is divided into very specific functional subgroups. Nowhere is this specificity better demonstrated than for the subgroups of the inferior olive that receive vestibular and visual information and project to the contralateral nodulus and flocculus of the cerebellum.[2-4] For example, the dorsal cap of the medial accessory olive is composed of about 2000 cells. The most caudal 600–800 of these cells are excited by horizontal optokinetic stimulation of the contralateral eye in the posterior-anterior direction[2,4,5] and project to both the nodulus and flocculus. Rostral to the caudal dorsal cap are olivary neurons that appear to code optokinetic stimulation in the coordinate system that corresponds roughly to the orientation of the anterior and posterior semicircular canals. These neurons project to different zones within the flocculus than do the caudal dorsal cap neurons.[4] Just below and medial to the dorsal cap is the β-nucleus. These olivary neurons receive vestibular information from the ipsilateral medial and descending vestibular. Rostral to the β-nucleus lies the dorsomedial cell column (dmcc) of the inferior olive.[6-9] Neurons within the dmcc and the β-nucleus project as climbing fibers onto discrete zones within the contralateral uvula-nodulus.[10-13]

In the present report we characterize the vestibularly related GABAergic innervation of the β-nucleus and the dmcc, and we compare the effects of natural vestibular stimulation on the response properties of these olivary neurons. Each neuron was characterized by its sensitivity to linear acceleration (otolithic stimulation) and angular acceleration (semicircular canal stimulation). We have found a systematic topographic representation of vestibularly mediated inputs to these two olivary subgroups. The β-nucleus receives both information from the vertical semicircular canals as well as the utricular otoliths. Stimulation in the plane of the ipsilateral anterior semicircular canal is encoded by neurons in the caudal β-nucleus. Stimulation in the plane of the ipsilateral posterior semicircular canal is encoded by neurons in the rostral nucleus. The dmcc contains neurons that appear to be activated by otoliths exclusively, and vestibular stimulation in the horizontal plane does not modulate the activity of any olivary neurons in the β-nucleus. Climbing fibers originating from the β-nucleus and dmcc may establish a postural reference system

[a]Address correspondence to Neal H. Barmack, Ph.D., R. S. Dow Neurological Sciences Institute, 1120 N.W. 20th Avenue, Portland, Oregon 97209. E-mail: barmackn@lhs.org

within the uvula-nodulus based upon vestibular information and acting upon axial musculature.

METHODS

GAD Immunocytochemistry

Four pigmented rabbits were deeply anesthetized with sodium pentobarbital (40 mg/kg) and perfused transcardially with physiological saline followed by a fixative consisting of 4% formaldehyde, 0.2% zinc salicylate, and 0.9% NaCl, pH 6.5. The brain stems between the rostral pole of the pons and the caudal pole of the inferior olive were removed, cryoprotected in 30% sucrose in saline, and cryosectioned at 20 μm in the transverse plane. The sections were processed for glutamic acid decarboxylase (GAD) immunochemistry with a double peroxidase–antiperoxidase protocol using a sheep-α-rat-GAD primary antibody.[14]

Vestibular Stimulation

Rabbits were anesthetized intravenously with α-chloralose (50 mg/kg) and urethane (500 mg/kg). The head of the rabbit was attached to a restraining bar through surgically implanted screws fixed with dental cement. The restraining bar held the head rigidly in the center of rotation of a three-axis vestibular rate table, with the plane of the horizontal semicircular canals maintained in the earth horizontal plane. The body of the rabbit was encased in foam rubber and fixed with elastic straps to a semicircular plastic tube aligned with the longitudinal axis. The rate table was sinusoidally oscillated about the vertical axis (yaw), about the longitudinal axis (roll) or about the interaural axis (pitch) (±10 deg, 0.02–0.80 Hz). During vestibular stimulation the vision of the rabbit was completely occluded.

Vestibular Null Technique

A "null technique" was used to characterize the peripheral origin of vestibularly modulated Purkinje cell activity in the uvula-nodulus. While the rabbit was rotated about the longitudinal axis, the angle of its head about the vertical axis was changed systematically until a minimum ("null plane") in the vestibularly modulated neuronal activity was detected. On either side of this null plane, the phase of the vestibularly modulated activity was shifted with respect to the sinusoidal vestibular forcing function by 180 deg. For each tested neuron, the null plane characterized the polarization vector of the hair cells of particular end organs that contributed to the modulated response. The null plane was orthogonal to the optimal response plane for a particular neuron.

Static Vestibular Sensitivity

A "static roll" test was used to determine whether the discharge of a Purkinje cell was related to otolithic stimulation. Low-frequency exponential steps were used to tilt the rabbit 5–10 deg about the longitudinal axis. After an adaptation period of 30 s, the average discharge frequency was measured for the next 30 s. The rabbit was then tilted in the opposite direction. A difference in mean discharge frequency for static roll-tilt in the two directions of more than 20% was taken as evidence for sensitivity to linear acceleration.

Optokinetic Stimulation

The rate table was located 55 cm from the center of a rear-projection tangent screen subtending 70 × 70 deg of visual angle. An optokinetic stimulus was rear-projected onto the screen by beaming the image of a random dot contour-rich pattern, projected by a 35-mm slide projector, off three first surface mirrors, two of which were mounted orthogonally on EEG pen motors. Appropriate voltage ramps to the pen motors generated constant velocity movement of the projected image on the tangent screen in the horizontal and vertical axes.

Microelectrode Recording

The floor of the fourth ventricle, rostral to the obex, was exposed by reflecting the muscles overlying the cisterna magna and slightly enlarging the dorsal aspect of the foramen magnum. The signal from the microelectrode was amplified (bandwidth 0.1–10,000 Hz), discriminated with a window discriminator–Schmitt trigger and then connected to a computer. The evoked single-unit activity was displayed on-line as a peristimulus histogram.

Histological Verification of Recording Sites

The location of each neuron from which recordings were obtained was marked electrolytically (-5 μA, 15 s). At the conclusion of the experiment each rabbit was deeply anesthetized with sodium pentobarbital (60 mg/kg) and perfused transcardially with 0.9% saline, followed by 10% paraformaldehyde. Serial frozen sections through the caudal brain stem were stained with neutral red. The location of each recorded neuron was reconstructed from the locations of the marking lesions and marked on schematic representations of the inferior olive at 0.3-mm rostro-caudal intervals.

Horseradish Peroxidase Histochemistry

In two rabbits we microinjected either the left posterior cerebellum (lobules 9 and 10) or the left flocculus with 2–4 μL of a 30% solution of horseradish peroxidase (HRP). The injections were done with a glass micropipette connected to a 1-μL syringe (Hamilton). The posterior cerebellar pressure injection was made after surgically exposing lobules 9a and b. The flocculus injection was made following a surgical approach through the middle ear. A 1-mm opening was made immediately rostral to the anterior semicircular canal.[15] A micropipette containing HRP was inserted through this opening directly into the flocculus. A diaminobenzidine (DAB)-stabilized, $CoCl_2$-intensified, tetramethylbenzidine reaction was used to demonstrate retrogradely transported HRP.[16,17]

RESULTS

GAD Immunochemistry

Although the entire inferior olive receives a GABAergic innervation,[18,19] two areas in particular stand out as receiving a distinct and relatively more dense innervation than other areas. These are the β-nucleus and the dmcc (FIG. 1). These areas of relatively dense GABAergic innervation are not depleted by lesions to the cerebellar nuclei, the origin of most of the GABAergic projection to the inferior olive.[18] Furthermore, the GABAergic innervation of both the β-nucleus and the dmcc is depleted following lesions to the medial and descending vestibular nuclei (Barmack, Mugnaini, and Fredette, unpublished observations). Anatomical tracer studies demonstrate that the β-nucleus and the dmcc receive projections from the ipsilateral medial and descending vestibular nuclei.[7,8,20]

Recordings from Neurons in the β-Nucleus

The activity of neurons in the inferior olive is related to both vestibular input from the vertical semicircular canals as well as the utricular otoliths because the activity can be modulated by static tilt as well as sinusoidal rotation about the longitudinal axis. In either instance, the essential result is the same. The activity of neurons in the β-nucleus decreases when the rabbit is rolled onto the ipsilateral side and increases when the rabbit is rolled onto the contralateral side. Roughly one-half of the neurons in the β-nucleus evince some static sensitivity. Such a statically sensitive neuron, recorded from the right β-nucleus, is illustrated in FIGURE 2A. Conversely, the other half of the population responds exclusively to transient stimulation in the plane of one of the two pairs of vertical semicircular canals (FIG. 2C). Such a transiently responding neuron, recorded from the left β-nucleus, is illustrated in FIGURE 2B.

The optimal response planes of transiently responding β-nucleus neurons not only correspond to the planes of pairs of vertical semicircular canals, but there is a definite topography of these neurons. In the caudal β-nucleus, neurons have optimal response planes that align with the ipsilateral anterior semicircular canal and the contralateral posterior semicircular canal (FIG. 2D,4–6). In the rostral β-nucleus, neurons have optimal response planes that align with the ipsilateral posterior semicircular canal and contralateral anterior semicircular canal (FIG. 2D,1–3).

Recordings from Neurons in the Dorsal Medial Cell Column

In contrast to neurons of the β-nucleus, the activity of neurons in the dmcc had a static vestibular sensitivity. During tilt onto the ipsilateral side, the activity of these neurons decreases, and during tilt onto the contralateral side it increases (FIG. 3). In a recorded population of 20 neurons recorded from the dmcc, 18 evinced a static vestibular sensitivity. During sinusoidal oscillation the vestibularly evoked activity discharges in phase with head position (FIG. 3A). The optimal response planes of these neurons do not align with either pair of vertical semicircular canals (FIG. 4).

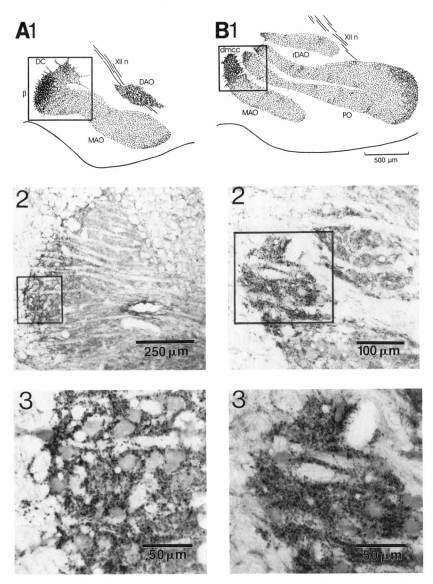

FIGURE 1. GABAergic innervation of the β-nucleus and dorsomedial cell column of the inferior olive. Illustration of the termination of glutamic acid decarboxylase-positive (GAD) fibers within β-nucleus, **A1,** and dorsomedial cell column, **B1.** Low- and higher-power photomicrographs demonstrate GAD-positive boutons within the β-nucleus, **A2,3,** and dorsomedial cell column, **B2,3.** Note the GAD-containing boutons surround olivary GAD-negative olivary cell bodies (**A3, B3**). β, β-nucleus; DAO and MAO, dorsal and medial accessory olive; DC, dorsal cap of Kooy; PO, principal olive; XII n, hypoglossal nerve.

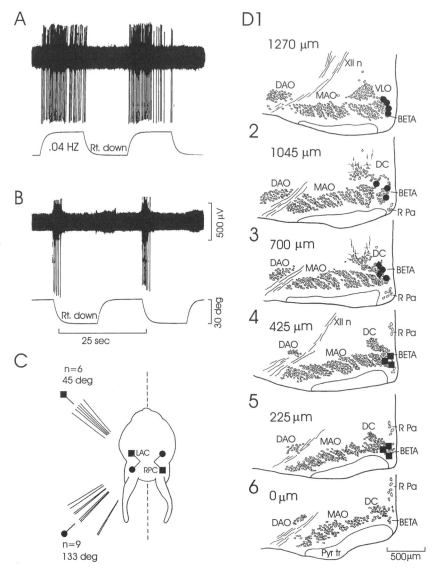

FIGURE 2. Activity of β-nucleus neurons evoked by vestibular stimulation about the longitudinal axis. Vestibular stimulation about the roll axis modulated the discharge of neurons within the β-nucleus. In both **A** and **B** the rabbit was rolled about the longitudinal axis (roll) using a 0.04 Hz, 20 deg exponential step with a time constant of 1.5 s. (**A**) Recording from an otolith-sensitive neuron located in the *right* β-nucleus. This neuron responded when the rabbit was rolled onto its left side and maintained its discharge for the duration of the step (0.04 Hz).

Differential Cerebellar Projections of Neurons in the β-Nucleus and Dorsal Medial Cell Column

Both the β-nucleus and the dmcc project onto uvula-nodulus of the cerebellum. HRP injections into the uvula-nodulus cause retrograde uptake of HRP by neurons in the β-nucleus, dmcc, dorsal cap, and some cells from the caudolateral aspect of the medial accessory olive (FIG. 5B). HRP injections into the flocculus label many more cells in the dorsal cap, but do not label any cells in either the β-nucleus or the dmcc. Interestingly, the flocculus-ventral paraflocculus injection labeled olivary neurons just below the dmcc in the rostral medial accessory olive, as well as from cells in the ventrolateral principal olive (vlPO) (FIG. 5A).

DISCUSSION

Vestibular stimulation activates olivary neurons located in the β-nucleus and dmcc. These olivary subnuclei receive a rich GABAergic projection from the medial and descending nuclei. This means that the vestibular control of olivary activity is mediated by an inhibitory pathway, accounting for the observation that activity of neurons in the β-nucleus and dmcc is decreased when the rabbit is rolled onto the ipsilateral side, and increased when the rabbit is rolled onto its contralateral side. This increased activity implies a release of inhibition (FIG. 6).

Both the vertical semicircular canals as well as the utricular otoliths are effective in modulating the activity of neurons in the β-nucleus and dmcc. In neither of these nuclei does horizontal vestibular stimulation modulate activity. These observations clearly contradict earlier reports of olivary neurons[21] and nodular climbing-fiber responses[22] that are driven by horizontal vestibular stimulation. In these instances, it is likely that horizontal (yaw) stimulation weakly modulated olivary activity due to stimulation of the vertical semicircular canals.

In addition to sharing a common transmitter-specific input, the β-nucleus and dmcc also project to a common cerebellar region, lobules 9 and 10. Vestibular stimulation evokes climbing-fiber responses from Purkinje cells in lobules 9c, d, and

---

FIGURE 2 *(continued).* (**B**) Recording from a vertical semicircular canal-sensitive neuron located in the *left* β-nucleus. This neuron responded transiently to roll steps onto the right side. Downward deflections of the stimulus traces indicated right-side down. (**C**) Optimal response planes were determined for 15 β-nucleus neurons that had no static sensitivity. The optimal response planes for these neurons clustered about the two axes that correspond to the anatomical axes of the two pairs of vertical semicircular canals. (**D1–6**) Locations of β-nucleus neurons with measured optimal response planes. The rostro-caudal location of each section is given in microns from the caudal pole of the β-nucleus, with the section of **D6** being the most caudal. These locations are represented as though all the recordings were made from the left β-nucleus. The *filled circles* indicate neurons with optimal response planes consistent with vestibular modulation originating from the left posterior–right anterior semicircular canals. The *filled squares* indicate the location of neurons with optimal response planes consistent with vestibular modulation originating from the left anterior–right posterior semicircular canals. The *filled diamonds* indicate the location of two neurons for which clearly defined optimal response planes could not be determined. Beta, β-nucleus; DAO, dorsal accessory olive; DC, dorsal cap; LAC and RPC, left anterior and right posterior semicircular canals; MAO, medial accessory olive; Pyr tr, pyramidal tract; R Pa, raphe pallidus nucleus; XII n, hypoglossal nerve.

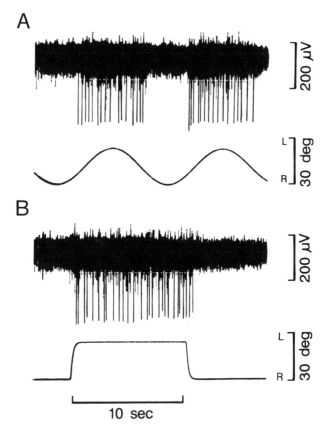

FIGURE 3. Vestibular stimulation of a neuron in the dorsomedial cell column during sinusoi-dal roll about the longitudinal axis. The activity of a neuron isolated in the right dorsal medial cell column was examined using both sinusoidal and exponential-step stimulation about the longitudinal (roll) axis. (**A**) Sinusoidal stimulation at 0.1 Hz ± 10 deg evoked an increased discharge when the rabbit was rolled onto its left side. This activity was modulated in phase with head position. (**B**) Step stimulation evoked an increased discharge when the rabbit was rolled onto its left side. This response to static roll indicates an otolithic origin of the evoked activity.

10.[23] More recently we have observed that this vestibular representation also extends to lobules 9a and b (Fushiki and Barmack, unpublished observations).

A major difference in the evoked activity of cells in the β-nucleus and the dmcc is that cells in the dmcc appear to receive an almost exclusive otolithic input. This may explain why centripetal acceleration of rats preferentially activates cells in the dmcc (as opposed to the β-nucleus), using an immunohistochemical stain for c-*fos* as a marker for cellular activity.[24]

Presently, we know more about the topography of the projection of the β-nucleus onto the uvula-nodulus than we do about the projection of the dmcc. In the β-nucleus, the vertical semicircular canals are mapped onto the caudal-rostral axis, and then, as climbing fibers, onto the medial-lateral axis in the uvula-nodulus.

Climbing-fiber responses that have an optimal vestibular plane corresponding to stimulation of the ipsilateral posterior and contralateral anterior semicircular canals project onto a medial strip of Purkinje cells in the uvula-nodulus.[23] Climbing-fiber responses that have an optimal plane corresponding to stimulation of the ipsilateral anterior and contralateral posterior semicircular canals activate a more lateral strip of Purkinje cells. This mediolateral gradient on the surface of the uvula-nodulus could modulate the control of skeletal muscles involved in maintenance of balance. It

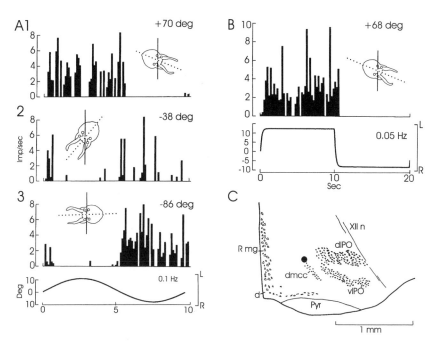

FIGURE 4. Peristimulus histograms of the activity of a neuron in the dorsomedial cell column evoked by vestibular stimulation about the longitudinal axis. Sinusoidal vestibular stimulation about the longitudinal (roll) axis was used to evoke activity of a neuron in the right dorsomedial cell column (dmcc). By shifting the head position about the vertical axis, during roll stimulation, it was possible to determine a null plane of vestibular stimulation, a plane of stimulation for which there was a minimal modulation of neuronal activity. Peristimulus histograms were constructed from 20 cycles of stimulation at 0.05 Hz ± 10 deg. The figurines in **A1–3** and **B** indicate the angle of the head (*dashed line*) relative to the axis of rotation (*solid line*). The null plane for this neuron corresponded to −22 deg, close to the head angle illustrated in **A2**. On either side of this null plane, **A1** and **A2,3,** the phase of the vestibularly evoked activity shifted by 180 deg relative to the sinusoidal stimulus. Orthogonal to the null plane was optimal response plane. This plane corresponded to the orientation of the head about the vertical axis that produced a maximal modulation of the neuronal activity during roll vestibular stimulation. For this particular neuron, the two optimal response planes were at 68 deg and −112 deg. Note that the neuron increased its discharge when the rabbit was rotated onto its left side. (**B**) Response of the same dmcc neuron to static roll about an optimal response plane. The static response indicates that this neuron received an otolithic input. (**C**) Illustration of the location within the dmcc of the recorded neuron. dIPO, vIPO, dorsolateral and ventrolateral principal olive; Pyr, pyramidal tract; R mg, nucleus raphe magnus.

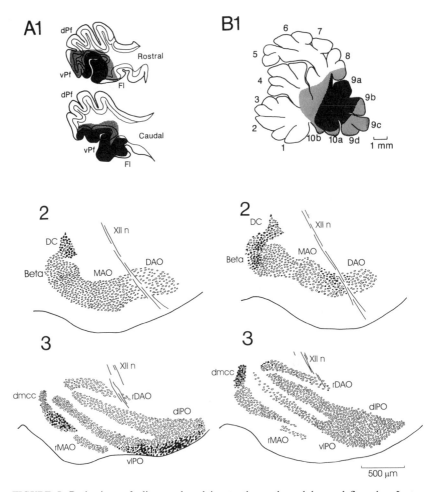

FIGURE 5. Projections of olivary subnuclei onto the uvula-nodulus and flocculus. In two separate experiments, horseradish peroxidase was microinjected into the left flocculus, **A,** and left nodulus, **B.** The locations of these injection sites are illustrated in **A1** and **B1.** The floccular injection produced retrograde labeling in the dorsal cap, **A2,** the ventral aspect of the rostral medial accessory olive, as well as the ventrolateral principal olive, **A3.** The uvula-nodulus injection produced retrograde labeling in the dorsal cap and β-nucleus, **B2,** as well as the dorsomedial cell column, **B3.** Beta, β-nucleus; DC, dorsal cap; dmcc, dorsomedial cell column; dlPO, vlPO, dorsolateral and ventrolateral principal olive; dPF, vPf, dorsal and ventral paraflocculus; DAO, MAO, dorsal and medial accessory olive; Fl, flocculus; Pyr, pyramidal tract; 9a-d, uvula; 10a-b, nodulus; XII n, hypoglossal nerve.

could selectively bias certain postural responses that would be appropriate following the activation of the otoliths and vertical semicircular canals. It remains to be seen whether these strips are anatomically fixed or whether their size might be dependent on vestibularly evoked olivary activity.

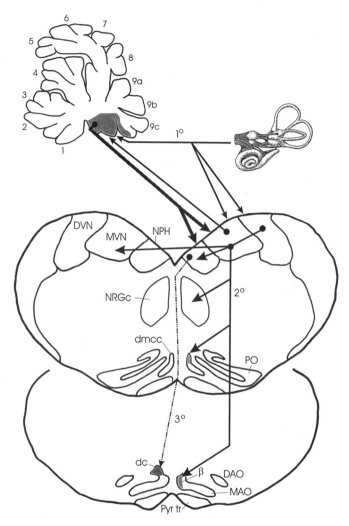

FIGURE 6. Functional connections of the β-nucleus and dmcc with the vestibular nuclei and cerebellum. Primary vestibular afferents project directly onto the ipsilateral uvula-nodulus and vestibular nuclei (*dark lines*). Lobules 9d and 10 are illustrated as shaded. The medial and descending vestibular nuclei (MVN, DVN) project as secondary vestibular afferents *bilaterally* to the nodulus and uvula (*dark line*). These same vestibular nuclei project as GABAergic secondary vestibular afferents onto the ipsilateral β-nucleus, dmcc, and nucleus reticularis gigantocellularis (*dark lines*). Tertiary vestibular GABAergic afferents project onto the *contralateral* dorsal cap (*dashed line*). The β-nucleus and dmcc send climbing-fiber projections to the contralateral uvula and nodulus. GABAergic Purkinje cells send a return projection onto the subjacent nucleus prepositus hypoglossi (NPH), MVN, and DVN (*shaded line*). The dorsal cap receives a visual projection from the contralateral eye via the nucleus of the optic tract and also receives a cholinergic input from the contralateral NPH. The dorsal cap projects to the contralateral flocculus and ventral aspect of the nodulus. β, β-nucleus; dc, dorsal cap; PO, principal olive; DAO, MAO, dorsal and medial accessory olive; NRGC, nucleus reticularis gigantocellularis; 1°, 2°, 3°, primary, secondary, and tertiary vestibular afferents; Pyr, pyramidal tract.

REFERENCES

1. KOOY, F. H. 1916. The inferior olive in vertebrates. Folia Neurobiol. **10:** 205–369.
2. ALLEY, K., R. BAKER & J. I. SIMPSON. 1975. Afferents to the vestibulo-cerebellum and the origin of the visual climbing fibers in the rabbit. Brain Res. **98:** 582–589.
3. BARMACK, N. H. & D. T. HESS. 1980. Multiple-unit activity evoked in dorsal cap of inferior olive of the rabbit by visual stimulation. J. Neurophysiol. **43:** 151–164.
4. LEONARD, C. S., J. I. SIMPSON & W. GRAF. 1988. Spatial organization of visual messages of the rabbit's cerebellar flocculus. I. Typology of inferior olive neurons of the dorsal cap of Kooy. J. Neurophysiol. **60:** 2073–2090.
5. BLANKS, R. H. I., I. S. CURTHOYS & C. H. MARKHAM. 1975. Planar relationships of the semicircular canals in man. Acta Otolaryngol. **80:** 185–196.
6. BARMACK, N. H., M. FAGERSON, B. J. FREDETTE, E. MUGNAINI & H. SHOJAKU. 1993. Activity of neurons in the beta nucleus of the inferior olive of the rabbit evoked by natural vestibular stimulation. Exp. Brain Res. **94:** 203–215.
7. GERRITS, N. M., J. VOOGD & I. N. MAGRAS. 1985. Vestibular afferents of the inferior olive and the vestibulo-olivo-cerebellar climbing fiber pathway to the flocculus in the cat. Brain Res. **332:** 325–336.
8. SAINT-CYR, J. A. & J. COURVILLE. 1979. Projection from the vestibular nuclei to the inferior olive in the cat: An autoradiographic and horseradish peroxidase study. Brain Res. **165:** 189–200.
9. WALBERG, F. 1974. Descending connections from the mesencephalon to the inferior olive: An experimental study in the cat. Exp. Brain Res. **21:** 145–156.
10. BALABAN, C. D. & R. T. HENRY. 1988. Zonal organization of olivo-nodulus projections in albino rabbits. Neurosci. Res. **5:** 409–423.
11. BRODAL, A. 1976. The olivocerebellar projection in the cat as studied with the method of retrograde axonal transport of horseradish peroxidase. II. The projection to the uvula. J. Comp. Neurol. **166:** 417–426.
12. KANDA, K-I., Y. SATO, K. IKARASHI & T. KAWASAKI. 1989. Zonal organization of climbing fiber projections to the uvula in the cat. J. Comp. Neurol. **279:** 138–148.
13. SATO, Y. & N. H. BARMACK. 1985. Zonal organization of the olivocerebellar projection to the uvula in rabbits. Brain Res. **359:** 281–291.
14. OERTEL, W. H., D. E. SCHMECHEL, M. L. TAPPAZ & I. J. KOPIN. 1981. Production of a specific antiserum to rat brain glutamic acid decarboxylase by injection of an antigen-antibody complex. Neuroscience **12:** 2689–2700.
15. BARMACK, N. H. & V. E. PETTOROSSI. 1985. Effects of unilateral lesions of the flocculus on optokinetic and vestibuloocular reflexes of the rabbit. J. Neurophysiol. **53:** 481–496.
16. OLUCHA, F., F. MARTINEZ-GARCIA & C. LOPEZ-GARCIA. 1985. A new stabilizing agent for the tetramethyl benzidine (TMB) reaction product in the histochemical detection of horseradish peroxidase (HRP). J. Neurosci. Methods **13:** 131–138.
17. RYE, D. B., C. B. SAPER & B. H. WAINER. 1984. Stabilization of tetramethylbenzidine (TMB) reaction product: Application of retrograde and anterograde tracing, and combination with immunohistochemistry. J. Histochem. Cytochem. **32:** 1145–1153.
18. FREDETTE, B. J. & E. MUGNAINI. 1991. The GABAergic cerebello-olivary projection in the rat. Anat. Embryol. **184:** 225–243.
19. NELSON, B. J., J. C. ADAMS, N. H. BARMACK & E. MUGNAINI. 1989. A comparative study of glutamate decarboxylase immunoreactive boutons in the mammalian inferior olive. J. Comp. Neurol. **286:** 514–539.
20. BARMACK, N. H., M. FAGERSON & P. ERRICO. 1993. Cholinergic projection to the dorsal cap of the inferior olive of the rat, rabbit and monkey. J. Comp. Neurol. **328:** 263–281.
21. ROBINSON, F. R., M. O. FRASER, J. R. HOLLERMAN & D. L. TOMKO. 1988. Yaw direction neurons in the cat inferior olive. J. Neurophysiol. **60:** 1739–1752.
22. PRECHT, W., J. I. SIMPSON & R. LLINÁS. 1976. Responses of Purkinje cells in rabbit nodulus and uvula to natural vestibular and visual stimuli. Pflugers Arch. Gesamte Physiol. **367:** 1–6.
23. BARMACK, N. H. & H. SHOJAKU. 1995. Vestibular and visual signals evoked in the uvula-nodulus of the rabbit cerebellum by natural stimulation. J. Neurophysiol. **74:** 2573–2589.
24. KAUFMAN, G. D., J. H. ANDERSON & A. BEITZ. 1991. Activation of a specific vestibulo-olivary pathway by centripetal acceleration in rat. Brain Res. **562:** 311–317.

Organization of the Vestibulocerebellum

JAN VOOGD, NICOLAAS M. GERRITS,
AND TOM J. H. RUIGROK

Department of Anatomy
Erasmus University Rotterdam
P. O. Box 1738
3000 DR Rotterdam, the Netherlands

The flocculo-nodular lobe and the corpus cerebelli are the two main subdivisions of the mammalian cerebellum.[55,57] Flocculus and nodulus are demarcated from the corpus cerebelli by the posterolateral fissure. This fissure is the first to appear during ontogeny of the mammalian cerebellum.[24] Usually the posterolateral fissure develops independently in the future vermis and the two hemispheres, and the merging of the three segments into a single fissure is the exception rather than the rule. In adult mammals the cortex between the nodulus and the uvula (lobules X and IX of the caudal vermis) and the flocculus and the paraflocculus usually is completely interrupted. A small cortical ridge, running along the attachment of the roof of the fourth ventricle, interconnects the cortex of the flocculus with the nodulus in marsupials and small bats, insectivores, and rodents. The cortices of the flocculus and the nodulus continue uninterruptedly into the cortices of the paraflocculus and the uvula, in the bottom of the posterolateral fissure.

The afferent and efferent connections of the flocculo-nodular lobe are chiefly with the vestibular nuclei, and, therefore, this subdivision of the cerebellum is often referred to as the vestibulocerebellum. On the afferent side the main connections of the cerebellar cortex are the mossy fibers. The output of the cerebellar cortex through the Purkinje cells is organized in a modular fashion: Purkinje cells that project to a specific cerebellar or vestibular nucleus are arranged in longitudinal zones and their olivocerebellar, climbing fiber afferents are distributed according to the same principle. Information processing in the cerebellum and the vestibular nuclei underlying gaze control recently was reviewed by Gerrits.[30] In our paper we will discuss the relevance of the afferent mossy fiber connections and the modular organization of the Purkinje cells for the concept of the vestibulocerebellum.

MOSSY FIBER PROJECTIONS TO THE CEREBELLUM: DISTRIBUTION OF VESTIBULOCEREBELLAR MOSSY FIBERS

Primary vestibulocerebellar mossy fibers from the vestibular nerve project profusely to the nodulus and the ventral uvula, but also terminate in lobules I and II of the anterior lobe and medially in the cortex in the bottom of the deep interlobular fissures. The primary vestibular projection to the vermis is ipsilateral, with some mossy fibers terminating on the contralateral side, next to the midline (FIG. 1). Vestibular root fibers do not terminate or are scarce in the flocculus.[10,35,49,53] Secondary vestibulocerebellar mossy fibers originate from all vestibular nuclei (FIG. 1), including groups x and y, but excluding the dorsal part of the lateral vestibular nucleus (Deiters' nucleus). They terminate bilaterally in the same regions as the primary vestibulocerebellar mossy fibers, but also in the flocculus and the adjoining

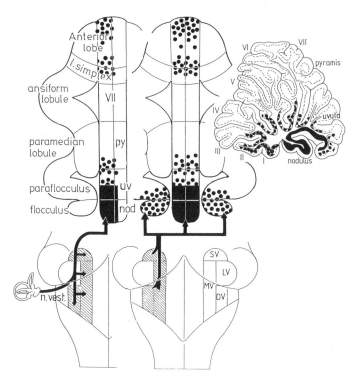

FIGURE 1. Diagram of the primary and secondary vestibulocerebellar mossy fiber projections. Vestibular nuclei that receive vestibular root fibers (*left*) and give rise to secondary vestibulocerebellar fibers (*right*) appear as hatched area. Dense projections to the nodulus/uvula are indicated in black; less heavy projections, with filled circles. Distribution in sagittal section of the cerebellum applies to both primary and secondary vestibulocerebellar projections. DV, descending vestibular nucleus; LV, lateral vestibular nucleus; MV, medial vestibular nucleus; n.vest, vestibular nerve; nod, nodulus; py, pyramis; SV, superior vestibular nucleus; uv, uvula; I–X, lobules I–X. (Based on data from Gerrits *et al.*[35] and Thunnissen *et al.*[76])

folia of the paraflocculus.[9,27,28,30,50,75] The distribution of mossy fibers from the perihypoglossal nuclei, including the nucleus prepositus hypoglossi in the squirrel monkey, is restricted to nodulus and uvula and flocculus and adjacent ventral paraflocculus, with a second focus in lobule VII and the adjacent ansiform lobule.[12] A more extensive distribution was reported for the cat.[51]

Is the distinction of the flocculo-nodular lobe as the vestibulocerebellum justified by the distribution of the vestibular mossy fibers? The answer can be both yes and no. Yes, for the profuse projections to the nodulus, when the adjoining ventral part of the uvula is included in it. Of the retrogradely labeled neurons in the brain stem, labeled from injections of retrograde tracers in the ventral uvula of the cat, 70–80% were located in the vestibular nuclei,[69] and for the nodulus this figure would be even higher. No, for the extension of the primary and secondary vestibular mossy fibers projecting into the ventral part of the anterior lobe and the bottom of the deep fissures and for the paucity of eighth nerve projections to the flocculus.

OVERLAP AND SEGREGATION OF MOSSY FIBER PROJECTIONS TO THE NODULUS/UVULA: TRANSVERSE ("LOBULAR") AND MEDIOLATERAL ("ZONAL") PATTERNS

The widespread distribution of vestibular mossy fibers in ventral parts of the cerebellum was accounted for in Ingvar's[44] division of the cerebellum into a vestibular "basement," consisting of nodulus/uvula, lingula and flocculus, a spinal "storey" comprising the anterior lobe and the pyramis, and a pontocerebellar "top floor" including lobules VI and VII. Ingvar's scheme suggests that the vestibular projections to the nodulus and the ventral uvula border on the spinocerebellar projections to the dorsal uvula and the pyramis. In the posterior lobe, spinocerebellar projections, indeed, terminate in the bottom of the secondary fissure between pyramis and uvula, and trigeminocerebellar mossy fibers are present in the dorsal uvula,[19,45,71,79,81] but the most prominent mossy fiber projection to the dorsal uvula arises from rostral and dorsal, presumably visual, areas of the basal pontine nuclei (FIG. 2).[18,29,32,33,36,80]

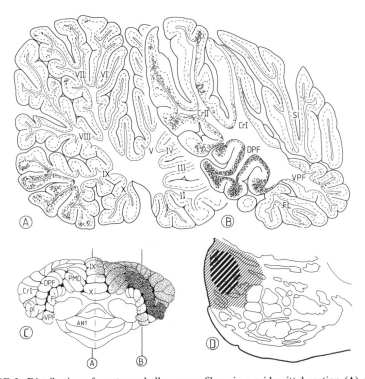

FIGURE 2. Distribution of pontocerebellar mossy fibers in a midsagittal section (**A**) and a section through the flocculus, the ventral paraflocculus, and the dorsal paraflocculus (**B**) of the cerebellum of *Macaca fascicularis*. The levels of the two sections and the distribution of the pontocerebellar fibers are indicated in the drawing of the ventral aspect of the cerebellum (**C**). In **D** the injection site of the axonal tracer (wheat germ–coupled horseradish peroxidase) in the dorsolateral pons is indicated. ANT, anterior lobe; CrI, CrI II, crus I, crus II; DPF, dorsal paraflocculus; FL, flocculus; pl, petrosal lobule; PMD, paramedian lobule; VPF, ventral paraflocculus; I–X, lobules I–X. (Modified from Glickstein *et al.*[36])

According to Sato et al.[69] the rostral pons accounts for 90% of the retrogradely labeled neurons after injections of the dorsal and ventrolateral uvula in the cat. In the anterior lobe the vestibulocerebellar mossy fibers overlap with the spinocerebellar projections from the central cervical nucleus that presumably subserve proprioceptive input from the neck.[61,62] The mossy fibers from the nucleus prepositus hypoglossi in the nodulus/uvula of the squirrel monkey,[12] the distributions of the spinocerebellar and trigeminocerebellar mossy fibers in the dorsal uvula, and the overlapping, secondary vestibulocerebellar and central cervical spinocerebellar projections to the anterior lobe display a mediolateral periodicity. Such a mediolateral periodicity is not observed for the termination of the primary and secondary vestibular mossy fibers and the pontocerebellar projections that terminate diffusely in the nodulus and the uvula.

MOSSY FIBER PROJECTIONS TO THE FLOCCULUS AND THE PARAFLOCCULUS

According to Sato et al.,[68] only 20% of the retrogradely labeled cells from injections of the flocculus in the cat are located in the vestibular nuclei, and the percentages of mossy fibers responding to vestibular stimulation in the primate flocculus[53] are even lower. The reticular and raphe nuclei (including the cell groups of the paramedian tracts of Büttner-Ennever and Horn, this volume) and the perihypoglossal nuclei provide most mossy fiber afferents to the flocculus in cat[68] and monkey.[53] In the monkey the basal interstitial nucleus of the cerebellum, which consists of cells in the roof of the fourth ventricle scattered between the flocculus and the nodulus, provides a sizable input to the flocculus.[53] Secondary vestibulocerebellar projections extend, across the posterolateral fissure, into the ventral paraflocculus. In the cat they occupy the folia of the medial extension (ME) of the ventral paraflocculus and the next, caudalmost folium of this lobule (FIG. 3A–D).[29] In the rabbit the secondary vestibulocerebellar mossy fibers appear to be mostly restricted to the flocculus but mossy fibers from the perihypoglossal nuclei also terminate in the folium of the ventral paraflocculus bordering on the flocculus (folium P[9,75,88]). The region of the primate paraflocculus that receives mossy fibers from the vestibular and perihypoglossal nuclei[12,53] is more extensive than in either cat or rabbit and includes the entire ventral paraflocculus.[a]

Differences in mossy fiber afferentiation between the flocculus proper, the adjoining folia of the paraflocculus (ME of the cat, folium P of the rabbit, and the primate ventral paraflocculus), and the rest of the paraflocculus thus far only have been documented for the basal pontine nuclei and the nucleus reticularis tegmenti pontis (NRTP). In the rabbit, retrograde labeling in the NRTP, including the processus tegmentosis lateralis, was only observed from injections of the flocculus.

---

[a] Ventral paraflocculus and flocculus originally were both included in the monkey flocculus by Larsell[56] and Madigan and Carpenter.[59] Larsell[57] later revised this opinion on the basis of the identification of the posterolateral fissure in fetal material of the rhesus monkey and then subdivided this region into the smaller flocculus proper and the ventral paraflocculus. In the experiments of Belknap and McCrea[12] in the squirrel monkey, the flocculus and the ventral paraflocculus were correctly identified. The experiments of Langer et al.[53] include retrograde tracer injections of both lobules. With respect to the vestibular nuclei and the nucleus prepositus hypoglossi, the distribution of the labeled neurons is a case where an injection of the flocculus proper (monkey Kaiser, their FIG. 2) and the ventral paraflocculus (monkey Franz, their FIG. 8) are roughly similar.

Labeling in the pontine nuclei was found after injections of folium P and the adjacent ventral paraflocculus.[88] Injections of antegrade axonal tracers in the rostral basal pontine nuclei in the cat spare the flocculus proper and the ME, but project profusely to the rest of the ventral paraflocculus and the dorsal paraflocculus.[33] Similarly, projections from the rostral dorsolateral pons in macaque monkeys spared the flocculus proper, but gave rise to a sparse projection to the ventral paraflocculus and a profuse projection to the petrosal lobule and the dorsal paraflocculus (FIG. 2[36]). The paucity of the pontine projections to the flocculus and the ME in the cat and the primate ventral paraflocculus contrasts with the strong projections to these lobules of the NRTP.[33,36] In the cat, the central part of the NRTP, the nucleus raphe pontis, and neurons from the processus tegmentosus lateralis project to the flocculus (FIG. 3E and G). The ME and the most caudal sublobule of the ventral paraflocculus receive a dense projection from neurons located near the medial edge of the medial lemniscus, next to the NRTP (FIG. 3F and H). This region also projects to the dorsal uvula.[33] The present evidence suggests that the main mossy fiber afferents of these lobules, be it pontine, reticular or vestibular, terminate diffusely, without signs of a zonal or patchy organization. However, indications for more restricted terminations of secondary vestibular, perihypoglossal and (reticulo)-pontine mossy fibers are contained in the publications of Yamamoto,[88] Gerrits *et al.,*[29,33] and Belknap and McCrea.[12]

MODULAR ("ZONAL") ORGANIZATION OF THE FLOCCULUS/PARAFLOCCULUS AND THE NODULUS/UVULA

The spatial arrangement of the afferent climbing fibers to the Purkinje cells and the efferent, corticonuclear, and corticovestibular projections of these cells is strikingly different from the organization of the mossy fibers. Purkinje cells with a projection to a specific cerebellar or vestibular target nucleus are distributed as one or more longitudinal zones, which are oriented perpendicular to the parallel fibers to the molecular layer and to the transverse, interfolial fissures. Purkinje cell zones and their target nucleus receive a projection from a particular subnucleus of the contralateral inferior olive, which terminates as climbing fibers on these Purkinje cells and as collaterals of the olivocerebellar fibers on the cells of the target nucleus.[17,37,38,82] This "modular" organization of the output system of the cerebellum is completed by the nucleo-olivary pathways that interconnect the cerebellar target nuclei with the olivary subnuclei. Purkinje cell zones sharing the same target nucleus often interdigitate with zones with different target nuclei. There appears to be little or no overlap in the connections of neighboring modules.

A modular organization also can be recognized in nodulus and uvula and in flocculus and paraflocculus. Different approaches can be used to study the modular organization of a lobule. In one approach the subdivision of the white matter of the lobule is studied. Efferent, Purkinje cell axons of a zone and its climbing fiber afferents occupy discrete compartments in the white matter of the cerebellum. At the borders of these compartments Purkinje cell axons are absent. Staining with Purkinje cell-specific antibodies reveals these narrow border zones as empty slits (FIG. 8B). With acetylcholinesterase staining the borders between the compartments are positively stained (FIGS. 4D and 8A).[42] The projections of the Purkinje cells can be

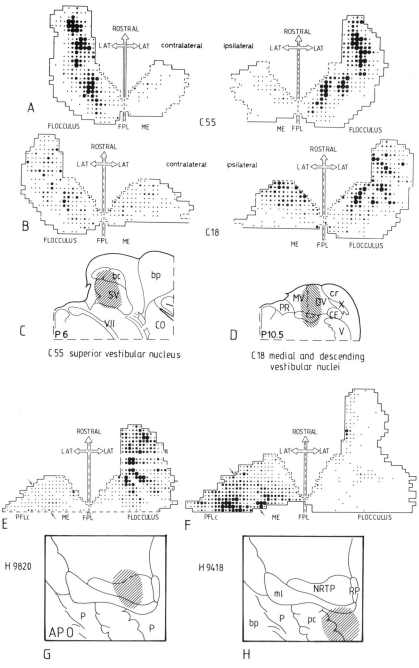

FIGURE 3.

studied with retrograde labeling from their target nuclei[82] or antegrade axonal labeling from small injections. Good results were obtained with injections of a few Purkinje cells with biocytin.[22,86] Climbing fiber projections can be studied with retrograde methods[43] or, preferably, with anterograde axonal labeling from injections of the subnuclei of the inferior olive.[31,37] Injection sites and axonal labeling can be correlated with the compartmental subdivision of the white matter of the lobules in adjacent AChE-stained sections and/or the electrophysiological properties of the climbing fibers and the results of microstimulation.[78]

WHITE MATTER COMPARTMENTS AND LONGITUDINAL ZONES OF THE FLOCCULUS OF THE RABBIT

Five compartments were delineated with AChE staining in the flocculus of the rabbit cerebellum (FIGS. 4 and 5).[72] The most lateral C_2 compartment continues into the paraflocculus and contains the posterior interposed nucleus. The other four are numbered laterally to medially as floccular compartments (FC) 1–4. The C_2 compartment and FC 1–3 continue into the white matter of folium P. Here FC 1 and FC 3 merge over the dorsal tip of FC 2. In the paraflocculus FC 1–3 are replaced by the D compartment, which contains the lateral cerebellar nucleus.[72] Olivocerebellar fibers from the caudal dorsal cap (DC) occupy the FC 2 and FC 4 compartment and terminate on Purkinje cells of the corresponding flocculus zones 2 and 4 (FIG. 5). Zone 4 is narrow and only present in the rostromedial flocculus; zone 2 extends to folium P. Climbing fibers of the rostral DC and the ventrolateral outgrowth (VLO) occupy the FC 1 and FC 3 compartments and terminate on zones 1 and 3, which interleave with the caudal DC-innervated zones, and extend to folium P. The olivocerebellar projection to the C_2 zone arises from the rostromedial accessory olive.[73]

Axons of Purkinje cells, which are located within a particular climbing fiber zone, collect in the corresponding white matter compartment. Axons were traced with wheat-germ-coupled horseradish peroxidase (HRP)[74] or, in more detail, from small injections of biocytin.[22] Purkinje cells of zones 1 and 3 projected to group y and the superior vestibular nucleus, and those of zones 2 and 4 to the magnocellular and parvicellular medial vestibular nucleus (FIG. 5). Purkinje cell axons from cells in zones 1 and 2 either enter the floccular peduncle, or arch through the dentate nucleus, where collaterals of zone 1 cells also terminate. Purkinje cell axons from zones 3 and 4 are restricted to the floccular peduncle. Zone C_2 projects to the lateral pole of the posterior interposed nucleus and group y. Similar results on the afferent and efferent projections of the Purkinje cells of the rabbit flocculus and folium P were obtained earlier by Yamamoto[87,89] and Balaban.[6]

←

FIGURE 3. Diagrams illustrating the distribution of labeled mossy fiber terminals in the floccular complex of the cat, after injections of tritiated leucine into the vestibular nuclei (**A–D**) and the region of the nucleus reticularis tegmenti pontis (**E–H**). Flocculus and adjacent paraflocculus [medial extension (ME) and caudal folium of the ventral paraflocculus (PFLc)] are projected upon a horizontal plane and unfolded along the bottom of the posterolateral fissure (FPL). Classes of increasing numbers of mossy fiber terminals are indicated with dots of increasing size. The concentrations of mossy fibers in the diagrams represent projections of the individual folia with their larger volume of granular layer, and are not due to differences in the overall density of the mossy fiber rosettes. (Based on data from Gerrits.[29,33])

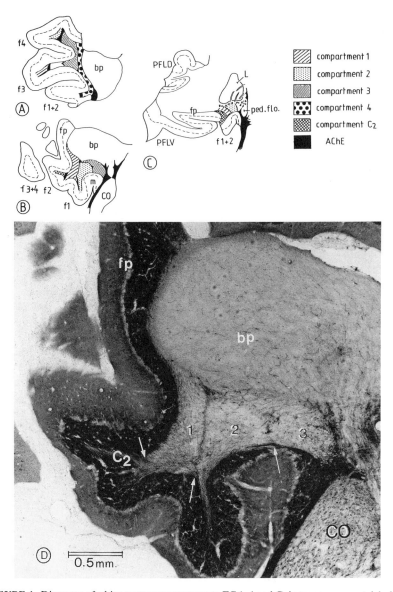

FIGURE 4. Diagrams of white matter compartments FC 1–4 and C_2 in transverse acetylcholinesterase-stained sections through the flocculus of the rabbit. (**A**) Most rostral section. (**D**) Photograph of section represented in **B**. Arrows in **D** indicate acetylcholinesterase-positive borders between the compartments. bp, brachium pontis; CO, cochlear nucleus; f1–4, folia 1–4; fp, folium p of the ventral paraflocculus; m, folium m; ped.flo., pedunculus flocculi; fp, folium P; PFLD, dorsal paraflocculus; PFLV, ventral paraflocculus. (Based on Tan *et al.*[72])

MODULAR ("ZONAL") ORGANIZATION OF THE FLOCCULUS/PARAFLOCCULUS IN CAT AND RAT. COMPARISONS WITH THE RABBIT

The pattern of connections of the Purkinje cells of the flocculus in cat (FIG. 6) and rat (FIG. 7) is very similar to that in rabbit. Gerrits and Voogd[31] distinguished a

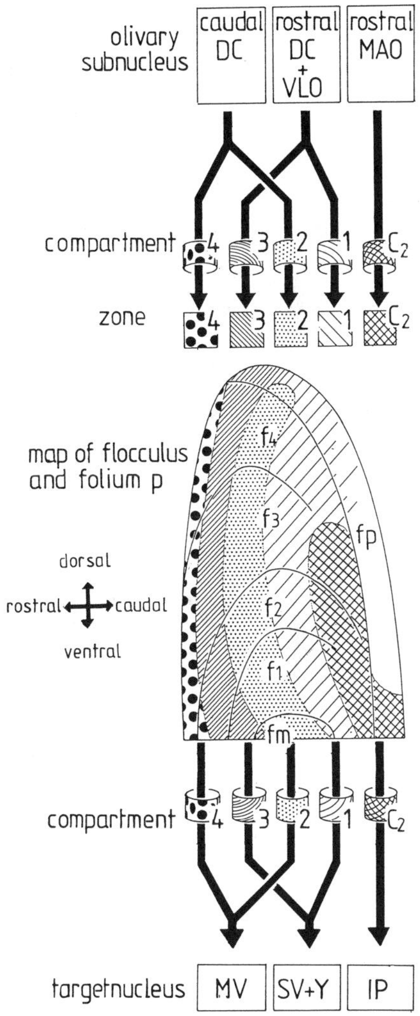

FIGURE 5. Diagram of the white matter compartments and zones 1–4 and C_2 of the rabbit flocculus. Olivocerebellar fibers innervating Purkinje cells of a particular zone and the Purkinje cell axons of the zone to their target nucleus occupy the same compartment. DC, dorsal cap; f1–f4 = folia 1–4; fm, folium m; fp, folium p; IP, posterior interposed nucleus; MAO, medial accessory olive; MV, medial vestibular nucleus; SV, superior vestibular nucleus; VLO, ventrolateral outgrowth; Y, group y. (Based on Tan et al.[73,74] and De Zeeuw et al.[22])

C_2 zone and seven floccular (F) climbing fiber zones in the flocculus and the ME of the cat. Their caudal DC-innervated zones F1 and F4 are clearly identical to the zones 4 and 2 of the rabbit flocculus of Tan et al.[73] The equivalents of the rostral DC/VLO-innervated zones 1 and 3 of the rabbit flocculus can be further subdivided in the cat,

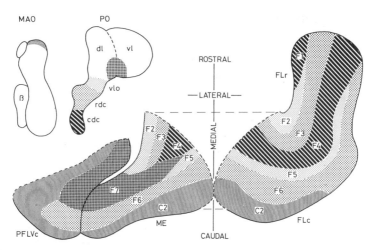

FIGURE 6. Diagram of the topographical relation between subdivisions of the inferior olive and the climbing fiber strips F1–F7 and C_2 of the flocculus (subdivided into caudal, FLc, and rostral, FLr, parts) and the medial extension (ME) and the caudal folium of the ventral paraflocculus (PFLVc) of the cat. Medial accessory and principal olive are represented as horizontal projections of these nuclei. Flocculus and ventral paraflocculus are unfolded (cf. FIG. 3). Corresponding climbing fiber strips and subdivisions of the inferior olive are indicated with the same symbols. Abbreviations for subdivisions of the inferior olive: β, group beta; cdc, caudal dorsal cap; dl, dorsal leaf principal olive; MAO, medial accessory olive; PO, principal olive; rdc, rostral dorsal cap; vl, ventral leaf of the principal olive; vlo, ventrolateral outgrowth. (From Gerrits and Voogd.[31] Reproduced with permission of *Neuroscience*.)

where they are represented by the zones F5 + 6 + 7 and F2 + 3, respectively. The medial subzones F2 and F5 of the cat are innervated by the VLO, the lateral subzones F3 and F6 by the rostral DC, and subzone F7, which is restricted to the ME and the next caudal folium of the ventral paraflocculus, receives its climbing fibers from the caudal principal olive.[31]

Climbing fiber responses to optokinetic stimulation were recorded as complex spike modulation of Purkinje cells of the flocculus of the rabbit by Kusonoki *et al*.[52] Cells that preferred horizontal movement were activated when a temporally to nasally moving optokinetic stimulus was presented to the ipsilateral eye (Ipsi F cells). These cells were located in a single, 1-mm-wide strip along the caudal part of the rostral one-third of the flocculus. Some Ipsi F cells were found scattered in folium P. A good correspondence is found between this strip and the projection of the caudal DC, which contains the vertical axis neurons of Leonard *et al*.,[58] to zone 2 of Tan *et al*.[73] The rostromedial, caudal DC-innervated zone 4 of Tan *et al*.[73] was not noticed in these electrophysiological studies.[52]

Most of the cells that preferred vertical optokinetic stimulation were excited by upward movement presented to the ipsilateral eye (Ipsi U cells) or downward movement presented to the contralateral eye (Contra D cells).[52] Cells with a preference for vertical movement were located in two strips, one rostral and one caudal to the Ipsi F cells. These two strips correspond to the zones 1 and 3 of the rabbit flocculus, which receive climbing fiber projections from the rostral DC and the VLO. The optokinetic stimulus activating the Ipsi U cells appears to be equivalent to the rotation that activated the posterior (135°) axis units in the VLO in the experiments of Leonard *et al.*[58] The Contra D stimulus probably was relayed by the anterior (45°) axis units of Leonard *et al.*[58] located in the rostral DC. There is a tendency for Ipsi U cells, innervated by the VLO, to be located more rostrally and medially in the flocculus than the Contra D cells, rostral DC-innervated zone (FIG. 10B and C of Kusonoki *et al.*[52]). This mediolateral gradient in the rostral DC/VLO innervated zone 1 of the rabbit flocculus is identical to the disposition of climbing fibers from the VLO and the rostral DC in the medial F5 and lateral F6 subzones of the flocculus of the cat, respectively, as described by Gerrits and Voogd.[31] The presence of these subzones in the flocculus of rabbit and cat may indicate that floccular zones can be further subdivided into microzones, as has been described for the B and C$_3$ zones of the anterior lobe of the cat.[1,26]

Corticonuclear projections of the individual floccular zones have not yet been studied in the rat, and data on the cat are still controversial. The distribution of the Purkinje cell axons of the flocculus as a whole has been extensively studied in both species. The flocculus projects to the central and dorsal part of the superior vestibular nucleus, and to the lateral part of the medial vestibular nucleus and the medial part of the spinal vestibular nuclei including group f. Deiters' nucleus and the rostral part of the magnocellular part of the medial vestibular nucleus are mostly spared. Projections to group y and the nucleus prepositus hypoglossi have been

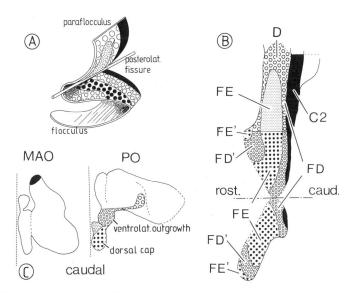

FIGURE 7. Diagram of the projection from the inferior olive to the flocculus and the ventral paraflocculus in the rat. Paraflocculus and flocculus (**A**) are unfolded in **B.** (**C**) The medial accessory olive (MAO) and the principal (PO) are drawn as diagrams of the unfolded inferior olive; the cortex of the flocculus and the ventral paraflocculus are unfolded. Corresponding climbing fiber zones and subdivisions of the inferior olive are indicated with the same symbols. The climbing fiber zones of the rat flocculus correspond to those in the rabbit (FIGS. 4 and 5). FD corresponds to zone 1 of the rabbit; FE to zone 2; FD′ to zone 3; and FE′ to zone 4. FD and FD′ continue as zone D of the paraflocculus. C$_2$, C$_2$ zone; caud, caudal; FD, FD′, FD (′) zone (projections of vlo and PO); FE, FE′, FE (′) zone (projections of dorsal cap); FLOd and v = dorsal and ventral surface of the flocculus; MAO, medial accessory olive; PO, principal olive; rost., rostral; vlo, ventrolateral outgrowth. (Modified from Ruigrok *et al.*[65])

occasionally mentioned. The flocculus projects to the caudolateral dentate nucleus; terminations in the posterior interposed nucleus only have been established for the rat.[2,13,24,77,80,90]

Sato and collaborators (reviewed by Sato and Kawasaki[67]) distinguished three zones in the flocculus of the cat. Their rostral zone is innervated from the rostral DC and the VLO and projects to the superior vestibular nucleus, and their middle zone receives climbing fibers from the caudal DC and projects to the medial vestibular nucleus. These zones closely correspond to floccular zones 2 and 3 of the rabbit[73,74] and to zones F2 + 3 and F4 of the cat.[31] The caudal DC/VLO innervated zone of Sato projects to group y and, sparsely, to the lateral cerebellar nucleus. Equivalents of the rostromedial floccular zone 4 of the rabbit (zone F1 of Gerrits and Voogd[31]) and of the C_2 zone in the caudal flocculus and a projection of the caudal zone to the superior vestibular nucleus were not identified by them in the cat.

MODULAR ("ZONAL") ORGANIZATION OF THE FLOCCULUS/PARAFLOCCULUS IN PRIMATES

Data on the zonal organization of the primate flocculus are scarce. The olivocerebellar projection to the flocculus in Galago[b,85] and the flocculus and the ventral paraflocculus of the rhesus monkey[16,53] appears to be similar to that in other mammals. The projection of the flocculus as a whole to the vestibular nuclei in Galago[b,40] and of the flocculus and the ventral paraflocculus in the rhesus monkey[54] is very similar to the projections of the flocculus in rat, rabbit, and cat. The y group in primates is much larger than in lower mammals and receives a dense projection from the flocculus and the ventral paraflocculus.[54] Langer et al.[54] also noticed a diffuse output of these lobules to the basal interstitial nucleus. Projections to the cerebellar nuclei in primates have not been reported.

Acetylcholinesterase staining of the macaque cerebellum revealed a compartmentation of the white matter of the flocculus and the paraflocculus.[42,83,84] Four compartments can be distinguished in the white matter of the flocculus and the ventral paraflocculus (FIG. 8). The lateral C_2 compartment continues, through the petrosal lobule into the dorsal paraflocculus, where it envelops the posterior interposed nucleus. The medial three compartments are restricted to the flocculus and the ventral paraflocculus. Their correspondence with compartments 1–3 of the rabbit flocculus is suggested by the fusion of the medial (1) and lateral (3) compartments over the dorsal tip of the middle (2) compartments, and by the localization of the olivocerebellar fibers in the middle compartment of the flocculus and the ventral paraflocculus in experiments with injections of tritiated leucine in the caudal DC in macaque monkeys.[83,84] The localization of retrogradely labeled Purkinje cells in a middle zone of these lobules after injections of retrograde tracers in the medial vestibular nucleus in primates[7,11] is in accordance with this interpretation. An equivalent of the caudal DC-innervated, medial vestibular nucleus-projecting, zone 4 of the rabbit flocculus appears to be lacking in primates.

---

[b]It is not known whether the flocculus of Galago, as described by Haines,[39] corresponds to the flocculus of lower mammals, or whether it includes a region corresponding to the ventral paraflocculus of primates.

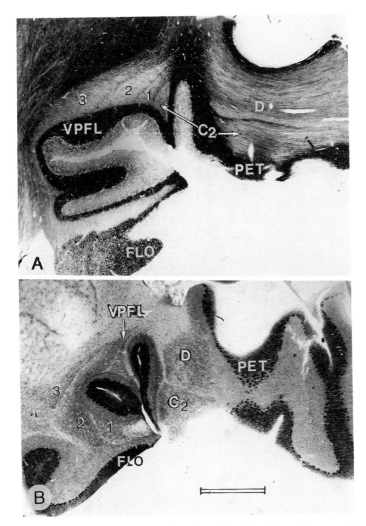

FIGURE 8. Photographs of transverse sections through the flocculus and the ventral parafloc-culus of *Macaca fascicularis*. (**A**) Acetylcholinesterase-reacted section, showing positive staining of the borders of compartments 1–3 and C_2 in the white matter of the ventral paraflocculus (VPFL) and the flocculus (FLO). C_2 extends into the petrosal lobule (PET), where compartments 1–3 are replaced by the compartment D. (**B**) Zebrin-I immunoreacted section with positive staining of all Purkinje cells and their axons. The borders between the compartments in the flocculus, the ventral paraflocculus, and the petrosal lobule remain unstained. Bar = 1 mm.

MODULAR ("ZONAL") ORGANIZATION OF THE NODULUS/UVULA. CLIMBING FIBER PROJECTIONS

The modular organization of the nodulus and the uvula has been studied in rabbit[5,8,27,28,48,66,73] and rat.[3,13,25] Data on the cat[14,37,46,70] and on primates[85] are scarce.

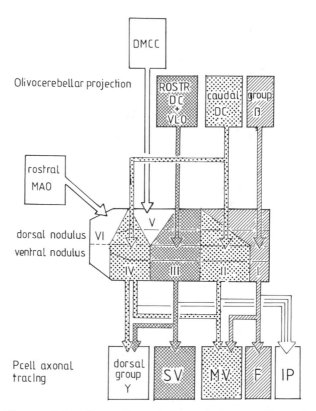

FIGURE 9. Diagram of the afferent olivocerebellar projection according to Katayama and Nisimaru,[48] Balaban and Henry,[8] and Tan *et al.*[73] and the efferent projection of the zones of the nodulus to the vestibular and cerebellar nuclei according to Wylie *et al.*[86] in the rabbit. β, group beta of the medial accessory olive (MAO); DC, dorsal cap of Kooy; F, fastigial nucleus; IP, posterior interposed nucleus; MV, medial vestibular nucleus; P cell, Purkinje cell; SV, superior vestibular nucleus; VLO, ventrolateral outgrowth; I–VI, zones of rabbit nodulus, numbered according to Katayama and Nisimaru.[48]

The projections of the nodulus and the uvula as a whole have been reported for most species. The projections of the nodulus to the vestibular nuclei are complementary to the projections of the flocculus.[2,40,80]

FIGURE 9 depicts the zonal arrangement in the terminations of the climbing fibers in the nodulus of the rabbit according to Balaban and Henry[8] and Katayama and Nisimaru.[48] Six climbing fiber zones were distinguished. A medial, group beta-innervated zone I and two caudal, DC-innervated zones II and IV, separated by the rostral DC-innervated zone III, were present on the ventral surface of the nodulus. On its dorsal surface the dorsomedial cell column (DMCC)-innervated zone V appears and the climbing fibers from the rostral medial accessory olive (MAO; zone VI) terminate along the lateral pole of the lobule. The pattern established by Tan *et al.*[73] differs only from this arrangement by the presence of an extension of the caudal DC-innervated zone IV between the DMCC- and rostral MAO-innervated zones V and VI on the dorsal surface of the nodulus. Olivocerebellar fibers that were located in compartments in the caudal flocculus (FC 3: rostral DC and VLO; FC 2: caudal DC) could be traced along the attachment of the roof of the fourth ventricle to the respective zones II, III, and IV of the nodulus.[73] This pathway may be related to the branching of olivocerebellar fibers from these subnuclei of the inferior olive that innervate both the flocculus and the nodulus.[47,52,60]

In the rabbit the projection of the DC and the VLO appears to be mostly restricted to the nodulus, but the climbing fibers from the group beta, DMCC, and the rostral MAO continue on the uvula.[8,66] The division of the uvula into a ventral, vestibular-dominated and a dorsal, nonvestibular part, which was so obvious for the mossy fiber projections, cannot be recognized in the map of the climbing fiber zones of the uvula of the rabbit.[66] The group beta-innervated zone of the uvula falls apart into medial and lateral strips that receive climbing fibers from the caudal and rostral group beta, respectively (FIG. 10). The DMCC- and ventral MAO-innervated zones extend from the dorsal nodulus into the lateral uvula. In between these zones, caudal MAO- and vlPO (ventral leaf of the principal olive)-innervated zones make their appearance in the uvula. An identical map of the olivocerebellar projection to the uvula was published for the cat.[46]

The climbing fiber zones of the nodulus and the uvula of the rat were studied with retrograde axonal transport methods by Eisenman,[25] Bernard,[13] and Apps.[3] Bernard[13] distinguished a medial, DC-innervated zone in the nodulus, flanked by a group beta/VLO-innervated zone, which moves to a medial position in the uvula (FIG. 11). The lateral uvula contains two strips, a medial one innervated by the DMCC and a lateral one innervated by the vlPO and the DM (dorsomedial subnucleus of the ventral leaf of the principal olive[4]). Apps[3] noticed a caudal MAO-innervated zone between the projections of the group beta and the DMCC,

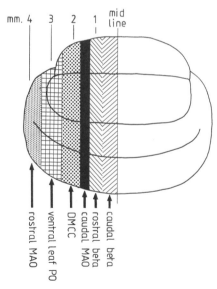

FIGURE 10. Diagram of the olivocerebellar projection to the uvula of the rabbit cerebellum. Based on experiments with retrograde tracer injections in the uvula. DMCC, dorsomedial cell column; MAO, medial accessory olive; PO, principal olive. (From Sato and Barmack.[66] Reproduced with permission of *Brain Research.*)

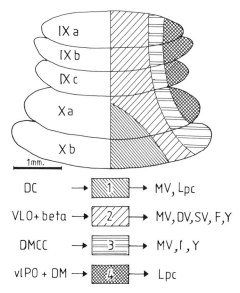

FIGURE 11. Diagram of the modular organization of the olivocerebellar and corticonuclear projections of the nodulus (lobule X) and uvula (lobule IX) of the rat. Based on experiments with injections of wheat germ–coupled horseradish peroxidase in the cerebellar cortex. The connections of the individual modules are indicated in the lower part of the diagram: olivocerebellar connections on the left, corticonuclear projections on the right. DC, dorsal cap; DM, dorsomedial subnucleus of ventral leaf of the principal olive; DMCC, dorsomedial cell column; DV, descending vestibular nucleus; F, fastigial nucleus; I, interposed nucleus; MV, medial vestibular nucleus; Lpc, parvocellular part of lateral cerebellar nucleus; SV, superior vestibular nucleus; VLO, ventrolateral outgrowth; vlPO, ventral leaf of the principal olive; Y, group y. (Modified from Bernard.[13])

and Eisenman[25] described a projection of the rostral MAO to the lateral border of the uvula.

In recent experiments on the rat (Voogd and Ruigrok, unpublished data), we combined anterograde axonal tracing with *Phaseolus vulgaris* leukoagglutinin from small injections into the inferior olive, with anti-zebrin immunoreactivity as a marker for zonally distributed Purkinje cells in the rat.[41] The results of these experiments are summarized in FIGURE 12. Most if not all Purkinje cells of the nodulus and the rostral half of the ventral surface of the uvula (i.e., the region receiving primary and secondary vestibulocerebellar mossy fibers) are zebrin-positive. Purkinje cells in lateral and medial regions of the dorsal nodulus and the ventral uvula are more strongly immunoreactive than the intermediate region, but a distinct zonation only appears more caudally in the uvula (FIG. 12, right). Here the characteristic zonal pattern (FIG. 13C)[41] can be recognized with a zebrin-positive band at the midline (P1+) and three, lateral zebrin-positive bands P2+, P3+, and P4+, separated by narrow, zebrin-negative slits (P1− to P3−).

The projections from the DC occupy medial and lateral zones in the nodulus (FIGS. 12 and 13A). In accordance with the observations of Bernard[13] and Balaban and Henry,[8] these climbing fibers medially border on the midline. The medial DC-innervated zone merges with a medial strip of climbing fibers from the caudal group beta, which extends over the dorsal surface of the nodulus, the entire uvula onto the pyramis, where it is displaced laterally.[25] In the uvula the medial, caudal beta-innervated strip is bisected, and occupies the ipsilateral half of P1+ and the medial half of P2+, sparing P1− (FIG. 12, left). Injections of the VLO label climbing fibers that occupy an intermediate position on the ventral and dorsal surface of the nodulus and the rostral half of the ventral surface of the uvula (FIG. 13B). The climbing fibers of the VLO are located in the middle of a wider climbing fiber zone, innervated from the rostral group beta. This zone extends over the entire uvula, where it is bisected and overlaps with the lateral half of P2+ and the medial half of P3+ (FIG. 13C–H). In the pyramis, climbing fibers from the rostral group beta innervate the lateral half of P2+. Climbing fibers from the DMCC terminate still more laterally in the lateral half of P3+. In the nodulus they are located along the lateral border of its dorsal surface. Purkinje cells of the zebrin-negative strips P2− and P3− receive climbing fibers from the caudal MAO and the DM, respectively (FIG. 13). Climbing fibers from the rostral MAO terminate in P4+.

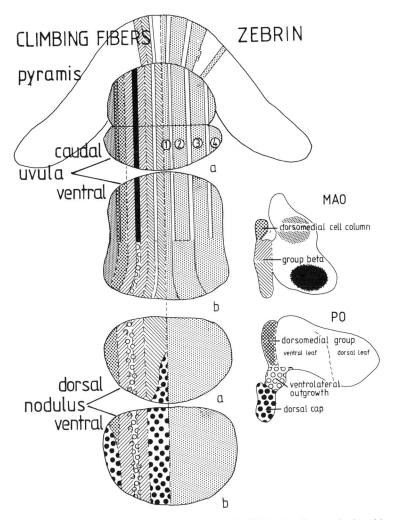

FIGURE 12. Diagram of the zebrin-positive and -negative Purkinje cell zones (*right side*) and the olivocerebellar climbing fiber zones (*left side*) of the nodulus and the uvula of the rat. Ventral and dorsal surface of the nodulus and ventral and caudal surface of the uvula are reconstructed from serial sections. Apex (a) and base (b) of the lobules are indicated. Shaded areas on the right indicate zebrin-positive Purkinje cells. The zebrin-positive zones P1+ to P4+ of Hawkes and Leclerc[41] are indicated with numbers. Subdivisions of the inferior olive indicated in the diagrams of the flattened principal (PO) and medial accessory (MAO) olives and the corresponding climbing fiber zones are indicated with the same shadings. (Ruigrok and Voogd, unpublished data.)

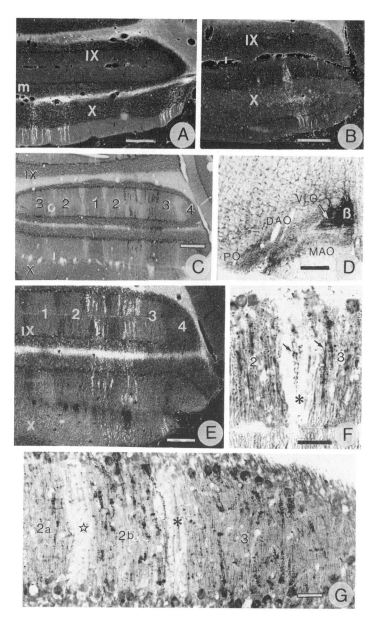

FIGURE 13. *Phaseolus vulgaris*-labeled climbing fibers, with projections to the nodulus/uvula of the rat, in sections reacted with an antibody against zebrin.[40] (**A**) Projection of the dorsal cap to medial and lateral strips in nodulus; darkfield. (**B**) Projection of ventrolateral outgrowth to intermediate nodulus; darkfield. No labeling in uvula **A** or **B**. (**C**) Climbing fibers from rostral group beta terminate in uvula on Purkinje cells of lateral zebrin band P2+ and medial P3+, sparing P2−; brightfield. (**D**) Injection site of rostral group beta. (**E**) Adjacent section to **C**; darkfield. Climbing fiber labeling extends on the nodulus. (**F**) Climbing fibers (*arrows*) from injection of caudal medial accessory olive occupy P2−. (**G**) Same case as **C, D,** and **E.** Climbing fiber labeling in lateral P2+ and medial P3+, sparing P2− (*asterisk*). An additional zebrin-negative strip separates medial and lateral P2+ (*star*) in this section, and on the right side in **C** and **E**. 1–4, zebrin-positive bands P1+ to P4+; β, group beta; DAO, dorsal accessory olive; m, midline; MAO, medial accessory olive; PO, principal olive; IX, uvula; X, nodulus. Bar = 300 μm in **A–E**; 50 μm in **F** and **G**.

This pattern in the olivocerebellar projection to the nodulus and the uvula, as revealed by antegrade tracing, roughly corresponds with Bernard's[13] data (FIG. 11). There is a close correspondence with Sato and Barmack's[66] diagram of the zonal arrangement in the olivocerebellar projection to the uvula of the rabbit (FIG. 10). Differences concern the bisection of the rostral and caudal group beta-innervated strips and the position of the caudal MAO and subnucleus DM (ventral leaf of the PO) innervated strips in rat and rabbit. A remarkable degree of congruity exists between the climbing fiber strips with bands of zebrin-positive and -negative Purkinje cells. Moreover, the borders between the caudal and rostral beta- and DMCC-innervated climbing fiber strips are located in the middle of the zebrin-positive P1+, P2+, and P3+ bands.

Few data are available on the olivocerebellar projection to the nodulus and the uvula in primates. Whitworth *et al.*[85] described a medial, DC/group beta-innervated zone, a middle DMCC-innervated zone, and a lateral zone receiving climbing fibers from the vlPO in the nodulus of the uvula of Galago, and Brodal and Brodal[15,16] traced projections to the uvula of the rhesus monkey from the group beta, the caudal MAO, and the DMCC. Injections of tritiated leucine were made in the inferior olive of several rhesus monkeys in this laboratory (Gerrits and Voogd, unpublished data). One of these cases, in which an injection was made in the DC and the caudal group beta on one side, as well as an injection in the VLO, the rostral group beta, and part of the rostral MAO on the other side, is illustrated in FIGURES 14 and 15. DC/caudal group beta-innervated strips are present, medially and laterally in the nodulus. The medial strip extends medially over the uvula. The injection in the VLO labels an intermediate strip in the nodulus that also continues on the uvula. The lateral pole of both lobules remains unlabeled. In analogy to the situation in rabbit and rat, the medial zone of the nodulus supposedly receives the projection from the caudal DC, which merges with a projection from the caudal group beta, extending into the uvula. The composition of the middle zone may be similar, with a projection of the VLO to the nodulus and the merging projection of the rostral group beta continuing onto the uvula. The lateral caudal DC/group beta-innervated zone is restricted to the nodulus and, thus, may represent a pure caudal DC projection zone. The lateral part of the uvula may contain climbing fibers from the DMCC and the vlPO.

MODULAR ("ZONAL") ORGANIZATION OF THE NODULUS/UVULA. CORTICO-NUCLEAR AND CORTICO-VESTIBULAR PROJECTIONS

The zonal organization of the corticonuclear and the corticovestibular projections of the caudal vermis is more difficult to study and has received much less attention. Bands or patches of Purkinje cells that were retrogradely labeled from injections of the medial and superior vestibular nuclei, and that extend from the nodulus into the uvula and the pyramis were reported by Balaban[5] and Epema[27,28] in the rabbit, and by Shojaku *et al.*[70] in the cat. Correlations between olivocerebellar projection zones and efferent projections of their Purkinje cells were made for the nodulus and the uvula of the rat[13] and for the ventral surface of the nodulus of the rabbit (Wylie *et al.*[86]). Wylie *et al.*[86] concluded that the caudal DC-innervated zones II and IV both project to the medial vestibular nucleus and the rostral DC/VLO-innervated zone III to the superior vestibular nucleus (FIG. 9). The medial zone I, which receives a climbing fiber projection from the group beta, projects to the fastigial and the medial vestibular nucleus. In addition, all four zones project to the posterior interposed nucleus, and zones III and IV to dorsal group y. The linkage of caudal DC afferents with a projection to the medial vestibular nucleus and of rostral

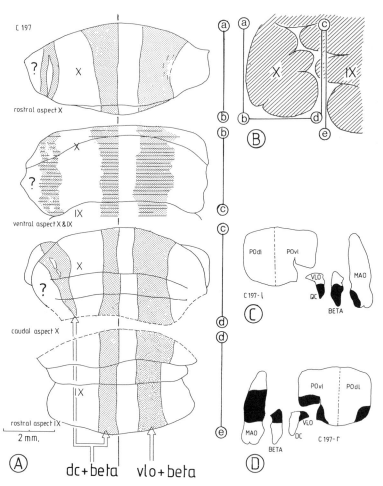

FIGURE 14. Diagram of the olivocerebellar projection to the nodulus of the rhesus monkey. (**A**) Reconstructions of the distribution of climbing fibers from serial transverse sections. Position of the reconstructed rostral (ab), ventral (bc), and caudal (cd) aspects of the nodulus, and the rostral aspect of the uvula (de) are shown in **B**. Injection sites of the antegrade tracer [³H]leucine in the inferior olive are indicated in black in diagrams of the flattened principal and medial accessory olive (**C** and **D**). The injection of the dorsal cap (DC) and the caudal group beta in **C** labels two bands of climbing fibers on the left side in **A**. The injection including the ventrolateral outgrowth (VLO) and the rostral group beta in **D** labels a single band of climbing fibers on the right side in **A**. (Gerrits and Voogd, unpublished data.)

DC/VLO afferents with a projection to the superior vestibular nucleus is similar to the flocculus. The projection of the caudal DC-innervated zone II to dorsal group y is not in accordance with its counterpart (zone 2) in the flocculus, and the diffuse projection to the posterior interposed nucleus is unexpected. Bernard,[13] similarly, observed projections from his DC-innervated zone to the medial vestibular nucleus, and from his VLO-innervated zone to the superior and inferior vestibular nuclei

(FIG. 11). The beta, DMCC, and vlPO-innervated zones of the uvula projected to the fastigial nucleus, the interposed nucleus, and the ventral leaf of the lateral nucleus with group y, respectively.

RECIPROCAL CONNECTIONS BETWEEN TARGET NUCLEI OF CEREBELLAR MODULES AND THE INFERIOR OLIVE. DIFFERENCES BETWEEN CEREBELLAR AND VESTIBULAR TARGET NUCLEI

Reciprocal connections between the cerebellar nuclei and the inferior olive, consisting of GABAergic, nucleo-olivary pathways, and collateral projections to the nuclei of the olivocerebellar climbing fiber paths, have been reported in many mammalian species (reviewed in ref. 64). Collateral projections of olivocerebellar pathways to the vestibular nuclei have been established for the climbing fiber pathway from the caudal dorsal accessory olive (the dorsal fold of the dorsal accessory olive of the rat[37]) to the B zone. This collateral projection terminates in Deiters' nucleus (cat;[37] monkey;[84] rat; Ruigrok, unpublished data). The reciprocal nucleo-olivary projection from Deiters' nucleus to the dorsal fold of the dorsal accessory olive thus far only has been demonstrated in the rat.[64] Collateral projections from the DC and the VLO to the medial and superior vestibular nuclei were traced by Balaban[5,6] in the rabbit, but have not been confirmed in other studies.

De Zeeuw *et al.*[20,21] proposed that the reciprocal connections of the target nuclei of the caudal DC- and rostral DC/VLO-innervated modules of the rabbit flocculus, with the inferior olive, are effectuated through other circuits. They showed that predominantly crossed, GABAergic pathways to the DC and the VLO in the rabbit take their origin from the nucleus prepositus hypoglossi and the ventral, parvocellular, lateral cerebellar nucleus with dorsal group y, respectively. The reciprocal connection from the VLO to the parvocellular lateral cerebellar nucleus exists in the rat,[65] but a collateral projection of the caudal DC to the nucleus prepositus

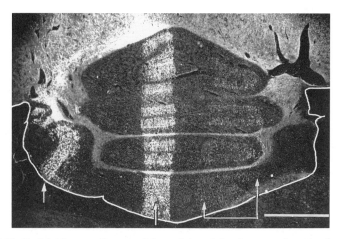

FIGURE 15. Darkfield autoradiogram of the nodulus of the rhesus monkey showing [^{3}H]leucine antegrade transport in climbing fibers (*arrows*) from injections including the caudal dorsal cap and group beta (*left*) and the ventrolateral outgrowth (*right*). Compare with FIGURE 14. Bar = 1 mm.

hypoglossi has not yet been demonstrated. The VLO/rostral DC-innervated floccular zone 1 projects profusely to dorsal group y, but only sparsely to the parvocellular dentate; the projection from the caudal DC-innervated zones 2 and 4 to the nucleus prepositus hypoglossi[90] is still disputed.

MODULAR ORGANIZATION AND THE CONCEPT OF THE VESTIBULOCEREBELLUM

Is it possible to reconcile the modular organization of flocculus, paraflocculus, nodulus and uvula with the concept of the vestibulocerebellum? Gerrits *et al.,*[34] in their study of projections of the vestibular nuclei to the inferior olive of the cat, pointed out that subnuclei that project to the flocculus (DC, VLO, and rostral MAO) do not receive their afferents from the vestibular nuclei, but from optokinetic centers in the mesencephalon (including the visually dominated subdivision of Darkschewitsch nucleus,[63] the nucleus prepositus hypoglossi and the group y[20,21]). The group beta, the DMCC, and the subnucleus b of the caudal MAO receive projections from the vestibular nuclei[34] (see also Kaufman, this volume).

In nodulus and uvula the nonvestibular, visually dominated DC and VLO-innervated zones alternate with vestibular (group beta and DMCC innervated) modules. The visually dominated zones are mainly restricted to the nodulus, but the beta- and DMCC-innervated zones extend far beyond the limits of the classical vestibulocerebellum into the dorsal uvula and the pyramis, where they interdigitate with strips receiving climbing fibers from the caudal MAO and the DM; that is, from subnuclei of the inferior olive dominated by afferents from somatosensory relay nuclei.

The major efferent connections of the DC and VLO-innervated zones of the flocculus and the nodulus, indeed, are to the vestibular nuclei. However, in these pathways, the vestibular nuclei function as premotor centers for the oculomotor nuclei and the spinal cord, and their vestibular afferentiation is of secondary importance. The modular organization of these lobules, therefore, does not justify their designation as the vestibulocerebellum.

CONCLUSIONS

Different combinations of modules occur in different lobules. Each module is probably linked to a specific motor system, and the combination of modules in any particular lobule thus determines its span of control over motor behavior. This differential output system can be activated by mossy fibers that terminate in the different lobules: vestibular mossy fibers in the nodulus and ventral uvula, pontocerebellar mossy fibers in the dorsal uvula, and reticular and perihypoglossal mossy fibers in the flocculus. The main orientation of the mossy fibers and the parallel fibers that constitute the next link in the pathway connecting them with the Purkinje cells is transverse, that is, perpendicular to the orientation of the modules. Access of a particular mossy fiber-parallel fiber system to a module may be determined by a process of selective activation by the climbing fibers.

The prefix "vestibulo" in the vestibulocerebellum is used in a double sense. It was derived from one particular mossy fiber input and from the anatomical designation used for one of its main output stations. The term is unfortunate because it obscures the differences in spatial organization of the mossy fiber-parallel fiber input and the multimodular output of the cerebellum, which is fundamental in the understanding of its integrative function.

ACKNOWLEDGMENTS

Histology was performed by Erika Sabel-Goedknegt; photography by Eddie Dalm. Secretarial assistance of Edith Klink is gratefully acknowledged. The antibody against zebrin II was a gift from Dr. R. Hawkes.

REFERENCES

1. ANDERSSON, G. & O. OSCARSSON. 1978. Climbing fiber microzones in cerebellar vermis and their projection to different groups of cells in the lateral vestibular nucleus. Exp. Brain Res. **32:** 565–579.
2. ANGAUT, P. & A. BRODAL. 1967. The projection of the "vestibulo-cerebellum" onto the vestibular nuclei in the cat. Arch. Ital. Biol. **105:** 441–479.
3. APPS, R. 1990. Columnar organization of the inferior olive projection to the posterior lobe of the rat cerebellum. J. Comp. Neurol. **302:** 236–254.
4. AZIZI, S. A. & D. J. WOODWARD. 1987. Inferior olivary nuclear complex of the rat: Morphology and comments on the principles of organization within the olivocerebellar system. J. Comp. Neurol. **263:** 467–484.
5. BALABAN, C. D. 1984. Olivo-vestibular and cerebello-vestibular connections in albino rabbits. Neuroscience **12:** 129–149.
6. BALABAN, C. D. 1988. Distribution of inferior olivary projections to the vestibular nuclei of albino rabbits. Neuroscience **24:** 119–134.
7. BALABAN, C. D., M. ITO & E. WATANABE. 1981. Demonstration of zonal projections from the cerebellar flocculus to vestibular nuclei in monkeys (*Macaca fuscata*). Neurosci. Lett. **27:** 101–105.
8. BALABAN, C. D. & R. T. HENRY. 1988. Zonal organization of olivo-nodulus projections in albino rabbits. Neurosci. Res. **5:** 409–423.
9. BARMACK, N. H., R. W. BAUGHMAN, F. P. ECKENSTEIN & H. SHOJAKU. 1992. Secondary vestibular cholinergic projection to the cerebellum of rabbit and rat as revealed by choline acyltransferase immunohistochemistry, retrograde and orthograde tracers. J. Comp. Neurol. **317:** 250–270.
10. BARMACK, N. H., R. W. BAUGHMAN, P. ERRICO & H. SHOJAKU. 1993. Vestibular primary afferent projection to the cerebellum of the rabbit. J. Comp. Neurol. **327:** 521–534.
11. BELKNAP, D. B. & R. A. McCREA. 1985. Anatomy and physiology of cerebellar efferents to the vestibular complex and nucleus prepositus hypoglossi of the squirrel monkey. Neurosci. Abstr. **11:** 1036.
12. BELKNAP, D. B. & R. A. McCREA. 1988. Anatomical connections of the prepositus and abducens nuclei in the squirrel monkey. J. Comp. Neurol. **268:** 13–28.
13. BERNARD, J-F. 1987. Topographical organization of olivocerebellar and corticonuclear connections in the rat. An WGA-HRP study. I. Lobules IX, X, and the flocculus. J. Comp. Neurol. **263:** 241–258.
14. BRODAL, A. 1976. The olivocerebellar projection in the cat as studied with the method of retrograde axonal transport of horseradish peroxidase. II. The projection to the uvula. J. Comp. Neurol. **166:** 417–426.
15. BRODAL, P. & A. BRODAL. 1981. The olivocerebellar projection in the monkey. Experimental studies with the method of retrograde tracing of horseradish peroxidase. J. Comp. Neurol. **201:** 375–393.
16. BRODAL, P. & A. BRODAL. 1982. Further observations on the olivocerebellar projection in the monkey. Exp. Brain Res. **45:** 71–83.
17. BUISSERET-DELMAS, C. & P. ANGAUT. 1993. The cerebellar olivo-corticonuclear connections in the rat. Prog. Neurobiol. **40:** 63–87.

18. BURNE, R. A., G. A. MIHAILOFF & D. J. WOODWARD. 1978. Visual cortico-pontine input to the paraflocculus: A combined autoradiographic and horseradish peroxidase study. Brain Res. **143:** 139–146.
19. CHOCKKAN, V. & R. HAWKES. 1994. Functional and antigenic maps in the rat cerebellum: Zebrin compartmentation and vibrissal receptive fields in lobule IXa. J. Comp. Neurol. **345:** 33–45.
20. DE ZEEUW, C. I., P. WENTZEL & E. MUGNAINI. 1993. Fine structure of the dorsal cap of the inferior olive and its GABA-ergic and non-GABAergic input from the nucleus prepositus hypoglossi in rat and rabbit. J. Comp. Neurol. **327:** 63–82.
21. DE ZEEUW, C. I., N. M. GERRITS, J. VOOGD, C. S. LEONARD & J. I. SIMPSON. 1994. The rostral dorsal cap and ventraolateral outgrowth of the rabbit inferior olive receive a GABAergic input from dorsal group Y and the ventral dentate nucleus. J. Comp. Neurol. **341:** 420–432.
22. DE ZEEUW, C. I., D. R. WYLIE, P. L. DiGIORGI & J. I. SIMPSON. 1994. Projections of individual Purkinje cells of identified zones in the flocculus to the vestibular and cerebellar nuclei in the rabbit. J. Comp. Neurol. **349:** 428–447.
23. DIETRICHS, E. & F. WALBERG. 1989. Direct bidirectional connections between the inferior olive and the cerebellar nuclei. *In* The Olivocerebellar System in Motor Control. Experimental Brain Research, Series 17. P. Strata, Ed.: 61–81. Springer-Verlag. Berlin.
24. DOW, R. S. 1942. The evolution and anatomy of the cerebellum. Biol. Rev. **17:** 179–220.
25. EISENMAN, L. M. 1984. Organization of the olivocerebellar projection to the uvula in the rat. Brain Behav. Evol. **24:** 1–12.
26. EKEROT, C-F., M. GARWICZ & J. SCHOUENBORG. 1991. Topography and nociceptive receptive fields of climbing fibres projecting to the cerebellar anterior lobe in the cat. J. Physiol. **441:** 257–274.
27. EPEMA, A. H. 1990. Connections of the vestibular nuclei in the rabbit. PhD thesis, University of Rotterdam, the Netherlands.
28. EPEMA, A. H., J. M. GULDEMOND & J. VOOGD. 1985. Reciprocal connections between the vestibular nuclei and the caudal vermis in the rabbit. Neurosci. Lett. **57:** 273–278.
29. GERRITS, N. M. 1985. Brainstem control of the cerebellar flocculus. PhD thesis, University of Leiden, the Netherlands.
30. GERRITS, N. M. 1994. Vestibular and cerebellar connections subserving eye movements. *In* Information Processing Underlying Gaze Control. J. M. Delgado-Garcia, E. Godaux & P-P. Vidal, Eds.: 341–350. Pergamon Press. Oxford.
31. GERRITS, N. M. & J. VOOGD. 1982. The climbing fiber projection to the flocculus and adjacent paraflocculus in the cat. Neuroscience **7:** 2971–2991.
32. GERRITS, N. M. & J. VOOGD. 1986. The nucleus reticularis tegmenti points and the adjacent rostral paramedian reticular projections: Differential projections to the cerebellum and the caudal brain stem. Exp. Brain Res. **62:** 29–45.
33. GERRITS, N. M., A. H. EPEMA & J. VOOGD. 1984. The mossy fiber projection of the nucleus reticularis tegmenti pontis to the flocculus and adjacent ventral paraflocculus in the cat. Neuroscience **11:** 627–644.
34. GERRITS, N. M., J. VOOGD & I. N. MAGRAS. 1985. Vestibular afferents of the inferior olive and the vestibulo-olivo-cerebellar climbing fiber pathway to the flocculus in the cat. Brain Res. **332:** 325–336.
35. GERRITS, N. M., A. H. EPEMA, A. VAN LINGE & E. DALM. 1989. The primary vestibulo-cerebellar projection in the rabbit: Absence of primary afferents in the flocculus. Neurosci. Lett. **290:** 262–277.
36. GLICKSTEIN, M., N. M. GERRITS, I. KRALJ-HANS, B. MERCIER, J. STEIN & J. VOOGD. 1994. Visual pontocerebellar projections in the macaque. J. Comp. Neurol. **347:** 1–22.
37. GROENEWEGEN, H. J. & J. VOOGD. 1977. The parasagittal zonation within the olivocerebellar projection. I. Climbing fiber distribution in the vermis of cat cerebellum. J. Comp. Neurol. **174:** 417–488.
38. GROENEWEGEN, H. J., J. VOOGD & S. L. FREEDMAN. 1979. The parasagittal zonation within the olivocerebellar projection. II. Climbing fiber distribution in the intermediate and hemispheric parts of cat cerebellum. J. Comp. Neurol. **183:** 551–602.

39. HAINES, D. E. 1969. The cerebellum of Galago and Tupaia. I. Corpus cerebelli and flocculonodular lobe. Brain Behav. Evol. **2:** 377–414.
40. HAINES, D. E. 1977. Cerebellar corticonuclear and corticovestibular fibers of the flocculonodular lobe in a Prosimian primate (*Galago senegalensis*). J. Comp. Neurol. **174:** 607–630.
41. HAWKES, R. & N. LECLERC. 1987. Antigenic map of the rat cerebellar cortex: The distribution of sagittal bands as revealed by monoclonal anti-Purkinje cell antibody mabQ113. J. Comp. Neurol. **256:** 29–41.
42. HESS, D. T. & J. VOOGD. 1986. Chemoarchitectonic zonation of the monkey cerebellum. Brain Res. **369:** 383–387.
43. HODDEVIK, G. H. & A. BRODAL. 1977. The olivo-cerebellar projections studied with the method of retrograde axonal transport of horseradish peroxidase. V. The projection to the flocculo-nodular lobe and the paraflocculus in the rabbit. J. Comp. Neurol. **176:** 269–280.
44. INGVAR, S. 1918. Zur Phylo-und Ontogenese des Kleinhirns. Folia Neurobiol. Lpz. **11:** 205–495.
45. JOSEPH, J. W., G. M. SHAMBES, J. M. GIBSON & W. WELKER. 1978. Tactile projections to granule cells in caudal vermis of the rat's cerebellum. Brain Behav. Evol. **15:** 141–149.
46. KANDA, K-I., Y. SATO, K. IKARASHI & T. KAWASAKI. 1989. Zonal organization of climbing fiber projections to the uvula in the cat. J. Comp. Neurol. **279:** 138–148.
47. KANO, M., M-S. KANO, M. KUSUNOKI & K. MAEKAWA. 1990. Nature of optokinetic response and zonal organization of climbing fiber afferents in the vestibulocerebellum of the pigmented rabbit. II. The nodulus. Exp. Brain Res. **80:** 238–251.
48. KATAYAMA, S. & W. NISIMARU. 1988. Parasagittal zonal pattern of olivo-nodular projections in rabbit cerebellum. Neurosci. Res. **5:** 424–428.
49. KORTE, G. & E. MUGNAINI. 1979. The cerebellar projection of the vestibular nerve in the cat. J. Comp. Neurol. **184:** 265–278.
50. KOTCHABHAKDI, N. & F. WALBERG. 1978. Cerebellar afferent projections from the vestibular nuclei in the cat: An experimental study with the method of retrograde axonal transport of horseradish peroxidase. Exp. Brain Res. **31:** 591–604.
51. KOTCHABHAKDI, N., G. H. HODDEVIK & F. WALBERG. 1978. Cerebellar afferent projections from the perihyoglossal nuclei: An experimental study with the method of retrograde axonal transport of horseradish peroxidase. Exp. Brain Res. **31:** 13–29.
52. KUSONOKI, M., M. KAN, M-S. KANO & K. MAEKAWA. 1990. Nature of optokinetic response and zonal organization of climbing fiber afferents in the vestibulocerebellum of the pigmented rabbit. I. The flocculus. Exp. Brain Res. **80:** 225–237.
53. LANGER, T., A. F. FUCHS, C. A. SCUDDER & M. C. CHUBB. 1985. Afferents to the flocculus of the cerebellum in the rhesus macaque as revealed by retrograde transport of horseradish peroxidase. J. Comp. Neurol. **235:** 1–25.
54. LANGER, T., A. F. FUCHS, M. C. CHUBB, C. A. SCUDDER, S. G. LISBERGER. 1985. Floccular efferents in the rhesus macaque as revealed by autoradiography and horseradish peroxidase. J. Comp. Neurol. **235:** 26–37.
55. LARSELL, O. 1937. The cerebellum. A review and interpretation. Arch. Neurol. Psychiatry **38:** 580–607.
56. LARSELL, O. 1953. Cerebellum of cat and monkey. J. Comp. Neurol. **99:** 135–200.
57. LARSELL, O. 1970. The Comparative Anatomy and Histology of the Cerebellum from Monotremes through Apes. J. Jansen Ed. University of Minnesota Press. Minneapolis, MN.
58. LEONARD, C. S., J. I. SIMPSON & W. GRAF. 1988. Spatial organization of visual messages of the rabbit's cerebellar flocculus. I. Typology of inferior olive neurons of the dorsal cap of Kooy. J. Neurophysiol. **60:** 2073–2090.
59. MADIGAN, J. C. & M. B. CARPENTER. 1971. Cerebellum of the Rhesus Monkey. Atlas of Lobules, Laminae, and Folia, in Sections. University Park Press. Baltimore, MD.
60. MAEKAWA, K., T. TAKEDA, M. KANO & M. KUSUNOKI. 1989. Collateralized climbing fiber projection to the flocculus and the nodulus of the rabbit. Exp. Brain Res. Ser. **17:** 30–45.
61. MATSUSHITA, M. & T. TANAMI. 1987. Spinocerebellar projections from the central cervical

nucleus in the cat, as studied by anterograde transport of wheat germ agglutinin-horseradish peroxidase. J. Comp. Neurol. **266:** 376–397.

62. MATSUSHITA, M. & C-L. WANG. 1987. Projection pattern of vestibulocerebellar fibers in the anterior vermis of the cat: An anterograde wheat germ agglutinin-horseradish peroxidase study. Neurosci. Lett. **74:** 25–30.

63. PORTER, C. M., P. L. E. VAN KAN, K. M. HORN, J. R. BLOEDEL & A. R. GIBSON. 1993. Functional divisions of cat rMAO. Soc. Neurosci. Abstr. **19:** 1216.

64. RUIGROK, T. J. H. & J. VOOGD. 1990. Cerebellar nucleo-olivary projections in the rat: An anterograde tracing study with *Phaseolus vulgaris*-leucoagglutinin (PHA-L). J. Comp. Neurol. **298:** 315–333.

65. RUIGROK, T. J. H., R-J. OSSE & J. VOOGD. 1992. Organization of inferior olivary projections to the flocculus and ventral para-flocculus of the rat cerebellum. J. Comp. Neurol. **316:** 129–150.

66. SATO, Y. & N. H. BARMACK. 1985. Zonal organization of olivocerebellar projections to the uvula in rabbits. Brain Res. **359:** 281–292.

67. SATO, Y. & T. KAWASAKI. 1991. Identification of the Purkinje cell/climbing fiber zone and its target neurons responsible for eye-movement control by the cerebellar flocculus. Brain Res. Rev. **16:** 39–64.

68. SATO, Y., T. KAWASAKI & K. IKATASHI. 1983. Afferent projections from the brainstem to the three floccular zones in cats. II. Mossy fiber projections. Brain Res. **272:** 37–48.

69. SATO, Y., K-I. KANDA, K. IKARASHI & T. KAWASAKI. 1989. Differential mossy fiber projections to the dorsal and ventral uvula in the cat. J. Comp. Neurol. **279:** 149–164.

70. SHOJAKU, H., Y. SATO, K. IKARASHI & T. KAWASAKI. 1987. Topographical distribution of Purkinje cells in the uvula and the nodulus projecting to the vestibular nuclei in cats. Brain Res. **416:** 100–112.

71. SOMANA, R., N. KOTCHABHAKDI & F. WALBERG. 1980. Cerebellar afferents from the trigeminal sensory nuclei in the cat. Exp. Brain Res. **38:** 57–64.

72. TAN, J., J. SIMPSON & J. VOOGD. 1995. Anatomical compartments in the white matter of the rabbit flocculus. J. Comp. Neurol. **356:** 1–22.

73. TAN, J., N. GERRITS, R. NANHOE, J. SIMPSON & J. VOOGD. 1995. Zonal organization of the climbing fiber projection to the flocculus and nodulus of the rabbit. A combined axonal tracing and acetylcholinesterase histochemical study. J. Comp. Neurol. **356:** 23–50.

74. TAN, J., A. EPEMA & J. VOOGD. 1995. Zonal organization of the flocculo-vestibular nucleus projection in the rabbit. A combined axonal tracing and acetylcholinesterase histochemical study. J. Comp. Neurol. **356:** 51–71.

75. THUNNISSEN, I. E. 1990. Vestibulocerebellar and vestibulo-oculomotor relations in the rabbit. PhD thesis, University of Rotterdam, the Netherlands.

76. THUNNISSEN, I. E., A. H. EPEMA & N. M. GERRITS. 1989. Secondary vestibulocerebellar mossy fiber projection to the caudal vermis in the rabbit. J. Comp. Neurol. **290:** 262–277.

77. UMETANI, T. 1992. Efferent projections from the flocculus in the albino rat as revealed by an autoradiographic orthograde tracing method. Brain Res. **586:** 91–103.

78. VAN DER STEEN, J., J. I. SIMPSON & J. TAN. 1994. Functional and anatomical organization of three-dimensional eye movements in rabbit cerebellar flocculus. J. Neurophysiol. **72:** 31–46.

79. VAN HAM, J. J. & CH. H. YEO. 1992. Somatosensory trigeminal projections to the inferior olive, cerebellum and other precerebellar nuclei in rabbits. Eur. J. Neurosci. **4:** 302–317.

80. VOOGD, J. 1964. The cerebellum of the cat. Structure and fiber connections. PhD thesis, University of Leiden, the Netherlands, Van Gorcum, Assen, the Netherlands.

81. VOOGD, J. 1967. Comparative aspects of the structure and fibre connections of the mammalian cerebellum. Prog. Brain Res. **25:** 94–134.

82. VOOGD, J. & F. BIGARE. 1980. Topographical distribution of olivary and cortico-nuclear fibers in the cerebellum: A review. *In* The Olivary Nucleus. Anatomy and Physiology. J. Courville *et al.,* Eds.: 207–234. Raven Press. New York.

83. VOOGD, J., D. T. HESS & E. MARANI. 1987. The parasagittal zonation of the cerebellar

cortex in cat and monkey. Topography, distribution of acetylcholinesterase and development. *In* New Concepts in Cerebellar Neurobiology. J. S. King, Ed.: 15. Liss. New York.

84. VOOGD, J., N. M. GERRITS & D. T. HESS. 1987. Parasagittal zonation of the cerebellum in Macaques: An analysis based on acetylcholinesterase histochemistry. *In* Cerebellum and Neuronal Plasticity. M. Glickstein, Ch. Yeo & J. Stein, Eds.: 15–39. Plenum Press. New York.

85. WHITWORTH, R. H., JR., D. E. HAINES & G. W. PATRICK. 1983. The inferior olive of a Prosimian primate, *Galago senegalensis*. II. Olivocerebellar projections to the vestibulocerebellum. J. Comp. Neurol. **219:** 228–240.

86. WYLIE, D. R., C. I. DE ZEEUW, P. L. DiGIORGI & J. I. SIMPSON. 1994. Projections of individual Purkinje cells of identified zones in the ventral nodulus to the vestibular and cerebellar nuclei in the rabbit. J. Comp. Neurol. **349:** 448–463.

87. YAMAMOTO, M. 1978. Localization of rabbit's flocculus Purkinje cells projecting to the cerebellar lateral nucleus and the nucleus prepositas hypoglossi investigated by means of the horseradish peroxidase retrograde axonal transport. Neurosci. Lett. **7:** 197–202.

88. YAMAMOTO, M. 1979. Topographical representation in rabbit cerebellar flocculus for various afferent inputs from the brain stem investigated by means of retrograde transport of horseradish peroxidase. Neurosci. Lett. **12:** 29–34.

89. YAMAMOTO, M. & I. SHIMOYAMA. 1977. Differential localization of rabbit's flocculus Purkinje cells to the medial and superior vestibular nuclei, investigated by means of the horseradish peroxidase retrograde axonal transport. Neurosci. Lett. **5:** 279–283.

90. YINGCHAROEN, K. & E. RINVIK. 1983. Ultrastructural demonstration of a projection from the flocculus to the nucleus prepositus hypoglossi in the cat. Exp. Brain Res. **51:** 192–198.

The Interaction of the Human Linear Otolith-Ocular and Angular Horizontal Vestibulo-Ocular Reflexes in Darkness

D. ANASTASOPOULOS, C. GIANNA, A. M. BRONSTEIN,
AND M. A. GRESTY

MRC Human Movement and Balance Unit
Institute of Neurology, National Hospital
Queen Square
London WC1N 3BG, England

Most natural head movements combine angular and linear components of head acceleration, and it is presumed that ocular compensation for the linear component of head motion is of otolithic origin (linear vestibulo-ocular reflex, LVOR). The nature of the interaction between canal and otolith components is, however, not clear, and it is not known whether the combined eye movement response is a linear summation of LVOR and angular (AVOR) reflexes.[1,2] In these experiments the LVOR obtained during combined angular and linear motion was estimated by subtracting the response to pure angular rotation (AVOR) from the response to combined angular and linear motion (ALVOR) obtained by rotation with the head eccentric. The result of this subtraction was then compared to the LVOR in response to isolated linear motion with a matched linear acceleration profile.

Subjects were seated upright on an electrically powered linear bogie. The motion stimuli were y-axis velocity ramps accelerating the subject to 0.25 g in less than 80 msec (FIG. 1). Responses in the dark (LVORd) were obtained immediately after the subject fixated a gray screen (120 cm × 120 cm) at a distance of 1.5 m. The room lights were extinguished, and after 1 sec the bogie moved. The subjects were then seated on a Barany chair with the head placed forwards 40 cm from the axis of rotation (ALVOR). Chair motion parameters were adjusted to provide, in addition to the angular component, a tangential acceleration acting along the interaural axis, similar to that delivered on the bogie (FIG. 1). Because of torque limitations, the tangential linear acceleration during the combined canal–otolith stimulation was of smaller magnitude for the first 130 msec after the onset of the movement (0.15 g at 80 msec). The ocular responses to isolated angular stimulation (AVOR) were obtained with the head of the subject centered on the axis of rotation using the same angular motion as during the eccentric head position. In order to standardize vergence angle, the subjects previewed the gray screen at 1.5 m in all conditions. Eye movements were recorded with bitemporal dc EOG with a flat response to 80 Hz. For each condition 12 healthy human subjects produced 10 responses for each right/left stimulus direction. The EOG signal was differentiated, and saccades were removed, interpolating a straight line between the beginning and the end of the saccade. The signals were averaged using stimulus onset for synchronization.

FIGURE 1, top record, shows the grand average (+1 SD) of eye displacement to isolated linear acceleration in darkness (LVORd). The average amplitude of the slow-phase eye movements reached 0.7 deg at 180 msec from stimulus onset. Eye velocity increased with time, approaching an asymptote of approximately 10 deg/sec at about 250 msec after stimulus onset. The velocity of the slow-phase eye movement responses to rotation closely matched the velocity of the stimulus (averages with 1 SD are shown in FIG. 1, upper records, ALVORd and AVORd) attaining a gain of approximately 0.8 at 60 msec after stimulus onset, when the head was centered, and of 1.2 with head eccentric.

The upper trace in FIG. 2 is the result of subtracting the grand average of slow-phase eye displacement during AVORd from that during ALVORd. The lower trace in FIGURE 2 is the average of the slow-phase eye movements recorded on the

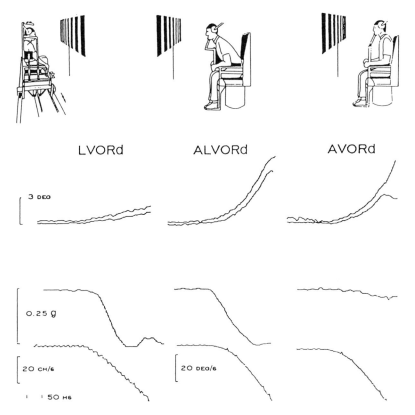

FIGURE 1. Grand averages +1 SD of the desaccaded eye movements of 12 subjects (upper records) recorded during pure linear acceleration (LVORd), combined angular–linear stimulation (ALVORd), and isolated angular stimulation (AVORd) in darkness. The two lower traces show the linear acceleration profile recorded from the subject's forehead and the chair linear and angular velocity.

bogie. The difference, in amplitude and velocity, between the responses during head eccentric and head centered (ALVORd-AVORd) was greater than that obtained on the bogie (LVORd), although only the first 200 msec after stimulus onset are considered. The former would be compensatory for a target set at 1.6 m, whereas the eye movement obtained during LVORd would compensate for a target at 2.9 m. This study has shown that the linear component of combined linear and angular VOR is stronger than the linear reflex tested in isolation. The results suggest a nonlinear

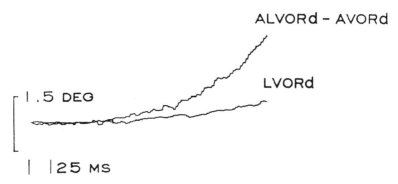

FIGURE 2. Comparison of the linear component of the response during combined canal–otolith stimulation (ALVORd-AVORd) with the response to linear acceleration on the bogie in darkness (LVORd).

addition of otolith and canal reflexes that would result in more efficient vestibulo-ocular compensation during combined angular–linear head movements.

REFERENCES

1. VIIRRE, E., D. TWEED, K. MILNER & T. VILIS. 1986. A reexamination of the gain of the vestibuloocular reflex. J. Neurophysiol. **56:** 439–450.
2. GRESTY, M. A., A. M. BRONSTEIN & H. BARRATT. 1987. Eye movement responses to combined linear and angular head movement. Exp. Brain Res. **65:** 377–384.

Otolith Directional Sensitivity and Ocular Torsion

JELTE E. BOS,[a] BERND DE GRAAF, AND ERIC GROEN

TNO Human Factors Research Institute
P.O. Box 23
3769 ZG Soesterberg, the Netherlands

It is generally accepted that the utricles are the principal y-direction accelerometers (i.e., sensitive along the interaural axis), and that otolith-induced ocular torsion (OT) is generated by the utricles. The basic idea discussed in this paper is that if this were true, OT in the normal upright position and in weightlessness should be equal, because the shear force exerted on the utricles in both cases is zero. This hypothesis is, however, falsified by results obtained in experiments with a tilt chair, a centrifuge, and during parabolic flight. For mere utricular function, we found a linear relationship between G-load and OT, whereas a different behavior is shown when saccular function is involved.

EXPERIMENTS AND RESULTS

A series of experiments was set up to obtain OT data from stimulation of the utricles solely and in combination with the saccules. Eye movements were recorded on videotape and analyzed off-line.[1] In all cases OT was determined with respect to the normal upright position (the force in the y-direction $F_y = 0$, and that along the subjects' z-axis $F_z = 1$G).

Tilt

Utricular and saccular function were examined in combined action during static tilt in roll (0–90°). Here, F_y increases from 0 to 1G with tilt, while F_z decreases from 1 to 0G. Mean OT of 20 subjects is presented in FIGURE 1 by upright triangles.

Centrifuge

To isolate the utricular function, subjects were exposed to hypergravity in a centrifuge. Subjects lay in a free-swinging gondola, with their right ear down to keep F_y aligned with the resultant of the gravitational and the centrifugal force. Here F_y is increased from 1 to 3G, while $F_z = 0$. Mean OT from 20 subjects is shown in the figure by upside down triangles.

Parabolic Flight

To extend our data with data under hypogravity ($F_y = F_z = 0$), subjects endured parabolic flight facing the flight direction in the upright and 90° tilted positions. In addition, in the 90° tilted position during pull-up and pull-out, hypergravity data

---

[a] E-mail: bos@tm.tno.nl

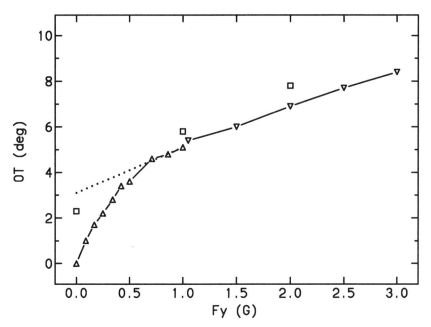

FIGURE 1. Average ocular torsion (OT) with respect to utricular shear force F_y. *Upright triangles* represent data obtained by tilting 20 subjects in the range from 0 to 90°, where $F_z = \sqrt{(1 - F_y^2)}$. *Upside down triangles* represent data obtained from 20 subjects in a centrifuge with $F_z = 0$. *Squares* represent data obtained from five subjects during parabolic flight with $F_z = 0$.

could be replicated. Mean OT during stable conditions from five subjects is given in the figure by squares.

DISCUSSION AND CONCLUSIONS

If only the utricles are responsible for OT, then OT should be equal in the normal upright position ($F_y = 0$, $F_z = 1$) and during weightlessness ($F_y = F_z = 0$). As indicated by the left-most square in the figure, this is shown to be not true (there is a significant statistical difference of 2–3°). Therefore, we conclude that the saccules do contribute to OT. Moreover, no difference was found between the assumed OT at 0G, as obtained by linear extrapolation of the centrifuge data (dotted line in Fig. 1), and the OT in true weightlessness. This suggests a linear relationship between the shear force exerted on the utricles and OT. In tilt at 1G, then, additional saccular function results in a nonlinear relationship.

Asymmetries between both eyes are yet concealed, but it may be inferred that the utricles generate cyclo-version, whereas the saccules generate cyclo-vergence. This idea is supported by binocular results obtained during z-axis centrifugation.

REFERENCE

1. BOS, J. E. & B. DE GRAAF. 1994. Ocular torsion quantification with video images. IEEE Trans. Biomed. Eng. **41:** 351–357.

The Physiological Basis of Imperfect Compensation by the VOR at High Frequencies of Rotation

DIANNE M. BROUSSARD[a] AND JOTINDER K. BHATIA

Playfair Neuroscience Unit
University of Toronto
Toronto, Canada

Human patients that have recovered from unilateral labyrinthectomy show an asymmetric VOR in response to sudden passive head movements.[1] This result was interpreted as reflecting the asymmetric responses of primary vestibular afferents. We have investigated the residual asymmetry after compensation for a unilateral horizontal canal block in cats. Our data suggest that central mechanisms may be responsible for the asymmetry.

METHODS

Four 4- to 7-month-old cats were used. First, the cat was conditioned to the apparatus. Then, a head holder was attached to the cranium by cortical screws, and a scleral search coil was implanted in one eye. For recording, the alert cat's head was centered in alternating vertical and horizontal magnetic fields and on the axis of rotation of a rate table. Two kinds of vestibular stimuli were delivered. First, short-velocity trapezoids, which accelerated in 90 msec to an overshoot followed by a plateau of 250 (cats W, H, and P) or 500 msec (cat C) were used. In some experiments we applied a second acceleration at the end of the plateau. The second type of stimulus was steady-state sinusoidal stimulation at a variety of frequencies and amplitudes.

After normal data were obtained using the various stimuli, the horizontal semicircular canal was plugged on one side (the left side in cat W and the right side in all other cats). Cats W and C showed postoperative nystagmus in darkness and other signs of vestibular damage in addition to the mechanical canal plug, but cats H and P had no nystagmus or other deficits, except for a low VOR gain. Recovery was monitored beginning one day after the canal plug and continued for up to 8 months post-plug.

RESULTS

Before the canal plug, the gain of the VOR as measured during the plateau of a short-velocity trapezoid (steady-state gain) was approximately 0.8 in all of our cats. After the horizontal semicircular canal was plugged on one side, the steady-state

---

[a]Address for correspondence: Dianne M. Broussard, MC 12-409, The Toronto Hospital, Western Division, Toronto, Ontario M5T 2S8, Canada.

gain recovered rapidly for 4 to 5 days, then more slowly to approach an asymptote of approximately 0.6 over a period of 20 to 30 days. The ratio of the peak to the steady-state eye velocity (dynamic index) revealed an asymmetry that persisted for at least 8 months. As illustrated in FIGURE 1, the dynamic index was higher for rotation contraversive to the canal plug than for rotation ipsiversive to the plug. This asymmetry was also evident for sinusoidal stimulation, when the peak velocity of the sinusoid was kept constant at 10 deg/sec, and frequency was varied between 0.05 and 15 Hz. It was frequency-dependent, with a maximum asymmetry between 5 and 10 Hz. Spectral analysis of the short trapezoids yielded similar results.

The low dynamic index of the ipsiversive response was not due to saturation. As FIGURE 2 illustrates, when the plateau velocity of the trapezoid was varied while keeping the time course constant, the response was linear over the range of 1 to 40

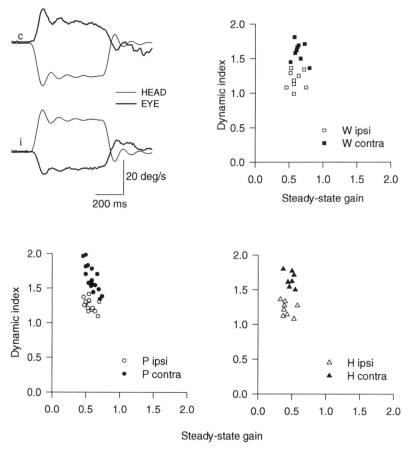

FIGURE 1. Response of the compensated VOR to fast trapezoids of head velocity. *Inset:* Head and eye velocity for rotation contraversive (c) and ipsiversive (i) to the plugged horizontal canal in cat C. The other three panels plot dynamic index as a function of gain for all responses obtained more than 30 days after surgery in cats W, P, and H. *Filled symbols* are responses to contraversive and *open symbols* to ipsiversive rotation with respect to the lesion.

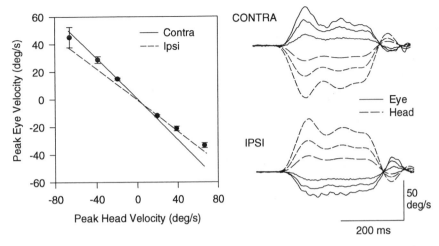

FIGURE 2. Asymmetry over a range of peak velocities and accelerations. *Inset*: Head and eye velocities. The amplitude of the stimulus, but not its time course, was varied. Peak eye velocity was linearly related to peak head velocity with little or no saturation. However, the slope was lower for ipsiversive rotation. Data from cat P, more than 30 days after the canal plug.

deg/sec except for a slight saturation in the contraversive response at high velocities (this could not, however, explain the asymmetry). The asymmetry was independent of the peak acceleration for sinusoids as well as for trapezoids; when acceleration was varied between 100 and 600 deg/sec, while keeping frequency constant at 8 Hz, the same asymmetry was seen at all accelerations. This suggested that the asymmetry was frequency-dependent. When frequency was varied (2–10 Hz) while keeping peak acceleration constant at 550 deg/sec^2, the asymmetry appeared only between 5 and 10 Hz.

DISCUSSION

A canal plug or labyrinthectomy removes all of the input signaling head rotation from one labyrinth, and the response of the VOR would be expected to reflect the properties of the afferents from the remaining labyrinth. Over the frequency range of 0.05–50 Hz, primary afferents deviate from this pattern, displaying an increasing gain and phase lead with respect to angular acceleration over the range of 1–8 Hz.[2] Thus, an angular acceleration signal is present in primary afferents above 1 Hz. Lisberger[3] found that in response to short trapezoids, most afferents display an overshoot, suggesting an acceleration sensitivity. The acceleration sensitivity is asymmetric due to saturation in the inhibitory direction.[4]

Our results suggest that the asymmetric responses to rapid accelerations reported here and in human patients[1] are frequency rather than acceleration dependent. Therefore, it appears likely that the source of the asymmetry is central. One possibility is that commissural pathways have a higher gain for frequencies below 5 Hz than for higher frequencies. This would be expected to reduce the responses of secondary neurons on the plugged side at frequencies above 5 Hz.

REFERENCES

1. HALMAGYI, G. M., I. S. CURTHOYS, S. T. AW, & M. J. TODD. 1993. The human vestibulo-ocular reflex after unilateral vestibular deafferentation: The results of high-acceleration impulsive testing. H. O. Barber & J. A. Sharpe, Eds.: 45–54. The Vestibulo-Ocular Reflex and Vertigo. Raven Press, NY.
2. GOLDBERG, J. M. & C. FERNANDEZ. 1971. Physiology of peripheral neurons innervating semicircular canals of the squirrel monkey. III. Variation among units in their discharge properties. J. Neurophysiol. **34:** 676–684.
3. LISBERGER, S. G. & T. A. PAVELKO. 1986. Vestibular signals carried by pathways subserving plasticity of the vestibulo-ocular reflex in monkeys. J. Neurosci. **6:** 346–354.
4. GOLDBERG, J. M. & C. FERNANDEZ. 1971. Physiology of peripheral neurons innervating semicircular canals of the squirrel monkey. I. Resting discharge and response to constant angular accelerations. *J. Neurophysiol.* **34:** 635–660.

Properties of Nucleus Incertus Neurons of the Cat Projecting to the Cerebellar Flocculus

GUY CHERON,[a,b] MARIE-PIERRE DUFIEF,
NICO GERRITS, AND EMILE GODAUX

[a] Laboratory of Neurosciences
University of Mons-Hainaut
Place du Parc
20 7000 Mons, Belgium

Department of Anatomy
Erasmus University of Rotterdam
the Netherlands

In the cerebellar flocculus, three longitudinal Purkinje cell zones have been described that respond selectively to large-field visual pattern movement. Purkinje cells in a centrally located zone control horizontal eye movements, whereas those in the flanking zones control vertical eye movements.[1] Stimulation of the horizontal zone was recently performed to enable antidromic identification of its mossy fiber inputs with an origin in the medial vestibular nucleus (MVN)[2] and the nucleus prepositus hypoglossi (NPH).[3] Although these two nuclei are two important sources of floccular mossy fibers,[4] several studies have shown that the pontine reticular formation (PRF) provide another mossy fiber input.[5]

The brain-stem region explored in the present study contains a variety of neurons, located in and around the mlb and the adjacent periaqueductal gray. Our attention was focused on a relatively unknown region: the nucleus incertus (NIC). Four adult cats were prepared for chronic recording of neuronal activity in the brain stem and the cerebellum, and for eye movement recording (magnetic search coil technique). The neuronal activity in the PRF was explored with glass micropipettes during bipolar stimulation of the middle zone of both flocculi (FIG. 1A). We focused our attention only on antidromically activated neurons for which collision tests were successful. Projection of these neurons onto the flocculus was verified with retrograde transport of horseradish peroxidase (HRP) after injections in the flocculus (FIG. 1B, E–G). A total of 57 neurons antidromically activated from either flocculus were located in the NIC (FIG. 1C,D). The majority of these neurons modulated their firing rate during spontaneous horizontal saccades in a burst-tonic fashion (BT-neurons). FIGURE 2 illustrates the spiking behavior of a representative BT neuron of the NIC activated antidromically from the contralateral flocculus. Before and during rapid eye movements, this neuron paused when the eyes moved towards the recording side and bursted when the eyes moved in the opposite direction (FIG. 2A,B). During intersaccadic fixation, the tonic discharge rate of this neuron increased with more eccentric (contralateral side) gaze position (FIG. 2C), but it did not change as a function of vertical eye position (FIG. 2D). During sinusoidal

[b] E-mail: GCHERON@RESULB.ULB.AC.BE

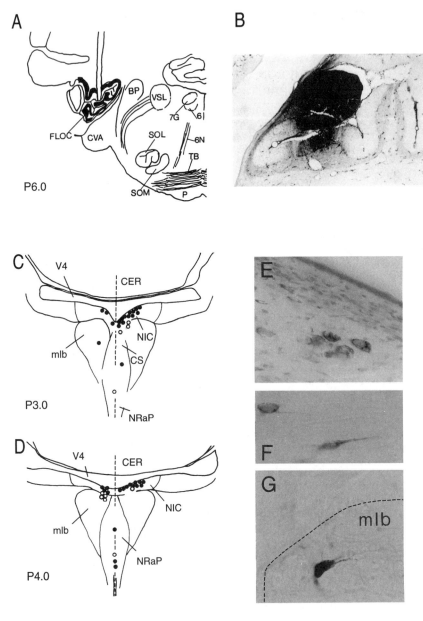

FIGURE 1

vestibular stimulation, the firing rate of this BT-neuron showed a type I sinusoidal modulation interrupted by burst-like increases and by pauses corresponding to the quick phases, directed away or towards the recording side, respectively (FIG. 2B). The BT neurons in the NIC that project to the flocculus showed a spiking behavior very similar to the BT neurons observed in the NPH[3] and the MVN,[2] which were also antidromically activated from the horizontal zone of the flocculus. The present study confirms the results of an earlier electrophysiological analysis of the PRF floccular projection in the anesthetized cat.[6] However, the BT neurons described in this latter study were not located in the NIC.

   In conclusion, the data presented in this study show that the majority of the horizontal BT neurons with a projection to the flocculus, recorded in the dorsolateral pontine tegmentum, are localized in a region hitherto not associated with the oculomotor system: the caudal part of the NIC. It remains to be determined whether the caudal NIC neurons are a subset of the paramedian tract cell groups associated with specific aspects of oculomotor behavior.[7] The absence of data on the precise connections of these neurons preclude conclusions concerning their functional role related to eye movements. Nevertheless, their high sensitivity for both eye position

FIGURE 1 (*facing page*). (A) Drawing of a sagittal section showing the track of the stimulation electrode that ends in the middle zone of the flocculus. Abbreviations: FLOC, flocculus; CVA, anteroventral cochlear nucleus; BP, brachium pontis; VSL, superior vestibular nucleus; SOL, lateral nucleus of the superior olive; SOM, medial nucleus of the superior olive; 7G, genu of the facial nerve; 6, abducens nucleus; 6N, abducens nerve; TB, trapezoid body; P, pyramidal tract. (B) Transverse section through the HRP injection site in the middle zone of the flocculus. (C,D) Localization of the floccular projecting neurons in the PRF. In the cat, the NIC is a collection of small- to medium-sized neurons with an oval to fusiform shape. They are located in the periaquaductal gray directly dorsal to the medial longitudinal bundle (mlb) between the stereotactic planes P 5.5 and P 1.5. Caudally, the NIC abuts on the supragenual nucleus capping the facial genu, but its lateral and rostral borders are indistinct. The horizontal BT neurons (*filled circles*) are mainly located in the NIC. Some of them are located in the nucleus raphe pontis (NRaP) and in the central superior nucleus of the raphe (CS). *Open circles* represent BT neurons with vertical eye movement sensibility, and they are located close to the medial longitudinal bundle (mlb) in the ventral part of the NIC. (E) Cluster of retrogradely labeled small neurons in the contralateral NIC (±P4, Nissl counterstain). (F) Retrogradely labeled small oval and fusiform neurons in the contralateral NIC (±P3). (G) Retrogradely labeled medium-sized polygonal neuron at the dorsomedial corner of the mlb (±P3.5).

FIGURE 2 (*see page 592*). (A,B) Behavior of a representative BT neuron of the NIC during spontaneous eye movements (A) and during the horizontal VOR (B). Abbreviations: ev: vertical eye position; eh: horizontal eye position; f.r.: firing rate; h: head position. Note that in this case the phase lead of the firing rate modulation is 18° with respect to eye position. (C)) scatter plot of mean instantaneous firing rate of the same BT neuron over horizontal eye position during intersaccadic fixation periods. The slope (Kf) of the linear regression between the horizontal eye position and the firing rate (r = 0.85) corresponds to the sensitivity to horizontal eye position (Kf = 6.05 spikes · sec^{-1}/deg). (D) Scatter plot of mean instantaneous firing rate of the neuron over vertical eye position. Note the absence of any significant relation. (E) Analysis of the eye velocity sensitivity (Rv) of this BT neuron. The slope of these different rate–velocity regressions (Rv) varied with eye position from 1.51 to 4.02 spikes · sec^{-1}/deg · sec^{-1}. For each of these lines, the firing rate at zero velocity, F(0), was calculated by interpolation. F: relationship between F(0) and horizontal eye position. The data points are well fitted by a linear regression line. The slope (Kv) of this line corresponds to the sensitivity of this neuron to eye position during the VOR (Kv = 4.52 spikes · sec^{-1}/deg).

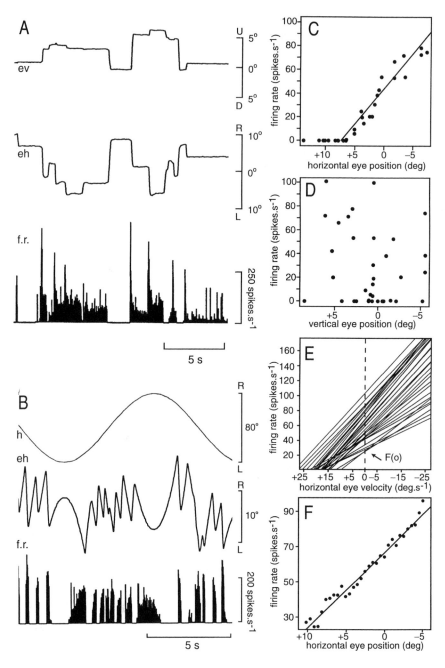

FIGURE 2

and eye velocity might indicate that they provide an efference copy of eye movement commands to the flocculus. The anatomical and physiological characteristics of the NIC neurons show a strong correspondence with the NPH floccular projecting neurons,[3] that is, the superficial localization, the specific projection to the horizontal floccular zone, and the spiking behavior. The convergence onto a single floccular zone of very similar eye-movement-related signals from different brain-stem nuclei could represent an important element in the signal processing of the flocculus.

REFERENCES

1. SATO, Y. & T. KAWASAKI. 1990. J. Neurophysiol. **64:** 551–564.
2. CHERON, G., M. ESCUDERO & E. GODAUX. 1996. J. Neurophysiol. In press.
3. ESCUDERO, M., G. CHERON & E. GODAUX. 1996. J. Neurophysiol. In press.
4. TAN, H. & N. M. GERRITS. 1992. Neuroscience **47:** 909–919.
5. SATO, Y., T. KAWASAKI & K. IKARASHI. 1983. Brain Res. **272:** 37–48.
6. NAKAO, S., I. S. CURTHOYS & C. H. MARKHAM. 1980. Brain Res. **183:** 291–299.
7. BUTTNER-ENNEVER, J. A. 1992. Vestibular and Brain Stem Control of Eye, Head and Body Movements. H. Shimazu & Y. Shinoda, Eds.: 323–330. Japan Scientific Societies Press. Tokyo/S. Karger, Basel.

Improvements of the Neural Network Simulation of the Vestibulo-Oculomotor Integrator

JEAN-PHILIPPE DRAYE,[a,b,c] GUY CHERON,[d,e]
GAËTAN LIBERT,[c] AND EMILE GODAUX[d]

[c] "Parallel Information Processing" Laboratory
Faculté Polytechnique de Mons
B-7000 Mons, Belgium

[d] Department of Neurosciences
Faculty of Medicine
University of Mons-Hainaut
Mons, Belgium

[e] Laboratory of Biomechanics
University of Brussels
Brussels, Belgium

Connectionist models, also refered to as artificial neural networks, have focused much attention for the last few years on the principle of parallel distributed processing in the brain. Nevertheless, the mean challenge of artificial neural networks simulation of real systems is to reach biological interpretability. For this purpose, the oculomotor system, particularly for its role in the horizontal vestibulo-ocular reflex (VOR), offers a number of simplifying features that are reasonably comprehensible.[1] In this system, the modifications to the vestibular signals by the vestibular nuclei (VN) and other neurons before they are transmitted to the motoneurons include a mathematical integration by the final neural integrator (NI); this one performs an essential function: the maintenance of position of both eyes in space. It has been localized in the nucleus prepositus hypoglossi (NPH).[2]

Several models of the NI were proposed, but to gain new insight into the nature of VN neurons, dynamic processing in the horizontal VOR was modeled using recurrent neural networks.[3–5] The first neural network approach of the NI was proposed by Cannon and Robinson.[3,4] Their hard-wired model can integrate a push–pull input signal without integrating the background rates and has the appealing property that localized lesions produced a decrease in the time constant of the entire network (a clinically observed phenomenon); the synaptic weights were explicitly specified. Later, Anastasio and Robinson proposed the first learning model for the NI[5]; nevertheless, this model lacks constraints on the synaptic weights (after training, it does not present the push–pull configuration that the real integrator has).

The purpose of the present investigation is not to develop a new model of the NI but rather to improve the biologically plausible features of the existing models. We based our work on the learning model of Anastasio-Robinson.[5] This model simulates

[a] Address for correspondence: Jean-Philippe Draye, Faculté Polytechnique de Mons, Laboratoire "Processus, Informatique, Parallélisme," Rue de Houdain, 9, B-7000 Mons, Belgium. E-mail: JPD@PIP.FPMS.AC.BE
[b] Research assistant of the Belgian National Fund for Scientific Research.

the horizontal NI in the particular case of the dynamic processing of the horizontal VOR. It presents two afferent inputs from the horizontal canals, a fully connected hidden layer of 16 inhibitory units and two output units that represent the motoneurons of the median and lateral rectus muscles of the left eye (see FIG. 1). The improvements that we bring to the model include strong constraints on the synaptic weights (in order to respect the biological Dale's principle) and the introduction of an artificial distance in our network (to define a notion of proximity). Because of these modifications (the constraints on the weights introduces singular points during training), a new learning process was needed, and we chose a learning algorithm based on a general supervisor. This algorithm trains the network to leakily integrate (in the sense of the Newtonian calculus) the push–pull eye-velocity signals provided by the semicircular canals without integrating the background rate of 100 spikes/sec.

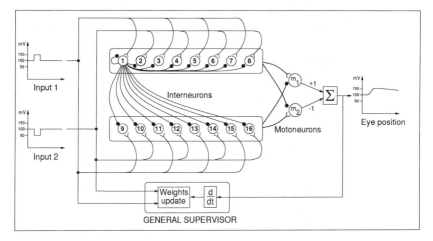

FIGURE 1. The modified artificial neural network for the modeling of the neural integrator. The 16 interneurons of the hidden layer are divided into two groups of eight and are fully connected with inhibitory connections (only the connections out of interneuron 1 are depicted). Each interneuron is connected to both motoneurons with a connection whose sign is given on the figure. The eye position is simply given by the difference between the motoneuron outputs. The general supervisor computes all the weight updates.

Once our network has been trained, we will be interested in the behavior of the hidden units of our model: Could the distribution of the artificial synaptic weights of these units be related to a particular organization depending on specific requirements? This task is not as simple as it might be; it is even widely assumed that the hidden units are of little use in illuminating the basic problem of how the brain processes signals. After training, we observed that the structure of the lateral connection weights of the hidden layer exhibits several clusters. The weights are obviously structured in conglomerates or groups of interneurons where the weights seem quite important. Other zones are quite flat and characterized by very low-value weights (see FIG. 2). The important thing is that the high-value weights are grouped in what we call clusters. A cluster can be defined as a particular group of adjoining interneurons that have strong and privileged connections with another neighborhood of interneurons (the notion of neighborhood has a clear meaning with respect to the introduction of a distance in the network).

From the biological point of view, microelectrode recordings have shown that neighboring neurons often disclose similar patterns of electrical activity corroborating the existence of a functional clustering of the NI. For example, the goldfish NI presents very clear nonoverlapping compartments with proper functions (eye position or eye velocity integrators).[6] Moreover, neurochemically defined clusters were

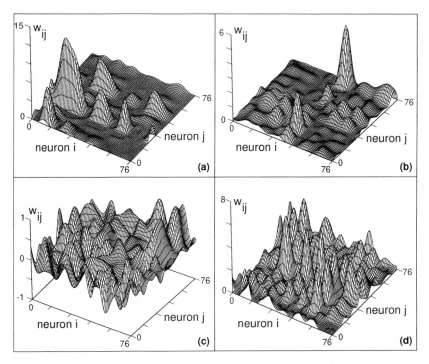

FIGURE 2. Surface plots of the weights distribution. The 16×16 weights surfaces were treated with cubic splines to get a better visualization. Values of the weights are plotted versus indexes i and j. Even if the lateral layer has inhibitory connections (except for **c**), the weights are plotted as positive values. (**a** and **b**) Two clustered structures of the weights distribution of our network. (**c**) The weight distribution of the Arnold-Robinson network trained with the general supervisor without any constraints on the sign of the weights (the sign can be positive or negative). (**d**) The weight distribution of the network where each interneuron has its own muscle.

found in the NPH of the cat. Like other iterated patterns of the brain circuitry (the columns and blobs in visual cortex, the barrels in the somatosensory cortex and the patches in the striatum, the clusters reflect one of the organizing principles of neural assemblies.[7] This type of organization could therefore be considered to be expressions of different kinds of biological constraints. These can be genetic, biochemical, developmental (synaptic growth), and/or due to the information processing in the network. Artificial neural networks give us an opportunity to analyze this latter hypothesis by means of a computational model using supervised learning to mimic the behavior of the NI. The spontaneous emergence of clusters in artificial neural networks, performing a well-defined physico-mathematical task (a temporal integration) is due to computational constraints, with a restricted space for solutions. Thus, information-processing constraints are a plausible factor in inducing the emergence of iterated patterns in biological neural networks.

REFERENCES

1. ROBINSON, D. A. 1992. Behav. Brain Sci. **15:** 644–655.
2. CHERON, G., E. GODAUX, J. M. LAUNE & B. VANDERKELEN. 1986. J. Physiol. (Lond.) **372:** 75–94.
3. CANNON, S. C. & D. A. ROBINSON. 1983. Biol. Cybern. **49:** 127–136.
4. CANNON, S. C. & D. A. ROBINSON. 1985. Biol. Cybern. **53:** 93–108.
5. ARNOLD, D. B. & D. A. ROBINSON. 1991. Biol. Cybern. **64:** 447–454.
6. PASTOR, A. M., R. R. DE LA CRUZ & R. BAKER. 1994. Proc. Natl. Acad. Sci. USA **91:** 807–811.
7. PURVES, D., D. R. RIDDLE & A.-S. LAMANTIA. 1992. Trends Neurosci. **15:** 362–368.

Mild Mal de Debarquement after Sailing[a]

HELEN COHEN

*Bobby R. Alford Department of Otorhinolaryngology
and Communicative Sciences
Baylor College of Medicine
One Baylor Plaza
Houston, Texas 77030*

After recreational boating many nonprofessional sailors report motion illusions that mimic the sensations of sailing. Similar, but unpleasant, post-sailing motion illusions are known as mal de debarquement.[1,2] Although common among sailors, little is known about these illusions. These motion illusions were studied under unique circumstances—the week-long annual sea trials of a restored nineteenth century square-rigged ship, the barque, *Elissa*. The ship is sailed each year in the waters around Galveston by professional officers, assisted by trained, amateur, volunteer crew.

METHODS

Officers, crew members, and guests who sailed during the first four days of the 1994 sea trials participated ($n = 59$). The number of participants varied each day depending on the number of people who sailed. Some people participated on more than one day. Several hours after disembarking, subjects filled out a self-administered survey about the intensity and quality of the sensations that they experienced.

RESULTS

Sailing conditions were relatively calm, although varying slightly each day. Because of the antique nature of the ship, accurate data on wind direction, sea conditions, and ship velocity were unavailable. Two of the three mates were interviewed daily about the wind and sea conditions; they had high interrater reliability. Over the four days, 20 to 41% of subjects reported motion illusions after disembarking (FIG. 1). No subjects became seasick during the voyage. No subjects reported nauseating or other noxious sensations. Subjects experienced the sensations for a mean of 1.8 hours (SD 2.3), with a mean onset 1.9 hours after disembarking. Approximately 80% of subjects reported mild sensations, usually a sense of rocking, usually while indoors, for example, in the workshop or in a shower stall, rather than outside on the pier or elsewhere in the vicinity (FIG. 2). None of the nine professional sailors reported these sensations. Of the crew members with no or minimal previous sailing experience, 39% reported the sensations; of the experienced crew 50% reported the sensations. These data are presented in greater detail

[a]This work was supported by the Clayton Foundation for Research.

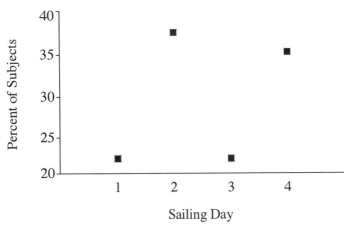

FIGURE 1. Percent of subjects who experienced motion illusions following each day's sail.

elsewhere.[3] Over the four days of the sea trials, crew members who sailed for two or more days varied in their reports from none to mild sensations.

DISCUSSION

These data suggest that nonnoxious sensations of motion after sailing, characterized by some resemblance to the motion of the vessel and usually occurring indoors within a short period after the cessation of sailing, are relatively common among nonprofessional sailors. These findings suggest that a kind of vestibular memory

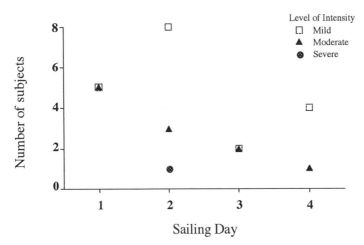

FIGURE 2. Intensity of motion illusions experienced by subjects following each day's sail.

stores vestibular sensations and subsequently generates these illusions, supporting Groen's concept of a vestibular system pattern generator.[4]

ACKNOWLEDGMENTS

This project was possible thanks to the generosity of the Texas Seaport Museum and the officers and crew of *Elissa*.

REFERENCES

1. MURPHY, T. P. 1993. Mal de debarquement syndrome: A forgotten entity? Otolaryngol. Head Neck Surg. **109:** 10–13.
2. BROWN, J. J. & R. W. BALOH. 1987. Persistent mal de debarquement syndrome: A motion-induced subjective disorder of balance. Am. J. Otolaryngol. **8:** 219–222.
3. COHEN, H. 1996. Vertigo after sailing a nineteenth century ship. J. Vestib. Res. **6:** 31–35.
4. GROEN, J. J. 1960. Problems of the semicircular canal from a mechanicophysiological point of view. Acta Otolaryngol. Suppl. **163:** 59–66.

Inhibitory Burst Neuron Activity Encodes Gaze, Not Eye, Metrics and Dynamics during Passive Head on Body Rotation

Evidence that Vestibular Signals Supplement Visual Information in the Control of Gaze Shifts

KATHLEEN E. CULLEN[a] AND DANIEL GUITTON

Aerospace Medical Research Unit and
The Montreal Neurological Institute
McGill University
Montreal, Quebec H3G 1Y6, Canada

Short lead inhibitory burst neurons (IBNs) project to the contralateral abducens and function together with ipsilaterally projecting excitatory burst neurons to drive saccadic eye movements. Our recent studies in the cat and monkey[1,2] have demonstrated that IBN discharges are best correlated, not with the metrics and dynamics of the movement of the eye in the head, but with the movement of the visual axis in space (gaze) during active coordinated eye and head gaze shifts. In the present study, IBN activity was studied during a different paradigm in which we passively generated rapid rotations of the animal's head on its body (PHBR). Previous studies of the coordination of eye and head movements during passive head on body rotations[3,4] have suggested that eye movements, and corresponding "gaze shifts" are driven by vestibular and/or neck proprioceptive inputs rather than retinal information. In the PHBR paradigm, the applied head movement typically evoked a compensatory vestibulo-ocular reflex during the first ~ 100 msec, after which the gaze trajectory was directed towards the ongoing movement of the head. During these gaze shifts, the eye's contribution to the ongoing movement was quite small; indeed, in some movements the eye was almost immobile. However, although the eye moved little during PHBRs, IBNs were active until gaze had completely stabilized. In order to determine the nature of the signal encoded by IBNs during shifts in gaze generated by PHBR, we have carried out both metric and dynamic analyses of IBN discharges and investigated the effect of momentarily halting the head movement (by a friction clutch) on IBN activity and eye (and gaze) movements.

METHODS AND RESULTS

IBNs were identified by (1) their location relative to the abducens nucleus, (2) their discharge during ipsilateral saccades made head-fixed and vestibularly driven quick phases, and (3) their lack of response during the slow phase of vestibular nystagmus (FIG. 1A and B). Analysis of IBN activity during head-fixed saccades and

---

[a] Address for correspondence: Kathleen E. Cullen, Aerospace Medical Research Unit, 3655 Drummond St., Montreal, Quebec H3G 1Y6, Canada.

PHBRs demonstrated that the number of spikes (NOS) generated during a burst was consistently best correlated with the horizontal gaze amplitude. In fact, NOS was on average as well correlated with gaze amplitude during PHBR as during head-fixed saccades (mean: r = 0.79 in both paradigms). Moreover, during PHBR, NOS was correlated with the horizontal head amplitude (mean: r = 0.64), but was poorly correlated with the horizontal eye amplitude (mean: r = 0.22). In addition, IBN burst duration was related to gaze duration during the PHBR paradigm as well as

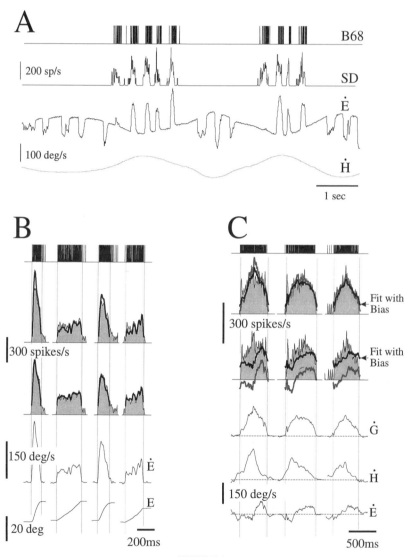

FIGURE 1

during head-fixed saccades (mean: $r = 0.90$ and 0.88, respectively). Burst duration was also strongly related to head movement duration (mean: $r = 0.78$) during PHBR.

The instantaneous firing frequency of IBNs also better encoded gaze, than eye, trajectories during the PHBR paradigm. RMS errors and parameter estimates were determined over 40 head-fixed saccades or gaze shifts for two velocity-based dynamic models: (1) $FR = b_l \cdot I$ and (2) $FR = b_l \cdot I + r$, where FR is unit firing rate; I is either eye, head, or gaze velocity; b_l is a gain term and r is the bias term. Firing rates were estimated using an eye-based model during head-fixed saccades (FIG. 1B) and eye-, head-, and gaze-based models during PHBR gaze shifts. The unit illustrated in FIG. 1C is typical in that, for PHBRs, gaze or head velocity-based models were significantly better at predicting IBN firing rate than eye velocity-based models. Estimated gain terms for gaze- and head-based models were significantly less during PHBR than during head-fixed saccades. Estimated bias terms for IBN head-fixed models (103) and PHBR models, based on gaze or head velocity, were comparable (mean bias = 80 and 106, respectively), while the bias term in eye-based PHBR models was significantly larger and not significantly different from the mean value of IBN firing rate ($p < 0.001$; 156 versus 162). These results were consistent with the observed relationships between movement amplitudes and NOS (FIG. 2A). (1) The slope of the relationship, NOS versus gaze amplitude, was consistently less during PHBR than during head-fixed saccades and (2) the intercept of this relationship was comparable during PHBR and head-fixed saccades. Furthermore, the intercept for the regression between NOS and head amplitude was comparable to those of the head-fixed and PHBR gaze relationships, while the intercept of the regression between NOS and eye amplitude was significantly higher (not shown).

The difference between the parameters estimated for head-fixed versus PHBR models suggested that head-fixed models should not be used to describe the discharge of IBNs during PHBR. This issue was directly addressed in the analysis illustrated in FIG. 2B. We used the parameters of the optimal head-fixed model (FIG. 1B) to analyze IBN firing rate during PHBR. When PHBR gaze velocity was the input, unit discharge was overestimated; whereas when eye velocity was the input, unit discharge was overestimated. The evident similarity between the head and gaze

←——————————————————————————————————————

FIGURE 1. (A) Example of the firing behavior of cat IBN (unit B68) during whole-body rotation in the head-fixed condition. **(B)** Examples of the same cell during head-fixed saccades in the ipsilateral direction. The fit of a simple model: firing rate α eye velocity, is superimposed (*heavy line*) on the actual firing rate (*shaded curve*) (*second panel*). The model fit is considerably improved when a bias term is added to the model (*heavy line, third panel*). **(C)** Examples of the same IBN during passive rotation of the cat's head on its body. Note that the applied head movement initially evoked a compensatory eye movement response, after which gaze moved in the same direction as the head, coincident with the onset of IBN activity. A simple dynamic model: $FR = b_l \cdot G$ (*second panel from top*), produced a significantly better fit (*gray heavy line*) of the actual firing rate (*shaded curve*) than the model: $FR = b_l \cdot E$ (*gray heavy line, third panel from top*). When a bias term was added ($FR = b_l \cdot I + r$) the goodness of the model fit remained significantly better when gaze, rather than eye velocity, was the input (I) to the model (*black heavy line, second and third panels*). Abbreviations: G, H, and E denote horizontal gaze, head and eye velocity, respectively. E denotes horizontal eye position. Dashed vertical lines indicate the onset and offset of the saccade using a 20 deg/sec eye velocity criterion. Dashed horizontal lines indicate 0 deg/sec. Spike density (SD) was obtained by replacing each spike by a gaussian of a 5 msec width.

trajectories in this paradigm suggested to us that IBN discharges were vestibularly driven. In order to investigate this further, head movement was halted (100 msec) by a friction clutch during a PHBR shift in gaze (FIG. 2C). IBN firing ceased immediately following the cessation of head movement (coincident with an accompanying stabilization of gaze) and only resumed once the brake was released. The striking

A

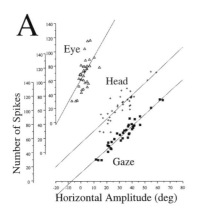

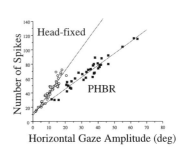

B

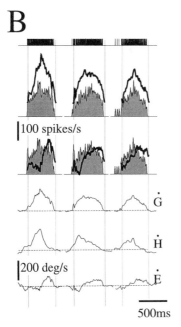

C

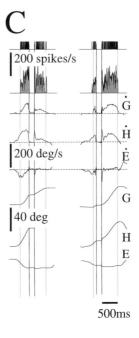

FIGURE 2

similarity between the time course of a head motion and IBN discharge during mechanical braking further suggests that IBNs themselves have access to vestibular information.

CONCLUSIONS

1. The total number of spikes in the burst was best correlated with gaze amplitude and was also well correlated with head amplitude, but was poorly correlated with eye amplitude. Similarly, dynamic analysis revealed that instantaneous IBN firing rate was better predicted on the basis of gaze than eye velocity trajectories. In addition, the bias term estimated for gaze and head velocity-based models during PHBR were comparable to those estimated for head-fixed saccades, whereas the bias term estimated for eye velocity-based models was significantly higher.

2. The eye movement trajectories in the passively generated gaze shifts could not generally be explained in terms of the firing behavior of IBNs during head-fixed saccades (as revealed through metric and dynamic analysis). Because IBNs project monosynaptically to abducens motor neurons, this suggests that other premotor inputs (e.g., vestibular/prepositus) to the motor neurons must be considered during passively generated gaze shifts.

3. When head motion was momentarily halted, gaze stabilized and IBN activity ceased during the brake period. Once the brake was released, the resumption of head movement and IBN activity were coincident. This striking similarity in the time course of a head motion and IBN discharge suggests that IBNs receive a vestibular input.

4. These results suggest that the previously proposed vestibular drive to brain-stem burst neurons is unmasked during the PHBR paradigm. We conclude that for visually triggered gaze shifts, it is likely that the brain-stem burst generator is under the influence not only of collicular signals but also of a head velocity input.

←

FIGURE 2. (A) Regression analysis relating the total number of spikes occurring in a burst and movement amplitude for neuron B68. *Left*: The relationship between the total number of spikes generated during a gaze shift and the amplitude of the gaze (*filled symbols;* slope = 1.7, r = 0.94), head (*crosses;* slope = 1.7, r = 0.87) and eye (*open symbols;* slope = 3.2, r = 0.61) movements for neuron B68 during the PHBR paradigm. *Right*: Relationship between the number of spikes and gaze amplitude for neuron B68. Data are shown for the active head-fixed (slope = 3.2, r = 0.94) and passive head rotation paradigms. Note that the slope of this relationship is less during the PHBR paradigm. (B) Parameter values (r, b_1) calculated for head-fixed saccades using the model: ($FR = b_1 \cdot E + r$) were used to predict the discharge of cat IBN (B68) during PHBR when eye and gaze velocity were the inputs to the model. For every IBN, a gaze velocity input to the model (*heavy line, second panel*) resulted in an overestimation of the unit discharge, while an eye velocity input to the model (*heavy line, third panel*) resulted in an underestimation of the unit discharge. (C) Example of the firing rate of cat IBN (B75) during two passively induced gaze shifts in which the head movement was halted by a friction clutch. When the head stopped (*first solid vertical line*) the neuron immediately ceased firing, and gaze velocity went to 0 deg/sec. When the brake was released (*second solid vertical line*), gaze velocity and unit discharge resumed coincidentally within 30 msec. Abbreviations: G, H, and E denote horizontal gaze, head and eye velocity, respectively.

REFERENCES

1. CULLEN, K. E., D. GUITTON, W. JIANG & C. G. REY. 1993. Gaze-related activity of putative inhibitory burst neurons in the head-free cat. J. Neurophysiol. **70:** 2678–2683.
2. CULLEN, K. E., C. G. REY & D. GUITTON. 1994. Downstream and upstream models of IBN activity during gaze shifts in the head-free cat and monkey. Soc. Neurosci. Abstr. **20.**
3. BARNES, G. R. 1979. Vestibulo-ocular function during co-ordinated head and eye movements to acquire visual targets. J. Physiol. (Lond.) **287:** 127–147.
4. GUITTON, D., R. M. DOUGLAS & M. VOLLE. 1984. Eye–head coordination in cats. J. Neurophysiol. **52:** 427–459.

Individual Purkinje Cell Axons Terminate on Both Inhibitory and Excitatory Neurons in the Cerebellar and Vestibular Nuclei

C. I. DE ZEEUW[a,c] AND A. S. BERREBI[b]

[a]Department of Anatomy
Erasmus University Rotterdam
P.O. Box 1738
3000 DR Rotterdam, the Netherlands

[b]Departments of Otolaryngology and Anatomy
P.O. Box 9200 HSCS
Morgantown, West Virginia 26506-9200

The cerebellar and vestibular nuclei consist of a heterogeneous group of inhibitory and excitatory neurons. A major proportion of the inhibitory neurons provides a GABAergic feedback to the inferior olive, while the excitatory neurons exert more direct effects on motor control via nonolivary structures (e.g., De Zeeuw *et al.*,[1] Fredette and Mugnaini,[2] De Zeeuw and Ruigrok[3]). It is not clear whether Purkinje cells innervate all types of neurons in the cerebellar and vestibular nuclei nor whether an individual Purkinje cell axon can innervate different types of neurons. In the present study, we studied the postsynaptic targets of Purkinje cell axons in the rat using a combination of postembedding GABA immunocytochemistry and preembedding immunolabeling of the Purkinje cell terminals by L7, a Purkinje cell specific marker.[4,5]

Electron microscopic analysis of the various cerebellar nuclei and vestibular nuclei indicated that L7-labeled terminals (1) were all GABA-positive, (2) usually included pleiomorphic vesicles, and (3) formed symmetric synapses. In a quantitative analysis of the postsynaptic distribution of Purkinje cells in the lateral and interposed cerebellar nuclei (see TABLE 1) we observed that (1) the majority was apposed to nonGABAergic structures (79%); and (2) that about half of the all Purkinje cell terminals contacted distal dendrites (51%). Both in the cerebellar and vestibular nuclei individual Purkinje cell terminals were found to innervate both the GABAergic and the larger nonGABAergic neurons (FIG. 1). In nonserial sections 2.6% of the Purkinje cell terminals made synaptic contacts with both structures. Following serial analysis of sets of about 50 ultrathin sections (with a thickness of 50 nm), this percentage increased to 9%. Frequently, we encountered individual Purkinje cell axons that contained more than one terminal in a particular set of serial sections. Therefore, the percentage of individual Purkinje cell axons that contacted both GABAergic and nonGABAergic structures was higher (13%) than that of individual terminals. Considering that the serial section analysis was performed on pieces of tissue not thicker than 3 μm and that individual Purkinje cell axons give off varicosities in the cerebellar and vestibular nuclei over hundreds of micrometers in

[c]E-mail: DeZeeuw@Anat.Fgg.Eur.Nl

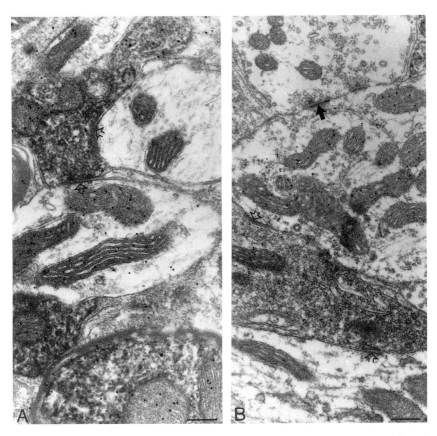

FIGURE 1. In both the vestibular (**A**) and cerebellar (**B**) nuclei, individual Purkinje cell terminals were found to innervate both GABAergic and nonGABAergic dendrites. Note that the GABAergic dendrite in B is contacted by both a L7-labeled GABAergic dendrite and an excitatory, nonGABAergic terminal with round vesicles and an asymmetric synapse. *Open arrows* indicate symmetric synapses and the *black arrow* indicates an asymmetric synapse. Scale bar in **A** indicates 0.19 μm and scale bar in **B** indicates 0.25 μm.

the rostrocaudal plane,[6] it can be concluded that most of the Purkinje cell axons probably innervate both GABAergic and nonGABAergic neurons.

The vast majority of the GABAergic neurons contacted by the Purkinje cells are probably neurons projecting to the inferior olive, since Fredette and Mugnaini[2] observed that at least 93% of GAD-positive neurons in the cerebellar nuclei are retrogradely labeled following injection of HRP in the inferior olive. This presumably monosynaptic input from the Purkinje cells onto the olivary projection neurons indicates that the olivocerebellar modules described by Voogd and Bigaré[7] are indeed formed by a three-element loop consisting of a specific olivary subnucleus, a specific cerebellar sagittal zone of Purkinje cells, and a specific cerebellar nucleus. Purkinje cell terminals were also found to form synapses with GABAergic neurons in group y, nucleus prepositus hypoglossi, and the descending and medial vestibular

TABLE 1. Tabulation of Postsynaptic Distribution of Purkinje Cell Terminals (L7+/GA+), other GABAergic Terminals (L7−/GA+), and NonGABAergic Terminals (L7−/GA−) in the Lateral Cerebellar Nucleus and Interposed Cerebellar Nucleus

	GABAergic			NonGABAergic		
	Cell Bodies	Prox. Den.	Dist. Den.	Cell Bodies	Prox. Den.	Dist. Den
L7+/GA+ (n = 986)	4%	8%	9%	8%	29%	42%
L7−/GA+ (n = 215)	4%	6%	9%	13%	29%	39%
L7−/GA− (n = 149)	3%	9%	10%	1%	20%	57%

NOTE: Of a total of 1350 terminals randomly collected from the most superficial sections of these nuclei 986 (73%) terminals contained GABA and L7, 215 (16%) contained GABA but were L7-negative, and 149 (11%) were nonGABAergic and L7-negative (FIG. 2). The postsynaptic structures are divided into GABAergic and nonGABAergic cell bodies, proximal dendrites, and distal dendrites. It should be noted that the percentages given above make 100% for each row. The percentages within a column cannot be compared unless the sample numbers of the various types of terminals are taken into account. Terminals that formed synapses with different postsynaptic structures and terminals that formed synapses with an axon hillock are not included in the analysis.

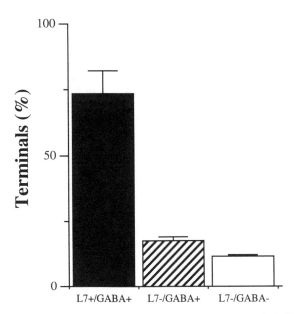

FIGURE 2. Histogram illustrating the percentages of Purkinje cell terminals (L7+/GABA+), GABAergic terminals of recurrent collaterals and/or interneurons (L7−/GABA+), and nonGABAergic terminals of predominantly climbing fiber and mossy fiber collaterals (L7−/GABA−), as collected randomly from the lateral cerebellar nucleus and the interposed cerebellar nucleus.

nucleus, which are known to project, respectively, to the ventrolateral outgrowth, dorsal cap, and β-nucleus of the inferior olive.[8,9] This finding suggests that the arrangement of the three-element modules also occurs in the vestibulocerebellum.

The observation that individual Purkinje cells innervate both GABAergic and nonGABAergic neurons in the cerebellar and vestibular nuclei indicate that the Purkinje cells control simultaneously the inhibitory feedback to the inferior olive, which is part of the closed, three-element, anatomical pathway, and the excitatory cerebellar output system, which is part of an open anatomical pathway through which the motor commands are finally influenced.[6] These combined inhibitory and excitatory effects of individual Purkinje cells may, therefore, be of crucial importance for the role of the cerebellum in controlling the timing of movements.[10,11]

REFERENCES

1. DE ZEEUW, C. I., J. C. HOLSTEGE, T. J. H. RUIGROK & J. VOOGD. 1989. An ultrastructural study of the GABAergic, the cerebellar and the mesodiencephalic innervation of the cat medial accessory olive: Anterograde tracing combined with immunocytochemistry. J. Comp. Neurol. **284:** 12–35.

2. FREDETTE, B. J. & E. MUGNAINI. 1991. The GABAergic cerebello-olivary projection in the rat. Anat. Embryol. **184:** 225–243.

3. DE ZEEUW, C. I. & T. J. H. RUIGROK. 1994. Olivary projecting neurons in the nucleus of Darkschewitsch in the cat receive excitatory monosynaptic input from the cerebellar nuclei. Brain Res. **653:** 345–350.

4. OBERDICK, J., F. LEVINTHAL & C. LEVINTHAL. 1988. A Purkinje cell differentiation marker shows a partial DNA sequence homology to the cellular sis/PDGF2 gene. Neuron **1:** 367–376 [Erratum **3:** 385].

5. BERREBI, A. S. & E. MUGNAINI. 1992. Characteristics of labeling of the cerebellar Purkinje neuron by L7 antiserum. J. Chem. Neuroanat. **5:** 235–243.

6. DE ZEEUW, C. I., D. R. WYLIE, P. L. DIGIORGI & J. I. SIMPSON. 1994. Projections of individual Purkinje cells of identified zones in the flocculus to the vestibular and cerebellar nuclei in the rabbit. J. Comp. Neurol. **349:** 428–448.

7. VOOGD, J. & F. BIGARÉ. 1980. Topographical distribution of olivary and corticonuclear fibers in the cerebellum. A review. In The Inferior Olivary Nucleus. J. Courville, C. de Montigny & Y. Lamarre, Eds.: 207–235. Raven. New York.

8. DE ZEEUW, C. I., P. WENTZEL & E. MUGNAINI. 1993. Fine structure of the dorsal cap of the inferior olive and its GABAergic and non-GABAergic input from the nucleus prepositus hypoglossi in rat and rabbit. J. Comp. Neurol. **327:** 63–82.

9. DE ZEEUW, C. I., N. M. GERRITS, J. VOOGD, C. LEONARD & J. I. SIMPSON. 1994. The rostral dorsal cap and ventrolateral outgrowth of the rabbit inferior olive receive a GABAergic input from dorsal group y and the ventral dentate nucleus. J. Comp. Neurol. **341:** 420–432.

10. WELSH, J. P., E. LANG, I. SUGIHARA & R. LLINÁS. 1995. Dynamic organization of motor control within the olivocerebellar system. Nature **374:** 453–457.

11. DE ZEEUW, C. I., D. R. WYLIE, J. S. STAHL & J. I. SIMPSON. Phase relations of Purkinje cells in the rabbit flocculus during compensatory eye movements. J. Neurophysiol. **74:** 2057–2064.

Vestibular Afferent Projections to the Brain Stem in Pigeons[a]

J. DAVID DICKMAN

Departments of Surgery (Otolaryngology) and Anatomy
University of Mississippi Medical Center
Jackson, Mississippi 39216

Pigeons, like many other animals, contain a large region in the brain stem that receives direct afferent input from the vestibular receptors and is involved in the processing of movement and positional information. The question of whether a differential distribution of vestibular afferent information to central nuclear neurons is present in pigeons was studied using neural tracer compounds.

METHODS

The animals were anesthetized (Nembutal), and the left labyrinth was surgically exposed under aseptic conditions. A single branch of the vestibular nerve that innervated a specific receptor crista or macula was isolated and cut immediately adjacent to the receptor neuroepithelium. Free crystals of either horseradish peroxidase (HRP) or a horseradish peroxidase/cholera-toxin mixture (HRP-CTP) were applied to the cut nerve stump. Next, bone wax was applied over the area, the wound sutured closed, and analgesic (Butorphanol) administered. Following a survival period of 48 to 96 hours, the animals were given an overdose of anesthetic and perfused transcardially with heparinized saline and aldehyde fixatives. Frozen serial sections were cut in either the transverse or parasagittal planes, then processed histochemically using either diamino benzidine (DAB) or tetramethyl benzidine (TMB) as a chromagen for the HRP and HRP-CTP tracing tissue. Afferent fibers and their terminal distributions were visualized and photographed using light microscopy, then drawn for comparison using either camera lucida and a digipad or direct video camera image tracing on a computer screen with reconstruction software. For delineation of possible tracer spread between the intended cut nerve branch and other vestibular organs, the receptor neuroepithelia were examined in several animals, with no evidence of tracer spread being observed.

RESULTS

In pigeons, like most animals, the afferents that innervate the different vestibular end organs project to the brain stem and cerebellum. When tracer compounds were applied to the horizontal semicircular canal nerve branch, the afferent terminal distribution was generally observed to be present in the central regions of the superior (S), ventral lateral (Lv), medial (M), and descending (D) vestibular nuclei,

[a]This work was supported in part by funds provided by the National Institutes of Health, NIDCD DC01092, and by the National Aeronautics and Space Administration, NAG2-786.

as illustrated in FIGURE 1. Horizontal canal afferents also terminated in the medial M, the cerebellar nuclei, and the cerebellar cortex; a few afferent fibers were observed to terminate in the dorsal lateral vestibular nucleus (Ld) and the prepositus hypoglossi (PH). The vertical semicircular canal afferents had projections to the

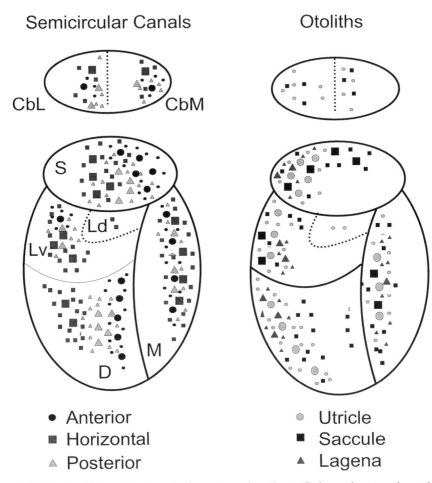

FIGURE 1. Vestibular afferent projection patterns into the vestibular nuclear complex and cerebellar nuclei in pigeons. Symbols represent terminal fields of the different receptor organs. CbL, lateral cerebellar nucleus; CbM, medial cerebellar nucleus; D, descending vestibular nucleus; Ld, dorsal lateral vestibular nucleus; Lv, ventral lateral vestibular nucleus; M, medial vestibular nucleus; S, superior vestibular nucleus.

central regions of the vestibular nuclei which partially overlapped with areas receiving horizontal canal terminations. However, the majority of the vertical canal afferents projected in a segregated fashion to the most medial regions of the vestibular nuclei. All of the semicircular canal organs had some fibers that projected to the cerebellar nuclei, the nodulus and uvula, and a few fibers were observed to terminate in the lateral paraflocculus. Afferent fibers innervating the otolith organs had a distinctly different termination pattern, as compared to the semicircular canal fibers. As represented in FIGURE 1, otolith afferents projected to the most lateral regions of the vestibular nuclei, as well as the cerebellar nuclei and posterior cortex. Utricular afferents also had terminal fields that overlapped those of the horizontal canal fibers in the central regions of the S, the Lv, and the D. Conversely, saccular afferents had separate terminal fields that overlapped those of the vertical canal afferents in the medial S, Lv, and D. Lagenar fibers projected primarily to the auditory nuclei, with other fibers projecting to regions that overlapped those of the utricle and saccule terminal fields.

CONCLUSION

Some regions of the vestibular nuclei appear to receive input from all receptor types, while other regions receive input from canal and otolith receptors with similar response vector orientations. This pattern may provide specificity for determination of the spatial–temporal response sensitivities of second-order neurons through specific patterns of otolith-canal convergence. How these different anatomical termination patterns affect nuclei neuron responsiveness remains a question of physiological interest, which should provide insight toward understanding vestibular motor function.

Role of Cerebellar Uvula-Nodulus in the Control of Head Orientation-Specific Eye Velocity in the Rabbit

P. ERRICO,[a] A. A. FERRARESI,[a] N. H. BARMACK,[b]
AND V. E. PETTOROSSI[c]

[a] Institute of Human Physiology
Catholic University S. Cuore
Largo F. Vito I
00168 Rome, Italy

[b] R. S. Dow Neurological Sciences Institute
Legacy Good Samaritan Hospital & Medical Center
1120 Northwest 20th Avenue
Portland, Oregon 97209

[c] Institute of Human Physiology
University of Perugia
Via del Giochetto
06100 Perugia, Italy

INTRODUCTION

A central problem in neurobiology is how sensory stimulation modulates ongoing rhythmic neural activity. Classic approaches to this problem have included investigations of cutaneous stimulation on the spatial localization of the "scratch reflex."[1,2] The vestibular system offers an excellent model for studying this problem, since it is possible to induce a rhythmic activity, ocular nystagmus, and then determine the effect of a controlled sensory input through natural vestibular stimulation on the functional manifestation of this rhythmic activity.

In the present report, we have induced horizontal nystagmus by prolonged optokinetic stimulation. Such optokinetic stimulation evokes an optokinetic after-nystagmus that lasts several hours. This nystagmus has been termed negative optokinetic after-nystagmus (negative OKAN),[3] since its slow phase is opposite to the direction of optokinetic stimulus that induces it. We have used this negative OKAN to characterize the influence of static tilt of the head of the rabbit about the interaural axis in the pitch plane. Because the cerebellar uvula-nodulus receives both visual and vestibular information concerned with spatial orientation, we have also investigated the influence of lesions of the uvula-nodulus on the ability of rabbits to alter the plane of negative optokinetic after-nystagmus as a consequence of changes in static tilt of the head in the pitch plane.

METHODS

Rabbits were restrained within an optokinetic drum rotating at angular velocity of 5°/sec in the horizontal plane. The head was fixed by a spring-loaded flexible coupling by means of head bolts previously implanted under anesthesia. The head was pitched downward by 15° relative to the stereotaxic horizontal position of 0°. In this position the horizontal semicircular canals were aligned in the horizontal plane. The alignment of the head was critical, since even slight misalignments could result in vertical as well as horizontal optokinetic stimulation.[4] Optokinetic stimulation lasted 48 hours and was interrupted every 8 hours to give food and water. At the end of the conditioning period, the rabbits were put in a turntable with the head restrained at stereotaxic 0°. The spatial orientation and velocity of negative OKAN was measured at different static pitch angles about the interaural axis. Eye movements were measured by an infrared light projection technique.[5] Eye velocity was obtained by digital differentiation of the eye position signal (sampled at 200 Hz) within horizontal and vertical orbital coordinates. The mean SPEV of both horizontal and vertical components was computed by averaging the velocity during the intersaccadic interval. In three rabbits we removed the nodulus and ventral uvula under Fluothane anesthesia and repeatedly tested the orientation and velocity of negative OKAN at 10, 30, and 90 days after the surgery. The extent of the lesions was measured histologically.

RESULTS

Like post-rotatory nystagmus, negative OKAN develops in the earth's horizontal plane and remains in this plane even while the head is pitched statically with respect to gravity by as much as ± 90°.[9] In rabbits that received optokinetic stimulation, negative OKAN reoriented toward horizontal with a gain of 0.89, over a range of ±90° (FIG. 1). Slow-phase eye velocity (SPEV) showed a progressive decrease when the head was pitched downward or upward from the position at which it was maintained during optokinetic stimulation. A second-order curve-fitting all velocity data showed that the peak SPEV occurred with the head pitched down about 20°. This corresponded approximately to the earth-horizontal head position maintained during optokinetic stimulation (FIG. 1). This indicates that the change in SPEV is not simply a function of the head tilt out of horizontal plane, but also depends on the head position during optokinetic stimulation.

In uvula-nodulus-lesioned rabbits, there was no change in the reorientation gain (0.89 and 0.97) (FIG. 2). Conversely, SPEV increased by a factor of 2. In lesioned rabbits, the influence of the head pitch in the velocity of nystagmus was remarkably modified (FIG. 2). Within head pitch angles of ±90°, a progressive increase of velocity from up to down was observed, rather than peaking at the approximate head position maintained during optokinetic stimulation. Linear regression lines fit to the normalized SPEV values with $r = 0.675$ and $r = 0.8743$.

CONCLUSION

Rabbits are capable of maintaining negative OKAN in an earth-horizontal plane during pitch angles of at least ±90°. This finding agrees with other findings obtained primarily from monkeys.[6,7] These combined findings stress the importance of the otoliths in maintaining a postural spatial reference of earth-horizontal.

In the rabbit, lesions of the uvula-nodulus do not disrupt the reorientation of

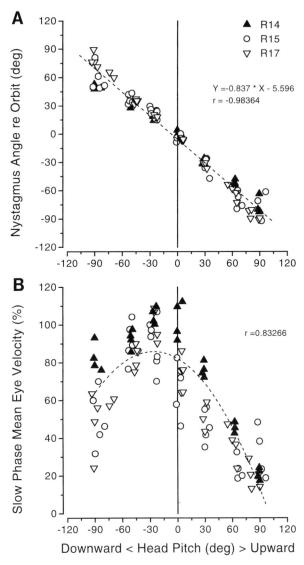

FIGURE 1. Orientation and velocity of negative optokinetic after-nystagmus in normal rabbits. (A) Relation between nystagmus orientation (re: orbit) and head pitch angle. Linear regression fits to all data from three normal rabbits. (B) Slow-phase mean eye velocity at different head pitch angles. A second-order curve is fitted to the normalized data.

negative OKAN. This observation contrasts with previous experiments on monkeys in which it is asserted that reorientation of post-rotatory nystagmus is dependent on the nodulus.[6,8] (See also Wearne, Cohen, and Raphan, this volume.)

Our principal finding is that lesions of the uvula-nodulus *do* influence the velocity of the slow phase of eye movements during negative OKAN at different head-pitch angles. Postoperatively, the velocity of the nystagmus was no longer maximal at the head orientation that accompanied optokinetic stimulation. Rather, the velocity of nystagmus increased linearly from upward to downward head tilt. This implies that the uvula-nodulus is part of a neural circuit providing a "remembered" head

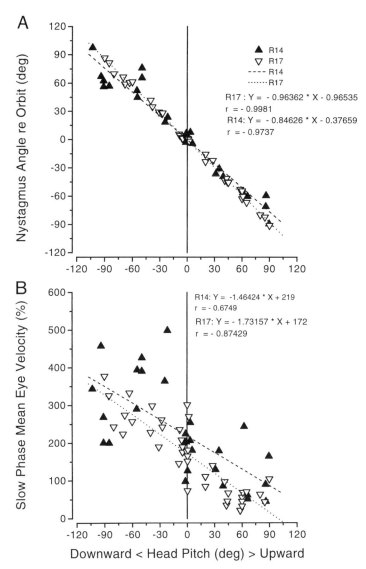

FIGURE 2. Orientation and velocity of negative optokinetic after-nystagmus in rabbits with lesions of the uvula-nodulus. (A) Relation between nystagmus orientation (re: orbit) and head pitch angle. Linear regressions lines are fitted to data from two rabbits with uvula-nodulus lesions. (B) Slow-phase mean eye velocity at different head pitch angles. The velocity of the nystagmus is altered relative to the velocity of nystagmus of normal rabbits. There is no longer a peak in velocity about the head position maintained during optokinetic stimulation.

reference angle relative to gravity. This circuit influences the velocity, but not spatial orientation of nystagmus.

REFERENCES

1. ADRIAN, E. D. 1939. The localization of activity in the brain. Proc. R. Soc. London (Biology) **126:** 433–449.
2. SHERRINGTON, C. S. 1906. The integrative action of the nervous system. Yale University Press. New Haven, CT.
3. BARMACK, N. H. & B. J. NELSON. 1987. Influence of long-term optokinetic stimulation on eye movements of the rabbit. Brain Res. **437:** 111–120.
4. BARMACK, N. H. & P. ERRICO. 1993. Optokinetically-evoked expression of corticotropin-releasing factor in inferior olivary neurons of rabbits. J. Neurosci. **13:** 4647–4659.
5. PETTOROSSI, V. E., P. ERRICO & R. M. SANTARELLI. 1995. Contribution of the maculo-ocular reflex to gaze stability in the rabbit. Exp. Brain Res. **83:** 366–374.
6. ANGELAKI, D. E. & B. J. M. HESS. 1995. Inertial representation of angular motion in the vestibular system of rhesus monkeys. II. Otolith-controlled transformation that depends on an intact cerebellar nodulus. J. Neurophysiol. **73:** 1729–1751.
7. MERFELD, D. M., L. R. YOUNG, G. D. PAIGE & D. L. TOMKO. 1993. Three dimensional eye movements of squirrel monkeys following postrotatory tilt. J. Vest. Res. **3:** 123–139.
8. ANGELAKI, D. E. & B. J. M. HESS. 1995. Lesion of the nodulus and ventral uvula abolish steady-state off-vertical axis otolith response. J. Neurophysiol. **73:** 1716–1720.
9. ERRICO, P., V. E. PETTOROSSI, F. DRAICCHIO & N. H. BARMACK. 1993. Influence of gravity on the plane of negative optokinetic after-nystagmus in the rabbit. Soc. Neurosci. Abstr. **19:** 345.

Three-Dimensional Human VOR in Acute Vestibular Lesions

M. FETTER[a] AND J. DICHGANS

Department of Neurology
Eberhard-Karls University
72076 Tübingen, Germany

The vestibuloocular reflex (VOR) has usually been studied one-dimensionally both in normals and in patients with vestibular lesions, by examining its horizontal, vertical, or, more recently, torsional component in isolation. In reality, however, the input and output of the VOR are not scalars but three-component vectors (the angular velocity vectors of the head and eye), and so a more complete characterization of the VOR requires a description, not only of the relative sizes of the eye and head velocities, but also of their relative directions, that is, the axes about which the eye and head spin.[1] In this study we used a description of the VOR in all three rotational degrees of freedom. This allows the calculation of the eye rotation axis during spontaneous nystagmus in head coordinates and the precise evaluation of the vestibular responses for stimulation in the different semicircular canal (SCC) planes.

Sixteen patients (10 male, 6 female, mean age 50.5 ± 13.6 years; 8 patients with lesions on the right and 8 with lesions on the left side) were tested with eyes open in complete darkness in a motor-driven 3-D rotating chair. Three-dimensional eye movements were measured using the magnetic field-search coil technique. After measuring spontaneous nystagmus in darkness, patients were rotated sinusoidally at 0.3 Hz with an amplitude of $\pm 20°$ and a maximum speed of about $41°/\text{sec}$ about fixed axes. The rotation axes were body-vertical (for horizontal rotation in yaw, stimulating mainly the horizontal SCCs) with the rotation axis being earth-vertical and in idealized planes of the vertical SCCs with the rotation axis being earth-horizontal.

The average amount and direction (in stereotaxic head coordinates) of the slow-phase eye velocities of spontaneous nystagmus in the dark was calculated during a period of 20 sec. FIGURE 1 shows two projections of the normalized average vectors of spontaneous nystagmus for all subjects. The rotation vectors clustered between the expected directions for a lesion of just the horizontal SCC or a combined lesion of the horizontal and anterior SCCs on one side. In none of our patients did spontaneous nystagmus direction indicate a combined lesion of the afferences of all SCCs on one side or a singular or combined lesion of just the vertical SCC. To quantify the amount of asymmetries for stimulation in the different planes, we calculated the magnitude of the average maximum eye velocity corrected for spontaneous nystagmus in each patient and determined the directional preponderance. FIGURE 2 shows the preponderance values for the different stimulation planes for all patients. Most patients showed asymmetries with significantly smaller eye velocities when the horizontal SCC or the anterior SCC on the lesioned side was excited.

In conclusion, both measurements suggest that vestibular neuritis does not lead to a complete unilateral vestibular lesion but may involve in general mainly the

---

[a] E-mail: michael.fetter@uni-tuebingen.de

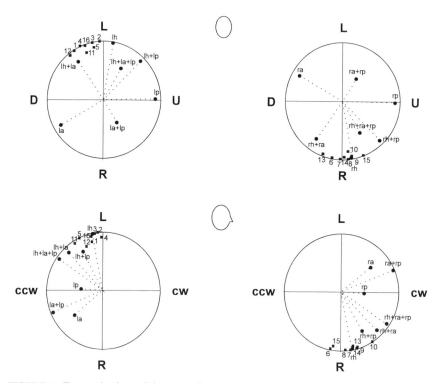

FIGURE 1. Two projections of the normalized average vectors of spontaneous nystagmus for all subjects with left-sided lesions in the left column and for right-sided lesions in the right column (to avoid clutter only the tips of the vectors are shown as filled squares; patients are identified with numbers). The upper row shows a behind view with the horizontal component on the ordinate and the vertical component on the abscissa and the lower row a right-side view with the torsional component on the abscissa. In addition the theoretical vectors of expected eye movements if one or more SCCs are missing are depicted (filled circles connected to the origin with dotted lines).

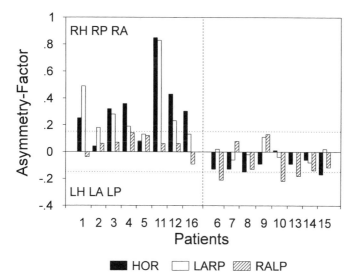

FIGURE 2. Asymmetry values for the different stimulation planes for the patients with left-sided lesions (left half of the figure) and with right-sided lesions. Dotted lines indicate the upper normal limits of a maximum preponderance of 15% as determined from our normal data. Positive values indicate better responses when one of the right-sided SCCs were excited (as in patients with left-sided lesions) and vice versa. In most cases with significant dynamic asymmetries, the analysis was suggestive for a combined unilateral lesion of the afferences of the horizontal and anterior SCC. In a few cases the analysis was suggestive for a lesion of just the anterior or horizontal SCC on one side, while the afferences of the posterior SCC seemed to be spared in all cases.

superior division of the vestibular nerve (including afferences from the anterior and horizontal canal). This confirms the earlier hypothesis that vestibular neuritis is only a partial lesion.[2]

REFERENCES

1. ROBINSON, D. A. 1982. Use of matrices in analyzing the three-dimensional behavior of the vestibulo-ocular reflex. Biol. Cybern. **46:** 53–66.
2. BÜCHELE, W. & T. BRANDT. 1988. Vestibular neuritis, a horizontal semicircular canal paresis? Adv. Oto-Rhino-Laryngol. **42:** 157–161.

Rotational Kinematics and Eye Position Dependence during Vestibular–Optokinetic Stimulation in the Monkey

M. A. FRENS,[a] K. HEPP, Y. SUZUKI, AND V. HENN

Neurology Department
University Hospital
CH-8091 Zürich, Switzerland

The vestibulo-ocular reflex (VOR) moves the eyes in order to compensate for movements of the head, thus stabilizing the image of the visual world on the retina. Although for rotational components about the yaw and pitch axes the gain of the VOR is close to the ideal value of one, the roll-gain is considerably less than unity, both in humans[1] and monkeys.[2]

It has been argued that roll-axis rotation has only a minor effect on the amount of retinal slip on the fovea[1] and that therefore no complete compensation is nescessary. This argument was further substantiated by the recent observation that the rotational kinematics of VOR slow phases of human subjects in the dark change with eye position.[3] Thus, the system seems to choose between a strategy that is a trade-off between minimizing retinal slip at the position of the fovea, optimizing Listing's law and possibly orbital mechanics.

This paper presents a similar analysis on the slow phases of rhesus monkeys that were rotated in the light, thus being subject to both vestibular and visual head movement information.

METHODS

Three rhesus monkeys (*Macaca mulatta*), having their head fixed, were rotated sinusoidally in the light with a frequency of 0.2 Hz and a peak–peak amplitude of 80 deg, symmetrically around the upright position. Rotation directions were in the roll, pitch, and yaw plane as well as in the right-anterior/left-posterior and left-anterior/right-posterior canal planes. During the stimulation the monkeys were freely making eye movements throughout the oculomotor range. Three-dimensional eye position was monitored using the dual scleral coil technique,[4] sampled at 833 Hz/channel, and stored on hard disk for off-line analysis, together with the sampled head-movement signal.

In order to compute the three-dimensional gain of the nystagmus velocity as well as the dependence of eye position, linear regression was calculated between the eye angular velocity ($\vec{e}$), the head angular velocity ($\vec{h}$), and mean eye position ($\vec{q}$), respectively. On the basis of these fits, the properties of the slow phases could be reconstructed systematically. See Misslisch *et al.*[3] for a detailed description of this methodological approach.

[a] E-mail: MFRENS@NEUROL.UNIZH.CH

RESULTS

Overall Gain

Calculation of the overall gain matrix G_{AV}, not taking the position of the eyes into account, showed an average gain of 0.77, 0.97, and 0.93 for the diagonal components in the torsional, vertical, and horizontal direction, respectively. Individual gain matrices of the monkeys were highly reproducible on a day-to-day basis. Cross-coupling components of G_{AV} were very small (<0.1), indicating that the direction of the eye rotation was about opposite to the direction of the head.

Influence of Eye Position

The position of the eye in the orbit had a systematic influence on the rotational kinematics of the eye. FIGURE 1 shows a graphical representation of gain matrices at several reconstructed eye positions of monkey CR. Note that several cross-coupling components clearly change with eye position.

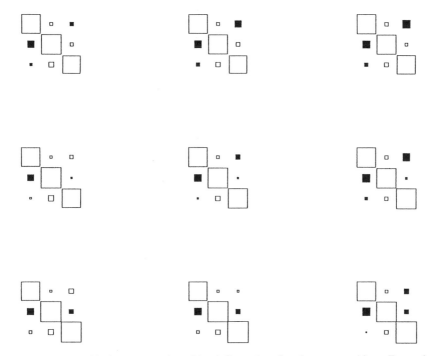

FIGURE 1. Graphical representation of local G-matrices for given eye positions. For each subfigure, *filled squares* indicate positive values, whereas *open squares* indicate negative. The surface of the square symbolizes the size of the component. Component order is torsional, vertical, horizontal. This graph shows the changes in the gains of monkey CR at each of the combinations of horizontal and vertical eye position components $\in$ [−20,0,20] deg. The torsional eye position component was chosen to be 0 deg in all cases. For instance, the left upper graph represents an eye position, looking left-upward at (−20,20) deg and the center graph represents the straight ahead position.

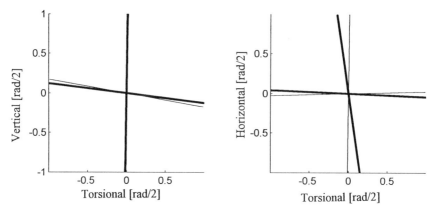

FIGURE 2. This figure shows how the changes in the local G-matrices affect the direction of $\vec{e}$. The left graph shows the eye velocity axes that result from pure roll and yaw-axis body rotations. *Thick lines* signify an eye position of 15 deg to the right, whereas *thin lines* indicate an eye position of 15 deg to the left. The right graph shows in a similar format responses to roll and pitch axis rotations, with eye positions 30 up (*thick*) and down (*thin*).

FIGURE 2 makes clear what the consequences of these changes are for the resulting eye movements. Although the dependence of eye velocity direction on eye position is qualitatively similar to human nystagmus, the changes are on the average much smaller.

DISCUSSION

In a qualitative way the data that are presented in this paper, concerning monkeys that were rotated in the light, are similar to the data that have been found previously in human subjects without visual input.[3]

However, quantitative differences were found:

1. In our experiments the overall gain matrix G_{AV} was more isotropic; that is, the three diagonal components were mutually more similar than in human VOR.

2. Changes of eye rotation directions as a result of changes in eye position were smaller.

Apart from interspecies differences, the fact that these experiments were carried out in the light may have increased the relative contribution of "optical flow" in the factors that determine the rotational kinematics of the eye during slow-phase movements. The observed strategy is more compatible with reducing slip on the whole retina.

REFERENCES

1. COLLEWIJN, H., J. VAN DER STEEN, L. FERMAN & T. C. JANSSEN. 1985. Exp. Brain Res. **59:** 185–196.
2. CRAWFORD, J. D. & T. VILIS. 1991. J. Neurophysiol. **65:** 407–423.
3. MISSLISCH, H., D. TWEED, M. FETTER, D. FISCHER & E. KOENIG. 1994. J. Neurophysiol. **72:** 2490–2502.
4. HESS, B. J. M., A. J. VAN OPSTAL, D. STRAUMANN & K. HEPP. 1992. Vision Res. **32:** 1647–1654.

Exploring Sites for Short-Term VOR Modulation Using a Bilateral Model

A. GREEN[a] AND H. L. GALIANA

Department of Biomedical Engineering
McGill University
Montreal, Quebec, Canada, H3A 2B4

Natural rotation of the head both translates and rotates the eyes relative to *near,* stationary visual targets. Thus, stable fixation of gaze requires modulation of the vestibulo-ocular reflex (VOR) gain with viewing distance, target eccentricity, and axis of rotation. Furthermore, VOR modulation must be distinct for each eye, requiring both conjugate and vergence changes to the reflex. Appropriate changes in the gain of the VOR are reported to actually *precede* target acquisition[1] and nearly perfect compensation is possible beyond the visual bandwidth.[2] This implies that central brain-stem signals rather than vision are used to adapt the reflex. Similar VOR gain modulation is observed during linear translation (LVOR),[3] suggesting the vestibular nuclei (VN) as a suitable site for VOR adaptation, since both canal and otolith (angular and linear) primary afferents converge there. We are exploring the VN as potential sites for modulation of the VOR gain. To this end, we have improved the structural and physiological relevance of a previous bilateral model of binocular control,[4] such that it now accounts for recently characterized central cell types in the VN, prepositus hypoglossi (PH), and cerebellar flocculus (CF) and allows for on-line VOR adaptation with behavioral context. This initial research has focused on the effects of modulating only the head-velocity sensitivity of one type of known premotor VN cell, using a combination of centrally available binocular internal eye position estimates (E*) and motor errors (me).

The geometrical relationship required for perfect gaze stabilization has been described by Viirre *et al.*[2] Ideal expressions for conjugate and vergence components of the VOR gain (VOR$_{conj}$, VOR$_{verg}$) as functions of target location, interocular distance (I), and radius of rotation (R) can hence be *approximated* by:

$$VOR_{conj} = -1 + \frac{R}{I} \frac{(\theta_L + \theta_R)}{2} (\cos \theta_R + \cos \theta_L)$$

$$VOR_{verg} = -\frac{R}{I} \frac{(\theta_L + \theta_R)}{2} (\cos \theta_R - \cos \theta_L)$$

VOR$_{conj}$ modulates about 1 while VOR$_{verg}$ adapts from zero, both increasing with radius of rotation and convergence.[1-3] Note that correct monocular responses require estimates of *monocular* angles.

The bilateral model structure is shown in FIGURE 1. Interconnections between the VN, PH, and CF on both sides give rise to two internal dynamic modes that can be directly related to the conjugate and vergence components of binocular responses. The model incorporates two known premotor cell types in the VN[5,6] (position-vestibular-pause cells (PVP) and floccular-target-neurons (FTN)) and gaze-velocity

[a] E-mail: andrea@eyebeam.biomed.mcgill.ca

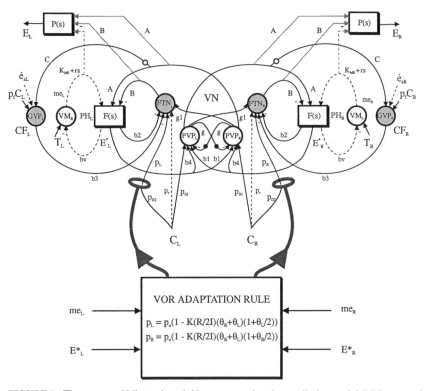

FIGURE 1. The proposed bilateral model interconnecting the vestibular nuclei (VN), preposi-tus hypoglossi (PH), and cerebellar flocculus (CF). Two known premotor cell types are incorporated in the VN: (1) Type I, position-vestibular-pause cells (PVP) and (2) eye-contraversive floccular target neurons (E-c FTNs)[5] that resemble eye-head-velocity (EHV)[6] cells during certain protocols and are Type II during VOR cancellation. Gaze velocity Purkinje (GVP) cells[7] in the CF make inhibitory connections on ipsilateral FTNs. The PH on each side are presumed to contain neural filters with dynamics similar to those of the eye plants (F(s) ∝ P(s)). They receive copies of all motoneural projections so that each PH provides a monocular eye position estimate (E^*_R, E^*_L), allowing for independent control over each eye despite the highly coupled nature of the structure. Dashed pathways are activated only with visual or cognitive goals; motor projections are shaded. Inputs include the following: vestibular afferent signals ($C_{R,L}$), monocular retinal slip ($e_{R,L}$), and monocular internal motor errors ($me_{R,L}$), which have both position and velocity components. The adaptation rule in the figure is a linear approximation of the equations in the text and is only applied to FTN primary sensitivities (see text). In the rule, θ variables represent internal eye position estimates (E^*) in the dark, or desired eye positions in the light ($\theta = E^* + me$); this allows VOR adaptation to precede executed changes in average eye position.

Purkinje cells (GVP)[7] in the CF. The distinct dynamic properties of each cell type are reproduced as a result of the cell's position in the loops and the weighting of its visual, vestibular, and tonic afferents. Both tonic PH cells and the tonic component of PVP cells in the model are monocular as has recently been confirmed experimen-tally.[8,9]

During rotation in the dark (previewing a far target) PVP, FTN, and GVP cells

Behavioral Responses

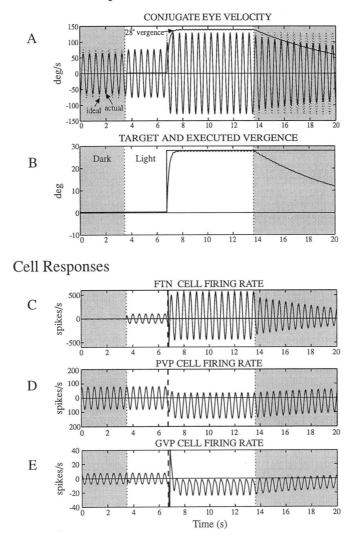

FIGURE 2. Simulated behavioral and central responses during short-term modulation of the VOR with a central target and rotation at 2 Hz (beyond model's visual bandwidth of 1 Hz). Shaded areas correspond to dark periods; target moves from a distance of 10 m to 12 cm (28 degrees of convergence) at the dashed line. **(A, B)** The changes in binocular responses are nearly ideal (see text). **(C)** FTN cells have a low head velocity sensitivity and are relatively tonic in the dark, but increase their modulation and are in phase with eye velocity in the light; in the converged state they show a disproportionately large change in their depth of modulation (five times larger) compared to the VOR gain change of 1.8. **(D)** PVP cells lag head velocity slightly and have a head velocity sensitivity close to one; they lower their set-point with convergence, but their depth of modulation does not reflect changes in VOR gain. **(E)** GVP cells are Type I, lead head velocity slightly, and show very little activity during VOR in the dark or in the light during far-target viewing, as reported; during near-target viewing, GVPs increase their modulation depth, show nonlinear profiles and phase shifts towards Type II behavior.[7]

operate with reference primary vestibular sensitivities p_{01}, p_{02}, and p_f, providing a pure conjugate response with a gain near one. By modulating the vestibular sensitivity of FTN cells about its reference value, p_{02}, the VOR gain for each eye is adjusted on-line with target position and axis of rotation. In general, application of the rule produces an imbalance in the FTN primary sensitivities on either side (p_R, p_L) resulting in both conjugate and vergence VOR components as required for target stabilization.

FIGURE 2 illustrates the results of simulations performed for rotation at 2 Hz, while viewing a central target. The conjugate VOR gain increases slightly (0.85 to 1) when the far target (10 m away) becomes visible and rapidly increases by about 80% when the near target appears (12 cm away). The increase in VOR gain precedes the executed change in vergence, as required.[1,3] When the light is extinguished, vergence angle and VOR gain decay in parallel with similar dynamics. Nearly perfect VOR correction is achieved despite a significant approximation in the adaptation rule. The eyes modulate independently as can be seen from the small ripple on the vergence position trace. The changes in modulation of the various cell types are illustrated in FIGURE 2 (see caption). Because of global dynamics and relative parametric weights in the model, the magnitude of any VOR gain change may or may not be reflected in any given cell's modulation. For example, vestibular sensitivities are only adapted on FTNs, yet changes in modulation are observed on both FTNs and GVPs. Similarly, a near doubling of the VOR gain is associated here with a fivefold change in FTN modulation depth. Such disproportionate changes in FTN response have been observed after long-term adaptation.[5]

CONCLUSION

Appropriate adaptation of any vestibular reflex in a binocular system requires access to both binocular and monocular information. Hence, bilateral models capable of binocular control are required to explore alternatives in reflex adaptation. Cell responses in the model for short-term modulation of the angular VOR are similar to those reported during LVOR (Tomlinson, personal communication) and long-term adaptation. We propose that all VOR adaptation may rely on the same central site.

REFERENCES

1. SNYDER, L. H., D. M. LAWRENCE & W. M. KING. 1992. Vision Res. **32:** 569–575.
2. VIIRRE, E., D. TWEED, K. MILNER & T. VILIS. 1986. J. Neurophysiol. **56:** 439–450.
3. PAIGE, G. D. 1991. Acta Otolaryngol. (Stockholm) Suppl. **481:** 282–286.
4. COVA, A. & H. L. GALIANA. 1995. Vision Res. **35:** 3359–3371.
5. LISBERGER, S. G., A. PAVELKO & D. M. BROUSSARD. 1994. J. Neurophysiol. **72:** 928–953.
6. SCUDDER, C. A. & A. F. FUCHS. 1992. J. Neurophysiol. **68:** 244–264.
7. LISBERGER, S. G., T. A. PAVELKO, H. M. BRONTE-STEWART & L. S. STONE. 1994. J. Neurophysiol. **72:** 954–973.
8. MCCONVILLE, K., R. D. TOMLINSON, W. M. KING, G. D. PAIGE & E.-Q. NA. 1994. J. Vest. Res. **4:** 391–400.
9. ZHOU, W. & W. M. KING. 1996. Ann. N. Y. Acad. Sci. This volume.

Eye Position Dependence of Innervation On-directions of Motoneurons in the Monkey[a]

K. HEPP, Y. SUZUKI, D. STRAUMANN, B. J. M. HESS, AND V. HENN

Neurology Department
University of Zürich
CH 8091 Zürich, Switzerland

We have recorded the firing patterns of motoneurons in the monkey during fixation with the head in different roll positions (whereby generating static eye positions with varying amount of torsion) and during passive head rotations about different axes. Average innervation on-directions are defined by multilinear regression of firing rate f as a function of eye rotation vector r. In a preliminary publication,[1] we have shown that these on-directions are closer to the sensitivity directions of the semicircular canals than to the geometric pulling directions of the extraocular muscles in periprimary position.

Here we report on the innervation on-directions and on their eye position dependence in Listing coordinates, generalizing the 2-D measurements by Hepp and Henn.[2] The analysis is based on 22 low-threshold motoneurons with a large number of evenly distributed data points, so that a quadratic regression

$$f_i = a + b^T * r_i + r_i^T * c * r_i + \text{noise} \qquad (*)$$

is well defined 20 degrees around the primary position, which allows us to compute local *innervation gradients* as $\nabla f = b + 2\,c^* r$. FIGURE 1 shows the best fit firing rate surface for a typical right MR motoneuron. In FIGURE 1A, f is plotted for eye positions in Listing's plane ($r_x = 0$), and in FIGURE 1B for horizontal-torsional eye positions ($r_y = 0$). From the orientation and curvature of these surfaces, one deduces that the innervation gradient lies approximately in the horizontal-torsional plane with a large positive horizontal and a small negative torsional component. The innervation gradient is expected to have a nontrivial eye position dependence. FIGURE 2 **A, B, C** shows the variation of the horizontal-torsional components of the innervation on-direction of this motoneuron for different eye positions in Listing's plane. One sees that, when the eye moves upward, the torsional component of the innervation on-direction becomes more positive, independent of the horizontal eye position.

A consistent pattern has been found in all motoneurons in our sample: In FIGURE 2D one sees how in the population average of MR and LR neurons the horizontal torsional components of the innervation gradients change when the eye moves from 20 degrees downwards to 20 degrees upwards as in FIGURE 2B. In FIGURE 2E the corresponding changes of the vertical-torsional components are shown for the vertical recti and obliques. In Listing coordinates the horizontal recti have their

[a] This work was supported by Swiss National Foundation Grant No. 31-42 373.94.

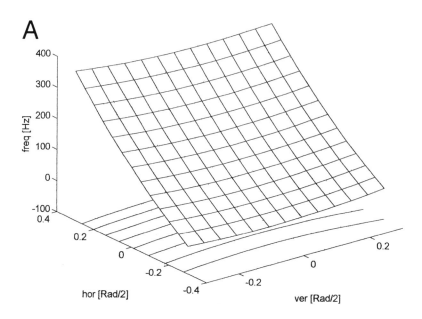

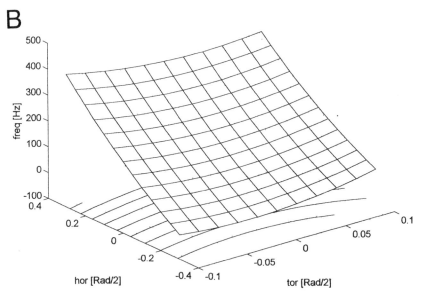

FIGURE 1. (A) Firing rate of a right MR motoneuron according to the formula (*) given in the text. The unit rad/2 for rotation vectors corresponds to about 100 degrees. In **A** f(r) is plotted in Listing's plane and in **B** for $r_y = 0$. The innervation gradient has positive horizontal and torsional components and is clearly eye position dependent.

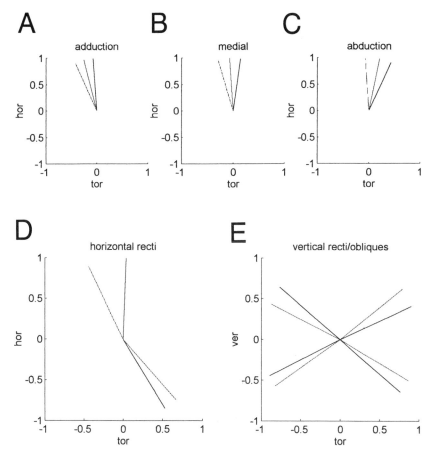

FIGURE 2. Eye position dependence of the horizontal-torsional components of the direction of the innervation gradient of the motoneuron shown in FIGURE 1, when the eye moves from 20 degrees up (*solid*) to 0 degrees (*dotted*) to 20 degrees down (*dash-dotted*) in 20-degree adduction (**A**), medial (**B**), and 20-degree abduction (**C**). In **D** the changes are shown for the population averages of MR and LR (positive resp. negative horizontal component) when the eye moves in the medial position from 20 degrees upwards (*solid*) to 20 degrees downward (*dash-dotted*). In **E** the corresponding changes in the vertical–torsional components are shown for the right vertical recti and obliques. The signs of these components are + + for IR, + − for SO, − − for SR, and − + for IO.

on-directions in the horizontal-torsional (z-x-) plane, and their innervation gradients rotate positively (by the right-hand rule) about the y-axis for upward changes of eye position (see FIG. 2D). The vertical recti and obliques have their on-directions in the vertical-torsional (y-x-) plane, and they rotate positively about the z-axis for rightward movements (see FIG. 2E). These patterns are antagonistic for LR-MR, SR-IR, and IO-SO. During eye movements in Listing's plane, the innervation planes of the horizontal recti and of the vertical recti and obliques stay fixed, as the horizontal-vertical components of the motoneuron innervation gradients do not change significantly.

We agree with Misslisch *et al.*[3] that the eye position dependence of visuo-vestibulo-oculomotor transformations cannot be simply explained by the geometry of orbital mechanics. In periprimary position the extraocular muscles have their insertions into the globe on the hemisphere opposite to their origin. For the right eye an upward rotation of the eye transports the insertion point of the MR such that the torsional component of its moment vector in head-fixed coordinates decreases, opposite to LR. Similarly, a rightward rotation of the eye increases the torsional components of the moments of SO and IR, antagonistic to IO and SR. This behavior is *opposite* of the corresponding changes of the innervation on-directions in FIGURE 2 and what has been found by electrical microstimulation of the trochlear nerve in alert rhesus monkeys.[4] It is intriguing that the eye position–dependent innervation pattern of the motoneurons and the tilt of the eye angular velocity axes during VOR[3,5] are qualitatively similar and opposite of the predictions from simple eye plant models.

It would be worthwhile to obtain dynamic 3-D recordings of the firing patterns of motoneurons for testing more elaborate models of the eye plant[6] and of the interface to preoculomotor structures.[7,8]

REFERENCES

1. SUZUKI, Y., D. STRAUMANN, K. HEPP & V. HENN. 1994a. Three-dimensional representation of position coding in extra-ocular motoneurons in the rhesus monkey. *In* Contemporary Ocular Motor and Vestibular Research—A Tribute to D. A. Robinson. A. F. Fuchs, T. Brandt, U. Büttner & D. S. Zee, Eds.: 528–536. Thieme Verlag. Stuttgart.
2. HEPP, K. & V. HENN. 1985. Iso-frequency curves of oculomotor neurons in the rhesus monkey. Vision Res. **25:** 493–499.
3. MISSLISCH, H., D. TWEED, M. FETTER, D. FISCHER & E. KOENIG. 1994. Rotational kinematics of the human vestibuloocular reflex III. Listing's law. J. Neurophysiol. **72:** 2490–2502.
4. SUZUKI, Y., D. STRAUMANN, K. HEPP & V. HENN. 1994b. Three-dimensional eye movements evoked by electrical micro-stimulation of the trochlear nerve in alert rhesus monkeys. Soc. Neurosci. Abstr. **20:** 1399.
5. FRENS, M. A., K. HEPP, Y. SUZUKI & V. HENN. 1996. Rotational kinematics and eye position dependence during vestibular-optokinetic stimulation in the monkey. Ann. N. Y. Acad. Sci. This volume.
6. MILLER, J. M. & J. L. DEMER. 1994. Biomedical analysis of binocular alignment. *In* Contemporary Ocular Motor and Vestibular Research—A Tribute to D. A. Robinson. A. F. Fuchs, T. Brandt, U. Büttner & D. S. Zee, Eds.: 18–25. Thieme Verlag. Stuttgart.
7. SCHNABOLK, C. & T. RAPHAN. 1994. Modelling three-dimensional velocity-to-position transformation in oculomotor control. J. Neurophysiol. **71:** 623–638.
8. TWEED, D., H. MISSLISCH & M. FETTER. 1994. Testing models of the oculomotor velocity to position transformation. J. Neurophysiol. **72:** 1425–1429.

Vestibular Influences on the Histaminergic and Cholinergic Systems in the Rat Brain

A. HORII,[a,b] N. TAKEDA,[b] A. YAMATODANI,[c]
AND T. KUBO[b]

[b]Department of Otolaryngology
[c]Department of Medical Physics
Faculty of Medicine
Osaka University
Osaka, Japan

Histamine H1-blockers and acetylcholine muscarinic blockers are used for treatment of nausea and vomiting associated with motion sickness or peripheral vestibular vertigo. These drugs are also effective in preventing motion sickness in an animal model using rats.[1] These findings suggest that the both histaminergic and cholinergic neuron systems are involved in the neuronal mechanisms of the vestibulo-autonomic reaction. To clarify the vestibular influences on these neuron systems, we investigated the effects of vestibular stimulation on the *in vivo* release of hypothalamic histamine and hippocampal acetylcholine (ACh) in urethan-anesthetized rats, using a brain microdialysis method. The results have been partially published elsewhere previously.[2–4]

A microdialysis probe was stereotaxically inserted into the anterior hypothalamus or CA1-CA3 region of hippocampus and was perfused with artificial cerebrospinal fluid at a flow rate of 1 μl/min. Perfusates were collected every 20 min, and the concentration of the neurotransmitters in the perfusate was measured by HPLC systems. Electrical stimulation of the round window evoked the releases of hypothalamic histamine and hippocampal ACh. These effects were inhibited by the blockade of second-order vestibular neurons by the pre-injection of DNQX, a non-NMDA glutamate receptor blocker, into the ipsilateral medial vestibular nucleus (FIG. 1). It is suggested that the electrical stimulation of the round window increased the releases of hypothalamic histamine and hippocampal ACh via the activation of the vestibular nucleus. Furthermore, caloric stimulation with both hot and cold water increased the releases of these neurotransmitters, whereas with 37°C-water caloric stimulation had no effect on the releases. These findings indicate that both histaminergic and cholinergic systems were activated by the vestibular stimuli.

We next examined the interaction between the histaminergic system and the cholinergic system. Depletion of neuronal histamine by α-fluoromethylhistidine (α-FMH), an irreversible inhibitor of histamine synthesis, did not suppress the vestibular-evoked release of hippocampal ACh. In contrast, vestibular stimulation failed to evoke hypothalamic histamine release in rats treated with ethylcholine aziridinium ion (AF64A), a putative cholinotoxin. In anatomical studies, main afferent connections of the hypothalamic tuberomammillary nucleus, which contain histaminergic cell bodies, arise from the limbic system. All these findings suggest that the vestibular stimuli activated the hypothalamic histaminergic system via the activation of the hippocampal cholinergic system. The hippocampal cholinergic

---

[a]Address for correspondence: A. Horii, M.D., Ph.D., Department of Otolaryngology, Osaka Teishin Hospital, 2-6-40 Karasugatsuji, Tennohji-ku, Osaka 543, Japan.

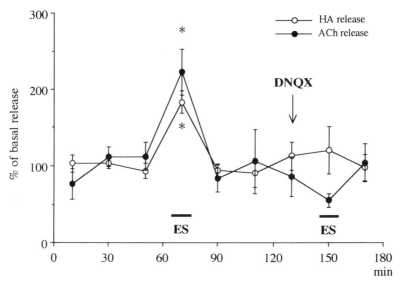

FIGURE 1. Effects of microinjection of DNQX, a non-NMDA glutamate receptor antagonist, into the ipsilateral medial vestibular nucleus on vestibular-evoked releases of hypothalamic histamine (*open circles*) and hippocampal ACh (*closed circles*). ES, electrical stimulation of the round window (1 Hz, 200 msec, 500 μA, 20 min). DNQX (10 nmol/0.2 μl) was injected 20 min before the second ES. Note that the second ES failed to evoke histamine and ACh releases. *$p < 0.05$ vs. release immediately before the evoked release.

system is reported to play a role in integrating ongoing sensory information and preserving past sensory experiences, suggesting that this system participates in the generation of neural mismatch signals. The central histaminergic system is suggested to be involved in the hypothalamic regulation of the autonomic nervous system.[5] Based on these findings, we suggest that the neural mismatch signals generated by vestibular information activate the septo-hippocampal cholinergic system, and that the signals from this system to the hypothalamic histaminergic neurons represent the symptomatic linkage in the development of the vestibulo-autonomic response.

REFERENCES

1. TAKEDA, N., M. MORITA, S. HASEGAWA, A. HORII, T. KUBO & T. MATSUNAGA. 1993. Neuropharmacology of motion sickness and emesis: A review. Acta Otolaryngol. (Stockholm) Suppl. **501:** 10–15.
2. HORII, A., N. TAKEDA, T. MATSUNAGA, A. YAMATODANI, T. MOCHIZUKI, K. OKAKURA-MOCHIZUKI & H. WADA. 1993. Effect of unilateral vestibular stimulation on histamine release from the hypothalamus of rats in vivo. J. Neurophysiol. **70:** 1822–1826.
3. HORII, A., N. TAKEDA, T. MOCHIZUKI, K. OKAKURA-MOCHIZUKI, Y. YAMAMOTO & A. YAMATODANI. 1994. Effects of vestibular stimulation on acetylcholine release from rat hippocampus: An in vivo microdialysis study. J. Neurophysiol. **72:** 605–611.
4. HORII, A., N. TAKEDA, T. MOCHIZUKI, K. OKAKURA-MOCHIZUKI, Y. YAMAMOTO, A. YAMATODANI & T. KUBO. 1995. Vestibular modulation of the septo-hippocampal cholinergic system of rats. Acta Otolaryngol. (Stockholm) Suppl. **520:** 395–398.
5. ONODERA, K., A. YAMATODANI, T. WATANABE & H. WADA. 1994. Neuropharmacology of the histaminergic neuron system in the brain and its relationship with behavioral disorders. Prog. Neurobiol. **42:** 685–702.

Altered Gravitational Conditions Affect the Early Development of the Static Vestibulo-Ocular Reflex in Lower Vertebrates[a]

EBERHARD R. HORN, CLAUDIA E. SEBASTIAN,
AND KONRAD EßELING

Department of Neurology
Section of Neurophysiology
University of Ulm
D-89081 Ulm, Germany

The demonstration of irreversible morphological and physiological changes after exposure of immature animals to altered stimulus conditions prompted the concept of a "sensitive period." Modifications of the sensory input included deprivation by manipulative surgery (eye or ear closure, cut of tactile hairs) or the presentation of noise (acoustic system). The general sensitivity of the developing gravity sensory systems to altered gravitational conditions (AGC) can be explored by exposing animals transiently to hypergravity (hg). This approach, however, cannot answer the question whether gravity is necessary for normal development. This problem requires a transient, but complete elimination of the sensory input. Lesion techniques are not useful for anatomical (vicinity of different sensory systems) and physiological (vestibular compensation) reasons. The method of first choice is a transient exposure of awake animals to microgravity (μg).

EXPOSURE TO MICROGRAVITY OR HYPERGRAVITY

Youngsters of the cichlid fish, *Oreochromis mossambicus,* and tadpoles of the clawed toad, *Xenopus laevis,* were exposed to microgravity aboard the space shuttle Columbia during the German spacelab mission D-2. They were transported by means of the STATEX-module, a closed survival system, which is equipped with a 1-g reference centrifuge. Hypergravity was produced by centrifugation. During AGC, the animals were kept in darkness; before and after AGC, they were reared under a 12:12 hr light–dark cycle.

BEHAVIORAL MEASUREMENTS

The efficiency of the developing otolith system was tested using the static vestibulo-ocular reflex (VOR). Between day 2 and day 4 (period 1) and day 9 and day 11 (period 2) after the end of AGC, the eye movements were videotaped during a stepwise 360° roll of the animals. The extent of the VOR was described by the

[a]This work was supported by DARA, Grant No. 01QV8925-5 to E. R. H.

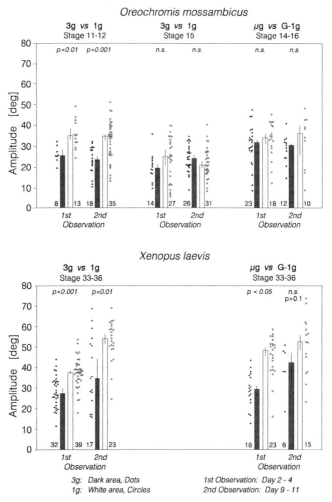

FIGURE 1. The early development of the static VOR in the fish *Oreochromis mossambicus* and the clawed toad *Xenopus laevis* after a transient exposure to AGC. The developmental stages of the animals at the beginning of AGC are indicated on the top of each column group of the specific experiment. Stages were selected according to the animal's ability to perform VOR. The extent of the static VOR was described by the peak-to-peak amplitude of the sinusoidal response characteristic (Amplitude). For each experimental group, two observations were performed. Generally, each animal from the second observation period (post-AGC days 9 to 11) was also tested during the first period (post-AGC days 2 to 4). For the left and middle part of the plot presenting the results from *Oreochromis*, the sample numbers for the second period are higher than those for the first because this species can switch off its static VOR for some, so far, unknown reasons. The figure presents the amplitude values obtained from the individual animals (*dots* for the 3-*g*- or μ*g*-exposed animals; *circles* for the 1-*g* controls) and the corresponding median values (*dark columns* for the 3-*g*- or μ*g*-exposed animals; *white columns* for the 1-*g* controls). In case of the μ*g*-experiment, the results of the ground control are given (G-1g). *Vertical bars*: Standard error of the medians. *Numbers at the column base:* numbers of animals. Levels of significances between the AGC-exposed samples and their 1-*g* controls were determined by the U-test and are indicated. n.s., non-significant ($p > 0.05$).

peak-to-peak amplitude of the VOR characteristics. Because of a VOR overshoot during a roll, all data were taken 7 sec after each 15° step.

THE EARLY VOR DEVELOPMENT

In the fish, the static VOR could be elicited at stage 13 for the first time. Its further development depended on the light conditions. In dark-reared fish, its amplitude increased to stage 22. In light–dark-reared fish a first increase was followed by a period of significant VOR depression that disappeared for older stages. In the clawed toad, the static VOR appeared in stage 41 for the first time. Its peak-to-peak amplitude increased during further development but, significantly retarded in the dark periods with respect to light–dark-reared tadpoles.

EXPOSURE TO MICROGRAVITY

Fish youngsters were exposed to μg for 10 days when they had reached stages 14 to 16, that is, after the first appearance of their static VOR. For both observation periods, no significant differences were found between the μg- and 1-g-exposed youngsters (period 1: 32.1° vs. 33.8°; period 2: 30.5° vs. 35.6°). Tadpoles were exposed

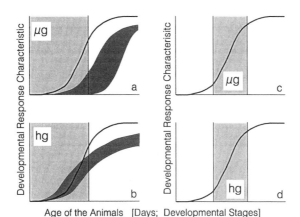

Age of the Animals   [Days; Developmental Stages]

FIGURE 2. A working hypothesis that describes the influence of transient AGC on the VOR development. The figure presents for both a transient microgravity (μg , i.e. gravity deprivation; cf. **a, c**) or hypergravity exposure (hg; cf. **b, d**) hypothetical developmental response characteristics that explain the results of the present post-AGC investigation. Significant differences from the standard development (*fat lines*) are expected if AGC started before (cf. **a, b**) but not after (cf. **c, d**) the first VOR appearance (*dark areas*). During μg exposure starting before VOR appearance (cf. **a**) either a delay or depression (lower or upper margin of the dark area, respectively) of the VOR development is likely. During hg exposure starting before VOR appearance (cf. **b**), either an augmentation or depression (upper or lower margin of the dark area, respectively) of the VOR development is likely. Both possibilities can lead to the depressed VOR expression during the post-AGC period found in the actual experiments (cf. Fig. 1). Reflex levels of AGC-exposed animals will differ from those of exclusively 1-g-reared ones permanently (cf. **a, b**) if a sensitive period exists, defined in the strictest way.

to μg for 10 days when they had reached stages 33 and 36; these tadpoles were unable to perform a static VOR. Their VOR amplitude was significantly lower than that obtained from 1-g-exposed controls during the first observation period (29.7° vs. 49.0°), but not for the second (42.9° vs. 53.0°) (FIG. 1).

EXPOSURE TO HYPERGRAVITY

Fish youngsters were exposed to 3 g for 9 days. Two groups were selected with respect to their ability to perform the static VOR. Group 1: a VOR could not be induced (stages 11 to 12). Group 2: their VOR could be induced (stage 15). For both observation periods, Group 1 showed significant lower VOR amplitudes than their 1-g-exposed controls (period 1: 25.4° vs. 35.1°; period 2: 23.5° vs. 34.7°), but not the youngsters from Group 2 (period 1: 19.3° vs. 25.0°; period 2: 24.1° vs. 20.8°). Tadpoles were exposed to 3 g for 9 days, beginning at stages 33 to 36, that is, immediately before hatching and the appearance of their static VOR. For both observation periods, they showed significantly lower VOR amplitudes than their 1-g-exposed controls (period 1: 27.3° vs. 37.6°; period 2: 34.7° vs. 54.3°) (FIG. 1).

CONCLUSION

It is concluded that (1) gravity influences the development of the gain frame of the static VOR; and (2) AGC affect the functional development of the vestibular otolith system only if they are imposed upon the animals before their static VOR has developed (FIG. 2).

Responses of Rat Primary Afferent Vestibular Neurons to Galvanic Polarization of the Labyrinth

J. F. KLEINE AND O.-J. GRÜSSER

Department of Physiology
Freie Universität
14195 Berlin, Germany

Galvanic polarization provides a handy tool for unilateral stimulation of the vestibular labyrinth. With separate low-frequency sine wave galvanic stimulation (0.1–1 Hz) of both labyrinths and a variable phase angle, the central vestibular integration can be studied. In man the perceived axis of apparent sine wave rotation and the corresponding oculomotor and skeletomotor responses changed with the phase angle of the galvanic stimuli.[1] To understand the neurophysiological mechanisms involved, we studied the responses of neurons of Scarpa's ganglion, the brain stem vestibular nuclei, and the cerebellar nuclei in anesthetized pigmented rats with unilateral and bilateral labyrinth galvanization (0.1–100 Hz, 1–250 μA amplitude). The following summarizes the results obtained from 76 Scarpa's ganglion neurons transmitting information from either the horizontal canal or one of the vertical canals or otolith receptors.

1. The responses to galvanic stimulation did not depend on the peripheral structures of origin (cupula receptors or otolith receptors), but a clear difference appeared in the respective "irregular" and "regular" units.[2]
2. Regularly and irregularly discharging neurons were easily discriminated by their spontaneous activity patterns, which were analyzed by interval histograms, average impulse rate $\overline{R}$, coefficient of variation c.v., first-order interval diagrams, and autocorrelation functions ("expectation density function") (FIGS. 1 and 2).
3. The galvanic sensitivity S_g, as measured with 1-Hz sine wave galvanic polarization of different amplitudes and expressed in [impulses $\cdot$ sec^{-1} $\cdot$ μA^{-1}], was higher in the irregular units, but the sensitivity ranges of the two categories overlapped considerably. Differences were greater when the *relative* galvanic sensitivity was determined ($S_g/\overline{R}$).
4. At stimulus frequencies between 0.1 and 10 Hz, the relationship between amplitude of the galvanic sine wave stimuli and the neuronal response amplitude was linear for regular units. For irregular units linearity was found up to stimulus amplitudes of 50 to 70 μA (FIGS. 1 and 2).
5. Between 0.1 and 10 Hz, the response gain remained relatively constant or increased slightly, and the slight phase lead of the neuronal response (re negative polarization maximum) did not change essentially in most units.
6. At higher stimulus frequencies (20–100 Hz), nonlinear response components became more prominent, consisting of the irregular units of discharge pauses during the inhibitory part of the stimulus cycle and phase locking of the action potentials (FIG. 1).
7. Although the responses of irregular units were adequately described by PSTHs, those of regular units require a more detailed analysis, for which the

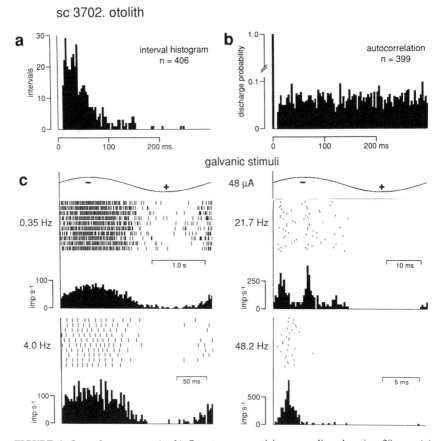

FIGURE 1. Irregular neuron. (a, b) Spontaneous activity, recording duration 20 sec. **(a)** Interval histogram. **(b)** Autocorrelation function of the neuronal discharges. **(c)** Responses to sinusoidal galvanization. Stimulus frequencies and amplitude as indicated. PSTHs were calculated by averaging the responses to 10 (0.35 Hz), 50 (4.0 Hz), 100 (21.7 Hz), and 200 (48.2 Hz) stimulus cycles; raster diagrams display the responses to 10 (*left side*) and 30 (*right side*) stimulus cycles.

continuous recordings of the instantaneous impulse rate were applied. Regular units frequently responded to low-amplitude, low- or medium-frequency sine wave stimuli with minute changes in the impulse intervals during part of the negative galvanic polarization phase.

8. Because the sensitivity ranges of the two unit categories overlapped considerably, the experimental approach in the squirrel monkey,[3] functionally segregating regular and irregular vestibular afferents by taking advantage of their different galvanic sensitivities, may not be simply transferable to other species.

CONCLUSION

During galvanic labyrinth polarization, primary afferent vestibular neurons were activated by ipsilateral negative electrical currents, whereby no systematic threshold

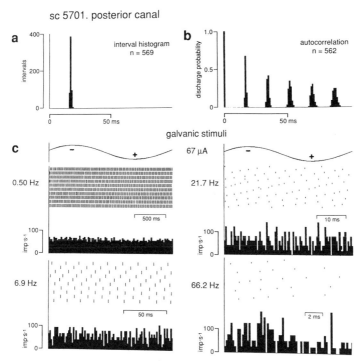

FIGURE 2. Regular neuron. (a, b) Spontaneous activity, recording duration 10 sec. **(a)** Interval histogram. **(b)** Autocorrelation function of the neuronal discharges. **(c)** Responses to sinusoidal galvanization. Stimulus frequencies and amplitude as indicated. PSTHs were calculated by averaging the responses to 10 (0.50 Hz), 50 (6.8 Hz), 100 (21.7 Hz), and 200 (66.2 Hz) stimulus cycles; raster diagrams display the responses to 10 (*left side*) and 30 (*right side*) stimulus cycles.

differences were found for the neurons transmitting signals from the semicircular canals or the otolith receptors. Galvanic threshold and sensitivity differences exist, however, for regularly and irregularly discharging neurons. The regularly discharging neurons are presumably the smaller nerve cells of the ganglion Scarpae, which are glutamate-positive and glycine-negative, while the irregularly discharging nerve cells are larger and positive for both transmitters.[4]

REFERENCES

1. GRÜSSER, O.-J. & J. F. KLEINE. 1995. The effect of bilateral galvanic labyrinth polarization in man. Soc. Neurosci. Abstr. **21(Pt. 1):** 135.
2. GOLDBERG, J. M., CH. E. SMITH & C. FERNANDEZ. 1984. Relation between discharge regularity and responses to externally applied galvanic currents in vestibular nerve afferents of the squirrel monkey. J. Neurophysiol. **51:** 1236–1256.
3. MINOR, I. B. & J. M. GOLDBERG. 1991. Vestibular nerve inputs to the vestibulo-ocular reflex: A functional ablation study in the squirrel monkey. J. Neurosci. **11:** 1636–1648.
4. REICHENBERGER, I., A. STRAKA & N. DIERINGER. 1994. Neuroactive amino acids in vestibular afferents. *In* Information Processing Underlying Gaze Control. J. M. Delgado, E. Godaux & P. P. Vidal, Eds.: 151–157. Pergamon. Oxford, England.

Dynamics of Visual Cue Control
over Head Direction Cells[a]

H. S. KUDRIMOTI, J. J. KNIERIM,
AND B. L. McNAUGHTON

ARL Division of Neural Systems, Memory, and Aging
University of Arizona
Tucson, Arizona 85724

Hippocampal neurons, known as "place" cells, show increased firing rates when a rat traverses a given location in the environment.[1,2] Some neurons in the anterior thalamus of the rat show increased firing rates as a function of head direction (H cells).[3] Place cells and H cells make up a tightly coupled system for spatial orientation and navigation.[4] These cells can be controlled by salient visual cues, in that rotation of the cues causes an equal rotation of the place field bearings and H-cell tuning curves.[5–7] Certain experimental manipulations can result in a loss of visual cue control over these cells, although the place cells and H cells remain tightly coupled to each other.[4] McNaughton *et al.*[8] proposed that H cells are driven primarily by self-motion (e.g., vestibular) cues, but that, during exploration, associations are found between cells representing the visual input at a given bearing and the H cells encoding that bearing. When error accumulates in the H-cell system, the visual input would correct this error by overriding the H cells and resetting the rat's internal compass. We investigated the dynamic properties of this reset process by giving the rat conflicting directional information between visual cues and vestibular cues. We then analyzed the time course over which the visual cue gained control over the place cells and H cells.

EXPERIMENTAL RESULTS AND CONCLUSIONS

Male Fischer-344 rats were trained to forage for chocolate pellets within a high-walled cylinder or square. Each apparatus contained a large visual cue card, covering 90° of the wall, which served as the only salient directional reference for the rat. The rats were implanted bilaterally with "tetrodes" (bundles of four closely spaced electrodes), positioned to encounter dorsal CA1 of the hippocampus in one hemisphere and the anterior thalamic nuclei in the other. In one experiment, rats were intentionally disoriented before and after each recording session. The cue card and apparatus were rotated between sessions. In approximately 75% of the sessions, place cells and H cells followed the rotation of the card. We divided the recording sessions into minute-long intervals to observe any temporal changes in the location of place fields and the tuning curves of H cells within a recording session. For most H cells, we determined a stable firing direction relative to the cue card over multiple sessions. In one-third of the 119 sessions, H cells rotated their firing directions by 30° to 130° within that session, usually in the first few minutes (FIG. 1). In 26 of 34 rotations, cells rotated from an "incorrect" direction and settled in the "correct,"

[a]This work was supported by the Office of Naval Research.

Min 1   Min 2   Min 3   Min 4   Min 5   Min 6

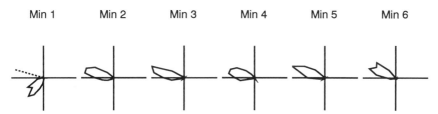

FIGURE 1. Tuning curves of a head direction cell constructed by dividing the number of spikes the cell fired when the rat faced a particular direction (in bins of 10°) by the amount of time the rat faced that direction. The H cell started off at an incorrect direction relative to the cue card (as determined by other recording sessions of the day) but rotated in the first 1 to 2 minutes to the correct direction (denoted by the dashed line). Axes, ±30 spikes/sec.

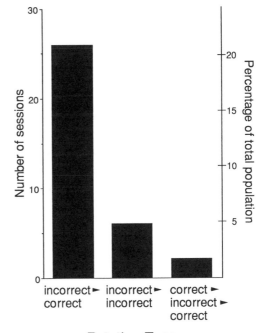

FIGURE 2. We could unambiguously identify a correct H-cell direction in 34 of the 38 sessions in which the H cells rotated. The numbers of sessions showing the different rotation patterns are shown here. It is important to note that H cells never rotated away from the correct direction without eventually returning to it.

stable direction. In six cases, cells rotated from an incorrect direction to another incorrect direction. In two cases, cells started at the correct direction, rotated away, but then returned to the correct direction. In no cases did a cell permanently rotate away from the correct direction (FIG. 2). In another experiment, rats were placed in the recording apparatus without disorientation. After a few minutes of random foraging, the whole apparatus (with the rat) was abruptly rotated 180°. In some sessions the H cells remained at the same direction relative to the external world. In other sessions, cells initially maintained their external firing directions, but then rotated 180°, apparently smoothly and directly, over a few minutes until they returned to the initial direction relative to the cue card. Thus, visual cues can correct for large errors in spatial orientation with a slow, steady rotation of the H cell system until it realigns with the cue. Apparently the internal dynamics of this network prevent direct realignment without passing through the intervening states.

REFERENCES

1. O'KEEFE, J. & J. DOSTROVSKY. 1971. Brain Res. **34:** 171–175.
2. WILSON, M. A. & B. L. MCNAUGHTON. 1993. Science **261:** 1055–1058.
3. TAUBE, J. S. 1995. J. Neurosci. **15:** 70–86.
4. KNIERIM, J. J., H. S. KUDRIMOTI & B. L. MCNAUGHTON. 1995. J. Neurosci. **15(3):** 1648–1659.
5. O'KEEFE, J. & D. H. CONWAY. 1978. Exp. Brain. Res. **31:** 573–590.
6. MULLER, R. U. & J. L. KUBIE. 1987. J. Neurosci. **77:** 1951–1968.
7. TAUBE, J. S., R. U. MULLER & J. B. RANCK, JR. 1990. J. Neurosci. **10:** 436–447.
8. MCNAUGHTON, B. L., L. L. CHEN & E. J. MARKUS. 1991. J. Cognit. Neurosci. **3:** 190–202.

Cell Proliferation in the Goldfish Ear

A BrdU Study[a]

P. J. LANFORD, J. C. PRESSON, AND A. N. POPPER

Department of Zoology
University of Maryland
College Park, Maryland 20742

Our laboratory has demonstrated the post-embyronic production of new hair cells in the ears of the teleost fish, *Astronotus ocellatus* (the oscar) and *Merluccius merluccius* (the hake).[1,2] As part of an ongoing comparative study of the inner ears of teleosts, we have extended our examination of post-embyronic cell proliferation in the teleost ear to an otophysan fish, the goldfish (*Carassius auratus*). The ear of otophysans is specialized for hearing by the presence of Weberian ossicles, a chain of bones that mechanically link the swim bladder to the primary auditory endorgan, the saccule. Sound pressure fluctuations are transmitted to the ear from the swimbladder via the ossicles in a manner thought to be analogous to that of the amniote middle ear (reviewed by Popper and Fay[3]). The otophysan fishes consequently have a broader range of hearing (50 to 3,000 Hz in the goldfish) than do nonhearing specialists.[4]

Platt[5] described the otic endorgans of the goldfish using scanning electron microscopy and indicated that the total number of hair cells may increase with increasing animal size. Consequently, we hypothesized that cell proliferation and hair cell addition occurs throughout the goldfish ear as it does in other teleosts, despite their specialized hearing capabilities. In this study, we used the mitotic S-phase marker bromodeoxyuridine (BrdU) to label proliferating cells in the goldfish ear. The specific aims of this study were to establish that cell proliferation occurs in the goldfish ear and to examine the distribution of proliferating cells within individual endorgans.

We injected goldfish (6 cm length, 7 gm body wt.) with a single dose (0.1 mg/g body wt.) of BrdU. After approximately three hours survival time post-injection, the animals were deeply anesthetized, decapitated, and their ears removed for immuno-histochemistry. Tissues were processed with the antibody against BrdU, using a peroxidase–anti-peroxidase visualization method (for procedure, see Stone & Cotanche[6]). The tissues were then preserved as whole mounts and examined on a Zeiss Axioplan with DIC optics. Proliferating cells were found within all of the end organs: the saccule, utricle, lagena, canal cristae, and macula neglecta. The presence of proliferating cells throughout the goldfish ear suggests that post-embryonic proliferative capacity is similar in otophysans and nonotophysans and is not necessarily related to the hearing capabilities of the animal.

REFERENCES

1. POPPER, A. N. & B. HOXTER. 1984. Growth of a fish ear I: Quantitative analysis of hair cell and ganglion cell proliferation. Hearing Res. **15:** 133–142.

[a]This work was supported by NIDCD Training Grant 1 T32 DC 00046 and NASA NAG 2 787.

2. LOMBARTE, A. & A. N. POPPER. 1994. Quantitative analyses of postembryonic hair cell addition in the otolithic endorgans of the inner ear of the European Hake, *Merluccius merluccius* (Gadiformes, Teleostei). J. Comp. Neurol. **345:** 419–428.
3. POPPER, A. N. & R. R. FAY. 1993. Sound detection and processing by fish: Critical review and major research questions. Brain Behav. Evol. **41:** 14–38.
4. JACOBS, D. W. & W. N. TAVOLGA. 1967. Acoustic intensity limens in the goldfish. Anim. Behav. **15:** 324–335.
5. PLATT, C. 1977. Hair cell distribution and orientation in goldfish otolith organs. J. Comp. Neurol. **172:** 283–297.
6. STONE, J. S. & D. A. COTANCHE. 1994. Identification of the timing of S-phase and the patterns of cell proliferation during hair cell regeneration in the chick cochlea. J. Comp. Neurol. **341:** 50–67.

The Mid-lateral Region of the Utricle Generates the Human Transaural Linear Vestibulo-Ocular Reflex

T. LEMPERT,[a] C. GIANNA, G. BROOKES, A. BRONSTEIN, AND M. GRESTY

MRC Human Movement and Balance Unit
National Hospital for Neurology and Neurosurgery
Queen Square
London WC1N 3BG, United Kingdom

The transaural linear vestibulo-ocular reflex (L-VOR) produces compensatory horizontal eye movements during lateral head accelerations and is a response to utricular stimulation. Unlike angular VORs, however, the directional organization of the L-VOR is still not well understood. Each utricular macula is sensitive to acceleration in both directions along the transaural axis because of the opposing orientations of its hair cells. The mid-lateral region of the utricle is activated by ipsilaterally directed acceleration, whereas the mid-medial region is excited by medially directed acceleration. To establish the contribution of these two clusters of hair cells to the L-VOR, we studied seven patients with only one functioning utricle in the acute stage after contralateral vestibular deafferentation.

Linear acceleration was provided in the dark by an electrically powered car running on a track. Patients were seated sideways on the car with their heads fixed by a bite board. The stimulus consisted of an acceleration step of $0.24\,g$ lasting 650 msec. Five stimuli to the left and to the right were applied in a random sequence. Horizontal eye movements were recorded by bitemporal electrooculography. The raw recordings were desaccaded and the resulting slow-phase eye position was averaged for each subject and direction. The L-VOR velocity was quantified from the slope of the position signal between 300 and 500 msec after onset of chair movement. Postoperative L-VORs were corrected by subtracting the slow-phase velocity of the spontaneous nystagmus (mean 2.4°/sec). Asymmetry of the L-VOR was calculated from the directional preponderance formula: $|R - L|/|R + L| \times 100$.

We investigated 21 healthy subjects and seven patients who underwent vestibular neurectomy for treatment of Meniere's disease (6) or acoustic neuroma (1). Patients were tested one day before ($n = 6$) and one week ($n = 7$) after surgery.

In normal subjects slow-phase velocities of the L-VOR ranged from 4.7 to 21°/sec (mean: 10.3°/sec). Asymmetries between leftward and rightward responses did not exceed 13% in any subject. Before surgery patients had L-VOR responses within the normal range of velocity. Mild asymmetries were observed in four patients. After surgery all patients had diminished, absent, or even reversed L-VORs when acceleration was directed towards the operated ear (mean: 2.8°/sec; range: −2.6 to 7.8°/sec). Responses were well preserved in the opposite direction (mean: 13.5°/sec; range: 7.1 to 18.5°/sec). Asymmetries invariably exceeded the normal limit of 13% (mean: 65%; range: 25 to 100%) (FIGS. 1 and 2).

[a] T. Lempert was supported by Deutsche Forschungsgemeinschaft.

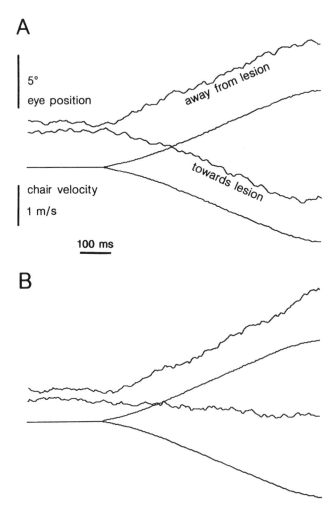

FIGURE 1. Averaged L-VOR responses from a patient with Meniere's disease illustrating postoperative loss of the L-VOR with acceleration towards the operated ear.

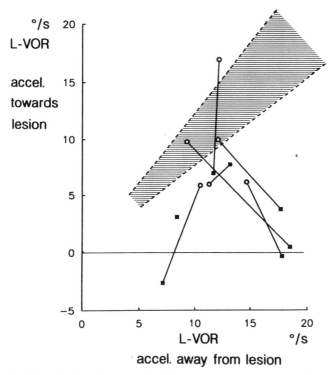

FIGURE 2. L-VOR velocities before and after surgery in seven patients. Responses are normalized with respect to the operated side. *Open circles*: preoperative; *filled squares*: postoperative. Hatched area indicates normal range.

In conclusion, early after unilateral vestibular loss the remaining utricle generates a normal L-VOR only when accelerated ipsilaterally. An explanation of this would be that L-VOR afferents originate from the mid-lateral sector of the utricular macula where hair cells are activated by ipsilateral translation. This agrees with observations in cats in which only stimulation of the mid-lateral region evokes horizontal eye movements.[1]

REFERENCE

1. FLUUR, E. & A. MELLSTRÖM. 1970. Utricular stimulation and oculomotor reactions. Laryngoscope **80:** 1701–1712.

Displacement Sensitivity of Mammalian Vestibular Transducers[a]

G. W. T. LENNAN,[b] G. S. G. GÉLÉOC,[c] AND C. J. KROS[b,d]

[b]School of Biological Sciences
University of Sussex
Falmer
Brighton BN1 9QG, United Kingdom

[c]Laboratoire de Neurophysiologie Sensorielle
INSERM U432
Place E. Bataillon
34095 Montpellier, France

INTRODUCTION AND METHODS

The generation of a transducer current, in response to displacement of the stereociliary bundle of the hair cell, is a primary event in vestibular function. Quantitative information about this process in the mammalian vestibulum has been lacking so far. For the first time, using a laser differential interferometer,[1,2] displacements of the tops of the stereocilia of mammalian vestibular hair cells have been measured simultaneously with transducer currents recorded under whole-cell voltage clamp.

Cultured utricular and saccular tissue from 1- to 2-day-old neonatal mice was maintained *in vitro* at 37°C for 1 to 4 days before transfer to a perfused chamber in which experiments took place at 22 to 25°C. Salts in the extracellular solution were (mM): 137 NaCl, 0.7 NaH$_2$PO$_4$, 5.8 KCl, 1.3 CaCl$_2$, 0.9 MgCl$_2$, 10 HEPES-NaOH, pH 7.5. Patch pipettes were filled with (mM): 140 CsCl, 0.1 EGTA-NaOH, 3.5 MgCl$_2$, 2.5 Na$_2$ATP, 5 HEPES-NaOH, pH 7.3. Stimuli were force steps delivered to the bundle by a fluid jet.[3,2] Conductance–displacement transfer functions, measured before the onset of any adaptation, were obtained at a holding potential of −84 mV.

RESULTS AND DISCUSSION

Forces that displaced the bundle in the direction of the kinocilium elicited transducer currents that saturated at 271 ± 87 pA (mean ± SD, $n = 4$). Assuming a reversal potential of +3 mV,[3] the maximum transducer conductance (g_{max}) was 3.1 ± 1.0 nS. At rest, 4.2 ± 1.3% of g_{max} was activated. The displacement sensitivity was 8.4 ± 6.1 pS/nm around rest and rose to a maximum of 24.5 ± 15.9 pS/nm at an excitatory displacement of 57 ± 40 nm. Fifty percent of g_{max} was activated at a displacement along the bundle's axis of bilateral symmetry of 104 ± 53 nm, and 90% at 325 ± 105 nm. A typical transfer function of a vestibular hair cell is shown in FIGURE 1.

[a]This work was supported by the Medical Research Council, the Hearing Research Trust, and Naturalia & Biologia (Paris). C. J. Kros is a Royal Society University Research Fellow.
[d]Corresponding author. E-mail: c.j.kros@sussex.ac.uk

The translational operating range is double that found in cultured cochlear (outer) hair cells.[2] However, the rotational operating range is similar because of the difference in bundle height (8–10 μm in vestibular, 3–5 μm in cochlear hair cells). For example, 90% of g_{max} was activated at about 2° for both. The maximum rotational sensitivity was 3.9 ± 2.0 nS/°, comparable to bullfrog saccular hair cells (1 nS/° to 2.4 nS/°).[4,5] For outer hair cells, where g_{max} was considerably larger (6.8 ± 1.7 nS, $n = 3$), the maximum sensitivity was 5.5 ± 1.3 nS/°.[2]

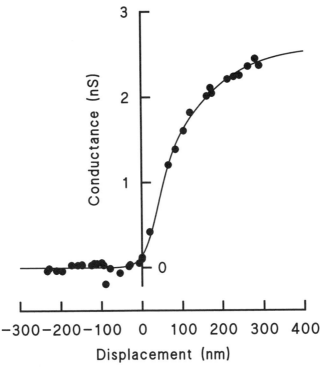

FIGURE 1. Transducer conductance of a vestibular hair cell as a function of bundle displacement, measured near the tips of the stereocilia (height 10 μm). The curve was the best fit to a second-order Boltzmann relation[2]:

$$g = \frac{g_{max}}{1 + \exp{(a_2(x_2 - x))}(1 + \exp{(a_1(x_1 - x))})}$$

where $a_1 = 0.049/nm$, $a_2 = 0.011/nm$, $x_1 = 45.7$ nm, $x_2 = 49.4$ nm, $g_{max} = 2.59$ nS.

Thus, in the neonatal mouse, vestibular hair cells appear to have fewer transducer channels than outer hair cells, assuming the same unitary conductance. We estimate from scanning electron micrographs that in neonatal mice there are some 30 tip-link sites in vestibular hair cells, compared to 100 in outer hair cells. The channels are gated over the same range of bundle rotations. A plausible explanation for the latter finding is that the transducer channels in vestibular and cochlear hair cells possess an identical intrinsic sensitivity to stretch of the tip links: a model of the hair bundle shows that tip-link stretch for a given bundle rotation is independent of bundle height.[6]

REFERENCES

1. KROS, C. J., A. RÜSCH, G. W. T. LENNAN & G. P. RICHARDSON. 1993. Voltage dependence of transducer currents in outer hair cells of neonatal mice. *In* Biophysics of Hair Cell Sensory Systems. H. Duifhuis, J. W. Horst, P. van Dijk & S. M. van Netten, Eds.: 141–148. World Scientific. Singapore.
2. KROS, C. J., G. W. T. LENNAN & G. P. RICHARDSON. 1995. Transducer currents and bundle movements in outer hair cells of neonatal mice. *In* Active Hearing. Å. Flock, D. Ottoson & M. Ulfendahl, Eds.: 113–125. Elsevier Science: Oxford.
3. KROS, C. J., A. RÜSCH & G. P. RICHARDSON. 1992. Proc. R. Soc. London B **249:** 185–193.
4. HOLTON, T. & A. J. HUDSPETH. 1986. J. Physiol. **375:** 195–227.
5. HOWARD, J. & A. J. HUDSPETH. 1987. Proc. Natl. Acad. Sci. USA **84:** 3064–3068.
6. PICKLES, J. O. 1993. Hearing Res. **68:** 159–172.

Immunohistochemical Study on the Distributions of AMPA Receptor Subtypes in Rat Vestibular Nuclear Complex after Unilateral Deafferentation[a]

HONGYAN LI,[b] TIMOTHY G. GODFREY,
DONALD A. GODFREY, AND ALLAN M. RUBIN

Department of Otolaryngology, Head and Neck Surgery
Medical College of Ohio
Toledo, Ohio 43699-0008

Glutamate has been suggested as an excitatory neurotransmitter in the vestibular nuclear complex (VNC).[1-3] Available evidence suggests involvement of α-amino-3-hydroxy-5-methyl-isoxazole-4-propionate(AMPA) receptors in excitatory transmission between the vestibular nerve and secondary VNC neurons[1-3] and in lesion-induced vestibular compensation.[4] However, the extents of involvement of the several subtypes of AMPA receptors[5] have not been determined.

Antibodies against COOH-terminal amino acid sequences of different AMPA receptor subtypes[6] were applied immunohistochemically to evaluate changes of their concentrations in rat VNC after unilateral vestibular ganglionectomy (UVG).[7] Density of neuronal immunoreactivity was measured via a computerized imaging system (NIH Image 1.44). Conditions were adjusted so that density measurements from all VNC regions were in the linear range. Variances among sections were corrected by reference to a calibrated standard density series (Kodak). Only neurons with visible nucleoli were measured.

Immunoreactivities for GluR2/3 (FIG. 1B) were much denser than those for GluR1 (FIG. 1A) and GluR4 (FIG. 1C) for both neurons (FIG. 1 **a, b, c**) and neuropil in all VNC regions, suggesting GluR2 and/or GluR3 as the major AMPA receptor subtype(s) in the rat VNC. Distributions of the immunoreactivities in other regions, such as cerebellum, were similar to a previous report.[6] Measurements in rats surviving 4, 7, 14, and 30 days after UVG suggested no significant differences in regional density of immunoreactivity between lesioned and unlesioned sides at any time for any of the antibodies. However, some bilateral asymmetry of GluR2/3 density in neuronal cytoplasm was found in most VNC regions (FIG. 2). Compared to the unlesioned side, small but significant decreases of GluR2/3 immunoreactivity on the lesioned side were revealed by 7 days after UVG in all VNC regions except the dorsal part of the medial vestibular nucleus (MVNd). Because these decreases occurred in VNC neurons shortly after removal of their excitatory vestibular nerve inputs, they are consistent with association of the GluR2/3 subtype of AMPA receptor with vestibular nerve synapses. The later disappearance of the bilateral differences in most VNC regions may represent recovery of symmetry in GluR2/3

[a]This work was supported by National Institutes of Health grant R01 DC02550.
[b]Corresponding author.

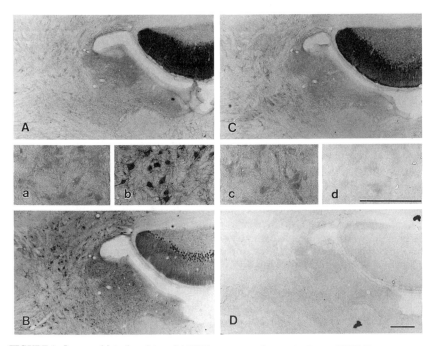

FIGURE 1. Immunohistochemistry of AMPA receptor subtypes in the rat VNC. Four consecutive brain sections (50 μm) from a control adult rat (Sprague-Dawley, male) were prepared for the immunohistochemical demonstration of different AMPA receptor subtypes (GluR1, GluR2/3, and GluR4), using antibodies and methods provided by Dr. Robert J. Wenthold.[6] Immunoreactivity to GluR1 is shown in **A,** GluR2/3 in **B,** and GluR4 in **C. D** shows the result when normal rabbit serum was substituted for primary antibody. Comparable regions of the lateral vestibular nucleus in **A** through **D** are shown at higher magnification in **a** through **d.** Exact locations can be discerned by comparing neuronal arrangements in high- and low-magnification photographs. Scale bars represent 0.5 mm.

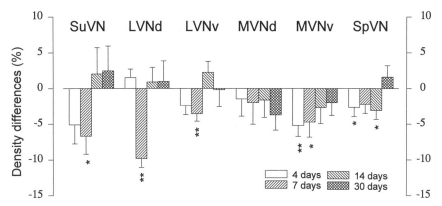

FIGURE 2. Changes of GluR2/3 immunoreactivity in the cytoplasm of VNC neurons after UVG. Differences in density of immunoreactivity between lesioned and unlesioned sides are expressed as percentages of those on the unlesioned side (mean ± SE). Negative values indicate lower density on the lesioned side. LVNd, dorsal part of lateral vestibular nucleus; LVNv, ventral part of lateral vestibular nucleus; MVNd, dorsal part of medial vestibular nucleus; MVNv, ventral part of medial vestibular nucleus; SpVN, spinal vestibular nucleus; SuVN, superior vestibular nucleus; *, $p < 0.05$; **, $p < 0.001$. Degrees of freedom for comparisons at 4, 7, 14, and 30 days are the following: 57, 57, 58, and 18 in SuVN; 284, 332, 263, and 50 in LVNd; 329, 467, 277, and 47 in LVNv; 93, 73, 88, and 28 in MVNd; 193, 140, 165, and 46 in MVNv; and 211, 209, 265, and 98 in SpVN.

expression during vestibular compensation. These results are generally consistent with those from our previous study of binding for non-*N*-methyl-D-aspartate (non-NMDA) receptors,[4] although the immunohistochemical changes were smaller. Possible changes of other AMPA receptor subtypes still need to be analyzed.

ACKNOWLEDGMENT

The antibodies used in this experiment were courtesy of Dr. Robert J. Wenthold, NIH/NIDCD.

REFERENCES

1. DARLINGTON, C. L., J. P. GALLAGHER & P. F. SMITH. 1995. In vitro electrophysiological studies of the vestibular nucleus complex. Prog. Neurobiol. **45:** 335–346.
2. DE WAELE, C., M. MÜHLETHALER & P. P. VIDAL. 1995. Neurochemistry of the central vestibular pathways. Brain Res. Rev. **20:** 24–46.
3. SMITH, P. F., C. DE WAELE, P. P. VIDAL & C. L. DARLINGTON. 1991. Excitatory amino acid receptors in normal and abnormal vestibular function. Mol. Neurobiol. **5:** 369–387.
4. LI, H., D. A. GODFREY & A. M. RUBIN. 1995. Changes of [³H]CNQX binding in rat vestibular nuclear complex and cochlear nucleus after unilateral deafferentation. Abstr. Assoc. Res. Otolaryngol. **15.**
5. KEINÄNEN, K., W. WISDEN, B. SOMMER, P. WERNER, A. HERB, T. A. VERDOORN, B. SAKMANN & P. H. SEEBURG. 1990. A family of AMPA-selective glutamate receptors. Science **249:** 556–560.
6. PETRALIA, R. S. & R. J. WENTHOLD. 1992. Light and electron immunocytochemical localization of AMPA-selective glutamate receptors in the rat brain. J. Comp. Neurol. **318:** 329–354.
7. LI, H., D. A. GODFREY & A. M. RUBIN. 1995. Comparison of surgeries for removal of primary vestibular inputs: A combined anatomical and behavioral study in rats. Laryngoscope **105:** 417–424.

A Quantitative Deoxyglucose Study of the Rat Vestibular End Organs

MICHAEL J. LYON[a] AND MICHAEL J. OLDS

Department of Otolaryngology
SUNY Health Science Center
750 East Adams Street
Syracuse, New York 13210

This study quantitated the local metabolic rate of glucose utilization (LMR_{glc}) for the vestibular end organs using a modification of the [^{14}C]deoxyglucose method[1] in awake adult rats ($n = 11$). Data are expressed as μmole/100 g per min $\pm$ SEM. Results (FIG. 1) show that the LMR_{glc} is similar within the saccule (40.3 ± 3.2) and utricle (41.2 ± 5.5) and significantly higher than that for the superior (20.1 ± 2.9), posterior (25.3 ± 6.8), or lateral canal (22.0 ± 2.6) ampullae. These differences in LMR_{glc} may be related to differences in the ratios of sensory to nonsensory cells, dark cell distributions, response to acoustic stimulation, and/or in activity levels during the experimental period.

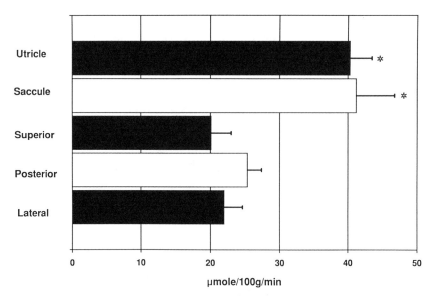

FIGURE 1. Bar chart displaying glucose utilization for the individual rat vestibular end organs. Data are expressed as μmole/100g/min. *denotes statistically significant difference from the superior, posterior, and lateral semicircular canal ampulla ($n = 11$).

[a] Corresponding author. E-mail: Lyonm@Vax.cs.HSCSYR.Edu

For the most part, LMR_{glc} and regional blood flow are directly linked in the CNS. Although some studies have correlated blood flow and glucose utilization in the cochlea,[2] evaluations of regional vestibular blood flow are very limited. Lyon and coworkers,[3,4] on the basis of capillary length/unit volume, speculated that the metabolic requirement for the utricle is greater than the posterior canal. Our data support this conclusion. Taken together, these studies bring up some interesting questions with regard to the coupling of vestibular blood flow and metabolism. If we assume that a mm^3 of end organ is equivalent to a mg wet weight, then the blood flow to the posterior canal ampulla is approximately 6 ml/g/min; three times the blood flow to the central nucleus of inferior colliculus[5] (2 ml/g/min), whereas the LMR_{glc} is only 17% that of the inferior colliculus. Blood flow greatly exceeds the need for delivery of glucose, suggesting that this is not a primary regulating factor for vestibular blood flow. Perhaps in this case a high blood flow rate is not for the delivery of metabolites but the removal of waste products, the maintenance of ion concentrations, pH, and/or temperature. These would all be of importance in the normal function of this system. In support of this, there are data showing that a pH change can alter membrane potential and ion conductance of transitional cells[6] and transepithelial transport of K^+ of dark cells.[7]

REFERENCES

1. SOKOLOFF, L., R. REIVICH, C. KENNEDY et al. 1977. The ^{14}C-deoxyglucose method for the measurement of local cerebral glucose utilization: Theory, procedure, and normal values in the conscious and anesthetized albino rat. J. Neurochem. **28:** 897–916.
2. RYAN, A. F. 1988. Circulation of the inner ear: II. The relationship between metabolism and blood flow in the cochlea. In Physiology of the Ear. A. F. Jahn & J. Santos-Sacchi, Eds.: 317–325. Raven Press. New York.
3. LYON, M. J. & H. H. WANAMAKER. 1993. Blood flow and assessment of capillaries in the aging rat posterior canal crista. Hearing Res. **67:** 157–165.
4. PAYMAN, R. & M. J. LYON. 1993. Rat utricular macula: Blood flow and stereological assessment of capillary morphology. Ann. Otol. Rhinol. Laryngol. **102:** 893–899.
5. GROSS, P. M., N. M. SPOSITO, S. E. PETTERSEN, et al. 1987. Topography of capillary density, glucose metabolism, and microvascular function within the rat inferior colliculus. J. Cereb. Blood Flow Metab. **7:** 154–160.
6. WANGEMANN, P. & N. SHIGA. Ba^{2+} and amiloride uncover or induce a pH-sensitive and a Na^+ or non-selective cation conductance in transitional cells of the inner ear. Pflügers Arch. **426:** 258–266.
7. WANGEMANN, P., J. LIU & N. SHIGA. 1995. The pH-sensitivity of transepithelial K^+ transport in vestibular dark cells. J. Memb. Biol. **147:** 255–262.

Nitric Oxide Synthase Localized in a Subpopulation of Vestibular Efferents with NADPH Diaphorase Histochemistry[a]

MARC SINGER AND ANNA LYSAKOWSKI[b]

Department of Anatomy and Cell Biology
University of Illinois College of Medicine
Chicago, Illinois 60612

Nitric oxide (NO) acts as a second messenger and as a neurotransmitter in diverse physiological systems.[1] One recent report[2] indicates that it may play an important role in the vestibular periphery. These authors have shown that NO-producing agents, such as sodium nitroprusside and nitroglycerin, inhibit a potassium current specific to type I vestibular hair cells. This potassium current ($I_{K,L}$) is activated at low voltages (> -90 mV), making the input resistance of these hair cells very low (15–50 MΩ). Previous reports have described the presence of diaphorase-positive vestibular ganglion cells[3,4] and boutons[3] throughout the crista. The presence of NOS in large numbers of ganglion cells but not in calyces, when 80% of all vestibular afferents in mammals are calyx-bearing, seemed inconsistent with previous morphological studies of afferent innervation in the chinchilla.[5] We decided to investigate the distribution of nitric oxide synthase (NOS) to clarify the role of NO in the vestibular periphery.

No known single neurotransmitter colocalizes with NOS. NADPH diaphorase histochemistry has been used to label NOS neurons because fixation of tissue with paraformaldehyde appears to inactivate all NADPH-dependent oxidative enzymes, except for NOS. Thus, the diaphorase stain selectively labels NOS neurons.[6–9]

METHODS

Twelve adult chinchillas (*C. laniger,* both sexes, 500–600 g) and four rats (*R. norvegicus,* both sexes, 250–300 g) were deeply anesthetized with Dial (diallylbarbituric acid) and perfused transcardially with heparinized isotonic saline followed by a fixative composed of 3.0% paraformaldehyde, 0.5% glutaraldehyde, and 1.0% acrolein in 0.1 M phosphate buffer. Vestibular end organs were dissected out, and the cristae reacted in an incubation solution consisting of 0.3 mM nitro blue tetrazolium, 3 mM NADPH, and 0.3% Triton X-100 in 0.1 M phosphate buffer for 18 ½ hours at 37°C. The end organs were dehydrated in a graded series of alcohols and propylene oxide and embedded in prepared Araldite capsules. The blocks were hardened in a 60°C oven for 48 hours. Five-micron serial sections were cut from the hardened

[a]This work was supported by grants DC-02521 and DC-02290, and the University of Illinois Campus Research Board.

[b]Author for correspondence: Department of Anatomy and Cell Biology, University of Illinois at Chicago, 808 South Wood Street, Chicago, IL 60612. E-mail: aLysakow@uic.edu

Araldite blocks using glass knives and mounted onto glass slides. Ultrathin sections were cut with a diamond knife (Delaware Diamond Knives) and collected on formvar-coated single-slot copper grids. Grids were examined in a JEOL 100CX electron microscope.

The brain stems of the animals were removed with the vestibular ganglia intact. Brains were post-fixed in 3% paraformaldehyde-30% sucrose fixative for 2 hours and cryoprotected in a 30% sucrose–0.1M phosphate buffer solution overnight. Thirty-micron frozen sections were cut on a sliding microtome, incubated in the NADPH diaphorase solution for 3 hours at 37°C, rinsed in 0.1 M phosphate buffer, mounted onto gelatinized slides, dried overnight, dehydrated in a graded series of alcohols and xylene, and coverslipped with Permount.

RESULTS

Results from the cristae only are presented, but they were qualitatively similar in the otolith end organs. Diaphorase-positive staining was observed in boutons at the basal end of hair cells and was markedly absent from calyces (FIG. 1) and ganglion cells (not shown). Staining was also present in some hair cells of both types (approx. 200 per crista, $\approx 10\%$), although the majority of stained hair cells ($81\% \pm 12\%$) were type I hair cells. Diaphorase labeling was also found in a randomly distributed subpopulation (20%) within the lateral vestibular efferent brain-stem group (FIG. 2). Like other cells in this lateral group, the diaphorase-positive neurons were multipolar, medium-sized neurons (about 26 ± 10 μm in diameter). In ultrastructural material, a particulate reaction product (not shown) was located in efferent boutons, rather than afferent boutons, and in the subcuticular plate region of some hair cells.

CONCLUSIONS

NADPH diaphorase histochemistry can be used to localize NOS in the vestibular end organs as well as in subpopulations of neurons in the brain stem.

In the chinchilla crista, NADPH diaporase staining was found in some hair cells and in boutons throughout the crista. It is likely that these stained boutons are efferent boutons, since they are found in both the central zone and the peripheral zone, whereas afferent bouton units are found only in the peripheral zones of the crista.[5] Furthermore, vestibular ganglion cells lacked diaphorase staining in all cases. If the labeled boutons were, in fact, afferents, then we would expect that the ganglion cells also contain diaphorase. Ultrastructural analysis of the neuroepithelium has confirmed that the boutons are efferents (not shown). The labeled boutons were filled with many small vesicles, and they contacted both type II hair cells and the calyces surrounding type I hair cells. The significance of diaphorase staining in a small subpopulation ($\approx 10\%$) of hair cells (mainly type I) is unclear at present. It could be a postsynaptic effect of NO in the efferents upon the hair cells. One notion is that NO, a gaseous transmitter synthesized in and released by the efferent boutons could diffuse across the calyx membrane and increase neurotransmitter output in the hair cell, thus acting as a retrograde messenger.[10] This could explain the effect of NO-producing agents that inhibit $I_{K,L}$, and its presence in both efferent boutons and in hair cells, particularly type I hair cells.

In the brain stem, NADPH diaphorase histochemistry defines a subpopulation ($\approx 20\%$) of the lateral vestibular efferent group. Other recent data from our

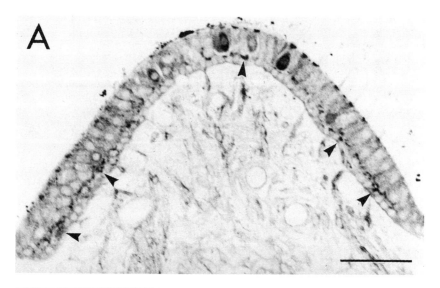

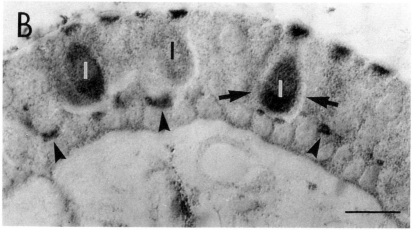

FIGURE 1. NADPH diaphorase staining in the crista. (A) Note the darkly stained NADPH diaphorase-positive boutons (*arrowheads*) at the basal ends of the hair cells. Such bouton labeling was found throughout the crista and otolith organs. Afferent boutons are present exclusively in the peripheral zones, while efferent boutons are found throughout. The distribution of labeled boutons shown above, particularly since they are found at the base of both type I and type II hair cells, suggests that the efferents are labeled. This data correlates with the absence of NOS in the vestibular ganglion cells (not shown). Scale bar represents 50 μm. **(B)** Higher magnification of the central portion of the sensory epithelium shown in **A.** The calyces that enclose type I hair cells (*arrows*) in calyx and dimorphic afferents are noticeably unstained. A small proportion (about 10%) of the total population of hair cells also stain with the diaphorase reaction. Of this 10%, approximately 80% are type I hair cells (*I*). Scale bar represents 10 μm.

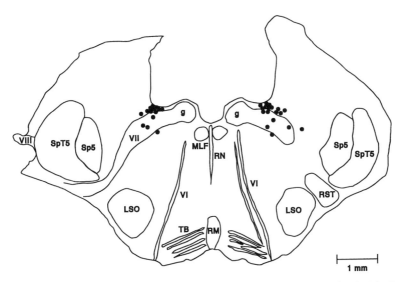

FIGURE 2. A camera lucida reconstruction of the chinchilla brain stem at the level of the facial colliculus. The NADPH diaphorase-positive neurons observed in a series of sections are plotted on this single illustration in order to approximate the location of the lateral efferent group, adjacent to the genu of the facial nerve (*g*). This lateral group was previously thought to be cholinergic and presumably homogeneous in function. However, total counts of such sections revealed NADPH diaphorase in approximately 20% of the neurons of the lateral vestibular efferent group. This histochemically defined subpopulation of neurons suggests the possibility of a functional subpopulation within the group. Such a group had not yet been demonstrated. In addition to this group, labeled neurons were also present in other groups such as the periolivary region and the parabrachial nucleus (not shown).

laboratory indicate that this distribution is also found in brain-stem sections with NOS immunohistochemical staining.[11]

The neurons of the lateral vestibular efferent group have previously been considered to be homogeneous in function. The present study suggests that the lateral group contains at least one subpopulation (NO-containing neurons) and presumably others. Such diversity in neurotransmitter content implies a diversity in function. Future experiments will distinguish these different subpopulations.

ACKNOWLEDGMENTS

We would like to thank Mr. Ashwin Patel and Mr. Steven Price for excellent technical assistance. We are also grateful to the Electron Microscopic Facility of the Research Resources Center of the University of Illinois at Chicago for providing equipment and assistance to conduct this study.

REFERENCES

1. BREDT, D. S. & S. H. SNYDER. 1992. Nitric oxide, a novel neuronal messenger. Neuron **8:** 3–11.

2. CHEN, W.-Y. & R. A. EATOCK. 1994. Nitric oxide inhibits a low-voltage-activated potassium conductance in mammalian type I hair cells. Biophys. J. **66:** A430.
3. LYON, M. J., D. GODIN & B. MAYER. 1994. Localization of nitric oxide synthase immunoreactivity and nicotinamide adenine dinucleotide phosphate diaphorase in the rat inner ear. Soc. Neurosci. Abstr. **20:** 969.
4. HARPER, A., W. R. BLYTHE, C. J. ZDANSKI, J. PRIZMA & J. C. PILLSBURY. 1994. Nitric oxide in the rat vestibular system. Otolaryngol. Head Neck Surg. **111:** 430–438.
5. FERNÁNDEZ, C., R. A. BAIRD & J. M. GOLDBERG. 1988. The vestibular nerve of the chinchilla. I. Peripheral innervation patterns in the horizontal and superior semicircular canals. J. Neurophysiol. **60:** 167–181.
6. HOPE, B. T., G. J. MICHAEL, K. M. KNIGGE & S. R. VINCENT. 1991. Neuronal NADPH diaphorase is a nitric oxide synthase. PNAS **88:** 2811–2814.
7. DAWSON, T. M., D. S. BREDT, M. FOTUHI, P. M. HWANG & S. H. SOLOMON. 1991. Nitric oxide synthase and neuronal NADPH diaphorase are identical in brain and peripheral tissues. PNAS **88:** 7797–7801.
8. MATSUMOTO, T., M. NAKANE, J. S. POLLOCK, J. E. KUK & U. FÖRSTERMANN. 1993. A correlation between soluble brain nitric oxide synthase and NADPH-diaphorase activity is only seen after exposure of the tissue to fixative. Neurosci. Lett. **155:** 61–64.
9. BREDT, D. S., P. M. HWANG, C. E. GLATT, C. LOWENSTEIN, R. R. REED & S. H. SNYDER. 1991. Cloned and expressed nitric oxide synthase structurally resembles cytochrome P-450 reductase. Nature **351:** 714–718.
10. BARINAGA, M. 1991. Is nitric oxide the "retrograde transmitter"? Science **254:** 1296–1297.
11. LYSAKOWSKI, A., M. SINGER & H. M. SHIN. 1996. Subpopulation of vestibular efferents identified as nitrosergic with NOS immunohistochemistry and NADPH diaphorase histochemistry. Bárány Society Abstr. Submitted.

Regional Distribution of Hair Cell Ionic Currents in Frog Vestibular Epithelium

S. MASETTO, G. RUSSO, AND I. PRIGIONI

Institute of General Physiology
University of Pavia
Via Forlanini 6
27100 Pavia, Italy

Current knowledge of the complement of voltage-dependent ion channels in hair cells of the acoustico-lateralis system derives from patch-clamp studies on enzymatically isolated sensory cells. Evidence has accumulated that hair cells express one type of Ca^{2+} channels[1] and several types of K^+ channels.[1-3] Basolateral channels in hair cells determine the receptor potential initiated by the transduction current, and functional differences among different sensory cells depend, at least in part, on the distribution of these channels. In this article we describe the distribution of voltage-dependent K^+ channels in frog semicircular canals by recording electrical activity from single hair cells *in situ*.[4] By using the whole-cell patch-clamp technique, evidence was obtained that there is a differential expression of K^+ conductances in hair cells located in the central isthmus and in the peripheral regions of the crista ampullaris.

RESULTS

Zero-current clamp method revealed that hair cells in the peripheral regions of the crista had an average resting membrane potential (Vz) of -46 mV, whereas cells from the central region had a more negative Vz (-58 mV). Hair cells from the two regions also differed in their response to voltage steps. Depolarization in cells from the peripheral regions (FIG. 1A) invariably produced outward currents characterized by a large transient component followed by a sustained component. By contrast, hair cells from the central region generated, upon depolarization, an initial small and rapidly decaying outward current followed by a slowly increasing component (FIG. 1B). Only the latter cells showed an inward rectification when hyperpolarized.

The outward current in cells from both regions could be separated pharmacologically into three distinct currents. In the presence of 12 mM 4-aminopyridine (4-AP), an A-type K^+ current (I_A) could be separated in hair cells from the peripheral regions (FIG. 2C). By contrast, the majority of hair cells from the central region were found to be insensitive to 4-AP. I_A was recruited close to cell resting membrane potential (~ -50 mV), showed a rapid time to peak (4 msec at 0 mV), a fast voltage-insensitive inactivation ($\tau_{decay} \sim 40$ msec), and $\sim 40\%$ of A-channels were in a noninactivated state at -50 mV. The 4-AP-resistant current (FIG. 2B and D) resembled the current recorded in normal Ringer from hair cells of the central region (FIG. 1B). After perfusion with a solution containing 4-AP plus cadmium (0.5 mM), hair cells from both regions exhibited a slowly activating outward current (FIG. 2E) showing features of a delayed rectifier K^+ current (I_K). This current activated close to $-50/-60$ mV, attained a maximal amplitude in about 100 msec at 0 mV and did not show significant inactivation. I_K in cells from the central region was

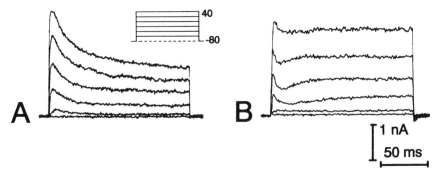

FIGURE 1. Typical outward K$^+$ currents elicited in hair cells from the peripheral regions (**A**) and from the central isthmus (**B**) of the crista ampullaris in response to the voltage protocol shown in the inset.

approximately twice as large as that generated by cells from the peripheral regions. When I$_K$ was subtracted from the 4-AP-resistant current, a calcium-sensitive current (IK$_{Ca}$) could be isolated (FIG. 2F). IK$_{Ca}$ was recruited close to −40 mV and rapidly inactivated to reach a steady level. The decay time constant was 4 msec at 0 mV. This behavior suggests the possible presence of two distinct populations of K$_{Ca}$ channels.

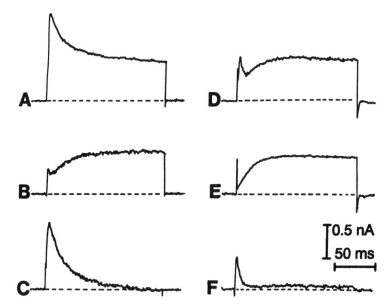

FIGURE 2. Isolation of A-type K$^+$ current (I$_A$), outward rectifier K$^+$ current (I$_K$) and calcium-sensitive K$^+$ current (IK$_{Ca}$) in hair cells from the peripheral regions. (**A**) control current; (**B**) and (**D**) currents after perfusion with 4-AP; (**C**) I$_A$ obtained by subtracting the tracing in **B** from the tracing in **A**; (**E**) I$_K$ isolated after treatment with 4-AP and Cd^{2+}. (**F**) IK$_{Ca}$ obtained by subtracting the tracing in **E** from the tracing in **D**. Currents were recorded in response to a single voltage step from −80 mV to 0 mV.

CONCLUSIONS

The present study provides the first information on the complement of hair cell ionic conductances *in situ*. We demonstrated that thin slices of frog crista ampullaris are a suitable preparation to study the electrical properties of hair cells by the patch-clamp method. The most important finding was that hair cells from different regions of the frog crista ampullaris differ in their complement of voltage-dependent K^+ conductances.[4] Cells from the peripheral regions, in fact, expressed a large I_A, an I_K, and an IK_{Ca}, whereas cells from the central region generated, besides an IK_{Ca}, a smaller I_K and little or no I_A. Moreover, only cells from the central region expressed an inward rectifier current. The different expression of K^+ conductances may allow hair cells located in discrete regions of the crista to encode the natural stimulus in different ways.

REFERENCES

1. FUCHS, P. A. 1992. Prog. Neurobiol. **39:** 493–505.
2. ASHMORE, J. F. 1991. Annu. Rev. Physiol. **53:** 465–476.
3. LANG, D. G. & M. J. CORREIA. 1989. J. Neurophysiol. **62:** 935–945.
4. MASETTO, S., G. RUSSO & I. PRIGIONI. 1994. J. Neurophysiol. **72:** 443–455.

Damage and Recovery of Otolithic Function following Streptomycin Treatment in the Rat[a]

G. MEZA,[b,f] B. BOHNE,[c] N. DAUNTON,[d]
R. FOX,[e] AND J. KNOX[e]

[b]Departamento de Neurociencias
Instituto de Fisiologia Celular
Universidad Nacional Autonoma de Mexico
04510 Mexico, D.F., Mexico

[c]Department of Otolaryngology
Washington University Medical School
Saint Louis, Missouri 63110

[d]Biomedical Research Division
NASA Ames Research Center
Moffett Field, California 94035-1000

[e]Department of Psychology
San Jose State University
San Jose, California 95192-0120

The toxic action of chronic administration of streptomycin sulfate (STP) on the vestibular hair cells of mammals is well documented.[1,3–6] Preliminary findings of our group in pigmented rats described severe alterations of motor abilities but an absence of deleterious effects on semicircular canal function (assessed with postrotatory nystagmus) or auditory function (assessed with evoked auditory potentials) after prolonged treatment with STP. These results suggest that STP specifically disrupts otolith organ function in the rat.[6,9]

Recently, we described gradual recovery of vestibular biochemistry and function in guinea pigs following chronic treatment with STP.[7] In a morphological study in guinea pigs treated with gentamicin rather than STP, hair cell stereocilia were regenerated after discontinuation of gentamicin injections.[2]

Because mature rodents are considered to have ceased production of sensory and neuronal elements, these findings are intriguing, and they encouraged us to investigate further the deleterious effects of STP and the possible mechanism involved in recovery after chronic administration of this antibiotic in the mammalian ear using the pigmented, Long-Evans rat as a model. The aim of our work is (a) to confirm an otolithic organ toxicity for STP, (b) to identify the cell type affected, and (c) to assess whether recovery occurs in the pigmented rat.

In this paper we report analysis of swimming behavior and morphology by optical microscopy of the sensory epithelium of the utricle in the pigmented rat during and following STP treatment.

[a]This project was financed in part by grant 400346-5-4712-N from CONACyT to G.M.
[f]E-mail: gmeza@ifcsun1.ifisiol.unam.mx

METHODOLOGY

Treatment Protocol

Twenty-day-old male Long-Evans rats were used in this study. Seventeen animals were injected daily intramuscularly for 48 to 57 days with 400 mg/kg body weight of STP (PISA Laboratories, Mexico) dissolved in physiological saline (SPS). Eleven rats served as controls and received SPS injections for the same time interval and conditions as their experimental comates. Three of the 57-day-treated rats and three of the SPS-injected animals were used to follow recovery for 8 to 12 weeks and did not receive any STP or SPS beyond the 48th day.

Swimming Analysis

Swimming behavior was assessed at approximately one-week intervals by placing the rats in a water tank at 27°C and recording, on videotape, swimming activity for 45 sec. Analysis and classification of swimming patterns were performed after the test.

TABLE 1. Percentage of Rats Displaying Each of the Disrupted Swimming Patterns

Experimental Condition	Swimming Characteristics			
	Vertical Swimming with Roll	Barrel Rolling	Corkskrew Swimming	Forward/Backward Looping
48 Days of Treatment	90	60	80	40
8 Weeks Post Treatment	100	0	33	0

Morphology

After completion of each experimental manipulation, two of the 48-day-treated rats and two of the treated and allowed to recover animals, plus two of the SPS injected rats were deeply anesthetized and transcardially perfused with aldehyde fixative. The auditory bullae were extracted and postfixed in 1% osmium tetroxide, dehydrated, and embedded in Araldite. Vestibular organs and half turns of cochlear duct were sectioned at 1-μm thickness, stained with methylene blue and azure II, and examined by brightfield microscopy.

RESULTS AND DISCUSSION

Abnormal swimming patterns consisting of vertical swimming with rolls, barrel rolling, corkscrew swimming, and forward and backward looping were observed with varying frequencies in rats treated with STP. None of these responses was observed in any test of control rats. Eight weeks post treatment, vertical swimming with rolls remained in all rats. One of the three rats showed corkscrew swimming, but no rat showed barrel rolling or looping. Hence, partial functional recovery was observed (see TABLE 1).

Histological examination of STP-treated rats revealed that in the utricular macula sensory cells presented fused stereocilia and pyknotic nuclei. In addition, some of these sensory cells were in the process of being extruded from the epithelium

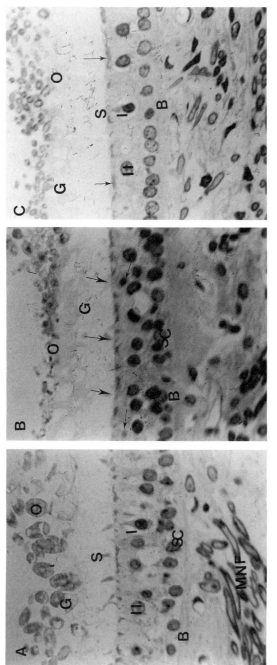

FIGURE 1. One-micron sections of utricular maculae cut perpendicular to endolymphatic surface. (**A**) Control (saline injected). Hair cell bodies are closely packed together, and stereocilia bundles occur at regular intervals above epithelial surface. (**B**) Streptomycin treated. Some stereocilia are fused (*big arrows*) and some hair-cell nuclei are pyknotic (*small, thin arrows*). (**C**) Streptomycin treated and "recovered." Sensory epithelium appears more uniform than in **B** but slightly atrophic. Hair cells have normal appearance, stereocilia are not fused, but density of bundles is reduced (*arrows*). O, otoconia; G, gelatinous layer of otolithic membrane; I, type I hair cell; II, type II hair cell; B, basal lamina; SC, supporting cells; MNF, myelinated nerve fibers.

(FIG. 1). In contrast, sections of the cristae and organ of Corti appeared normal. In STP-treated and "recovered" animals, neither fused macular hair cell stereocilia nor pyknotic nuclei were observed, but bundle density was reduced. Thus, a partial recovery of sensory epithelium morphology also occurred.

The abnormal swimming behavior observed in rats chronically treated with STP is identical to that observed in congenitally otolith-deficient mice and supports our postulation of otolith organ-specific toxicity of STP in the rat. This is confirmed by our observation that degeneration of hair cells is restricted to the macular organs of antibiotic-treated rats. The partial reversibility of abnormal swimming behavior in animals eight weeks following treatment is in accord with our observations of partial morphological recovery in the same animals. These results show that hair cell and functional recovery can occur in a mammal subjected to prolonged treatment with a clinically relevant toxic agent.

ACKNOWLEDGMENT

Thanks are due to Mrs. Edith Ramos for valuable secretarial assistance.

REFERENCES

1. DUVALL, A. J. & J. WERSALL. 1964. Acta Otolaryngol. (Stockholm) **57**: 581–598.
2. FORBES, A., L. LI, J. T. CORWIN & G. NEVILL. 1993. Science **259**: 1616–1619.
3. FUTAKI, T. & I. KAWABATA. 1983. Adv. Otorhinolaryngol. **30**: 264–267.
4. KROESE, A. B. A. & J. BERCKEN. 1980. Nature **283**: 395–397.
5. LINDEMAN, H. H. 1969. Acta Otolaryngol. (Stockholm) **67**: 177–189.
6. MEZA, G., I. LOPEZ, M. A. PAREDES, Y. PENALOZA & A. POBLANO. 1989. Acta Otolaryngol. (Stockholm) **107**: 406–411.
7. MEZA, G., L. SOLANO-FLORES & A. POBLANO. 1992. Intl. J. Dev. Neurosci. **10**: 407–411.
8. MEZA, G., N. DAUNTON, L. LOPEZ-GRIEGO & M. SALAS. 1993. Soc. Neurosci. Abstr. **19(2)**: 989.
9. MEZA, G., N. DAUNTON, R. FOX, L. LOPEZ-GRIEGO, H. PRATT & H. ZEPEDA. 1994. Collegium Otorhinolaryngol. Abstr. **57**.

Human Cortical Activity during Vestibular- and Drug-Induced Nausea Detected Using MSI[a]

ALAN D. MILLER,[b] HOWARD A. ROWLEY,[c]
TIMOTHY P. L. ROBERTS,[c] AND JOHN KUCHARCZYK[d]

[b]Department of Neurophysiology
Rockefeller University
New York, New York 10021

[c]Department of Neuroradiology
University of California, San Francisco
San Francisco, California 94143

[d]Department of Neuroradiology
University of Minnesota
Minneapolis, Minnesota 55455

Although it is well known that unusual or noxious stimulation of the vestibular system can lead to nausea (e.g., motion sickness,[1] Meniere's disease[2]), the cortical region(s) that produces the sensation of nausea is unknown. In contrast, the mechanisms underlying the production of vomiting have received greater study and are better understood. In the present study, noninvasive magnetic source imaging (MSI)[3] was used to determine if a localized cortical area is activated during nausea induced by two different kinds of stimuli. On separate occasions, subjects either were exposed to vestibular stimulation (side-to-side head movements during yaw-axis rotation) or ingested syrup of ipecac (5–10 ml), after which the magnitude of nausea was continuously scored by the subject using a 10-point scale. MSI data were recorded using a 37-channel superconducting biomagnetometer (Magnes, Biomagnetic Technologies Inc., San Diego, CA) and analyzed for the occurrence of transient bursts of focal high-amplitude activity (>400 fT). The locations of waveforms meeting these criteria were determined using a single equivalent current dipole model and superimposed on anatomic magnetic resonance images of the subject's brain. During nausea, current dipoles indicative of neuronal activation were detected in a 2- to 3-cm diameter region of cortex in the inferior frontal gyrus. Source localizations were the same when nausea was induced by either stimulus (FIGS. 1 and 2). A greater number of dipoles was observed during intense nausea than during milder nausea. The specificity of this cortical response to nausea was further supported by the lack of dipoles in this brain region at baseline or during control sessions involving speech, finger movements, or exaggerated respiratory movements. These findings are consistent with previous reports of changes in electroencephalographic (EEG) activity recorded from the temporo-frontal region during motion sickness.[4] The inferior frontal gyrus appears to be important for the sensation of nausea and may represent a new cerebral cortical target for anti-nausea pharmaceu-

[a]This work was supported by grant NS20585 from the National Institute of Neurological Disorders and Stroke.

670

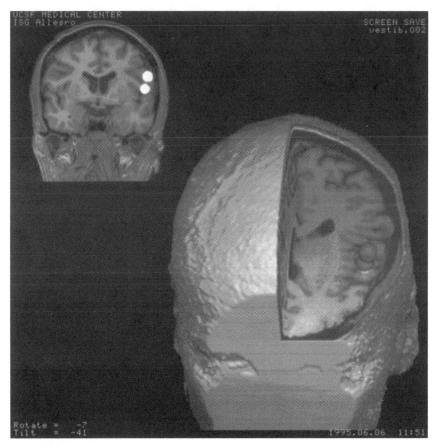

FIGURE 1. Locations of current dipoles, indicative of neuronal activation, in the inferior frontal gyrus in a subject made nauseous by prior vestibular stimulation (head movements made during yaw-axis rotation). The unilateral representation of the dipoles reflects magnetic source imaging of only one side of the head during a recording session.

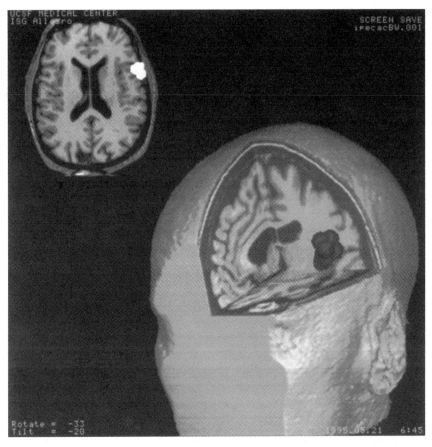

FIGURE 2. Dipoles were detected in the same location in the inferior frontal gyrus when the same subject was made nauseous by oral ingestion of syrup of ipecac (5 ml).

tical intervention. Furthermore, the MSI technique provides a quantitative means for assessing the efficacy of different pharmacological agents.

REFERENCES

1. MONEY, K. E. 1970. Motion sickness. Physiol. Rev. **50:** 1–39.
2. BALOH, R. W. & V. HONRUBIA. 1979. Clinical Neurophysiology of the Vestibular System. F. A. Davis Co. Philadelphia, PA.
3. GALLEN, C. C., D. F. SOBEL, J. D. LEWINE, J. A. SANDERS, B. L. HART, L. E. DAVIS & W. W. ORRISON, JR. 1993. Neuromagnetic mapping of brain function. Radiology **187:** 863–867.
4. CHELEN, W. E., M. KABRISKY & S. K. ROGERS. 1993. Spectral analysis of the electro-encephalographic response to motion sickness. Aviat. Space Environ. Med. **64:** 24–29.

Low-Frequency Stimulation Abolishes the High-Frequency Induced Long-Term Effects in Rat Medial Vestibular Nuclei

SILVAROSA GRASSI,[a,c] VITO ENRICO PETTOROSSI,[a]
AND MAURO ZAMPOLINI[b]

[a] Institute of Human Physiology
University of Perugia
Via del Giochetto
I-06100 Perugia, Italy

[b] Rehabilitation Centre
Hospital of Trevi
I-06039 Perugia, Italy

INTRODUCTION

Our recent experiments on rat brain-stem slices provide conclusive evidence for glutamate N-methyl-D-aspartate (NMDA)-mediated long-term modifications of synaptic efficacy in the medial vestibular nuclei (MVN).[1] In fact, high-frequency stimulation (HFS) of the primary vestibular afferents can induce an NMDA-mediated, long-lasting increase in the monosynaptic (N1) component of the field potentials elicited in the ventral portion (Vp) and a long-lasting decrease of the polysynaptic (N2) component in the dorsal portion (Dp) of the MVN. The N1 enhancement in the Vp can be considered a typical long-term potentiation (LTP), taking place at the level of glutamatergic excitatory synapses between the vestibular afferents and the secondary vestibular neurons. Conversely, N2 depression in the Dp results from an LTP of glutamatergic excitatory synapses on inhibitory GABAergic interneurons. The presence of a single phenomenon (LTP), however, responsible for both long-lasting potentiation and depression in the MVN, requires a cancellation mechanism to prevent saturation. As in hippocampus, the potentiated responses are reduced by low-frequency stimulations (LFS)[2]; therefore, we tested whether LFS can induce LTD and/or depotentiation of vestibular responses in the Vp and Dp of MVN.

METHODS

In rat transverse brain-stem slices, the ipsilateral vestibular afferents were stimulated at their entrance into the MVN (40–100 μA intensity, 0.07-msec duration). The extracellular field potentials recorded in the Vp or Dp of MVN, with 2M NaCl filled micropipettes (3–10 MΩ), showed a positive wave (P) at a latency of 0.2 ± 0.05 msec followed by two negative waves at 0.52 ± 0.18 msec (N1) and 1.51 ± 0.3 msec (N2). In the Vp, the N2 component was not clearly detectable. Stimulus intervals shorter than 4 msec and Ca^{2+}-free solution caused the N1 and N2 waves to

[c] E-mail: isfisuma@umipg.it

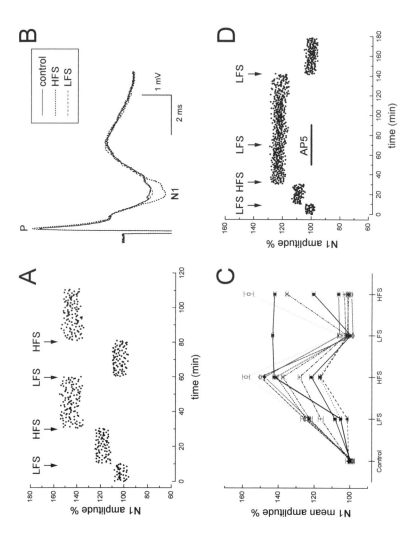

FIGURE 1. Effect of LFS before and after HFS on the N1 component of the vestibular field potentials recorded in Vp. (**A**) N1 amplitude (percentage of the baseline) plotted as a function of time. The arrows indicate the HFS and LFS delivery times. (**B**) Averaged field potentials (10 sweeps) recorded before (control) and after HFS and LFS. (**C**) HFS and LFS effects in 10 experiments. Each point is the mean ±SD of the N1 amplitude evaluated in each experiment within 5-min intervals. (**D**) Effect of AP5 on the induction of the LFS cancellation phenomenon. The horizontal bar represents the AP5 perfusion time.

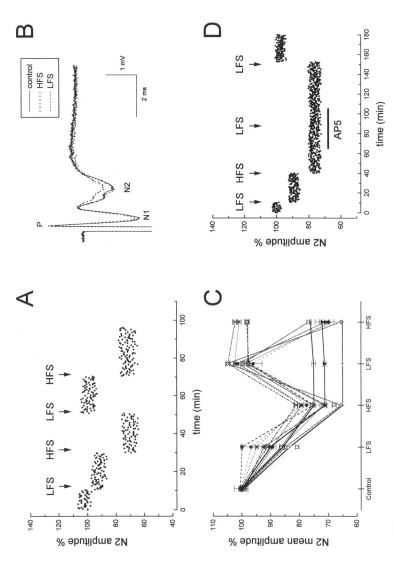

FIGURE 2. Effect of LFS before and after HFS on the N2 component of the vestibular field potentials recorded in Dp. Everything as in the legend of Figure 1.

disappear, leaving the P wave unaffected. High-frequency stimulation (HFS) consisted of four bursts at 100 Hz applied with alternated polarity for 2 sec with a 5-sec interval. Low-frequency stimulation (LFS) consisted of a stimulation at 1 to 5 Hz for 1 min. The NMDA receptor antagonist D, L-2-amino-5-phosphonovalerate (DL-AP5, Sigma, 100 μM) was used. The stimulus test was delivered every 15 sec. Peak amplitude of the evoked N1 and N2 waves was measured and expressed as a percentage of the baseline.

RESULTS

HFS of the ipsilateral primary vestibular afferents induced a long-lasting increase in the N1 component of the field potentials recorded in the Vp. The N1 amplitude was enhanced to 138.94 ± 5.63% ($n = 10$). The possibility that LFS could reduce the HFS-potentiated responses was tested by delivering LFS 20 min after the HFS effect induction. LFS caused a long-lasting (> 40 min) reduction of the N1 wave to reach the control values (102.35 ± 1.92%) in 9 out of 10 slices (FIG. 1 A–C). In many cases the N1 was potentiated again, by a subsequent HFS. The LFS effect was mediated by the NMDA receptor activation, since it was not induced during AP5 perfusion (FIG. 1D). Conversely, LFS delivered before HFS did not reduce the N1 wave, but increased it to 113.11 ± 4.45% (FIG. 1 A,C).

In the Dp, where HFS caused a long-lasting decrease of the N2 wave to 73.59 ± 2.05% ($n = 13$), the following LFS increased the N2 amplitude to the control values (100.07 ± 3.16%) in 10 out of 13 slices (FIG. 2 A–C). Also in the Dp, LFS effect was a long-term phenomenon, and it was blocked by AP5 (FIG. 2 D). Furthermore, LFS provoked a slight depression of the N2 wave to 89.34 ± 1.54% ($n = 13$), when applied before HFS (FIG. 2 A,C).

CONCLUSIONS

Unlike other brain structures, LFS does not seem to induce any long-term depression in the MVN, but it can only reproduce HFS effects, even if of minor extent. Thus, it seems that there is no way to provoke a long-term effect opposite to that elicited by HFS in unconditioned synapses. Conversely, LFS provoked an opposite long-term effect, which canceled that induced by HFS, when applied after HFS. Therefore, the MVN is provided with a mechanism preventing saturation and allowing further plastic changes.

REFERENCES

1. CAPOCCHI, G., G. DELLA TORRE, S. GRASSI, V. E. PETTOROSSI & M. ZAMPOLINI. 1992. NMDA receptor-mediated long term modulation of electrically evoked field potentials in the rat medialvestibular nuclei. Exp. Brain Res. **90:** 546–550.
2. BASHIR, Z. I. & G. L. COLLINGRIDGE. 1994. An investigation of depotentiation of long-term potentiation in the CA1 region of the hippocampus. Exp. Brain Res. **100:** 437–443.

Dendritic Growth and Changes in Electrophysiological Properties during Development of Chick Vestibular Neurons[a]

KENNA D. PEUSNER AND CHRISTIAN GIAUME

Department of Anatomy and Cell Biology
George Washington University
School of Medicine
Washington, DC 20037

Vestibular sensory neurons are the first brain elements that relay signals originating from vestibular end-organs to influence the motor neurons controlling eye movements and neck musculature. This basic vestibular reflex is highly conserved during vertebrate phylogeny.[1] Whereas the chick vestibular system contains the standard vestibular circuitry, it also offers several advantages to investigate development of neuronal physiology.[2] In avians the tangential nucleus (TN) is considered to be part of the lateral vestibular complex in the medulla. The principal cell (PC) population of this nucleus (80% of total) is composed of neurons whose axons may bifurcate in the contralateral medial longitudinal fasciculus and then innervate both oculomotor and cervical spinal cord motor neurons. The focus of this work is to correlate the morphological and electrophysiological ontogeny of PCs.

Brain slices were prepared from chick embryos staged at 13 days (E13), 15 to 16 days (E15–16), and also from hatchlings of 1 to 2 days (H1–2). Intracellular recordings and injections were performed on slices (350–500 μm thickness) incubated in an interface-type recording chamber (30–31°C) and perfused with standard saline solution.[3] Intracellular microelectrodes contained 1.5% biocytin in 2M potassium acetate and had resistances of 150 to 200 MΩ. Slices containing biocytin-injected cells were fixed, resectioned at 100-μm thickness, and reacted immunocytochemically to visualize staining before reconstructing their morphology using a camera lucida drawing tube attached to a light microscope.

At the three stages studied, the typical PC oval somata are constant in size ($\approx 27 \pm 1 \times 17 \pm 2$ μm, $n = 32$, m ± SEM) while the dendrites grow out. At E13, dendrites are beginning to form from somata covered by thin processes or filopodia that radiate in all directions (FIG. 1A$_1$). At E15–16 the dendrites continue to grow mainly in the medial and lateral directions parallel to the primary vestibular afferents (FIG. 1B$_1$). By H1–2 the dendrites have increased in total length as compared to E15–16, mostly by extending in the dorsoventral axis (FIG. 1C$_1$).

When comparing electrical properties of PCs at the three stages, the resting membrane potentials averaged -60 mV, while input resistances decreased from 60 ± 12 MΩ ($n = 4$) at E13 to 44 ± 12 MΩ ($n = 12$) at H1–2. Membrane responses were investigated by applying depolarizing currents of 400-msec duration with intensities ranging up to 1 nA. At E13, all the investigated cells ($n = 4$) responded with a single-action potential (AP) to maximum current. At E15–16, similar current

[a] This study was supported by National Institutes of Health grant DC00970.

produced either a single spike ($n = 3$) or in six other cells the firing of several APs. This firing was irregular in number and time interval between APs and occurred with an average discharge rate of 32 APs/sec. At H1–2, PCs responded to the same depolarizing current (1 nA) by repetitive firing with a discharge rate of 68 APs/sec with regularly spaced intervals ($n = 7$). Previous investigations[3] have suggested that firing of the largest diameter vestibular fibers, the colossal fibers, results in glutamatergic excitatory postsynaptic potentials (EPSPs) in PCs. Whereas the latency and the rise time of the EPSP remained in the same range, its duration measured just under the spike shortened with age (E13: 90 ± 34 msec, $n = 4$; E15–16: 25 ± 4 msec,

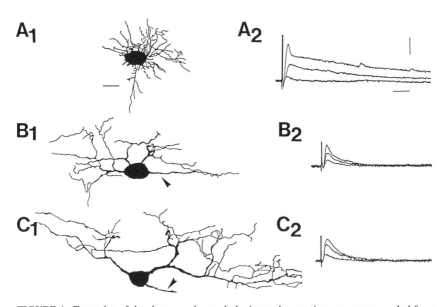

FIGURE 1. Examples of developmental morphologies and synaptic responses recorded from principal cells. Three critical ages were studied: 13-day (A_1–A_2) and 15- to 16-day (B_1–B_2) embryos and 1- to 2-day-old hatchlings (C_1–C_2). *Left side*: camera lucida drawings of biocytin-injected PCs (*arrowhead* indicates axon; scale = 20 μM). *Right side*: intracellular recordings of PC responses to increasing vestibular stimulation strength. In all cases, the highest amplitude EPSPs were obtained just under spike initiation (calibration bars = 10 mV, 10 msec).

$n = 18$; H1–2: 21 ± 3 msec, $n = 10$), and its decay half time was reduced (E13: 13 ± 9 msec, $n = 4$; E15–16: 6 ± 1 msec, $n = 20$; H1–2: 6 ± 1 msec, $n = 10$) (FIG. 1 A_2, B_2, C_2).

In conclusion, these results indicate that during the perinatal period PCs undergo rapid and extensive dendritic growth. Parallel to this dendritic morphogenesis, PCs show an increase in membrane excitability associated with changes in the pattern of synaptic responses to vestibular stimulation. Altogether, these observations suggest that, during development, these second-order vestibular neurons may receive more synaptic inputs and acquire electrical properties that allow them to follow vestibular stimuli characterized by high frequency of discharge.[4]

ACKNOWLEDGMENTS

We wish to thank Drs. B. Hamon and J. Hirsch for their helpful comments on the manuscript and Mrs M. Kelemen for excellent technical assistance.

REFERENCES

1. BAKER, R. 1991. A contemporary view of the history of eye muscles and motoneurons. *In* Vestibular and Brain Stem Control of Eye, Head and Body Movements. Shimazu & Shinoda, Eds. Springer Verlag. Berlin.
2. PEUSNER, K. D. 1992. Development of vestibular brainstem nuclei. *In* Development of Auditory and Vestibular Systems 2. Romand, Ed.: 489–518. Elsevier Science Publishers. Amsterdam.
3. PEUSNER, K. D. & C. GIAUME. 1994. Neuroscience **58:** 99–113.
4. GOLDBERG, J. M., C. E. SMITH & C. FERNANDEZ. 1984. J. Neurophysiol. **51:** 1236–1256.

Regional Distributions of Efferent Neurons in the Semicircular Canals in the Gerbil[a]

I. M. PURCELL AND A. A. PERACHIO[b]

Department of Otolaryngology
University of Texas Medical Branch
Galveston, Texas 77555

The linear and angular acceleration-sensitive receptors in the gerbil vestibular labyrinth receive direct bilateral innervation from two groups of efferent somatae in the medullary brain stem. The larger of the two groups is a collection of choline acetyltransferase (ChAT), acetylcholinesterase (AChE), calcitonin gene–related peptide (CGRP), and met-enkephalin (m-ENK) immunoreactive cells, located dorsolateral to the genu of the seventh nerve, ventral and medial to the vestibular nuclei. The smaller group, staining ChAT, AChE, CGRP, and m-ENK negative, is located immediately ventral to the genu.[1] The axons of these relatively few retrogradely labeled somatae travel in the inferior vestibular nerve, passing through Scarpa's ganglion to innervate both canal and otolith end organs. Upon entering the sensory neuroepithelium, the efferent axons ramify such that few parent axons give rise to extensive collateralized innervation. Regional variations of efferent innervation have been identified in the mammalian crista ampullares. In the chinchilla, the synaptic profiles of efferent boutons were identified making direct contact with type II hair cells and type I calyx endings.[2] In that species, there was no regional variance in the number of efferent-type II hair cell synaptic profiles; however, it was noted that the number of efferent-calyx synaptic profiles declined slightly from the peripheral zone to the central zone. In the rat,[3] no remarkable regional variations in the localization of CGRP immunolabeling were noted in any of the vestibular end organs examined. In squirrel monkey,[4] GABA-like immunoreactivity was found uniformly across the sensory epithelia of the maculae. However, in the cristae, labeling was more concentrated in the peripheral than the central areas. The purposes of the present study were to label the efferent projections into the vestibular labyrinth and to describe the patterns of innervation within the sensory neuroepithelia of the semicircular canals arising from individual ipsilateral and contralateral brain-stem efferents.

Extracellular injections made in the contralateral dorsal *group-e,* with solutions of the anterograde tracer biocytin, revealed labeled axons bifurcating in the stroma and forming a massive collateral network upon entering the sensory neuroepithelium of all the end organs. This has confirmed the prediction that individual efferent neurons have a divergent pattern of innervation in the vestibular end organs. The large number of identified preterminal and terminal processes tended to travel between

[a] This work was supported in part by National Institutes of Health grant DC00385 and NASA grants NAG 2-26 and NGT 50748.

[b] Author to whom correspondence should be sent at the following address: Department of Otolaryngology, 7.10R M.R.B., University of Texas Medical Branch, Galveston, TX 77555-1063. E-mail: perachio@beach.utmb.edu

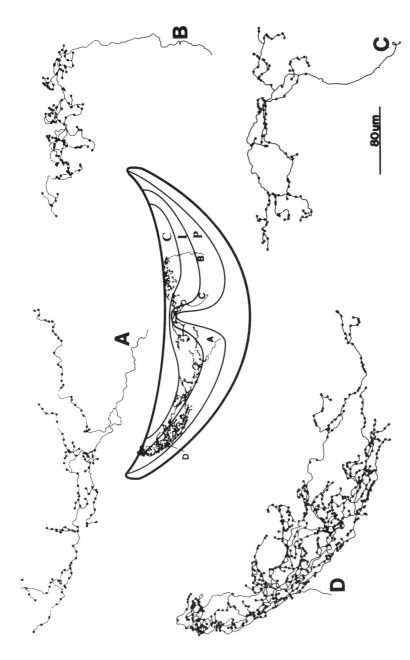

FIGURE 1. Reconstructions of labeled efferent neurons representative of the peripheral type (**A** and **C**), the planum semilunarum type (**D**), and the apical type (**B**). *Inset*: Side view of a modified standard surface schematic drawing of a crista indicating the location of the terminal fields within the sensory neuroepithelium. The sensory surface is divided into central (C), intermediate (I), and peripheral (P) zones.

the hair cell and supporting cell layer and appeared to make contact with both type II hair cell and type I calyx endings by multiple *bouton en passant* type swellings. Three-dimensional reconstruction and analysis of the labeled neurons' terminal fields in the sensory neuroepithelium of the lateral, anterior, and posterior cristae was performed (FIG. 1). Contralaterally projecting efferent terminal fields were found to innervate the peripheral nonapical regions of the sensory neuroepithelium. Those neurons have at least two patterns of innervation in the sensory neuroepithelium: (1) The planum–semilunarum type, which possesses the largest terminal field, innervates the hood of the planum and crosses the long axis of the crista to reach the lateral slopes. (2) The peripheral type enters the root of the crista to innervate the portions of the lateral slope between both planar regions confined within the intermediate and peripheral zones (FIG. 1).[2] Some of those cells, unlike the planum type, extend for short distances across the short axis of the crista but do not cross the long axis. Ipsilaterally projecting efferents were examined in animals that had previously received a saggital transection of the cerebellum and medulla. After a 14-day survival, the contralaterally projecting efferents were assumed to have degenerated. Extracellular injections of the anterograde tracer biotinylated dextran amine (10,000 MW) were then made into the ipsilateral *group-e*. Ipsilaterally projecting efferent terminal fields were found in the apical and/or peripheral regions of the sensory neuroepithelium. The distribution of efferent innervation in the crista suggests a relationship between the region of innervation and afferent sensitivity and implies a more complex role for the vestibular efferents than previously suspected.

REFERENCES

1. PERACHIO, A. A. & G. A. KEVETTER. 1989. Identification of vestibular efferent neurons in the gerbil: Histochemical and retrograde labeling. Exp. Brain Res. **78:** 315–326.
2. GOLDBERG, J. M., A. LYSAKOWSKI & C. FERNANDEZ. 1990. Morphophysiological and ultrastructural studies in the mammalian cristae ampullares. Hearing Res. **49:** 89–102.
3. TANAKA, M., N. TAKEDA, E. SENBA, M. TOHYAMA, T. KUBO & T. MATSUNAGA. 1988. Localization of calcitonin gene-related peptide in the vestibular end organs in the rat: An immunohistochemical study. Brain Res. **447:** 175–177.
4. USAMI, S., M. IGARASHI & G. C. THOMPSON. 1987. GABA-like immunoreactivity in the squirrel monkey vestibular endorgans. Brain Res. **417:** 367–370.

The Effect of Neomycin on Organotypic Cultures of the Adult Guinea-Pig Utricle[a]

E. QUINT, C. M. HACKNEY, AND D. N. FURNESS

Department of Communication and Neuroscience
Keele University
Keele, Staffordshire ST5 5BG
United Kingdom

It has been suggested that hair cells from the guinea-pig inner ear may be replaced following ototoxic insult *in vitro*[1] and *in vivo*.[2,3] In order to explore whether the process of hair cell degeneration, repair, or replacement in the guinea-pig vestibular system might provide a relevant model for the processes underlying the behavioral recovery that we have observed in the guinea-pig auditory system,[4] we are investigating the effects of aminoglycoside antibiotics on utricular explants maintained as organotypic cultures.

MATERIALS AND METHODS

Utricles from 18 adult pigmented guinea pigs were explanted and maintained as organotypic cultures using a protocol modified from Warchol *et al.*[1] After 24 hours in culture, half of the explants were transferred to medium containing 1 mM neomycin for a 48 h period. Following treatment with neomycin, the explants were returned to neomycin-free medium. Either 3 or 8 days after explantation, the utricles were fixed and processed for scanning electron microscopy[5] (SEM) or light microscopy (LM). Explanted utricles from 16 animals plus two controls (i.e., not cultured) were viewed in a S-4500 Hitachi field emission SEM to determine the comparative densities of hair bundles of two different types: tall hair bundles (THB), as defined by the arrangement of the stereocilia in serried rows, and small hair bundles (SHB), as defined by uniformity in stereociliary height, and/or a central kinocilium. Explanted utricles from two animals plus one control were embedded in Spurr resin and serial sections (1–2 μm thick) taken in a direction perpendicular to the striolar axis. The sections were stained with 1% toluidine blue, and the nuclear densities within the sensory epithelium estimated at 50-μm intervals along the length of each utricle. Nuclei were regarded as belonging to hair cells if they did not lie immediately above the basal lamina, had a rounded morphology, and the chromatin did not form a central dense patch. All other nuclei (referred to as non–hair cell nuclei hereafter) were classified as belonging to supporting cells.

RESULTS

At 3 and 8 days post-explantation, the densities of THBs and hair-cell nuclei were significantly lower in both the neomycin-treated and the untreated cultures, although

[a]This work was supported by the BBSRC, Hearing Research Trust, and Wellcome Trust.

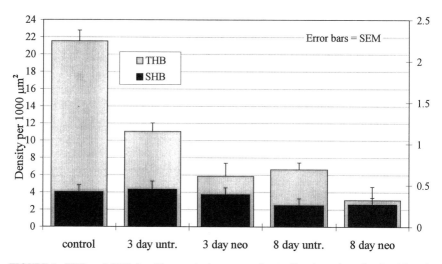

FIGURE 1. THB and SHB densities: control versus explants. Graph to show the densities of control, untreated, and neomycin-treated THBs (*left ordinate*) and SHBs (*right ordinate*) (untr. = untreated; neo = neomycin treated). Both the treated and untreated THB densities are significantly lower than those in the controls at 3 and 8 days (Mann-Whitney U-test, $p <$ 0.05); however, the SHB densities do not differ significantly from the controls.

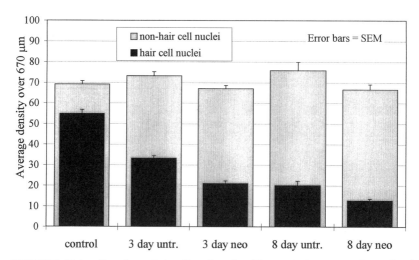

FIGURE 2. Hair-cell and non–hair cell nuclear densities: control versus explants. Graph to show the hair-cell and non–hair cell nuclear densities of control, untreated, and neomycin-treated explants (untr. = untreated; neo = neomycin treated). The nuclear densities of the treated and untreated hair cells 3 and 8 days after explantation are significantly lower than in the control, whereas the nuclear densities of non–hair cells are not significantly different from the control (Mann-Whitney U-test, $p < 0.05$).

the reduction was greater following neomycin treatment. The SHB densities and non–hair cell nuclear densities remained relatively stable (FIGS. 1 and 2). Evidence of cellular degeneration was observed in all explants, for example, fusion of the stereocilia, ejection of cuticular plates, depression of the bundles beneath the level of the reticular lamina, and a disruption of the usual bilayer arrangement of upper hair cells and lower supporting cells.

DISCUSSION

It is apparent that the culture regime employed here acts as a "stressor" on the utricular system, resulting in significant THB and hair cell loss even without treatment with ototoxic drugs, possibly due to a loss of innervation following explantation. According to Forge *et al.*[3] the characteristics of SHBs suggest that they are immature and may belong to newly regenerated hair cells. However, the apparent difference in the vulnerability of SHBs and THBs to insult reported here suggests that it is important to assess their absolute density rather than the relative proportion of the two types when investigating hair bundle loss and possible replacement. Further investigations are needed, however, using transmission electron microscopy to determine the exact identity of some apparently non–hair cell nuclei that were difficult to categorize by location and morphology; such cells may be either hair cells or supporting cells, or could even be hair-cell precursors.

REFERENCES

1. WARCHOL, M. E., P. R. LAMBERT, B. J. GOLDSTEIN, A. FORGE & J. T. CORWIN. 1993. Science **259:** 1619–1622.
2. NICOL, K. M. M., C. M. HACKNEY, E. F. EVANS & S. R. PRATT. 1992. Hearing Res. **61:** 117–131.
3. FORGE, A., L. LI, J. T. CORWIN & G. NEVILL. 1993. Science **259:** 1616–1619.
4. GOLDSTEIN, B. J., M. Y. HUANG & J. T. CORWIN. 1994. 17th Midwinter Research Meeting of the Association for Research in Otolaryngology Florida, Abstr. **524:** 131.
5. FURNESS, D. N. & C. M. HACKNEY. 1985. Hearing Res. **18:** 177–188.

Error Signals in Horizontal Gaze Velocity Purkinje Cells under Stimulus Conditions That Cause Learning in the VOR

JENNIFER L. RAYMOND[a] AND STEPHEN G. LISBERGER

Department of Physiology and
W. M. Keck Foundation Center for Integrative Neuroscience
University of California, San Francisco
Box 0444
San Francisco, California 94143

We are investigating the mechanism of motor learning in the vestibulo-ocular reflex (VOR). Our approach has been to characterize the dependence of learning on the temporal properties of the adapting stimuli and thereby place constraints on the neural signals capable of inducing plasticity in VOR pathways. The simple spikes (SSs) and complex spikes (CSs) of Purkinje cells have been suggested as signals that might contribute to the induction of plasticity in the cerebellar cortex and/or brainstem VOR pathways[1,2]; however, these hypotheses have been based on relatively limited data about the responses of the relevant neurons during learning. We examined the SS and CS responses to adapting stimuli with a range of temporal properties to look for consistent error signals that could be used to guide learning.

First, we established the effectiveness for inducing learning in the VOR of sinusoidal vestibular and visual stimuli of frequencies from 0.5 Hz to 10 Hz. Rhesus monkeys were adapted for 3 hours with passive head turns and optokinetic stimuli that mimicked the effects of magnifying ($\times 2$) or miniaturizing ($\times 0$) spectacles. Adaptation with stimuli at frequencies up to 5 Hz induced large, adaptive changes in the amplitude of the VOR. Adaptation with frequencies of 8 or 10 Hz resulted in smaller and less consistent changes in the VOR. These behavioral studies also revealed what appeared to be two components of learning in the VOR that were differentially induced by low- and high-frequency stimuli. Adaptation at a low frequency (e.g. 0.5 Hz) induced changes that were biggest in the low-frequency components of the VOR, whereas adaptation at a high frequency (e.g. 5 Hz) induced changes that were similar in amplitude across test frequency.

Next, we recorded SS (FIG. 1) and CS (FIG. 2) responses in horizontal gaze velocity Purkinje cells (HGVPs) to $\times 0$ and $\times 2$ sinusoidal stimuli at a range of frequencies from 0.5 to 10 Hz. As reported previously,[3,4] at low frequencies (e.g. 0.5 Hz), SS responses were in phase with ipsiversive head velocity for $\times 0$ stimuli and in phase with contraversive head velocity for $\times 2$ stimuli. Therefore, the phase of the SS responses relative to head velocity could be used at low frequencies to discriminate conditions in which the gain needed to decrease from conditions in which the gain needed to increase. At low frequencies, the phase of the CS responses relative to head velocity also differed for $\times 0$ and $\times 2$ stimuli. CSs were in phase with contraversive head velocity for $\times 0$ stimuli and in phase with ipsiversive head velocity for $\times 2$

---

[a] E-mail: jraymond@phy.ucsf.edu

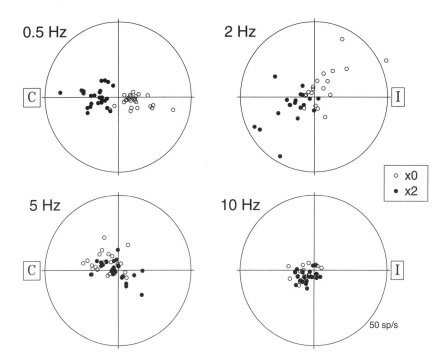

FIGURE 1. Simple spike responses to ×0 (*open symbols*) and ×2 (*filled symbols*) adapting stimuli at a range of frequencies from 0.5 to 10 Hz. Each point represents the SS response of a single HGVP averaged over 1 min. The responses are plotted in polar coordinates. Distance from the origin represents the amplitude of the response. Phase is plotted relative to head velocity; responses in phase with ipsiversive head velocity are plotted to the right of the origin and responses in phase with contraversive head velocity are plotted to the left of the origin, with clockwise rotation representing increased phase lead.

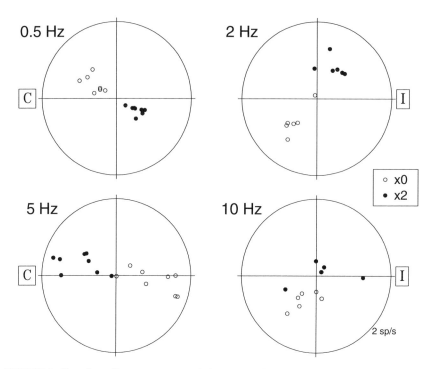

FIGURE 2. Complex spike responses to ×0 (*open symbols*) and ×2 (*filled symbols*) adapting stimuli at a range of frequencies from 0.5 to 10 Hz. Each point represents the CS response of a single HGVP averaged over 1 min. Axes as in FIGURE 1.

stimuli. Thus, at low frequencies, the correlation of either the SSs or the CSs and the vestibular stimulus contained information that could be used to determine whether the gain of the VOR should increase or decrease.

Our preliminary results indicate that the relationships between SS and CS responses and the vestibular stimulus observed at low frequencies do not hold at higher frequencies. At high frequencies (e.g. 5 Hz), the SS responses appeared to contain little information about the direction of the required changes in the VOR: responses were in phase with contraversive head velocity for both ×0 and ×2 stimuli. For CSs, the results at higher frequencies were more complex. At 5 Hz, CS responses were in phase with ipsiversive head velocity for ×0 stimuli and in phase with contraversive head velocity for ×2 stimuli. These phases were the opposite of those observed at 0.5 Hz. At each frequency tested, the CS responses were different for ×0 and ×2 stimuli and could therefore in principle determine whether the gain of the VOR should increase or decrease. For a particular visual condition (×0 or ×2), however, the phase shift between the CS response and the vestibular stimulus varied with frequency. Therefore, any mechanism that uses the correlation of CSs and vestibular signals to guide learning across the range of effective frequencies must compensate for this relative phase shift with frequency. An alternative hypothesis is that different mechanisms guide learning at high and low frequencies and that complex spikes have different roles in the induction of learning at different frequencies.

REFERENCES

1. ITO, M. 1982. Cerebellar control of the vestibulo-ocular reflex—around the flocculus hypothesis. Annu. Rev. Neurosci. **5:** 275–298.
2. MILES, F. A. & S. G. LISBERGER. 1981. Plasticity in the vestibulo-ocular reflex: A new hypothesis. Annu. Rev. Neurosci. **4:** 273–299.
3. LISBERGER, S. G. & A. F. FUCHS. 1978. Role of primate flocculus during rapid behavioral modification of vestibuloocular reflex. I. Purkinje cell activity during visually guided horizontal smooth-pursuit eye movements and passive head rotation. J. Neurophysiol. **41:** 733–763.
4. MILES, F. A., J. H. FULLER, D. J. BRAITMAN & B. M. DOW. 1980. Long-term adaptive changes in primate vestibuloocular reflex. III. Electrophysiological observations in flocculus of normal monkeys. J. Neurophysiol. **43:** 1437–1476.

A Delayed Rectifier Conductance Shapes the Voltage Response of Type I Hair Cells[a]

A. J. RICCI,[b,c] K. J. RENNIE,[b] AND M. J. CORREIA[b,d,e]

[b]Department of Otolaryngology
[d]Department of Physiology and Biophysics
University of Texas Medical Branch at Galveston
Galveston, Texas 77555-1063

Whole-cell ruptured and perforated patch recordings from dissociated type-I vestibular hair cells indicate that the dominant conductance is a potassium-selective delayed rectifier, termed I_{KI},[1] whose steady-state activation properties allow the conductance to be activated upon depolarization positive to -90 mV[1-3] and whose whole-cell activation kinetics show an exponential voltage dependence.[3] Together, these properties impart a low-input resistance (IR) (mean $<$ 100 MΩ), a fast time constant, and a hyperpolarized zero-current potential (V_z about -70 mV).[1-4] Current-clamp data from gerbil crista suggest that type I cells exhibit a low gain over a broad bandpass with no resonance about their V_z.[4] In addition, when I_{KI} was reduced, the membrane voltage demonstrated an initial peak response followed by a relaxation.[4]

FIGURE 1A–C presents examples of a pigeon type I hair cell's membrane voltage response to a series of current pulse injections. Initially, the membrane voltage response showed no relaxation; however, as current magnitude was increased, a peak voltage was seen that increased in magnitude with increasing stimuli. The extent of the voltage relaxation also increased with increasing stimuli. This response was typical for type I hair cells with IRs greater than 100 MΩ ($n = 13$). Current–voltage plots for each pulse protocol (A–C), showing peak depolarizing and steady-state responses, are given in FIGURE 1D–F. In each case the peak response appears linear, while the steady-state response shows rectification. The linearity in the peak voltage suggests that the response was a function of the cell's IR, established by the steady-state activation properties of I_{KI} and the slow activation time constant of I_{KI}. This is supported by the protocol of FIGURE 1B, where the cell was hyperpolarized to a potential where I_{KI} was deactivated; the cell time constant was increased to greater than 2 msec from less than 1 msec, and the peak response as well as the IR were much greater than those about the cell's V_z (FIG. 1A–C). Further substantiation comes from the plot of FIGURE 1G ($n = 6$), where peak voltage was plotted against predicted voltage (based on Ohm's law, with resistance being equivalent to the instantaneous IR). Each cell showed a linear response with a slope near 1 and an intercept near the cell's V_z. Similarly, a plot of steady-state voltage measured against predicted voltage, again using Ohm's law, was linear. In this case, the resistance was

[a]This work was supported by National Institutes of Health grant DC01273 (to M.J.C.). A.J.R. is a NASA Research Associate, K.J.R. is an NIH NRSA recipient, and M.J.C. is an NIH Clause Pepper investigator.
[c]Current address: Department of Neurophysiology, University of Wisconsin, 1300 University Avenue, Madison, WI 53706.
[e]Corresponding author.

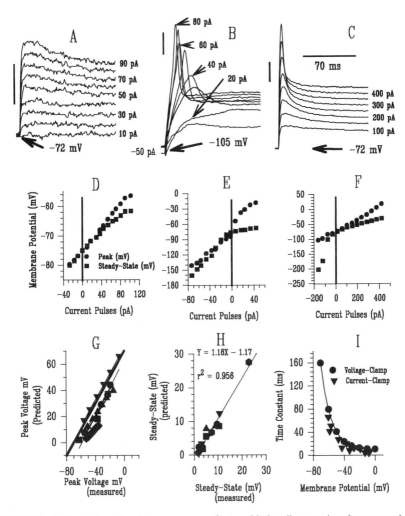

FIGURE 1. Perforated patch voltage responses of a type I hair cell to a series of current pulses are given in **A–C**. Pulse magnitudes are indicated at the end of each trace or for the dc level (**B**) at the start of the pulse. Scale bars represent 10 mV. Voltage–current plots are given for each of the pulse protocols (**D–E**), in which the circles represent the peak depolarizing voltage and the squares represent the steady-state value. Both **G** and **H** plot the measured voltage, either peak or steady-state, respectively, against the predicted voltage level assuming an Ohm's law linear relationship. For the peak response, the instantaneous voltage–current relationship (see text for protocol) was used to calculate resistance, while for the steady-state level the predicted input resistance was reduced based on the recruited conductance as estimated from the slope conductance in voltage-clamp. The relaxation rate of the voltage response, measured as the time constant from the fit to a single exponential decay, is plotted against peak membrane voltage (**I**). Also plotted versus voltage in FIGURE 1I is the time constant, estimated from the second-order Hodgkin–Huxley kinetic scheme fitted to the voltage-clamp activation acquired in voltage-clamp, from a pulse protocol that held the cell at -90 mV and pulsed in 10-mV increments from -110 mV to 0 mV.

estimated as the difference between IR and the resistance drop due to recruited conductance. Recruited conductance was estimated from the slope conductance of the current–voltage plot acquired in voltage clamp, from a pulse protocol that held the cell at its V_z and used 10-mV incremental pulses from -90 mV to $+30$ mV.

The time course of relaxation, measured from the peak voltage change to the steady-state level, became faster with depolarization (FIG. 1A–C). The activation of I_{KI} was best fit by a second-order Hodgkin–Huxley-type equation. A plot of the time constant of activation from the fitted data against membrane voltage demonstrates the exponential voltage dependence of the whole-cell activation kinetics. Superimposed on this plot is the relaxation time constant measured in current-clamp. The similarity in the plots suggests that the whole-cell activation kinetics are, for the most part, responsible for the time course of the membrane relaxation.

REFERENCES

1. RENNIE, K. J. & M. J. CORREIA. 1994. J. Neurophysiol. 71: 317–329.
2. CORREIA, M. J. & D. G. LANG. 1990. Neurosci. Lett. 119: 1106–1111.
3. RICCI, A. J., K. J. RENNIE & M. J. CORREIA. 1995. Assoc. Res. Otolaryngol. 18: 162.
4. RENNIE, K. J., A. J. RICCI & M. J. CORREIA. 1996. J. Neurophysiol. 75(5). In press.

Perception and Eye Movement during Low-Frequency Centripetal Acceleration[a]

S. H. SEIDMAN[b] AND G. D. PAIGE

Department of Neurology
University of Rochester Medical Center
Rochester, New York 14642

The otolith organs are acceleration sensors, and thus transduce linear forces due to both tilt and translation. Because the compensatory ocular-motor and postural responses to these two types of accelerations must differ, the ambiguity in otolith input must somehow be resolved. One hypothesis of how this differentiation may occur involves frequency-selective processing, with high-frequency signals conveying translation and low-frequency signals conveying tilt. This hypothesis is supported by studies of the linear vestibulo-ocular reflex (LVOR), which show that the ocular response to head translation exhibits high-pass characteristics,[1] and by studies of ocular counterrolling in response to interaural linear acceleration, which exhibits low-pass characteristics.[2] Low-frequency naso-occipital acceleration is similar to interaural, but results in perception of pitch tilt, illusory vertical movement of the horizon (the elevator illusion),[3] and vertical eye movements.[4,5] However, the frequency characteristics of these pitch effects have not been quantified.

We investigated the responses to low-frequency naso-occipital accelerations (0.005–0.025 Hz) in five human subjects. A rotating linear sled was employed to exploit centripetal acceleration. Subjects were seated and oriented with the naso-occipital axis aligned with the sled's motion axis. The sled was then accelerated to a constant angular velocity of 128°/sec. After perrotatory nystagmus and angular vection ended, sled position was slowly oscillated sinusoidally over ±50 cm eccentricity. This produced a peak acceleration of 0.25 g, which summed with the gravitational vector to produce a resultant pitch-tilt of 14°. Subjects viewed a small laser spot aligned with the viewing eye, which was projected onto a head-fixed screen in an otherwise dark room, and were instructed to keep the spot on the perceived horizon by using a joystick to control the vertical position. Alternatively, two subjects were also instructed to keep their eyes on the horizon in complete darkness without the presence of the laser spot, while eye movements were recorded using video oculography (Elmar, Toronto, Canada). Sled position, joystick position, and eye position were sampled at 100 Hz and stored for off-line analysis. Gains and phases (reported pitch tilt with respect to resultant tilt) of the responses (joystick and eye position) were calculated using a Welch periodogram technique.

Typical raw records of both the joystick task and the eye movement task are shown in FIGURE 1. During stimulation, subjects perceived a tilt and an illusory movement of the horizon and responded by smoothly adjusting the laser spot or gaze

[a]This work was supported by National Institutes of Health grant AG06442 (GDP), T32-EY07125 (Ctr. Vis. Sci.), RR06853, Resource for the Study of Neural Models of Behavior, and Research to Prevent Blindness.

[b]Address for correspondence: S. H. Seidman, University of Rochester Medical Center, Department of Neurology, Box 605, 601 Elmwood Ave., Rochester, NY 14642. E-mail: seidman@cvs.rochester.edu

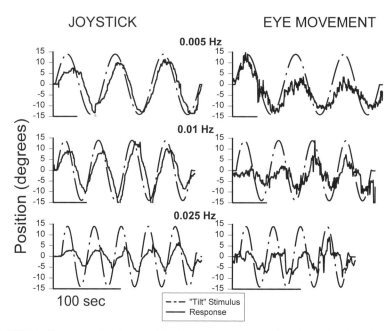

FIGURE 1. Raw records of one subject's responses to centripetal acceleration along the naso-occipital axis. Responses during the joystick task are on the left, and responses during the eye movement task are on the right. *Solid lines* show the subject's responses, and *interrupted lines* show the stimuli, expressed as the effective pitch-tilt angle resulting from the summation of the centripetal tilt vector with gravity. As stimulus frequency increases, both the joystick responses and eye movement responses diminish in size and develop increasing phase lags. All time bars show 100 seconds.

vertically to compensate. Laser spot or gaze position was adjusted upward when subjects perceived a forward tilt. This occurred near the peak of forward (nose-out) eccentricity, when peak acceleration was directed occipitally. Similarly, the spot or eye position was directed downward (while subjects perceived a backward tilt) when they were near the peak of backward eccentricity. Although intersubject variability was high, joystick response gain decreased as a function of frequency in four out of five subjects, with median values of 0.63 at 0.005 Hz (range 0.27–1.01) and 0.30 at 0.025 Hz (range 0.05–0.61). For all subjects, phase lag increased as a function of frequency, with median values of $-25.8°$ at 0.005 Hz (range, $-8.0°$ to $-45.4°$) and $-55.1°$ at 0.025 Hz (range $-29.0°$ to $-104.0°$). This difference was found to be significant ($p < 0.05$, Wilcoxin rank-sum test).

Subjects reported the eye movement task in darkness to be more difficult than the joystick task, and responses were accordingly more variable and less coherent. A comparison between the two tasks is shown in FIGURE 2B for a typical subject. Although gains for the two cases tended to differ, the phase relationships were nearly the same.

In conclusion, the dynamics of the pitch-tilt responses to low-frequency centripetal acceleration show low-pass characteristics. This is true of both the perceptual response as indicated by the joystick task and the reflexive response as shown by the eye movement task. All subjects showed a consistent phase lag, which increased as a

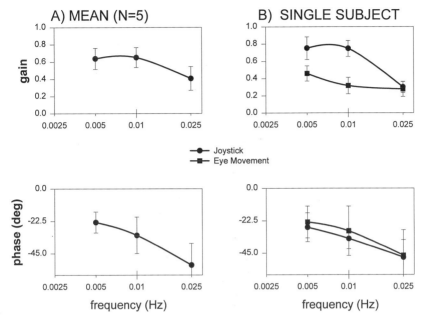

FIGURE 2. Frequency characteristics of the response to centripetal acceleration. (**A**) Gain and phase data showing the mean joystick responses for all five subjects. As stimulus frequency increases, gain decreases and phase lag increases. (**B**) Comparison of one subject's responses to the joystick task (*circles*) and eye movement task (*squares*). Although gain differences are observed, phase characteristics are nearly the same for the two tasks. Error bars in **A** are standard errors. Error bars in **B** are 95% confidence intervals as computed by the Welch periodogram technique.

function of frequency. Phase lags were apparent even at 0.005 Hz. These responses are consistent with previously reported responses to interaural acceleration,[2] which were carried out at frequencies an order of magnitude higher than those employed here. Both are consistent with the notion that tilt responses exhibit low-pass behavior.

REFERENCES

1. PAIGE, G. D. & D. L. TOMKO. 1991. J. Neurophysiol. **65:** 1170–1182.
2. LICHTENBERG, B. K., L. R. YOUNG & A. P. ARROTT. 1982. Exp. Brain Res. **48:** 127–136.
3. COHEN, M. M. 1973. Percept. Psychophys. **14:** 401–406.
4. BRANDT, U. & E. FLUUR. 1967. Acta Otolaryngol. **63:** 564–578.
5. BRANDT, U. & E. FLUUR. 1967. Acta Otolaryngol. **63:** 489–502.

NADPH-Diaphorase Histochemical Staining in the Rat Vestibular Nuclei during Postnatal Development[a]

JENNIFER L. SHAER,[b]

PILAR FERNANDEZ-RODRIGUEZ,[c]

GIORGIO P. MARTINELLI,[d] AND GAY R. HOLSTEIN[b,e,f]

[b]*Department of Neurology*
[c]*Department of Anesthesiology*
[d]*Department of Surgery*
[e]*Department of Cell Biology/Anatomy*
Mount Sinai School of Medicine
New York, New York 10029

Nitric oxide (NO) is currently regarded as a novel neuronal messenger. It is produced through the conversion of L-arginine into L-citrulline by a constitutive form of nitric oxide synthase (NOS), which is a Ca^{2+}/calmodulin-dependent enzyme (for reviews, see refs. 1–3). Nicotinamide adenine dinucleotide phosphate (NADPH)-diaphorase can be used as a reliable histochemical marker for neuronal NOS since such activity, but not that of related enzymes, is resistant to aldehyde fixation.[4,5] In the adult rat vestibular system, NOS has been reported in fibers of the vestibular ganglion and nerve,[6] and in some cells and processes is present in the vestibular nuclei.[7] The purpose of the present study was to visualize the distribution of NOS in the vestibular nuclei during early postnatal development, using NADPH-diaphorase histochemical staining in rats.

Sprague-Dawley rat pups, ranging in age from newborn (P0) to 30 days old (P30), as well as adults, were deeply anesthetized with pentobarbital and then perfused through the abdominal aorta with saline immediately followed by 4% paraformaldehyde/0.35% glutaraldehyde in phosphate buffer (pH 7.4). The brains were removed, post-fixed in 4% paraformaldehyde for 90 min, and then transferred to phosphate-buffered saline (PBS). Tissue blocks containing the vestibular nuclei were placed in an agarose support and Vibratome-sectioned in sagittal or coronal plane into wells containing Tris buffer (TB). Sections were then transferred to a solution of 0.4 mg/ml nitroblue tetrazolium, 1 mg/ml NADPH, and 0.2% Triton X-100 in TB and incubated for 45 min at room temperature in the dark on a clinical rotator. The histochemical reaction was stopped by two TB-saline rinses and one PBS rinse and stabilized by immersion for 30 sec in 0.1% osmium tetroxide.

In newborn rats, NADPH-diaphorase histochemical staining is apparent in small groups of vestibular neurons (FIG. 1A). Although the stain is spread diffusely through the somata of these cells, no processes are visible. In contrast, small, stained puncta appear to encapsulate these cell bodies, suggesting the presence of NO-positive

[a]This research was supported in part by research grant Nos. 5 RO1 DC 01705-04 from the National Institute on Deafness and Other Communication Disorders, and AM 07420 from the National Institutes of Health.

[f]Address for correspondence: Dr. G. R. Holstein, Department of Neurology, Box 1140, Mount Sinai School of Medicine, One Gustave L. Levy Place, New York, NY 10029.

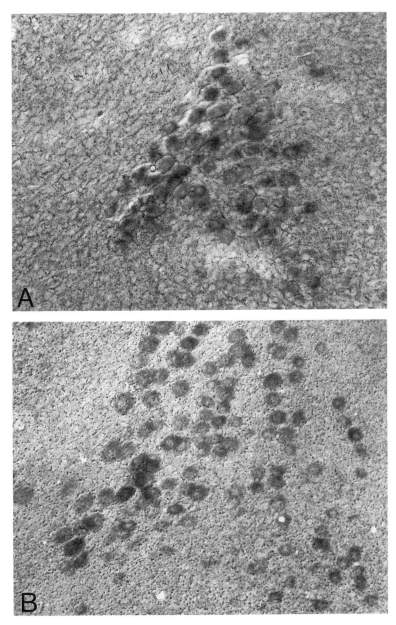

FIGURE 1. NADPH-diaphorase histochemical staining of neurons in the vestibular nuclei of newborn (**A**) and five-day-old (**B**) rat pups. Nomarski differential optics. (Magnification: 225×.)

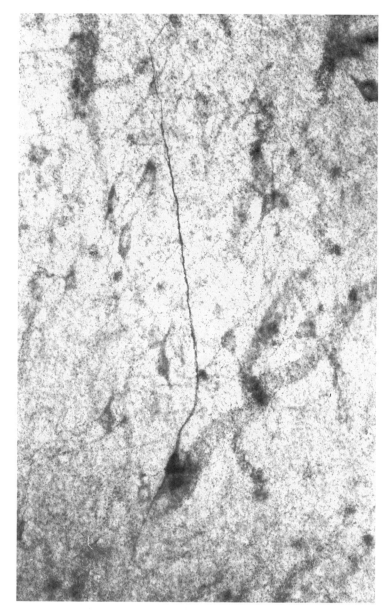

FIGURE 2. NADPH-diaphorase histochemical staining of a neuron in the medial vestibular nucleus of an adult rat. The long stained process of the cell is directed ventrally. Nomarski differential optics. (Magnification: 450×.)

afferent boutons. By P3, more intense staining is apparent in the perikarya of vestibular neurons. In addition, some cell processes are stained, particularly in fusiform neurons. By P5–6, more vestibular nucleus neurons appear to be stained (FIG. 1**B**). These are globular, rather than fusiform, and the processes are not visible. Puncta are more rod-like and pervade the neuropil. By P23, the perikarya and processes of globular and fusiform vestibular neurons are stained; and by P30 the number, size, and shape of the stained cells appear like adult cells.

Neurons of the adult rat vestibular nuclei, with robust and radiating processes, stain darkly using NADPH-diaphorase histochemistry (FIG. 2). Multipolar, fusiform, and globular neurons are apparent, particularly in the medial and descending vestibular nuclei. Long processes extend from many of these cells and course primarily in a ventral or medial direction. Comparatively few stained puncta are present in the neuropil or surrounding labeled or unlabeled neurons.

Our results indicate that NOS activity in the vestibular nuclei of newborn rats is different from that of adult animals. Most notably, processes of vestibular nucleus neurons are not stained in newborn animals, although small, labeled puncta surround these neurons. It is possible that these puncta represent extrinsic afferent inputs to these second-order vestibular neurons.

ACKNOWLEDGMENTS

The authors are grateful to Rosemary Lang and Barbara Royal for technical assistance.

REFERENCES

1. GARTHWAITE, J. 1991. Trends Neurosci. **14:** 60–67.
2. BREDT, D. S. & S. H. SNYDER. 1994. Annu. Rev. Biochem. **63:** 175–195.
3. VINCENT, S. R. & H. KIMURA. 1992. Neuroscience **46:** 755.
4. HOPE, B. T., G. J. MICHAEL, K. M. KNIGGE & S. R. VINCENT. 1991. Proc. Natl. Acad. Sci. USA **88:** 2811–2814.
5. DAWSON, T. M., D. S. BREDT, M. FOTUHI, P. M. HWANG & S. H. SNYDER. 1991. Proc. Natl. Acad. Sci. USA **88:** 7797–7801.
6. HARPER, A., W. R. BLYTHE, C. J. ZDANSKI, J. PRAZMA & H. C. PILLSBURY III. 1994. Otolaryngol. Head Neck Surg. **111**(4)**:** 430–438.
7. RODRIGO, J., D. R. SPRINGALL, O. UTTENTHAL, M. L. BENTURA, F. ABADIA-MOLINA, V. RIVEROS-MORENO, R. MARTINEZ-MURILLO, J. M. POLAK & S. MONCADA. 1994. Philos. Trans. R. Soc. London B **345:** 175–221.

Brain-stem Integrative Sites for Vestibulo-Sympathetic Reflexes[a]

B. C. STEINBACHER JR.[b] AND B. J. YATES

Departments of Otolaryngology and Neuroscience
University of Pittsburgh
Pittsburgh, Pennsylvania 15213

The vestibular system is known to participate in cardiovascular control[1,2] (see chapter by Yates in this volume). A vestibulo-sympathetic response is elicited by nose-up pitch stimulation of otolith receptors. When vestibular inputs are removed in an animal, there is a decreased ability to maintain normal blood pressure during nose-up tilt (i.e., orthostatic hypotension).[2] Therefore, the vestibular system may play a critical role in making immediate compensatory changes in blood pressure during postural adjustments. The known brain-stem circuitry necessary for producing the vestibulo-sympathetic response involves part of the medial vestibular nucleus, adjacent inferior vestibular nucleus, and the rostral ventrolateral medulla (RVLM). The RVLM sends excitatory projections to sympathetic preganglionic neurons in the intermediolateral zone (IML) of the thoracic spinal cord.[3] Synaptic activation of sympathetic preganglionic neurons causes peripheral vasoconstriction, which results in an increase in systemic blood pressure.[4]

Electrophysiological studies have shown that signals are sent from the vestibular nuclei to the RVLM via a multisynaptic pathway.[5] The purpose of this study was to identify which brain-stem interneurons relay labyrinthine signals to the RVLM. Experiments were performed in paralyzed, decerebrate cats. Lesions were made with the neurotoxin kainic acid in brain-stem areas known to influence cardiovascular regulation. These areas include the nucleus of the solitary tract (NTS), the parabrachial nucleus (PBN), the lateral tegmental field (LTF), and the caudal ventrolateral medulla (CVLM). Cells in the NTS receive afferent input from carotid sinus stretch receptors.[6] This information concerning arterial wall stretch is then sent, in part, from the NTS to the CVLM. Neurons in the CVLM, in turn, send inhibitory projections to the RVLM.[7] Thus, when CVLM neurons are active the excitatory drive to IML neurons drops and peripheral vasoconstriction decreases. The PBN relays signals from higher brain centers, such as the amygdala and lateral and paraventricular areas of the hypothalamus (which are known to participate in cardiovascular regulation), to the RVLM.[8] The LTF provides tonic input to cells in the RVLM and partially regulates certain rhythm components of sympathetic nerve discharge.[9,10]

Responses were recorded from the splanchnic nerve (a major sympathetic nerve that innervates the gut) following bipolar electrical stimulation of the vestibular nerves. The sciatic nerve was also stimulated to determine if lesions that affected vestibulo-sympathetic reflexes also altered somato-sympathetic responses. The results of these lesion studies suggest that neurons located in the lateral reticular

[a]This work was supported by National Institutes of Health grant DC00693.

[b]Address for correspondence: Bernard C. Steinbacher Jr., University of Pittsburgh, Dept. of Otolaryngology, Eye and Ear Institute Bldg., 203 Lothrop St., Room 113, Pittsburgh, PA 15213. E-mail: steinb@pop.pitt.edu

formation caudal to the obex, including the CVLM, are critically involved in producing the vestibulo-sympathetic reflex.[11] Lesions of this area greatly (between 75 and 100%) attenuate the amplitude of the sympathetic response elicited by vestibular stimulation (FIG. 1A). These lesions also produced a marked decrease in the amplitude of excitatory components of somato-sympathetic reflexes, while the inhibitory components of these responses usually persisted (FIG. 1A). Lesions made in the NTS, parabrachial area, and areas of the LTF rostral to the obex did not significantly alter the response characteristics of either the vestibulo- or somato-sympathetic reflexes.

This evidence suggests that neurons in the caudal and lateral reticular formation are essential for relaying vestibular signals to the RVLM. The effects of these lesions were due specifically to removal of vestibular signals to medullary neurons that influence the sympathetic nervous system and not to a reduction in the spontaneous activity of the sympathetic nervous system. This is suggested by the fact that spontaneous activity in the splanchnic nerve was detected following the lesions and that the inhibitory components of the somato-sympathetic reflex persisted. The finding that the excitatory components of somato-sympathetic reflexes were signifi-

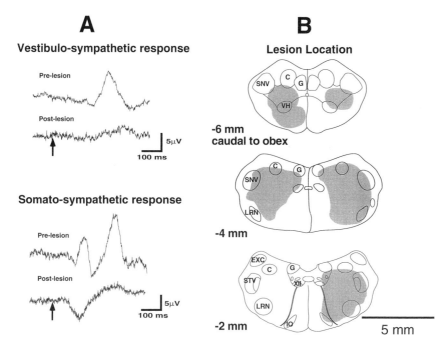

FIGURE 1. Column **A** shows the effects of brain-stem lesions made with kainic acid on both the vestibulo- and somato-sympathetic responses recorded from the splanchnic nerve. The left vestibular nerve was stimulated with five shocks at 150 μA, to elicit the vestibulo-sympathetic response. *Arrows* mark start of shock train. Note the persistence of the inhibitory component in the somato-sympathetic response (elicited by sciatic nerve stimulation, five shocks at 2.0 mA) after the lesion. Column **B** illustrates the location of the lesion that was effective in attenuating the response amplitude of the vestibulo- and somato-sympathetic reflexes in **A**. *Abbreviations*: C, cuneate n.; EXC, external cuneate n.; G, gracile n.; IO, inferior olivary n.; LRN, lateral reticular n.; SNT, spinal trigeminal tract; SNV spinal trigeminal n.; XII, hypoglossal n.

cantly attenuated by the same lesions provides evidence that caudal areas of the reticular formation integrate somatosensory and vestibular signals.[12,13] Neurons in the caudal and lateral reticular formation may serve to process somatic and vestibular inputs relating to body position and relay these integrated signals to the RVLM, which sends bulbospinal projections that influence blood pressure.

REFERENCES

1. YATES, B. J. 1992. Vestibular influences on the sympathetic nervous system. Brain Res. Rev. **17:** 51–59.
2. DOBA, N. & D. J. REIS. 1974. Role of the cerebellum and vestibular apparatus in regulation of orthostatic reflexes in the cat. Circ. Res. **34:** 9–18.
3. DAMPNEY, R. A., L. CZACHURSKI, J. DEMBOWSKY, K. GOODCHILD & A. K. SELLER. 1987. Afferent connections and spinal projections of the pressor region in the rostral ventrolateral medulla of the cat. J. Autonom. Nerv. Syst. **20:** 73–86.
4. LOEWY, A. D. & K. M. SPYER, EDS. 1990. Central Regulation of Autonomic Functions. Oxford University Press. New York.
5. YATES, B. J., T. GOTO & P. S. BOLTON. 1993. Responses of neurons in the rostral ventrolateral medulla of the cat to natural vestibular stimulation. Brain Res. **601:** 255–264.
6. RODER, S. & J. CIRIELLO. 1993. Convergence of ventrolateral medullary and aortic baroreceptor inputs in nucleus of solitary tract. Can. J. Physiol. Pharmacol. **71:** 365–373.
7. MASUDA, N., N. TERUI, N. KOSHIYA & M. KUMADA. 1991. Neurons in the caudal ventrolateral medulla mediate the arterial baroreceptor reflex by inhibiting barosensitive reticulospinal neurons in the rostral ventrolateral medulla in rabbits. J. Autonom. Nerv. Syst. **34:** 103–118.
8. AGARWAL, S. K. & F. R. R. CALARESU. 1993. Supramedullary inputs to cardiovascular neurons of rostral ventrolateral medulla in rats. Am. J. Physiol. **265:** R111–R116.
9. BARMAN, S. M. & G. L. GEBER. 1987. Lateral tegmental field neurons of cat medulla: A source of basal activity of ventrolateral medullospinal sympathoexcitatory neurons. J. Neurophysiol. **57:** 1410–1424.
10. BARMAN, S. M. & G. L. GEBER. 1993. Lateral tegmental field neurons play a permissive role in governing the 10-Hz rhythm in sympathetic nerve discharge. Am. J. Physiol. **265:** R1006–R1013.
11. STEINBACHER, B. C. & B. J. YATES. 1995. Brainstem interneurons necessary for vestibular influences on sympathetic outflow. Soc. Neurosci. Abstr. **21:** 892.
12. ISHIKAWA, T. & T. MIYAZAWA. 1980. Sympathetic responses evoked by vestibular stimulation and their interactions with somato-sympathetic reflexes. J. Autonom. Nerv. Syst. **1:** 243–254.
13. ZANZINGER, J., J. DOUTHEIL, J. CZACHURSKI & H. SELLAR. 1994. Excitatory somato-sympathetic reflexes are relayed in the caudal ventrolateral medulla in the cat. Neurosci. Lett. **179:** 71–74.

Acetylcholine Enhances Optokinetic Modulation of Floccular Purkinje Cells

H. S. TAN AND J. VAN DER STEEN[a]

Department of Physiology
Faculty of Medicine
Erasmus University Rotterdam
P.O. Box 1738
3000 DR Rotterdam, the Netherlands

Microinjection of the cholinergic agonist carbachol into the cerebellar flocculus of the rabbit strongly enhances the optokinetic and vestibulo-ocular reflexes.[1] To account for this effect, we hypothesized a positive modulatory action of acetylcholine (ACh) on cerebellar neurotransmission.[2] The present study is a search for such action at the level of the floccular Purkinje cells.

Extracellular recordings of Purkinje cells in the left cerebellar flocculus were made in three Dutch belted rabbits under Hypnorm sedation (0.25 ml/kg). Three-barreled glass micropipets with a tip diameter of 5 to 8 μm were used, containing 2M NaCl (2–6 MΩ) for recording, 0.5M for iontophoretic drug application (pH 4.5; 10–20 MΩ) and 2M NaCl for current balance (2–6 MΩ). Optokinetic stimulation was delivered around an axis oriented at earth vertical (vertical axis; VA) or an axis lying in the horizontal plane at 135° azimuth (horizontal axis; HA). Purkinje cells that were sensitive to optokinetic stimulation were subjected to iontophoretic application of ACh (90 nA) during continuous sinusoidal optokinetic stimulation (0.2 Hz, 10° peak-to-peak) while recording the simple spike activity.

Of 63 Purkinje cells that were sensitive to optokinetic stimulation, 39 reacted to ACh with enhancement of simple spike modulation. Examples of simple spike modulation by optokinetic stimulation about the VA and HA are shown in FIGURE 1. Before application of ACh, the simple spike activity of the Purkinje cell responsive to VA stimulation was sinusoidally modulated by, in this case, a depth of approximately 80 spikes/sec. During the application of ACh, modulation depth increased considerably to about 135 spikes/sec. For the HA cell, modulation depth changed from 60 spikes/sec before to 80 spikes/sec during ACh application. For both VA and HA cells, basal firing rate (= spike frequency during zero surround velocity) showed on average a slight increase, although it did not change in a consistent pattern.

The lower panels of FIGURE 1 depict the relation between spike frequency and velocity of the optokinetic stimulus. For the VA cell, a roughly linear relationship exists for optokinetic stimulation in the excitatory direction with a speed sensitivity of about 10 spikes/sec per degree/sec. In the inhibitory direction the relationship is still linear, but speed sensitivity is much lower. During ACh application the increase in velocity sensitivity is stronger in the excitatory direction.

For the HA cell, spike frequency is linearly related for surround velocities between + and −2°/sec. For higher surround velocities in both directions, the simple spike frequency saturates.

FIGURE 2 shows the time course of modulation depth of the same VA cell depicted in FIGURE 1. During iontophoresis of ACh, modulation depth increases

[a] Corresponding author. E-mail: steen@fys1.fgg.eur.nl

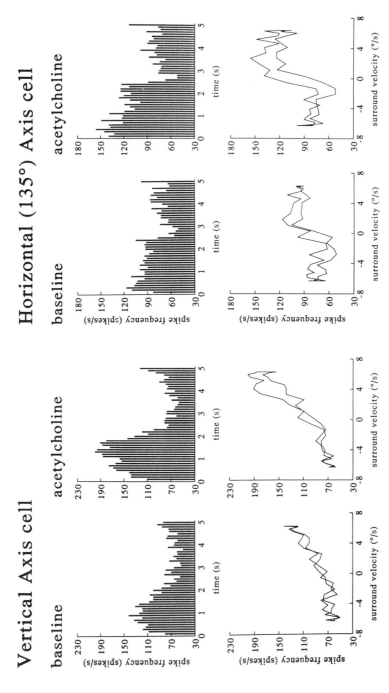

FIGURE 1. Upper panels: Peri-stimulus histograms of typical examples showing simple spike modulation by optokinetic stimulation before and during ACh application in a VA and a HA cell as averaged over 10 stimulus cycles. Lower panels: Plot of simple spike frequency as a function of optokinetic stimulus velocity. Positive velocity values around the VA correspond with movement of the optokinetic stimulus in the nasal-temporal direction of the ipsilateral (*left*) eye. Positive values around the HA correspond with clockwise optokinetic stimulation about an axis lying in the horizontal plane at 135° azimuth ipsilateral to the recorded (*left*) flocculus.

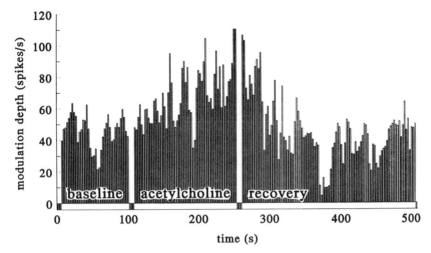

FIGURE 2. Time course of modulation depth of the same VA cell depicted in FIGURE 1. Modulation depth in this figure is defined as the difference between the sum of simple spikes during optokinetic stimulation in one direction and the sum of simple spikes during stimulation in the opposite direction. Each pair of bars thus represents one cycle of sinusoidal stimulation. Modulation depth increases gradually during ACh application and returns to baseline value after cessation.

gradually, with a gradual recovery towards baseline value after cessation of the application.

From these results, we conclude that in the cerebellar flocculus ACh acts as a positive neuromodulator at the level of the Purkinje cell. Our findings agree with recent studies showing that ACh positively modulates Purkinje cell responses to glutamate[3] and GABA.[4] In this light, the enhancing effects on optokinetic responses obtained by microinjection of carbachol in the flocculus can be interpreted as an amplification of optokinetic signals mediated through the flocculus. The exact mechanism remains to be determined, but a mechanism acting via muscarinic receptors and a slow after-hyperpolarization, as found among others in hippocampus and neocortex, remains one of the possibilities (see discussion of ref. 2).

REFERENCES

1. TAN, H. S. & H. COLLEWIJN. 1991. Cholinergic modulation of optokinetic and vestibulo-ocular responses: A study with microinjections in the flocculus of the rabbit. Exp. Brain. Res. **85:** 475–481.
2. TAN, H. S. & H. COLLEWIJN. 1992. Cholinergic and noradrenergic stimulation in the rabbit flocculus have synergistic facilitatory effects on optokinetic responses. Brain Res. **586:** 130–134.
3. ANDRE, P., O. POMPEIANO & S. R. WHITE. 1993. Activation of muscarinic receptors induces a long-lasting enhancement of Purkinje cell responses to glutamate. Brain Res. **617:** 28–36.
4. ANDRE, P., F. FASCETTI, O. POMPEIANO & S. R. WHITE. 1994. The muscarinic agonist, betanechol, enhances GABA-induced inhibition of Purkinje cells in the cerebellar cortex. Brain Res. **637:** 1–9.

The Vestibulo-Ocular Reflex during Horizontal Axis Eccentric Rotation and Near Target Fixation

E. S. VIIRRE AND J. L. DEMER

Jules Stein Eye Institute and
Departments of Ophthalmology and Neurology
University of California, Los Angeles
Los Angeles, California 90095

During a head rotation paradigm about an axis centered on the eye (oculocentric rotation), the eye experiences only angular acceleration. During rotation about an eccentric axis, the eye experiences both linear and angular acceleration. When a near visual target is viewed during eccentric rotation, the gain of the oppositely directed vestibulo-ocular reflex (VOR) must be increased in order to prevent slip of the retinal image of the near target. In monkeys and in humans, increased VOR gain has been observed for eccentric rotations about a vertical axis during near target fixation.[1-5] This increased VOR gain must be the result of interpretation of head linear acceleration inputs from the otolith apparatus in context of target distance. We wished to study the possibility of using eccentric rotation in pitch as a test of otolith function.[6] To eliminate the possible influences of visually guided reflexes, we statistically examined gain of compensatory eye movements within 80 msec of onset of sudden, random accelerations.

METHODS

Three female and five male normal volunteers, aged 19 to 22 years, were strapped securely into a chair that could be rotated about a horizontal axis that was either oculocentric or 15 cm behind the eyes (eccentric). Sinusoidal and sudden random impulsive accelerations of the chair were provided by a servomotor (108 ft-lb). Sinusoidal rotations were delivered with constant angular velocities of 30°/sec at frequencies of 0.8, 1.2, 1.6, and 2.0 Hz. Pseudorandom impulses were delivered with peak accelerations of the head of 700 to 1200°/sec/sec. Eye and head movements were measured with magnetic search coils on contact lenses and a bite appliance or head band. Two subjects wore scleral search coils on both eyes. Subjects fixated a near (**N**) target at 0.1 m from the eyes or a far (**F**) target at 3.0 m. The visually guided VOR (VVOR) was studied during rotations in the light while VOR measures were in darkness with a remembered target. No subject complained of diplopia while viewing a near target. The gains during sudden impulses were calculated in the epoch 25 to 80 msec from movement onset, less than the latency of pursuit or saccadic tracking.

RESULTS

During eccentric sinusoidal rotation, gain with an remembered **F** target was about 0.75, but increased to 0.90 with a visible target (FIG. 1). With a visible **N** target, there was a marked increase in VVOR gain to as much as 1.8 at low frequency, but gain enhancement decreased with increasing frequency to about 1.5 at 2.0 Hz (FIG. 1). With a remembered N target, VOR gain was significantly increased relative to the F target, although the magnitude of the effect was modest (0.65 to 0.85). For the N target, all gain values were below the ideal value of 2.5. Although there should theoretically be no effect of target distance during oculocentric rotation, a small decrease in VOR and VVOR gain was observed when viewing the N versus the F target.

During impulsive eccentric accelerations, both VOR and VVOR gain were increased by N target viewing even during the initial 25 to 80 msec following rotation onset (FIG. 2). During this interval, VVOR gain with the N target was 1.8, while VOR gain was 1.3. In contrast to sinusoidal rotations, the VVOR gain increased during oculocentric rotation when going from an F to an N target. This increase would not serve to stabilize gaze.

During sinusoidal VVOR trials, vergence was maintained as appropriate to target distance. In darkness, however, vergence was variable and often changed independently of VOR gain.

DISCUSSION

The increase in VVOR gain during the early portion of the impulses indicates that an internal target distance estimate and an estimate of the linear acceleration of the head act to the vertical VOR gain pathways. Although the synergistic effect of visual tracking might produce much of the VVOR gain enhancement observed during sinusoidal eccentric rotation with N target fixation, nonvisual mechanisms must instead be active to produce the large VVOR gain enhancement observed for

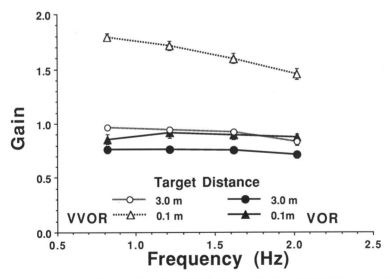

FIGURE 1. Average vestibulo-ocular reflex (VOR) (*filled symbols*) and VVOR (*empty symbols*) gains during pitch rotation with the axis of rotation 15 cm behind the center of the eyes. *Circles* indicate target distances of 3.0 m, and *triangles* indicate target distances of 0.1 m. Error bars are ±1.0 standard error of the mean. Note the strong gain enhancement during VVOR with a 0.1-m target.

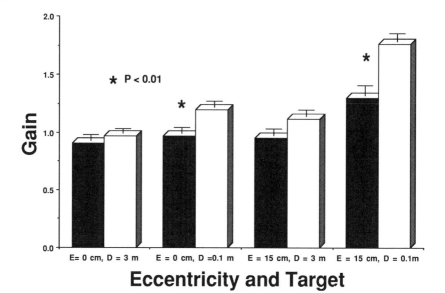

Eccentricity and Target

FIGURE 2. VOR (*filled bars*) and VVOR (*empty bars*) gains during the interval 25 to 80 msec after the onset of eye movement in response to a pseudorandom, sudden head acceleration. E indicates the eccentricity of the axis of rotation in cm and D indicates the target distance in m. An *asterisk* indicates a significant change (*t*-test) in VVOR gain from the control condition of $E = 0$ cm and $D = 3.0$ m. Error bars are ± 1.0 standard error of the mean. Note the VVOR gain enhancement with targets at 0.1 m during oculocentric ($E = 0$ cm) and eccentric ($E = 15$ cm) rotation.

the initial response to sudden accelerations. It is proposed that the greater enhancement of VVOR as compared with VOR gain under such conditions reflects the greater salience of a visible as compared with a remembered target. It is possible that the internal estimate of target position tends toward to a distant value in darkness.

The increase in VVOR gain with near target fixation during sudden eccentric accelerations at the levels used in this experiment may be robust enough for clinical testing of patients with suspected loss of otolith function.[1] Such a test would exploit the salience of a visible target but nevertheless test the vestibular system before visually guided reflexes have time to become active.

The lack of correspondence between VOR gain changes and vergence angle changes suggests that vergence may not be directly driving the gain changes observed during eccentric rotation.[4] Alternatively, an internal estimate of target distance may have different influences on both the signals driving vergence and the signals driving the VOR.

REFERENCES

1. GRESTY, M. A., A. M. BRONSTEIN & H. BARRATT. 1987. Exp. Brain Res. **65:** 377–384.
2. HINE, T. & F. THORN. 1987. Vision Res. **27:** 1639–1657.
3. SARGENT, E. W. & G. D. PAIGE. 1991. Exp. Brain Res. **87:** 75–84.
4. SNYDER, L. H. & W. M. KING. 1992. J. Neurophysiol. **67:** 861–874.
5. VIIRRE, E., D. TWEED, K. MILNER & T. VILIS. 1986. J. Neurophysiol. **56:** 439–450.
6. TAKEDA, N., M. IGARASHI, I. KOIZUKA, S. Y. CHAE & T. MATSUNAGA. 1991. Acta Otolaryngol. Suppl. **481:** 27–30.

Changes in Otolith VOR to Off Vertical Axis Rotation in Infants Learning to Walk

Preliminary Results of a Longitudinal Study[a]

S. R. WIENER-VACHER,[b] A. LEDEBT,[b,c] AND B. BRIL[c]

[b]Hôpital Robert Debré Département O.R.L.
Laboratoire d'Analyse du Mouvement et de la Posture chez l'Enfant
48, Bd Sérurier
75019 Paris, France

[c]Ecole des Hautes Etudes en Sciences Sociales
Apprentissage, Cognition et Contexte
54, Bd Raspail
75006 Paris, France

Although the vestibular organs are anatomically mature at birth, the characteristics of their responses are rather different from those obtained in adults. Previous studies of functional development of the vestibular system in children have focused on semicircular canal vestibulo-ocular reflexes (VOR). Otolith VOR has been neglected for the lack of a test practical for children. In our department, we have adapted the off-vertical axis rotation test (OVAR) for small children to evaluate its potential for eventual clinical applications. However, to establish the standard range of the responses to the test in normal children, we are first studying the otolith vestibulo-ocular reflex as a function of age and posturo-motor development. In our previous work, we have shown that in pooled data from toddlers learning to walk, the modulation of otolith VOR changes over time (the modulation of the slow-phase velocity of the horizontal component of the VOR increases, while this measure for the vertical component decreases significantly[1,2]). In order to better understand the correlation between changes in otolith VOR and the developmental stages of learning to walk (defined by Bril and Brenière[3,4]), we studied longitudinally a group of children from the age of 8 months through the first year of independent walking. We have shown that during the first year of walking experience, the gait parameters undergo a first phase of rapid changes (for about 20 weeks). During this period there are marked decreases in the amplitude of head and trunk rotations and also in the head-trunk angle in the roll and pitch planes.[5] These measures correspond to an increase in head-trunk stiffness, which is thought to represent a strategy for stabilizing gaze. We present here the changes of otolith VOR occurring during the same first period of independent walking for three of these children.

[a]This work was supported by grants from C.R.E. INSERM (#910207), CNES, Fondation pour la Recherche Médicale, La Fondation de France, Institut Electricité et Santé.

METHODS

For each child tested, otolith VOR was evaluated with OVAR while posturo-motor control was measured by analysis of gait parameters, with a video system and a force plate.[5] The OVAR test was applied in complete darkness, with a computer-driven rotating chair that could also be inclined. The child sat on the lap of an adult who was secured to the chair; the adult firmly held the head and body of the child during rotation by means of special supports. Vertical and horizontal eye movements were recorded with conventional EOG electrodes. The stimulation was a "rotation-tilt" paradigm (that is, a constant velocity rotation at 60°/sec about a vertical axis followed by an off-vertical axis rotation at an inclination of 13°). The rotations were made clockwise then counterclockwise at a 5- to 10-min interval. The VOR parameters presented here were the amplitude of the modulation of the slow-phase velocity of the horizontal and vertical components of the otolith response. Because of the large interindividual variability in the age of onset of independent walking, we analyzed the changes of the otolith vestibulo-ocular response parameters to OVAR as a function of time relative to the onset of walking. Two statistical analyses evaluated the significance of changes in the parameters: linear regression and two tailed t-tests comparing the data obtained before versus after the onset of walking.

RESULTS

During the first 20 to 40 first weeks of walking experience, for the three children tested longitudinally, the amplitude of the modulation of the slow-phase velocity of the otolith VOR underwent marked changes. These results are illustrated in FIGURE 1. Because of the wide range of intersubject variability in the gain of the VOR for the same stimuli,[1,2] we normalized the data and expressed them as a percentage of the maximum value measured during the observation period for each individual.

The top graph shows for the horizontal component of the otolith VOR that the lowest amplitudes of the modulation occur for the three children before the onset of walking (time = 0), whereas the highest values are obtained after the onset of walking. The graph below shows for the vertical component of the otolith VOR that the highest amplitudes of modulation occur at the onset of walking, in the three children, whereas the lowest are found 15 to 35 weeks after onset of walking. The statistical analyses applied to the pooled data from the three children show a significant increase (t-test, $p < 0.0001$) in the modulation of the slow phase of the horizontal component and a significant decrease (t-test, $p = 0.0085$) in the modulation of the slow phase of the vertical component; these changes both occurred upon the onset of independent walking and during the 20 to 40 first weeks of independent walking experience.

DISCUSSION

The preliminary results of this longitudinal study indicate that in individuals the development of otolith VOR parameters follow the same pattern we have described previously in pooled data of single observations from a group of 26 toddlers.[1,2] The characteristics of the otolith VORs change dramatically with the onset of independent walking: the modulation of the horizontal component increases and the modulation of vertical component decreases.

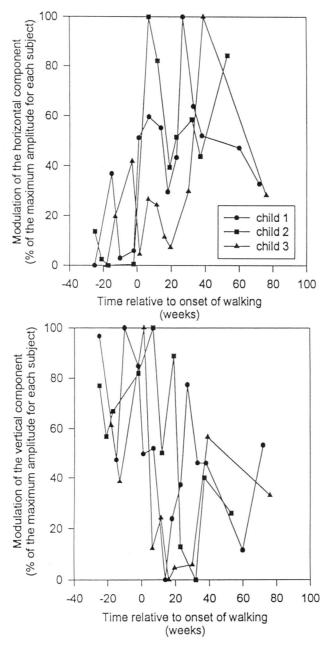

FIGURE 1. Longitudinal measures of the modulation of the slow-phase velocity of the otolith VOR in three children (amplitude of the modulation of the slow-phase velocity for the horizontal component in the top graph and for the vertical component in the bottom graph). Data have been normalized to permit comparisons of developmental trends between children. The time zero corresponds to the onset of independent walking, that is, the first steps without falling.

If we assume that OVAR gives an accurate indication of the global responsiveness of the otolith system, the changes in the characteristics of the otolith VOR found here could be interpreted as an index of the availability of otolith information for the central nervous system pathways involved in the processes of learning to walk. It is during the same first weeks of independent walking that the changes in responsiveness of the otolith system are observed and that the stabilization of the head and trunk increase by means of an increase in the head-neck stiffness.[5] This provides further evidence that otolith information may be essential in the process of learning to walk and may be involved in the organization of the head-trunk stiffness, a basic posturo-motor control strategy used to increase head stability and gaze stabilization in older children[6] and in adults.[7]

ACKNOWLEDGMENTS

The authors wish to acknowledge F. Toupet for her help administering the tests.

REFERENCES

1. WIENER-VACHER, S. R., A. LEDEBT & B. BRIL. 1994. Soc. Neurosci. Abstr. **20:** 1108.
2. LEDEBT, A., S. WIENER-VACHER & B. BRIL. 1994. Relation between vestibular and gait development. *In* Posture and Gait: Vestibular and Neural Front. K. Taguchi, M. Igarashi & S. Mori, Eds.: 155–158. Elsevier Science Publishers. Amsterdam.
3. BRIL, B. & Y. BRENIÈRE. 1992. J. Motor Behav. **24:** 105–116.
4. BRIL, B. & Y. BRENIÈRE. 1993. Posture and independent locomotion in early childhood. *In* The Development of Coordination in Infancy. G. J. P. Savelsbergh, Ed.: 337–358. Elsevier Science Publishers. Amsterdam.
5. LEDEBT, A., B. BRIL & S. R. WIENER-VACHER. 1995. Trunk and head stabilization during the first months of independent walking. Neuroreport **6:** 13–18.
6. ASSAIANTE, C. & B. AMBLARD. 1992. Head-trunk coordination and locomotion equilibrium in 3- to 8-year-old children. *In* The Head-Neck Sensory Motor System. A. Berthoz, W. Graf & P.-P. Vidal, Eds.: 121–125. Oxford University Press. Oxford. England.
7. POZZO, T., A. BERTHOZ & L. LEFORT. 1990. Exp. Brain Res. **82:** 97–106.

Normalization Effects of Vision on the Compensatory VOR after Canal Plugging[a]

SERGEI YAKUSHIN,[b,c,f] JUN-ICHI SUZUKI,[d] MINJIA DAI,[c] THEODORE RAPHAN,[c,e,f] AND BERNARD COHEN[c]

[c]Department of Neurology
Mount Sinai School of Medicine
New York, New York, 10029

[d]Department of Otolaryngology
Teikyo University
Tokyo, Japan

[e]Departments of Computer and Information Science
[f]Department of Experimental Psychology
Brooklyn College
Brooklyn, New York 11210

The vestibulo-ocular reflex (VOR) combines with vision to compensate for head movement in light. Vision can also adapt the VOR during long-term visual-vestibular conflict. How vision might modify the VOR after inactivation of individual semicircular canal pairs is unknown and was studied by recording eye movements during sinusoidal rotation in light and in darkness before and after canal plugging.

Experiments were performed on six cynomolgus monkeys (*Macaca fascicularis*) that had individual canals plugged. In two animals, the lateral canals were plugged (VC animals), and in four animals only one anterior and the contralateral posterior canals were intact (LARP-RALP animals). The techniques and methods of collection and analysis of data have been described in detail elsewhere.[1-3] Animals were sinusoidally rotated for 10 cycles at 0.2 Hz, peak velocity 60°/sec, about a spatial vertical axis while tilted in 10° increments forward or backward in pitch up to 90°. Horizontal, vertical, and torsional eye movements were recorded with search coils implanted on one eye. The gain was defined as the peak-to-peak eye velocity divided by peak-to-peak head velocity for the individual cycle of rotation (FIG. 1). Mean gains as a function of a tilt angle are shown in the graphs of FIGURE 2 (spatial curves).

When normal animals were rotated in darkness in the upright position (FIG. 1A), the induced eye velocities were predominantly horizontal. When the animals were tilted forward or backward, the horizontal component decreased, and the torsional component increased (FIG. 2E, G). The maximal gains of the horizontal (0.87) and torsional (0.52) components were calculated from the best sinusoidal fit through the spatial curves (FIG. 2). For normal monkeys, the maximal horizontal gain occurred when the animals were tilted forward by 11° (spatial phase). Torsional gain was zero in the upright position (2° tilt backward).

[a]This work was supported by grants NS00294 and EY04148.
[b]Address for correspondence: Sergei Yakushin, Department of Neurology, Box 1135, Mount Sinai School of Medicine, 1 East 100th Street, New York, NY 10029. E-mail: syakush@smtplink.mssm.edu

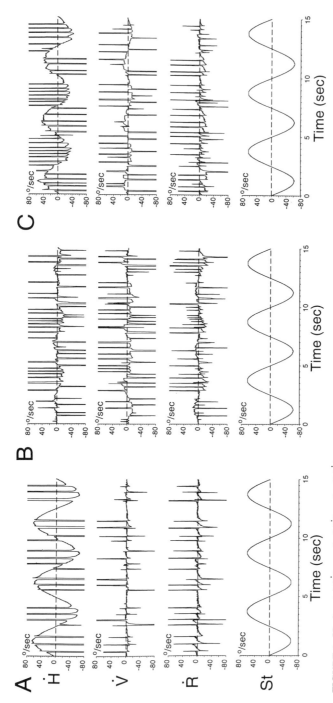

FIGURE 1. Horizontal ($\dot{\mathbf{H}}$), vertical ($\dot{\mathbf{V}}$) and roll ($\dot{\mathbf{R}}$) eye velocity of an animal before and after surgery during sinusoidal rotation about a vertical axis (**St**, stimulus) in darkness at a frequency of 0.2 Hz with a peak velocity ±60°/sec. (**A**) When the animal was upright before surgery, its eye velocity was predominantly horizontal. (**B**) After both lateral canals and the left anterior, right posterior, or right anterior and left posterior canals were plugged (RALP animal), rotation in dark while upright induced only small horizontal, vertical, and torsional velocities. (**C**) During the same rotation in light, however, the response was close to the preoperative response in darkness.

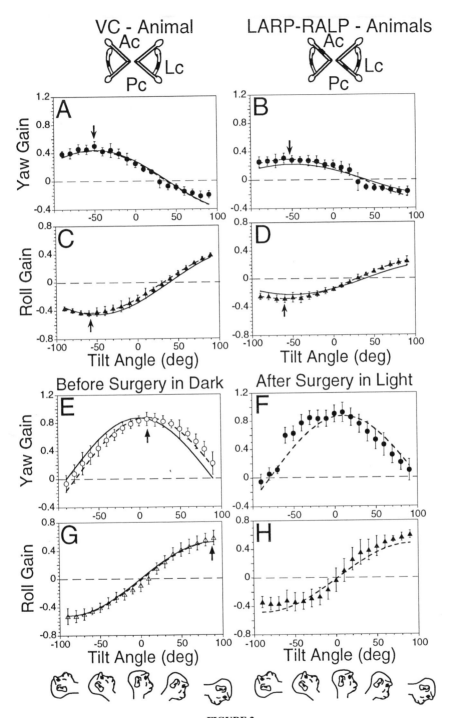

FIGURE 2

FIGURE 2 (*see page 715*). Averaged gains as a function of head tilt of the yaw and roll components from normal (**E, G**) and from canal-plugged monkeys who were tested in darkness (**A–D**) and in light (**F, H**). (**A, C**) Two monkeys had both lateral canals plugged. (**B, D**) Four monkeys had both lateral canals and one anterior and the contralateral posterior canal plugged. The *circles* represent mean value of the horizontal eye velocities; *triangles,* mean value of the torsional velocities. *Filled symbols* are value obtained after surgery; *unfilled,* before surgery. *Solid lines* are the model prediction for the data. *Dashed lines* are the best sinusoidal fits. The data were not fitted in **F** and **H**. In these graphs, the dashed line represents the best fit for the normal data in **E** and **G**. Negative values on the ordinate axis represent gains of eye velocities that were in phase with the stimulus. *Arrows* point to the tilt position with maximal gain response. The inserts below show head positions corresponding to the graphs above.

In VC animals, spatial curves of the horizontal and torsional components had maxima when the animals were tilted backward 52° and 58°, respectively, with peak gains of 0.43 for horizontal and 0.44 for the torsional components (FIG. 2A, C). The horizontal gains of VC animals agreed with previous findings.[4] In LARP-RALP animals, the horizontal and torsional gain peaked at 0.29 when the animals were tilted backward 54° and 61°, respectively (FIG. 2B, D). In contrast to normal animals, the spatial phases of the horizontal and torsional components were 180° out of phase with each other in the plugged animals. Therefore, the horizontal[5] and torsional components of the VOR recorded in darkness after surgery were anticompensatory at some tilt angles.

The data were compared ($p < 0.05$) to a model that projects the head velocity vector onto the normals of the canals according to the rotation of the canal plane within the head frame. It was assumed that each canal pair contributes independently to the eye movement response. The parameters of the model were taken from the normal data with the assumption that anterior, posterior, and lateral canals contribute equally to the roll and horizontal VOR, and that only the anterior and posterior canals contribute to the vertical VOR. The goodness of fit between the data and the model predictions were evaluated using an F statistic.[3] The model predicted the experimental data for the normal (FIG. 2E, G), the VC (FIG. 2A, C), and the LARP-RALP (FIG. 2B, D) animals without changes in parameters.

In each of the animals after canal plugging, vision caused the spatial phases to return to those recorded in the normal animals in darkness (FIG. 2F, H). The maximal horizontal gain for canal-plugged animals in light occurred at 10° forward and gains of 0.60 occurred for roll at 90° tilt forward. This can be compared to the data from the normal animals ($p < 0.05$).

These results indicate that both the vertical and lateral canals contribute a horizontal and torsional component to the VOR in the monkey according to the vector projection of head velocity onto the normals of the individual canals. The innate coordinate frame with regard to the head is not altered in adult animals by lesions of the individual canals. When the operated animals were tested in light, the gains, peak values, and spatial phases of eye velocity returned to the preoperative values, regardless of the type of surgery performed. Therefore, vision compensates for the lack of spatial adaptation of the response planes after peripheral lesions, converting a noncompensatory, direction-fixed response with regard to the head to an appropriate compensatory response.

REFERENCES

1. COHEN, B., J. I. SUZUKI & T. RAPHAN. 1983. Role of the otolith organs in generation of horizontal nystagmus: Effects of selective labyrinthine lesions. Brain Res. **276:** 159–164.

2. RAPHAN, T., B. COHEN & V. HENN. 1983. Nystagmus generated by sinusoidal pitch while rotating. Brain Res. **276:** 165–172.
3. YAKUSHIN, S., M. DAI, J. SUZUKI, T. RAPHAN & B. COHEN. 1995. Semicircular canal contributions to the three-dimensional vestibulo-ocular reflex: A model-based approach. J. Neurophysiol. **74:** 2722–2738.
4. BÖHMER, A., V. HENN & J. I. SUZUKI. 1985. Vestibulo-ocular reflex after selective plugging of the semicircular canals in the monkey—response plane determinations. Brain Res. **326:**291–298.
5. BAKER, J. F., J. GOLDBERG, B. W. PETERSON & R. SCHOR. 1982. Oculomotor reflexes after semicircular canal plugging in cats. Brain Res. **252:** 151–155.

Effects of Microinjection of Muscimol in the Vestibular Nuclei on Velocity Storage and Estimation of Head Velocity by the Otolith Organs[a]

JUN-ICHI YOKOTA,[b,c] HARVEY REISINE,[c]
THEODORE RAPHAN,[d] AND BERNARD COHEN[c]

[b]Department of Neuro-Otology
Saitama Medical College
38, Morohongo, Moroyama, Iruma-Gun
Saitama, Japan

[c]Departments of Neurology and Physiology
Mount Sinai School of Medicine
One Gustave L. Levy Place
New York, New York 10029

[d]Computer and Information Sciences
Brooklyn College
Brooklyn, New York 11210

INTRODUCTION

Velocity storage in the angular vestibulo-ocular reflex (aVOR) contributes activity that produces slow-phase eye velocity during vestibular nystagmus, optokinetic nystagmus (OKN), and optokinetic after-nystagmus (OKAN). It is also responsible for the bias component of nystagmus during off-vertical axis rotation (OVAR). As yet, the neural circuits that produce velocity storage remain unclear. Recently, we demonstrated that microstimulation of the vestibular nuclei (VN) elicited nystagmus and after-nystagmus related to velocity storage.[1] Active sites for eliciting such horizontal nystagmus were found mainly in dorsal parts of central MVN just caudal to the abducens nuclei. Injections of muscimol and bicuculline into VN[5] and of parenteral baclofen[4] indicate that GABA plays an important role in inhibitory control of velocity storage. From these and other data, we have concluded that neurons in VN are responsible for implementing velocity storage and that GABA is an important neurotransmitter controlling its dynamics.

From analysis of nystagmus during off-vertical axis rotation (OVAR), it has further been shown that otolith inputs drive the velocity storage integrator to produce compensatory eye movements for head velocity in space.[2] It is postulated that signals from the utricular macula are processed in a 'head velocity estimator'[3] before activating the velocity storage integrator, though there is no direct experimental evidence for this estimator yet.

In the present study, we recorded single units and electrically stimulated VN of alert monkeys implanted with scleral search coils. When sites where nystagmus related to velocity storage were induced, 0.5 µl of muscimol, a GABA$_A$ agonist, was

[a]This work was supported by grants NS00294, EY04148, and EY01867.

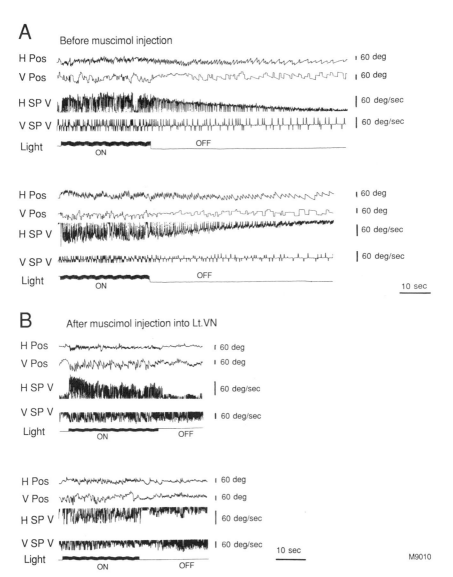

FIGURE 1. Comparison of OKN and OKAN before (**A**) and after (**B**) injection. (**A**) OKN and OKAN before injection. Shown are horizontal and vertical eye position and eye velocity. The bottom trace (Light) is a photocell recording of the passage of stripes. At the end of the **ON** period, the lights were extinguished (**OFF**). The time constant of OKAN was in the range of 30 sec before injection (**A**). After injection (**B**) OKAN was lost.

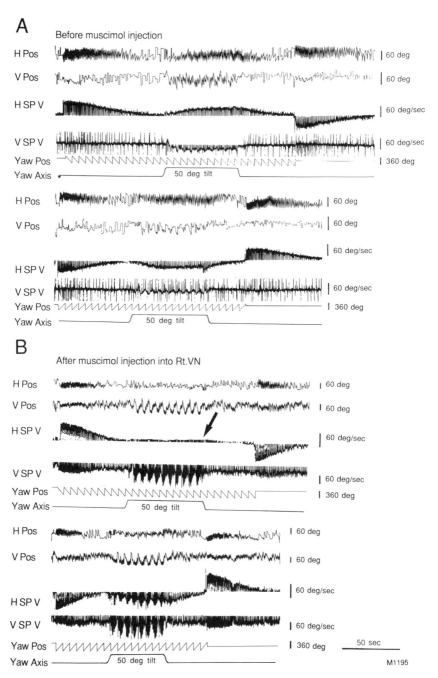

FIGURE 2

←

FIGURE 2. Comparison of nystagmus induced by off-vertical axis rotation (OVAR) before (**A**) and after (**B**) injection of muscimol into the region of otolith-input neurons in the right vestibular nuclei. In this paradigm, the animal was in darkness throughout. It was rotated with a step of velocity at 60°/sec around a vertical axis (Yaw Pos) until nystagmus slow-phase velocity had declined to zero (left side of each panel). (The sawtooth nature of the Yaw Pos curve was due to a position potentiometer that reset every 360°). Then the axis of rotation (Yaw Axis) was tilted 50° while rotation continued. This induced OVAR-nystagmus with a slow rise in slow-phase velocity to a steady-state level. The axis of rotation was then tilted back to the upright, and the nystagmus slow-phase velocity declined over the time course of velocity storage. (**A**) Shows characteristic OVAR nystagmus before injection. (**B**) After injection, the bias component of OVAR with slow-phase velocity ipsilateral to the side of injection was lost. The vertical component of spontaneous nystagmus was strongly modulated according to head position with regard to gravity after injection, demonstrating that otolith information was being processed, despite the loss of steady-state velocity to the ipsilateral side. OVAR slow-phase velocities to the contralateral side were preserved (**B**, *bottom panel*).

injected. In general, these injection sites were at locations where "vestibular-only" (VO) neurons[e] were located.[1] Further description of techniques is given elsewhere.[1] We also recorded and made injections of muscimol into regions where neurons related to otolith processing were located. This relationship was demonstrated by noting the sensitivity of the neurons to static head position with regard to gravity. None of the otolith neurons had evidence of velocity storage in their firing rates, and nystagmus with characteristics of velocity storage was never evoked by electrical stimulation in these regions. The results of injections at these different sites were different and will be considered separately.

RESULTS

Injection at Sites Where Velocity Storage Was Evoked

Before muscimol injection, there was no spontaneous nystagmus. Horizontal VOR gains were between 0.9 and 1.0, and horizontal time constants ranged between 20 and 40 sec. An example of optokinetic nystagmus (OKN) and after nystagmus (OKAN) in one of these monkeys is shown in FIGURE 1A. Slow-phase eye velocity jumped to close to the velocity of the surround at the onset of stimulation and was held until the lights were extinguished. This was followed by OKAN, which was symmetrical to the two sides. The falling time constant of the OKAN was approximately 30 sec. The gain of the angular VOR (aVOR) to steps of velocity was close to unity, and the time constants were similar but slightly longer than the OKAN time constants (FIG. 2A). During off-vertical axis rotation (OVAR), the animals developed a bias component that built over a time constant of several seconds at the onset of tilt of the axis of rotation and decayed over the dominant time course of the aVOR when the axis of rotation was tilted back to the upright (FIG. 2A).

---

[e]VO neurons change their activity in association with the envelope of slow-phase eye velocity during per- and post-rotatory nystagmus.[6] They are activated over the rising time course of the slow component of OKN and the fall in their discharge rates parallels the decline in slow-phase velocity during OKAN.[7] They have no activity related to eye movement, and they are insensitive to momentary losses of eye velocity due to drowsiness. Therefore, they have the appropriate characteristics to activate velocity storage.

Following injection of muscimol into the left vestibular nuclei, prominent spontaneous nystagmus developed with ipsilateral, downward, and rotatory slow phases. The downward component of the spontaneous nystagmus, which can be seen in the vertical slow-phase velocity traces of FIGURE 1**B**, was influenced by head position with regard to gravity. The slow-phase velocity of the nystagmus was minimal with the head tilted 90° ipsilateral side down and maximal when the contralateral side was down. The animals were unable to hold gaze stable after such injections, and the eyes drifted back toward the midposition after eccentric saccades. Thus, as previously reported,[5] the velocity-position integrator was affected by the VN injections.

A striking finding was that there was bilateral reduction in the time constant of the aVOR and of OKAN, suggesting bilateral loss of velocity storage. This is shown by the changes in OKN and the absence of OKAN in FIGURE 1**B**. Eye velocity rose rapidly at the onset of stimulation, as before injection (FIG. 1**A**), but was not well maintained (FIG. 1**B**). At the end of OKN, eye velocity dropped back to the level of spontaneous nystagmus, and there was no after nystagmus in either direction (FIG. 1**B**). Consistent with the loss of velocity storage, the bias component or steady-state velocity of nystagmus induced by OVAR was lost, and the aVOR time constant, evaluated by a step of velocity, fell to about 5 sec. The gain of the aVOR, measured from the initial jump in eye velocity at the onset and end of the steps of angular rotation, was maintained, however.

Injections at Sites Where Otolith Neurons Were Recorded

Injections were also made into regions of VN where neurons responded to otolith input by changing their firing rates as a function of head position with regard to gravity. Before muscimol injection, the animal had normal responses to angular rotation about vertical and off-vertical axes (FIG. 2**A**). After injection, the animal also had prominent vertical (downward) but little horizontal spontaneous nystagmus (FIG. 2**B**). Again, the spontaneous nystagmus was influenced by head position with regard to gravity: the position at which the vertical slow-phase velocity was minimal when the head was tilted 90° ipsilateral side down. It was maximal when the contralateral side was down. In contrast to the results of injection into the "VO" neuron areas, the time constants of the VOR and of OKAN were preserved (FIG. 2**B**), after the "otolith" region injections, indicating that velocity storage was intact. However, other aspects of vestibular control of velocity storage were disrupted. Despite the preservation of velocity storage, there was no bias (steady-state) slow-phase velocity when the slow phases were directed to the ipsilateral side (FIG. 2**B**, *upper panel, arrow*). The vertical velocity, which was related to the spontaneous nystagmus, was strongly modulated as a function of head position with regard to gravity. The loss was unilateral, and OVAR nystagmus with contralateral slow phases had a normal bias component (FIG. 2**B**, *bottom panel*). When the axis of rotation was tilted to the upright so that the animal rotated around a vertical axis, the bias component decayed back to zero over the dominant time constant of the aVOR. This confirms that velocity storage was intact to the contralateral side and that velocity estimation could couple to the velocity storage integrator in this direction.

CONCLUSIONS

These results are consistent with the postulate that velocity storage is generated in the vestibular nuclei. The loss of velocity storage in both directions after unilateral injections suggests that crossed input is important for producing the dominant time constant of the aVOR and OKAN as well as the slow component of OKN and the bias component of OVAR nystagmus. In addition, regions of the vestibular nuclei associated with otolith activity appear to be critical for producing estimates of head velocity that generate the bias component during OVAR. These regions are not directly involved in generating the time constants of velocity storage, but they appear to produce otolith-related activity that couples to it.

REFERENCES

1. YOKOTA, J., H. REISINE & B. COHEN. 1992. Nystagmus induced by electrical stimulation of the vestibular and prepositus hypoglossi nuclei in the monkey: Evidence for site of induction of velocity storage. Exp. Brain Res. **92:** 123–138.
2. REISINE, H. & T. RAPHAN. 1992. Neural basis for eye velocity generation in the vestibular nuclei of alert monkeys during off-vertical axis rotation (OVAR). Exp. Brain Res. **92:** 209–226.
3. RAPHAN, T. & C. SCHNABOLK. 1988. Modeling slow phase velocity generation during off-vertical axis rotation. Ann. N.Y. Acad. Sci. **545:**29–50.
4. COHEN, B., D. HELWIG & T. RAPHAN. 1987. Baclofen and velocity storage: A model of the effects of drug on the vestibulo-ocular reflex in the rhesus monkey. J. Physiol. **393:** 703–725.
5. STRAUBE, A., R. KURZAN & U. BUETTNER. 1991. Differential effects of bicuculline and muscimol microinjections into the vestibular nuclei on similar eye movements. Exp. Brain Res. **86:** 347–358.
6. WAESPE, W. & V. HENN. 1977. Neuronal activity in the vestibular nuclei of the alert monkey during vestibular and optokinetic stimulation. Exp. Brain Res. **27:** 523–538.
7. WAESPE, W. & V. HENN. 1977. Vestibular nuclei activity during optokinetic afternystagmus (OKAN) in the alert monkey. Exp. Brain Res. **30:** 323–330.

Ocular Selectivity of Units in Oculomotor Pathways[a]

WU ZHOU[b,c,d] AND W. M. KING[c]

[b]Neuroscience Program & Center for Visual Science
University of Rochester Medical Center
Rochester, New York 14642

[c]University of Mississippi Medical Center
Departments of Neurology and Anatomy
Jackson, Mississippi 39216-4505

During linear motion in space, the translational-vestibulo-ocular reflex (TVOR) produces disjunctive eye movements whose amplitude and direction depend on the spatial location of the subject's fixation point, as well as the vestibular sensory signal.[1] The processing of vestibular and eye movement signals in the pathways used to produce the TVOR have not been systematically studied in primates. To begin such a study, we have returned to the basic question of how eye position and speed are encoded by neurons in vestibulo-oculomotor pathways. The salient new issue is how left and right eye position and speed are encoded during the TVOR when these parameters may be different. Recent behavioral studies suggest that some premotor pathways (e.g., the TVOR[1] and smooth pursuit[2]) may generate disjunctive eye movement commands independently of the classical vergence system. Thus units in these pathways might encode *monocular* eye position and speed rather than *binocular* conjugate and vergence position and speed.

METHODS

Single-unit discharge patterns were recorded in monkeys trained to track visual targets that moved in three-dimensional space. Movements of each eye were recorded with scleral search coils. Target trajectories were selected to generate conjugate and disjunctive eye movement patterns that dissociated the positions and speeds of the two eyes (FIG. 1), so that any changes in a unit's discharge could be related selectively to the movements of either eye. Eye movement data and unit discharges were averaged over 50-msec intervals during fixation and smooth pursuit and were analyzed using multiple regression techniques to evaluate the relationship between firing rate and eye movement parameters. Ocular selectivity was defined as the extent to which a unit's firing rate was correlated with the movements of one or the other eye. Ocular selectivity indices were computed for eye position, OSK [equal to $(K_r - K_l)/(K_r + K_l)$, where K_r and K_l are unit discharge sensitivities to right or left eye position], and eye velocity, OSR [equal to $(R_r - R_l)/(R_r + R_l)$, where R_r and R_l are unit discharge sensitivities to right or left eye velocity]. According to these

[a]This work was supported by National Institutes of Health grant R01EY04045 and Office of Naval Research grant N00014 to Dr. King.

[d]Address for correspondence: Wu Zhou, Department of Anatomy, University of Mississippi Medical Center, 2500 North State Street, Jackson, MS 39216-4505. E-mail: wuz@cvs.rochester.edu

Abducens Unit12_1   Prepositus H. Unit10_7

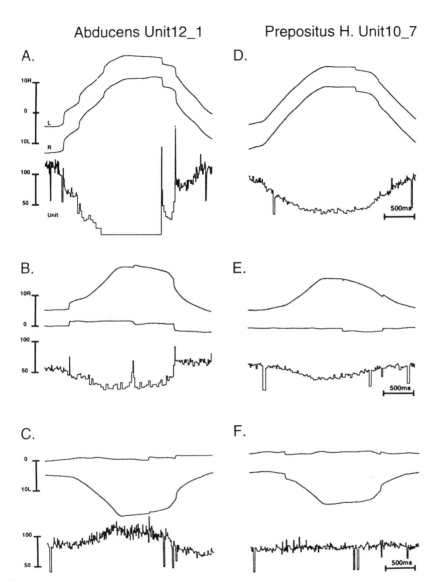

FIGURE 1. Responses of a binocular left burst-tonic abducens unit (**A–C**) and a monocular left tonic prepositus unit (**D–F**) during smooth pursuit of a visual target that moved in three-dimensional space. Panels **A** and **D** show unit responses during conjugate pursuit. Panels **B, C, E,** and **F** show unit responses during asymmetric pursuit (one eye is stationary). The abducens unit's firing rate was modulated regardless of which eye moved. However, the prepositus unit's firing rate was modulated only when the left eye moved. In each panel, the top trace is left eye position (deg), the middle trace is right eye position (deg), and the lower trace is unit firing rate (sp/sec).

definitions, a unit will be related monocularly to the right eye if ocular selectivity is 1 and monocularly to the left eye if ocular selectivity is -1. If the ocular selectivity is 0, then the unit's discharge is equally related to movements of either eye (binocular unit). Ocular selectivity was studied in burst-tonic or tonic neurons located in the abducens nuclei, nucleus prepositus hypoglossi, and the cerebellum.

RESULTS

FIGURE 1 shows examples of a binocular unit recorded in the abducens nucleus (panels A–C) and a monocular unit in the prepositus hypoglossi nucleus (panels D–F). The discharge of the abducens unit was modulated during conjugate movements (A), and during asymmetric tracking with the right (B) or the left (C) eye. The ocular selectivity indices were 0.04 for position and 0.23 for velocity, indicating that this was a binocular unit with a firing rate related to movements of both eyes. In contrast, the discharge of the prepositus unit was modulated only in relation to movements of the left eye as can be seen by comparing FIGURES 1E and F. The ocular selectivity indices of this unit were -1.0 for both eye position and velocity. FIGURE 2 shows the distribution of ocular selectivity indices for 74 abducens units (A), 18 prepositus units (B), and 27 cerebellar units (C). Abducens neurons could be divided into three nonoverlapping groups ($F(2, 69) = 397.4, p < 0.0001$) according to ocular selectivity for eye position: monocular left (OSK $= -0.87$, 47% of units), monocular right (OSK $= 1.0$, 9.7%), and binocular units (OSK $= -0.15$, 43.1%). In contrast, the majority of prepositus and cerebellar units were monocular (prepositus, 77.8% of units; cerebellum, 66.7% of units). Similar groups could be defined using the ocular selectivity indices for velocity.

DISCUSSION

These data suggest that unit discharges in oculomotor pathways may selectively influence the movements of one or the other eye. In an earlier study, we showed that position-vestibular-pause (PVP) cells in the vestibular nuclei also exhibit monocular eye position sensitivity,[3] suggesting that monocular ocular selectivity is a common feature of premotor eye movement pathways. These data imply that an analysis of ocular selectivity could provide a physiological means to identify premotor pathways associated with the production of motor commands for each eye. Identification of such pathways (reminiscent of the classically described three-neuron vestibulo-ocular reflex pathways) would be a crucial step in understanding how the TVOR produces disjunctive eye movements dependent on target location and eye position. The ocular sensitivity analysis also suggests that monocular pathways converge on abducens neurons, since many of these cells are binocular. It is likely that the physiological division of abducens units into subpopulations of monocular and binocular units does not correspond to the anatomical division of abducens units into subpopulations of motoneurons and internuclear neurons. Thus, motoneurons may be monocular or binocular. We speculate that significant convergence of left and right eye movement pathways on abducens cells might be present at birth. During the early development of conjugate eye movements, these convergent connections could be reinforced selectively on some neurons by synchronous activation of synapses in left/right monocular pathways during conjugate movements, but weakened on other neurons during disjunctive eye movements. Thus, the distribution of ocular selectiv-

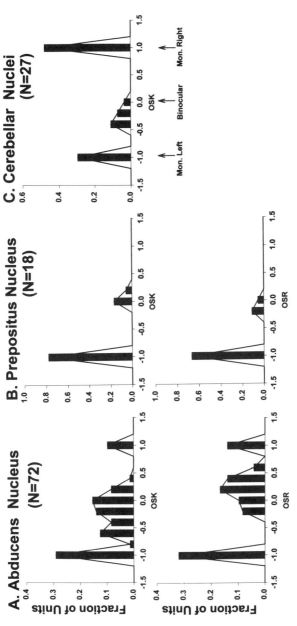

FIGURE 2. Distribution of ocular selectivity indices for 74 abducens neurons (**A**), 18 prepositus neurons (**B**), and 27 cerebellar neurons (**C**). Each population can be divided into statistically different and nonoverlapping groups according to ocular selectivity.

ity in the abducens nucleus may result from the same mechanism that produces ocular dominance columns in visual cortex. We further speculate that ocular selectivity will be altered by surgical, optical, or pharmacological treatments that disrupt binocular alignment during later life.

REFERENCES

1. PAIGE, G. D. & D. L. TOMKO. 1991. Eye movement responses to linear head motion in the squirrel monkey. II. Visual-vestibular interactions and kinematic considerations. J. Neurophysiol. **65:** 1183–1196.
2. KING, W. M. & W. ZHOU. 1995. Initiation of disjunctive smooth pursuit in monkeys: Evidence that Hering's law of equal innervation is not obeyed by the smooth pursuit system. Vision Res. **35:** 3389–3400.
3. McCONVILLE, K. M. V., R. D. TOMLINSON, W. M. KING, G. D. PAIGE & E. Q. NA. 1994. Eye position signals in the vestibular nuclei: Consequences for models of integrator function. J. Vest. Res. **4:** 391–400.

Subject Index

Index of Contributors